diFIORE'S ATLAS
OF HISTOLOGY
WITH FUNCTIONAL
CORRELATIONS

Victor P. Eroschenko, PhD

Professor Emeritus of Anatomy • WWAMI Medical Program
University of Idaho • Moscow, Idaho

 Wolters Kluwer | Lippincott Williams & Wilkins
Health

Philadelphia • Baltimore • New York • London
Buenos Aires • Hong Kong • Sydney • Tokyo

Acquisitions Editor: Crystal Taylor
Product Manager: Julie Montalbano
Marketing Manager: Joy Fisher-Williams
Designer: Terry Mallon
Compositor: SPi Global

12th Edition

Library of Congress Cataloging-in-Publication Data
Eroschenko, Victor P.
  diFiore's atlas of histology with functional correlations / Victor P. Eroschenko. — 12th ed.
    p. ; cm.
  Atlas of histology with functional correlations
  Includes index.
  ISBN 978-1-4511-1341-9
  1. Histology—Atlases. I. Fiore, Mariano S. H. di. II. Title. III. Title: Atlas of histology with functional correlations.
    [DNLM: 1. Histology—Atlases. 2. Tissues—physiology—Atlases.   QS 517]
    QM557.F5513   2013
    611'.018—dc23

2011027297

DISCLAIMER
Care has been taken to confirm the accuracy of the information present and to describe generally accepted practices. However, the authors, editors, and publisher are not responsible for errors or omissions or for any consequences from application of the information in this book and make no warranty, expressed or implied, with respect to the currency, completeness, or accuracy of the contents of the publication. Application of this information in a particular situation remains the professional responsibility of the practitioner; the clinical treatments described and recommended may not be considered absolute and universal recommendations.

The authors, editors, and publisher have exerted every effort to ensure that drug selection and dosage set forth in this text are in accordance with the current recommendations and practice at the time of publication. However, in view of ongoing research, changes in government regulations, and the constant flow of information relating to drug therapy and drug reactions, the reader is urged to check the package insert for each drug for any change in indications and dosage and for added warnings and precautions. This is particularly important when the recommended agent is a new or infrequently employed drug.

Some drugs and medical devices presented in this publication have Food and Drug Administration (FDA) clearance for limited use in restricted research settings. It is the responsibility of the health care provider to ascertain the FDA status of each drug or device planned for use in their clinical practice.

To purchase additional copies of this book, call our customer service department at (800) 638-3030 or fax orders to (301) 223-2320. International customers should call (301) 223-2300.

Visit Lippincott Williams & Wilkins on the Internet: http://www.lww.com. Lippincott Williams & Wilkins customer service representatives are available from 8:30 am to 6:00 pm, EST.

9 8 7 6 5 4 3 2 1

Dedicated
To those who matter so much

Ian
McKenzie
Sarah
Shannon

> *and*
> *Diane*
> *Kathryn*
> *Tatiana*
> *Sharon*

>> *and*
>> *Todd*
>> *Shaun*
>> *Chadwick*

>>> *and most especially and always*
>>> *Elke*

PREFACE to the 12th Edition

As in other previous editions, the author has carefully evaluated the very constructive comments that were provided by numerous reviewers of this atlas. Many of these suggestions that fit the design and purpose of the atlas were implemented. As a result, the atlas, while maintaining its main features, was improved in terms of improved text material, new artwork, and additional micrographs.

Basic Approach

The traditional approach to studying histology has been significantly altered. However, regardless of how histology is presented to the students, histology still remains one of the fundamental science courses that is essential in understanding and interpreting new scientific discoveries. Although most of the new advances in science remain submicroscopic, the final expectations of these findings will be eventually evaluated on their effects on individual cells, tissues, and organs of an organism.

In preparing the 12th edition of the atlas, the author maintained its unique and traditional approach, namely, providing the student with improved, realistic full-color composite and idealized illustrations of histologic structures. In addition, many of these illustrations are accompanied by actual light and transmission electron photomicrographs. This unique approach has become a popular trademark of the atlas. In addition, the morphology of these structures is directly correlated with their essential functions. This approach allows the student to learn different histologic structures and their major functions at the same time. This approach and the presentation format have served the needs of undergraduate, graduate, medical, veterinary, and biologic science students in numerous previous editions. The present and improved edition of the atlas continues to address the needs of histology students.

Changes in the 12th Edition

Several significant changes that have been incorporated into this atlas are presented in detail below.

- A new feature of the 12th edition is the addition of two brand new chapters.
  - The first chapter summarizes the histologic methods for different histological techniques, stain characteristics of the nine most commonly used stains, and pertinent photomicrograph examples for each stain.
  - The second chapter describes in detail the cell cycle, accompanied by both drawings and representative photomicrographs of the main stages in the cell cycle during mitosis.
- All chapters and functional correlations have been updated and expanded to reflect new scientific information and interpretations. All of the functional information is presented in an organized and informative way so as not to overwhelm or intimidate the student.
- Another brand new feature of this atlas is the online inclusion of multiple-choice exams designed for undergraduate, graduate, medical, and veterinary students that correspond to each chapter (except the methodology chapter).
- As in the previous edition, each chapter is followed by a comprehensive summary in the form of an easy-to-follow outline that has also been expanded to reflect new content.
- Some chapters in the atlas have been moved, renamed, renumbered, and subdivided into different sections for easier reading and comprehension of the topics.
- New images in the atlas have been replaced with original, digitized color illustrations.
- In addition, about 44 new photomicrograph images, including light and transmission electron micrographs, have been added to the atlas.

Online Ancillaries

Online Atlas

Currently, there is an increased use of various computer-based technologies in histology instruction. As a result, the 12th edition of the atlas allows the student access via a code to an interactive online atlas and a histology image library with each copy of the book. The interactive atlas is specifically designed to allow the students to further test their knowledge of histologic illustrations and photomicrographs that are found in the atlas. Specific features of the online atlas include a labels on/labels off feature, rollover "hot spots," and rollover labels. In addition, a self-testing feature allows the students to practice identifying the features on the images.

In addition to the interactive atlas, the students will have access to a histology library that contains more than 475 digitized histology photomicrographs. All histology images have been separated into chapters that match those in the atlas, with each chapter containing an average of 20 images. The library images are specifically designed for use by the students to reinforce the material that was previously learned in laboratory or lecture. An icon is placed at relevant points throughout the text, signaling to the reader that a collection of corresponding "real" micrographs is available online for comparison and contrast with the illustrated versions found in the book. Consequently, these images do not have any labels and are identified only by a figure number for each chapter.

For instructors, a separate histology image library has been prepared, with more than 950 improved and digitized photomicrograph images. These images have also been separated into corresponding chapters, with each image identified with abbreviations only. There are no labels on the images and each image can be imported into Microsoft PowerPoint and labeled by the instructors to provide necessary information during lectures or laboratory exercises. Because there are multiple images of the similar structures, instructors can use different images for lectures or laboratories of the same structures without repetition.

Additional Online Features

New for the 12th edition, an online e-book will also be included on thePoint as well as an interactive quiz bank for students with over 380 multiple-choice questions and answers.

Thus, the current edition of the atlas should serve as a valuable supplement in histology laboratories where traditional histology is taught either with microscopes and glass slides, or where computer-based images are used as a substitute for microscopes, or in which a combination of both techniques are used interchangeably.

ACKNOWLEDGMENTS

As in previous editions, the association with numerous professional individuals and their gracious contribution of different images greatly improved the contents of this atlas, for which the author is very grateful. The incorporation of these new images has greatly expanded the scope of the 12th edition of the atlas.

Dr. E. Roland Brown (earlrolandbrown@gmail.com), a freelance artist, has prepared again all of the new computer-generated histology illustrations.

Sonja L. Gerard of Oei Graphics, Bellevue, Washington, corrected or improved the lead-in art and color for each chapter of the atlas.

Dr. Mark DeSantis, a longtime colleague and Professor Emeritus of the WWAMI Medical Education Program and Department of Biology, University of Idaho, Moscow, Idaho, provided constructive suggestions for the last couple of editions and provided numerous transmission electron micrographs of nervous tissue for the current edition.

A beautiful immunohistochemical preparation of a mammalian pancreatic islet has been graciously provided by Dr. Ernest Adeghate, Professor and Chairman, Department of Anatomy, Faculty of Medicine and Health Sciences, UAE University, Al Ain, United Arab Emirates.

Dr. Rex A. Hess, a longtime colleague and Professor Emeritus, Comparative Biosciences, College of Veterinary Medicine, University of Illinois, Urbana, Illinois, provided numerous transmission electron micrographs for the last edition and again for different chapters in the present edition of the atlas.

Mr. Carter Rowley, Fort Collins, Colorado, a friend and a colleague of many years, graciously provided the transmission electron micrographs of the skeletal muscles from his own personal collection.

Finally, the assistance, cooperation, and professionalism of the editorial staff of the publisher made a significant contribution to the successful revision and publication of the newest edition of this atlas. I acknowledge the most able assistance of Crystal Taylor (acquisitions editor for numerous past editions), Julie Montalbano (product manager), and Jennifer Clements (art director) of Lippincott Williams & Wilkins. A special appreciation is extended to Kelly Horvath for her dedication and hard work as the freelance editor in preparing this atlas for the second time. The efforts of these wonderful individuals in working with me and assisting me in many different ways for preparing the best 12th edition of this atlas are sincerely appreciated.

Victor P. Eroschenko, PhD
Professor Emeritus of Anatomy
Moscow, Idaho
February, 2011

REVIEWERS

Faculty

Ernest Adeghate
United Arab Emirates University
Al Ain, United Arab Emirates

Brian R. MacPherson
University of Kentucky College of Medicine
Lexington, KY

Joan Witkin
Columbia University College of Physicians and Surgeons
New York, NY

Mark Kaminski
University of Western States
Portland, OR

Students

Michelle Walter
Bastyr University
Seattle Washington

Rachel Meyer
Mount Sinai School of Medicine
New York, NY

Meena Hasan
Michigan State University College of Human Medicine
East Lansing, MI

Low Liying
University of Glasgow
Glasgow, UK

CONTENTS

PART IV Systems

CHAPTER 11 Immune System 239

CHAPTER 12 Integumentary System 261

CHAPTER 17 Respiratory System   389

CHAPTER 18 Urinary System   417

CHAPTER 19 Endocrine System 451

CHAPTER 20 Male Reproductive System 477

CHAPTER 21 Female Reproductive System 505

PART I

Introduction

CHAPTER 1

Histologic Methods

SECTION 1 Tissue Preparation and Staining of Sections

Tissue Preparation—Light Microscopy

Histology is a visual, as well as a very colorful, science that is studied with the aid of a light microscope. The prepared specimens for examination are thinly sliced, placed on a glass slide, stained with a variety of stains, and examined with a light microscope via a light beam that passes through the tissues that are fixed on the slide. Most of the illustrations in this atlas are taken from slides that have been prepared by the methods described in the text that follows.

Fixation

To preserve a section of tissue or organ for histologic examination, the first step is prompt immersion and **fixation** of the specimen with different chemical solutions. Fixation is essential in order to permanently preserve the structural and molecular composition of the specimen. To further accelerate the penetration and proper fixation process, the tissue specimen is first cut into small pieces and then immersed into the fixative. Fixation hardens the specimen for sectioning and causes **cross-linkage** of **macromolecules** within the cells. This process reduces the cellular degeneration, preserves the integrity of cells and tissues, and increases their affinity to take up different stains. The most commonly used fixative for light microcopy is the neutral-buffered **formaldehyde**.

Postfixation

After the tissue specimen is fixed, which is usually overnight, water must first be removed from the fixed specimen by passing it through a series of ascending **alcohol** (ethanol) concentrations, usually from 70% to 100% ethanol. Before the specimen can be embedded in a **paraffin** (wax) medium for cutting, it must be cleared of alcohol by passing it through several changes of such clearing agents as **xylene**, which is miscible with both alcohol and paraffin.

Once the specimen is impregnated with the clearing agent xylene, it is then placed in a warm mold containing melted paraffin. Once removed from the heat source, the paraffin in the mold cools, solidifies, and encases the specimen. The paraffin block is then trimmed to the size of the specimen and mounted in an instrument called a **microtome**. The microtome precisely advances the paraffin block so that the sections are cut at specific and predetermined increments with a steel knife. For histologic examination of the specimen, the sections are normally cut at 5 to 10 μm thickness. The thin paraffin sections are then collected and floated in a warm water bath and placed onto a glass slide that has been covered with a thin layer of **albumen**, which serves as an adhesive medium for the specimen.

Staining of Sections

There are numerous stain-specific cell organelles, different cell types, fibers, tissues, and organs. Usually, the paraffin sections on the glass slide are colorless. In order to see the structural details in a given section, the section needs to be stained. To stain the specimen in the sections, paraffin must first be dissolved from the specimen with solvents, such as **xylene**, and the sections rehydrated with a series of decreasing **alcohol** concentrations. The hydrated sections can then be stained with a variety of water-soluble stains, which selectively stain various components of the specimen and allow visual differentiation between the different cellular and tissue components. After staining, the specimen is again dehydrated and immersed in xylene, after which a suitable mounting medium and a protective glass coverslip is placed over the specimen on the slide. The coverslip allows for viewing of the stained specimen on the glass slide with the light microscope.

Most of the stains used for histologic slide preparations act like acidic or basic compounds. Structures in the specimen that stain most readily with basic stains are called **basophilic**, and those that stain with acidic stains are called **acidophilic**. The most common stains that are used for histologic sections are **hematoxylin** and **eosin** stains.

Tissue Preparation—Other Methods: Transmission and Scanning Electron Microscopy

This atlas also contains a number of images obtained by using the transmission and scanning electron microscopes. A brief description of their methodology is now presented.

Examining the tissue sections with a **transmission electron microscope (TEM)** allows for much higher magnification and greater resolution. The principles used in the preparation of tissues for TEM are essentially the same as those used for light microscopy. However, the tissue sections are cut into very small pieces to allow for rapid fixation. In addition, the fixatives are different from those of the histologic slide preparation. The specimen that is to be collected is either previously perfused with the fixative in the body or removed and directly immersed in the fixative. The primary fixatives for TEM specimens include cold-buffered **gluteraldehyde**, in which the specimens are first immersed. Following gluteraldehyde fixation, the specimens are rinsed in several buffers and then postfixed in cold **osmium tetroxide**, which reacts with phospholipids. Osmium tetroxide imparts an electron density to the cells and tissues because of its heavy metallic property. This allows for image formations for viewing with TEM. Following fixation and postfixation, the tissues are embedded in epoxy resin, which then polymerizes and forms a hard plastic tissue block. From these plastic blocks, ultrathin sections are cut with a special instrument called an ultramicrotome, using either a diamond knife or special glass knives. The thin sections are collected on small copper grids and stained with **urinal acetate** and **lead citrate**. Using the TEM, the electron beams pass through the stained specimens and form high-resolution and high-contrast black-and-white images for viewing on the screen and recording.

In contrast to TEM, the **scanning electron microscope (SEM)** uses solid pieces of tissue, instead of ultrathin sections. Solid pieces of tissues that are normally larger than those for TEM are collected. The collected tissue samples are fixed in the same fixatives as those used for TEM. The specimens are first dehydrated by **critical point** drying, using liquid carbon dioxide, then attached to aluminum stubs, and finally coated with evaporated **gold palladium**. When viewing the prepared specimen with the SEM, the electron beams do not pass through the specimen, but instead the specimen is scanned along its surface. The electrons that are reflected from the surface of the prepared specimen are then collected by detectors and processed as three-dimensional, black-and-white images of the surface of the specimen. The image is then visible on the monitor.

SECTION 2 Histologic Slide Interpretation

Appearance of Histologic Sections Prepared by Different Types of Stains

Interpretation of histologic sections is greatly aided by the use of different stains, which selectively stain certain specific properties in different cells, tissues, and organs. The most prevalent stain that is used for preparation of histology slides is the hematoxylin and eosin stain. Most of the images prepared for this atlas were taken from slides that were stained with hematoxylin and eosin stain. To show other and more specific characteristic features of different cells, tissues, and organs, other stains are also used.

Listed on following pages and illustrated in Figures 1.1 through 1.9 are the descriptions of nine different stains that were used to prepare slides for this atlas, their specific staining characteristics, and selected histologic photomicrographs to illustrate the appearance of the stained structures.

Hematoxylin and Eosin Stain

- Nuclei stain blue
- Cytoplasm stains pink or red
- Collagen fibers stain pink
- Muscles stain pink

FIGURE 1.1 ■ Kidney cortex with renal corpusle and different convoluted tubules.

Masson Trichrome Stain

- Nuclei stain black or blue-black
- Muscles stain red
- Collagen and mucus stain green or blue
- Cytoplasm of most cells stains pink

FIGURE 1.2 ■ Skeletal muscle sectioned in the longitudinal plane and a cross section with surrounding blue-staining connective tissue.

Periodic Acid–Schiff Reaction

- Glycogen stains deep red or magenta
- Goblet cells in intestines and respiratory epithelia stain magenta red
- Basement membranes and brush borders in kidney tubules stain positive, or pink

FIGURE 1.3 ■ Villus of small intestine with brush border, columnar epithelium, and goblet cells.

Elastic Tissue Stain

- Elastic fibers stain jet black
- Nuclei stain gray
- Remaining structures stain pink

FIGURE 1.4 ■ Section of a wall from the aorta, showing the presence of dark-staining elastic fibers and the pink smooth muscles.

Mallory–Azan Stain

- Fibrous connective tissue, mucus, and hyaline cartilage stain deep blue
- Erythrocytes stain red-orange
- Cytoplasm of liver and kidney stains pink
- Nuclei stain red

FIGURE 1.5 ■ Intramembranous ossification in skull bones showing the blue connective tissue, red blood cells, and blood vessels with blood cells.

Wright/Giemsa Stain

- Erythrocyte cytoplasm stains pink
- Lymphocyte nuclei stain dark purple-blue with pale blue cytoplasm
- Monocyte cytoplasm stains pale blue, and the nucleus stains medium blue
- Neutrophil nuclei stain dark blue
- Eosinophil nuclei stain dark blue, and the granules stain bright pink
- Basophil nuclei stain dark blue or purple, cytoplasm pale blue, and granules deep purple
- Platelets stain light blue

FIGURE 1.6 ■ Blood smear with different cells and platelets.

Cajal and Del Rio Hortega Methods (Silver and Gold Methods)

- Myelinated and unmyelinated fibers and neurofibrils stain blue-black
- General background is nearly colorless
- Astrocytes stain black
- Depending on the methods used, the end product can stain black, brown, or gold

FIGURE 1.7 ■ Cross section of the spinal cord showing the gray and white matter.

Osmic Acid (Osmium Tetroxide) Stain

- Lipids in general stain black
- Lipids in the myelin sheath of nerves stain black

FIGURE 1.8 ■ Cross section of a peripheral nerve, showing the myelin sheath of the axons.

Iron Hematoxylin and Alcian Blue Stain

- Connective tissue fibers stain dark blue
- Smooth muscles stain light pink
- Nuclei stain dark and cytoplasm light pink

FIGURE 1.9 ■ Small artery and veins, showing blood cells and the surrounding connective tissues.

Interpretation of Histologic Sections

One of the most challenging and difficult aspects of histology that students encounter is the interpretation of what the two-dimensional histology sections represent in three dimensions. **Histologic sections** are thin, flat slices of fixed and stained tissues or organs mounted on flat glass slides. Such sections are normally composed of cellular, fibrous, and tubular structures that are cut in different planes. As a result, a variety of shapes, sizes, and layers may be visible, depending on the plane of section. **Fibrous** structures are solid and are found in connective, nervous, and muscle tissues. **Tubular** structures are hollow and represent various types of blood vessels, lymph vessels, glandular ducts, and glands of the body.

In tissues and organs, the cells, fibers, and tubes have a random orientation in space and are part of a three-dimensional structure. During the preparation of histology slides, the thin sections cut from the specimen do not show much depth. In addition, the plane of a section does not always bisect these structures in exact transverse or cross section. As a result, this produces a variation in the appearance of the cells, fibers, and tubes, depending on the angle of the plane of section. Consequently, it becomes difficult to correctly perceive the true three-dimensional structure of the specimen from which the sections were prepared on a flat slide. Therefore, correct visualization and interpretation of these sections in their proper three-dimensional perspective on the slide becomes an important criterion for understanding and mastering histology images. Figures 1.10 and 1.11 illustrate how the appearance of cells and tubes changes with different planes of section. Figure 1.12 is an actual histology slide of an organ that is filled with tubular structures that are highly convoluted. This section illustrates how the appearance of such tubular structures in the testis changes when they are sectioned in different planes.

 Supplemental micrographic images are available at **www.thePoint.com/Eroschenko12e** under Cell and Cytoplasm.

FIGURE 1.10 | Planes of Section of a Round, Solid Object

To illustrate how the shape of a three-dimensional cell can be altered in a histologic section, a hard-boiled egg has been sectioned in longitudinal and transverse (cross) planes. The composition of a hard-boiled egg serves as a good example of a cell, with the yellow yolk representing the nucleus and the surrounding egg white (pale blue) representing the cytoplasm. Enclosing these structures are the soft eggshell membrane and a hard eggshell (red). At the rounded end of the egg is the air space (blue).

The **midline** sections of the egg in the **longitudinal (a)** and **transverse planes (d)** disclose its correct shape and size, as they appear in these planes of section. In addition, these two planes of section reveal the correct appearance, size, and distribution of the internal contents within the egg.

Similar but more **peripheral** sections of the egg in the **longitudinal (b)** and **transverse planes (e)** still show the external shape of the egg. However, because the section was cut peripherally and below the midline, the internal contents of the egg are not seen in their correct size or distribution within the egg white. In addition, the size of the egg appears smaller.

The tangential **plane (c and f)** of the section grazes or only passes through the outermost periphery of the egg. This section reveals that the egg is an oval (c) or a small, round (f) object. The egg yolk is not seen in either section because it was not located in the plane of section. As a result, such tangential sectioning does not reveal sufficient detail for correct interpretation of the egg size or of its contents or their distribution within the internal membrane.

Thus, in a histologic section, individual structure's shape and size vary depending on the plane of section. Some cells may exhibit full cross sections of their nuclei, and they appear prominent in the cells. Other cells may exhibit only a fraction of the nucleus, and the cytoplasm appears large. Still other cells may appear only as clear cytoplasm, without any nuclei. All these variations are attributable to different planes of section through the nuclei. Understanding these variations in cell and tube morphology becomes important in interpreting different histologic sections.

FIGURE 1.10 ■ Planes of sections through a round object, a hard-boiled, solid egg.

FIGURE 1.11 | Planes of Section Through a Hollow Structure or a Tube

Tubular structures are often seen in histologic sections. Tubes are most easily recognized when they are cut in transverse (cross) sections. However, if the tubes are sectioned in planes other than transverse, their appearance is different. To be recognized as a hollow tube, they must first be visualized as three-dimensional structures. To illustrate how a blood vessel, duct, or a hollow glandular structure may vary in appearance in a histologic section, a curved tube with a simple (single) epithelial cell layer is sectioned in longitudinal, transverse, and oblique planes.

A **longitudinal** (**a**) plane of section that cuts the tube in the midline produces a U-shaped structure. The sides of the tube are lined by a single row of cuboidal (round) cells around an empty lumen, except at the bottom, where the tube begins to curve; in this region the cells appear multilayered.

Transverse (**d** and **e**) planes of section of the same tube produce round structures lined by a single layer of cells. The variations that are seen in the cytoplasm of different cells are related to the planes of section through the individual cells, as explained above. A transverse section of a straight tube can produce a single image (e). The double image (d) of the same structure can represent either two tubes running parallel to each other or a single tube that has curved in the space of the tissue or organ that is sectioned.

A **tangential** (**b**) plane of section through the tube with a single layer of cells produces a solid, multicellular, oval structure that does not resemble a tube. The reason for this is that the plane of section has grazed the outermost periphery of the tube as it made a turn in space; the lumen was

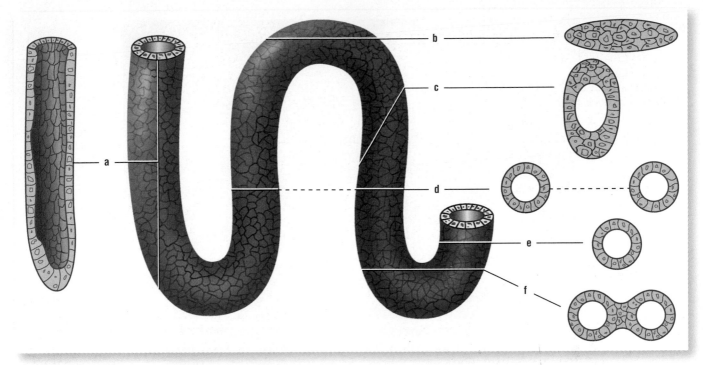

FIGURE 1.11 ■ Planes of section through a hollow object, a tube.

not present in the plane of section. An **oblique** (**c**) plane of section through the same tube and its single layer of cells produces an oval structure that includes an oval lumen in the center and multiple cell layers at the periphery.

A **transverse** (**f**) section in the region of a sharp curve in the tube grazes the innermost cell layer and produces two round structures connected by a multiple, solid layer of cells. These sections of the tube also contain round lumen, indicating that the plane of section passed perpendicular to the structure.

Figure 1.12 shows a section from the testis. This organ is filled with numerous and convoluted (twisted) tubular structures, the seminiferous tubules. Careful examination of this figure shows how individual tubular structures can change shape and appearance, depending on the plane of section through the tubules. Similar structural alteration is possible in solid structures, such as muscle fibers, connective tissue fibers, or nerve fibers.

FIGURE 1.12 | Hollow Tubules of the Testis in Different Planes of Section

Organs such as the testes and kidneys consist primarily of highly twisted or convoluted tubules. When flat sections of such organs are seen on a histology slide, the cut tubules exhibit a variety of shapes because of the plane of section. To show how twisted tubules appear in a histologic slide, a portion of a testis was prepared for examination. Each testis consists of numerous, highly twisted seminiferous tubules that are lined by multilayered or stratified germinal epithelium.

A **longitudinal plane** (**1**) through a seminiferous tubule produces an elongated tubule with a long lumen. A **transverse plane** (**2**) through a single seminiferous tubule produces a round tubule. Similarly, a **transverse plane through a curve** (**3, 5**) of a seminiferous tubule produces two oval structures that are connected by solid layers of cells. An **oblique plane** (**4**) through a tubule produces an oval structure with an oval lumen in the center and multiple cell layers at the periphery. A **tangential plane** (**6**) of a seminiferous tubule passes through its periphery. As a result, this plane produces a solid, multicellular, oval structure that does not resemble a tube because the plane of section passed below the lumen.

1 Longitudinal plane

2 Transverse plane

3 Transverse plane through curve

4 Oblique plane

5 Transverse plane through curve

6 Tangential plane

FIGURE 1.12 ■ Tubules of the testis in different planes of section. Stain: hematoxylin and eosin (plastic section). ×30.

PART II

Cell and Cytoplasm

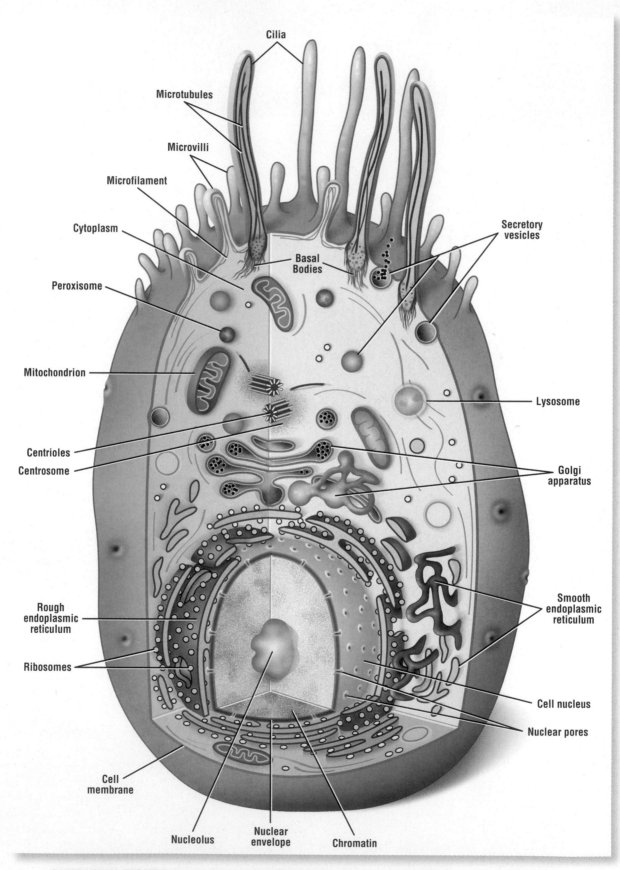

Cilia

Microtubules

Microvilli

Microfilament

Cytoplasm

Peroxisome

Mitochondrion

Centrioles

Centrosome

Rough
endoplasmic
reticulum

Ribosomes

Cell
membrane

Basal
Bodies

Secretory
vesicles

Lysosome

Golgi
apparatus

Smooth
endoplasmic
reticulum

Cell nucleus

Nuclear pores

Nucleolus

Nuclear
envelope

Chromatin

OVERVIEW FIGURE 2.1 ■ Composite illustration of a cell, its cytoplasm, and its organelles.

CHAPTER 2

Light and Transmission Electron Microscopy

Histology, or microscopic anatomy, is a visual, colorful science. The light source for the early microscopes was sunlight. In modern microscopes, an electric light bulb with a tungsten filament serves as the main light source.

With the simplest light microscopes, examination of mammalian cells showed a nucleus and a cytoplasm, surrounded by some sort of a border or cell membrane. As microscopic techniques evolved, the use of various histochemical, immunocytochemical, and staining techniques revealed that the cytoplasm of different cells contained numerous subcellular elements called **organelles**. Although much initial information in histology was gained by examining tissue slides with a light microscope, its resolving power was too limited. To gain additional information called for increased resolution.

With the advent of transmission electron microscopy, superior resolution, and higher magnification of cells, the examination of the contents of the cytoplasm became possible. Histologists are now able to describe the ultrastructure of the cell, its membrane, and the numerous organelles that are present in the cytoplasm of different cells.

The Cell

All living organisms contain a multitude of cell types, whose main functions are to maintain a proper **homeostasis** in the body, which is maintaining the internal environment of the body in a relatively constant state. To perform this task, the cells possess certain structural features in their cytoplasm that are common to all. As a result, it is possible to illustrate a cell in a more generalized, composite form with various cytoplasmic organelles. It is essential to remember, however, that the quantity, appearance, and distribution of the cytoplasmic organelles within a given cell depend on the cell type and its function.

The Cell Membrane

Except for mature red blood cells, all mammalian cells contain a **cytoplasm** and a **nucleus**. In addition, all cells are surrounded by a **cell** or **plasma membrane**, which forms an important barrier or boundary between the internal environment and the external environment. Internal to the cell membrane is the **cytoplasm**, a dense, fluid medium that contains numerous **organelles**, microtubules, microfilaments, and membrane-bound secretory granules, or ingested material.

The membrane that surrounds the cell consists of a **phospholipid bilayer**, a double layer of **phospholipid molecules**. Interspersed within and embedded in the phospholipid bilayer of the cell membrane are the **integral membrane proteins** and **peripheral membrane proteins**, which make up almost half of the total mass of the membrane. The integral membrane proteins are incorporated within the lipid bilayer of the cell membrane. Some of the integral proteins span the entire thickness of the cell membrane. These are the **transmembrane proteins**, and they are exposed on the outer and inner surfaces of the cell membrane. The membrane proteins participate in transporting molecules across the lipid bilayer, serve as membrane receptors for different hormones, attach to and support the internal cytoskeleton of the cell membrane, and possess specific enzyme activity. The peripheral proteins do not protrude into the phospholipid bilayer and are not embedded within the cell membrane. Instead, they are associated with the cell membrane on both its extracellular (outer) and intracellular (inner) surfaces. Some of the peripheral proteins are anchored to the network of tiny **microfilaments** of the cytoskeleton of the cell and are held firmly in place. Also present within the plasma membrane is the lipid molecule **cholesterol**. Cholesterol stabilizes the cell membrane, makes it more rigid, and regulates the fluidity of the phospholipid bilayer.

Located on the external surface of the cell membrane is a delicate, fuzzy cell coat called the **glycocalyx**, composed of carbohydrate molecules that are attached to the integral proteins of the cell membrane and that project from the external cell surface. The glycocalyx is seen primarily with electron microscopic images of the cells. The glycocalyx has important roles in cell recognition, cell-to-cell attachments or adhesions, and as a receptor or binding site for different blood-borne hormones.

Molecular Organization of the Cell Membrane

The lipid bilayer of the cell membrane has a fluid consistency, and, as a result, the compositional structure of the cell membrane is characterized as a **fluid mosaic model**. The phospholipid molecules of the cell membrane are distributed as two layers. Their **polar heads** are arranged on both the inner and outer surfaces of the cell membrane. The **nonpolar tails** of the lipid layers face each other in the center of the membrane. Images of cell membrane viewed with the transmission electron microscope, however, appear as three distinct layers, consisting of outer and inner electron-dense layers and a less dense or lighter middle layer. This discrepancy is due to the osmic acid (osmium tetroxide) that is used to fix and stain tissues for electron microscopy. Osmic acid binds to the polar heads of the lipid molecules in the cell membrane and stains them very densely. The nonpolar tails in the middle of the cell membrane remain light and unstained.

Cell Membrane Permeability and Membrane Transport

The phospholipid bilayer of the cell membrane is permeable to certain substances and impermeable to others. This property of the cell membrane is called **selective permeability**. Selective permeability forms an important barrier between the internal and external environments of the cell, which then maintains a constant intracellular environment.

The phospholipid bilayer is permeable to such molecules as oxygen, carbon dioxide, water, steroids, and other lipid-soluble chemicals. Other substances, such as glucose, ions, and proteins, cannot pass through the cell membrane and cross it only by specific **transport mechanisms**. Some of these substances are transported through the integral membrane proteins using pump molecules or through protein channels that allow the passage of specific molecules. A process called **endocytosis** performs the uptake and transfer of molecules and solids across the cell membrane into the cell interior. In contrast, the process of releasing material from the cell cytoplasm across the cell membrane to the exterior is called **exocytosis**.

Pinocytosis is the process by which cells ingest small molecules of extracellular fluids or liquids. **Phagocytosis** refers to the ingestion or intake of large solid particles, such as bacteria, worn-out cells, or cellular debris, by specialized cells. Examples of such cells are the neutrophils in the blood and macrophages or monocytes in the extracellular connective tissues. **Receptor-mediated endocytosis** is a highly selective form of pinocytosis, or phagocytosis. In this process, specific molecules in the extracellular fluid bind to receptors on the cell membrane and are then taken into the cell cytoplasm. These receptors cluster on the cell membrane, and the membrane indents at this point to form **coated pits** that are lined with peripheral membrane proteins called **clathrin**. The pit pinches off and forms a clathrin-coated vesicle that enters the cytoplasm. The clathrin molecules then separate from the coated vesicle and recycle back to the cell membrane to form new coated pits. Examples of receptor-mediated endocytosis include uptake of low-density lipoproteins and insulin from the blood.

Cellular Organelles

Each cell cytoplasm contains numerous organelles, each of which performs a specialized metabolic function that is essential for maintaining cellular homeostasis and cell life. A membrane similar to the cell membrane surrounds such cytoplasmic organelles as nuclei, mitochondria, endoplasmic reticulum, Golgi complexes, lysosomes, and peroxisomes. Organelles that are not surrounded by membranes include ribosomes, basal bodies, centrioles, and centrosomes.

Mitochondria

Mitochondria are round, oval, or elongated structures whose variability and number depend on cell function. Each mitochondrion (singular) consists of an outer membrane and an inner membrane. The inner membrane exhibits numerous folds called **cristae**, which contain respiratory chain enzymes that produce the energy molecule **adenosine triphosphate (ATP)**. In protein-secreting cells, these cristae project into the interior of the mitochondria as **shelves**. In steroid-secreting cells, such as the adrenal cortex or interstitial cells in the testes, the mitochondria cristae are **tubular** and contain enzymes for steroidogenesis (production of steroids).

Endoplasmic Reticulum

The **endoplasmic reticulum** in the cytoplasm is an extensive network of sacs, vesicles, and interconnected flat tubules called **cisternae**. The endoplasmic reticulum may be rough or smooth. Its predominance and distribution in a given cell depends on cell function.

Rough endoplasmic reticulum (RER) is characterized by numerous flattened, interconnected cisternae, whose cytoplasmic surfaces are covered or studded with dark-staining granules called **ribosomes**. The presence of ribosomes distinguishes the RER, which extends from the outer membrane of the nuclear envelope to sites throughout the cytoplasm. In contrast, **smooth endoplasmic reticulum (SER)** is devoid of ribosomes, and it consists primarily of anastomosing or connecting tubules. In most cells, SER, which is less abundant than the RER, is also continuous with RER.

Golgi Apparatus

The **Golgi apparatus** is also composed of a system of membrane-bound, smooth, flattened, stacked, and slightly curved **cisternae**. These cisternae, however, are separate from those of endoplasmic reticulum. In most cells, there is a polarity in the Golgi apparatus. Near the Golgi apparatus, numerous small vesicles with newly synthesized proteins bud off from the RER and move to the Golgi apparatus for further processing. The Golgi cisternae nearest the budding vesicles are the forming, convex, or the *cis* **face** of the Golgi apparatus. The opposite side of the Golgi apparatus is the maturing inner concave side or the *trans* **face**. Vesicles from the endoplasmic reticulum move through the cytoplasm to the *cis* side of the Golgi apparatus and bud off from the *trans* side to transport proteins to different sites in the cell cytoplasm.

Ribosomes

The **ribosomes** are small, electron-dense granules found in the cytoplasm of the cell; a membrane does not surround ribosomes. In a given cell, there are both **free ribosomes** and **attached ribosomes,** as seen on the endoplasmic reticulum cisternae. Ribosomes have an important role in **protein synthesis** and are most abundant in the cytoplasm of protein-secreting cells. Ribosomes perform an essential role in decoding or translating the **coded genetic messages** from the nucleus for the amino acid sequence of proteins that are then synthesized by the cell. The unattached or free ribosomes synthesize proteins for use within the cell cytoplasm. In contrast, ribosomes that are attached to the membranes of the endoplasmic reticulum synthesize proteins that are packaged and stored in the cell as lysosomes or are released from the cell as secretory products. Ribosomal subunits and associated proteins are first synthesized in the nucleolus and then transported to the cytoplasm via the nuclear pores.

Lysosomes

Lysosomes are cytoplasmic organelles that contain many hydrolyzing or digestive enzymes called **acid hydrolases**. Lysosomal hydrolases are synthesized in the RER and transferred to the Golgi apparatus, where they are modified and packaged into membrane-bound lysosomes. They are highly variable in appearance and size. To prevent the lysosomes from digesting the cytoplasm and cell contents, a membrane separates the lytic enzymes in the lysosomes from the cell cytoplasm. The main function of lysosomes is the **intracellular digestion** or **phagocytosis** of substances taken into the cells. Lysosomes digest phagocytosed microorganisms, cell debris, cells, and damaged, worn-out, or excessive cell organelles, such as RER or mitochondria. During intracellular digestion, a membrane surrounds the material to be digested. The membrane of the lysosome then fuses with the ingested material, and their hydrolytic enzymes are emptied into the formed vacuole. After digestion of the lysosomal contents, the indigestible debris in the cytoplasm is retained in large membrane-bound vesicles called **residual bodies**. Lysosomes are very abundant in such phagocytic cells as tissue macrophages and specific white blood cells (leukocytes) such as neutrophils.

Peroxisomes

Peroxisomes are cell organelles that appear similar to lysosomes but are smaller. They are found in nearly all cell types. Peroxisomes contain several types of **oxidases**, which are enzymes that oxidize various organic substances to form **hydrogen peroxide**, a highly cytotoxic product. Peroxisomes also contain the enzyme **catalase**, which eliminates excess hydrogen peroxide by breaking it down into water and oxygen molecules. Because the degradation of hydrogen peroxide takes place within the same organelle, peroxisomes protect other parts of the cells from this cytotoxic product. Peroxisomes are abundant in the cells of the liver and kidney, where much of the toxic substances are removed from the body. They detoxify, degrade alcohol, oxidize fatty acids, and metabolize various compounds.

The Cytoskeleton of the Cell

The **cytoskeleton** of a cell consists of a network of tiny protein filaments and tubules that extend throughout the cytoplasm. It serves as the cell's structural framework. Three types of filamentous proteins, microfilaments, intermediate filaments, and microtubules, form the cytoskeleton of a cell.

Microfilaments, Intermediate Filaments, and Microtubules

Microfilaments are the thinnest structures of the cytoskeleton. They are composed of the protein **actin** and are most prevalent on the peripheral regions of the cell membrane. These structural proteins shape the cells and contribute to cell movement and movement of the cytoplasmic organelles. The microfilaments are distributed throughout the cells and are used as anchors at cell junctions. The actin microfilaments also form the structural **core** of microvilli and the **terminal web** just inferior to the plasma membrane. In muscle tissues, the actin filaments fill the cells and are associated with **myosin** proteins to induce muscle contractions.

As their name implies, the **intermediate filaments** are thicker than microfilaments and are more stable. Several cytoskeletal proteins that form the intermediate filaments have been identified and localized. The intermediate filaments vary among cell types and have specific distribution in different cell types. Epithelial cells contain the intermediate filaments **keratin**. In skin cells, these filaments terminate at cell junctions, **desmosomes** and **hemidesmosomes**, where they stabilize the shape of the cell and their attachments to adjacent cells. **Vimentin** filaments are found in many mesenchymal cells. **Desmin** filaments are found in both smooth and striated muscles. **Neurofilament** proteins are found in the nerve cells and their processes. **Glial filaments** are found in astrocytic glial cells of the nervous system. **Nuclear lamin** intermediate filaments are found on the inner layer of the nuclear membrane.

Microtubules are found in almost all cell types except red blood cells. They are the largest elements of the cytoskeleton. Microtubules are hollow, unbranched cylindrical structures composed of two protein subunits, α and β **tubulin**. All microtubules originate from the microtubule-organizing center, the **centrosome** in the cytoplasm, which contains a pair of **centrioles**. In the centrosome, the tubulin subunits polymerize and radiate from the centrioles in a starlike pattern from the center. Microtubules determine cell shape and function in the intracellular movement of organelles and secretory granules such as axoplasmic transport in neurons. Microtubules are also essential in cell mitosis, where they form spindles that separate the duplicated chromosomes and remodel the cell during mitosis. These tubules are most visible and are predominant in **cilia** and **flagella**, where they are responsible for their beating movements. Microtubules also form the basis of the centrioles and basal bodies of the cilia.

Centrosome and Centrioles

The **centrosome** is an area of the cytoplasm located near the nucleus. It is the major microtubule forming the center and the site for generating new microtubules and mitotic spindles. The centrosome consists of two small cylindrical structures called **centrioles** and the surrounding matrix; the centrioles are oriented at right angels to each other. Each centriole consists of nine evenly spaced clusters of three sets of fused microtubules arranged in a circle or a ring. The microtubules exhibit longitudinal orientation and are parallel to each other.

Before mitosis, the centrioles in the centrosome replicate and form two pairs. During mitosis, each pair moves to the opposite poles of the cell, where they become microtubule-organizing centers for **mitotic spindles** that control the distribution of chromosomes to the daughter cells. Beneath the cell membrane, the centrioles induce the formation of **basal bodies** and organize the development of the microtubules in cilia and flagella.

Cytoplasmic Inclusions

The **cytoplasmic inclusions** are temporary structures that accumulate in the cytoplasm of certain cells. **Lipids**, **glycogen**, **crystals**, **pigment**, or byproducts of metabolism are inclusions and represent the nonliving parts of the cell.

The Nucleus, Nuclear Envelope, and Nuclear Pores

The **nucleus** is the largest organelle of a cell. Most cells contain a single nucleus, but other cells may exhibit multiple nuclei. Skeletal muscle cells have multiple nuclei, whereas mature mammalian red blood cells do not have a nucleus, or are "nonnucleated."

The nucleus consists of **chromatin**, one or more **nucleoli** (singular, nucleolus), and **nuclear matrix**. The nucleus contains the cellular genetic material **deoxyribonucleic acid (DNA)**, which encodes all cell structures and functions. A double membrane called the **nuclear envelope** surrounds the nucleus, whereas the nucleolus is not surrounded by a membrane. Both the inner and outer layers of the nuclear envelope have a structure similar to that of the lipid bilayer of the cell membrane. The outer nuclear membrane is studded with ribosomes and is continuous with the RER. The inner nuclear membrane lacks ribosomes and is in contact with the nuclear chromatin.

At intervals around the periphery of the nucleus, the outer and inner membranes of the nuclear envelope fuse to form numerous **nuclear pores**. These pores function in controlling the movement of metabolites, macromolecules, and ribosomal subunits between the nucleus and the cytoplasm.

 Supplemental micrographic images are available at **www.thePoint.com/Eroschenko12e** under Cell and Cytoplasm.

Extracellular fluid

Peripheral
proteins

Cholesterol

Glycolipids

Carbohydrate

Glycoprotein

Phospholipid
bilayer

Filaments
of cytoskeleton

Transmembrane
proteins

Channel

Peripheral
protein

Cytoplasm (intercellular fluid)

OVERVIEW FIGURE 2.2 ■ **Composition of the cell membrane.**

FIGURE 2.1 | **Internal and External Morphology of Ciliated and Nonciliated Epithelium**

A low-magnification electron micrograph shows the internal morphology and surfaces of ciliated and nonciliated cells in the epithelium of the efferent ductules of the testis. The numerous **cilia** **(2)** in the ciliated cells are attached to the dense **basal bodies (8)** at the cell apices, from which they extend into the **lumen (1)** of the duct. In contrast to cilia, the **microvilli (7)** in the nonciliated cells are much shorter and have a different internal structure than the cilia (see Figure 2.5 for details and comparison).

Note also the dense structures in the apices between the adjacent epithelial cells. These are the **junctional complexes (3, 9)** that hold the cells tightly together. Distinct **cell membranes (10)** separate the individual cells. Located in the cytoplasm of these cells are numerous, elongated or rod-shaped **mitochondria (4, 11)** and numerous light-staining **vesicles (6)**. Each cell also contains various-shaped **nuclei (12)** with dispersed, dense-staining nuclear **chromatin (5)** that is arranged around the nuclear periphery.

1 Lumen

2 Cilia

3 Junctional complex

4 Mitochondria

5 Nuclear chromatin

6 Vesicles

7 Microvilli

8 Basal bodies

9 Junctional complex

10 Cell membranes

11 Mitochondria

12 Nuclei

FIGURE 2.1 ■ Internal and external morphologies of ciliated and nonciliated epithelium. ×11,000.

FIGURE 2.2 | Junctional Complex Between Epithelial Cells

A high-magnification electron micrograph illustrates a junctional complex between two adjacent epithelial cells. In the upper or apical region of the cells, the opposing cell membranes fuse to form a **tight junction** or **zonula occludens (2a)**, which extends around the cell peripheries like a belt. Inferior to the tight junction (2a) is another junction called the **zonula adherens (2b)**. It is characterized by a dense layer of proteins on the inside of the plasma membranes of both cells, which attach to the cytoskeleton filaments of each cell. A small intercellular space with transmembrane adhesion proteins separates the two membranes. This type of junction also extends around the cells like a belt. Below the zonula adherens is a **desmosome (2c)**. Desmosomes (2c) do not encircle the cells but are spotlike structures that have random distribution in the cells. The cytoplasmic side of each desmosome exhibits dense areas composed of attachment proteins. Transmembrane glycoproteins extend into the intercellular space between opposing cell membranes of the desmosome and attach the cells to each other.

Note also in the micrograph the distinct **cell membranes (3)** of each cell, the numerous **mitochondria (1)** in cross section, and a variety of **vesicular structures (6)** in their cytoplasm. Visible on the cell apices are sections of **cilia (5)** with a core of **microtubules** and a few **microvilli (4)**.

FUNCTIONAL CORRELATIONS 2.1 | Junctional Complex

Junctional complexes have a variety of functions, depending on their morphology, shape, and location. In the epithelium that lines the stomach, intestines, and urinary bladder, the **zonulae occludentes,** or tight junctions, are the most apical junctions that prevent the passage of corrosive chemicals or waste products between cells and into the bloodstream. The tight junctions consist of **transmembrane proteins** called **claudins** that fuse the outer membranes of adjacent cells. In this manner, the cells form a tight epithelial barrier. Similarly, the **zonula adherens** or adhering junctions assist these cells in resisting separation, such that the transmembrane proteins attach to the cytoskeleton proteins and bind adjacent cells. **Actin filaments** attach zonula adherens. **Desmosomes** are spotlike structures that are most commonly seen in the epithelium of the skin and in cardiac muscle fibers. Here, the cells are subjected to great mechanical stresses. In these organs, desmosomes prevent skin cells from separating and cardiac muscle cells from pulling apart during the powerful heart contractions. The desmosomes are bound to **intermediate filaments** and form strong attachment sites between the adjacent cells.

Other junctional complexes are **hemidesmosomes** and **gap junctions**. Hemidesmosomes are one half of the desmosome and are present at the base of epithelial cells. Here, hemidesmosomes anchor the epithelial cells to the basement membrane and the adjacent extracellular connective tissue. The basement membrane consists of a basal lamina and reticular fibers of the connective tissue (see Figure 2.4).

Gap junctions are also spotlike in structure. The plasma membranes at gap junctions are closely apposed, and tiny fluid channels called **connexons** connect the adjacent cells. Molecules, ions, and low-resistance electrical communication occurs through these connexons between adjacent cells. These fluid channels are vital in cardiac muscle cells and nerve cells, where fast impulse transmission through the adjacent cells or axons is essential for synchronization and coordination of normal functions.

FIGURE 2.3 | Basal Regions of Epithelial Cells

A medium-magnification electron micrograph illustrates the appearance of the basal region or the base of epithelial cells. Note that the basal regions of the cells are attached to a thin, moderately electron-dense layer called the **basal lamina (3)**. Deep to the basal lamina (3) is a **connective tissue (2)** layer of fine reticular fibers. The basal lamina (3) is seen only with the electron microscope. Basal lamina (3) and the reticular fibers of connective tissue (2) are seen under the light microscope as a basement membrane.

Inferior to the epithelial cells is an elongated, spindle-shaped **fibroblast (4)** with its **nucleus (4)** and dispersed **chromatin (5)**, surrounded by numerous connective tissue fibers (2) produced by the fibroblasts. In the cytoplasm of one of the epithelial cells is also seen a **nucleus (8)**, dispersed **chromatin (9)**, and a dense, round **nucleolus (7)**. **Cisternae** of **RER (11)**, elongated **mitochondria (14)**, and various types of **dense bodies (6)** are visible in different cells. Between the individual epithelial cells is a distinct **cell membrane (1, 10)**. Hemidesmosomes are not illustrated (see Figure 2.4) but attach the basal membrane of the cells to the basal lamina (3).

FIGURE 2.2 ■ Junctional complex between epithelial cells. ×31,200.

FIGURE 2.3 ■ Basal regions of epithelial cells. ×9,500.

FIGURE 2.4 | Basal Region of an Ion-Transporting Cell

A medium-magnification electron micrograph illustrates the basal region of a cell from the distal convoluted tubule of the kidney. In contrast to the basal regions of epithelial cells, the basal regions of cells in convoluted kidney tubules are characterized by numerous and complex **infoldings** of the **basal cell membrane (5)**. These infoldings then form numerous **basal membrane interdigitations (11)** with the similar infoldings of the neighboring cell. Numerous and long **mitochondria (4, 10)** with vertical or apical–basal orientations are located between the cell membrane infoldings. Also, numerous, dark-staining spotlike **hemidesmosomes (6, 12)** attach the highly infolded basal cell membrane to the electron-dense **basal lamina (7, 13)**.

A portion of a large **nucleus (1)** is visible with its dispersed **chromatin (9)**. Surrounding the nucleus is a distinct **nuclear envelope (2)**, which consists of a double membrane. Both the outer and inner membranes of the nuclear envelope (2) fuse at intervals around the periphery of the nucleus to form numerous **nuclear pores (3)**.

FUNCTIONAL CORRELATIONS 2.2 | Infolded Basal Regions of the Cell

The deep **infoldings** of the basal and lateral cell membranes are seen only with electron microscopy. These infoldings are found in certain cells of the body, whose main function is to transport **ions** across the cell membrane. The cells in the tubular portions of the kidney (proximal convoluted tubules and distal convoluted tubules) selectively absorb useful or nutritious components from the glomerular filtrate and retain them in the body. At the same time, these cells eliminate toxic or nonuseful metabolic waste products, such as urea and drug metabolites.

Because these cells transport numerous ions across their membranes, increased amounts of energy are needed, which is generated by **Na$^+$/K$^+$ ATPase (sodium pumps)** embedded in the infolded basal and lateral cell membranes. To perform these vital functions, numerous long **mitochondria** that are located in these basal infoldings continually supply the cells with the energy source (ATP) that operates these pumps for membrane transport. Similar basal cell membrane infoldings are seen in the striated ducts of the salivary glands. These glands produce saliva, which is then modified by selective transport of various ions across the cell membrane as it moves through these ducts to the larger excretory ducts.

FIGURE 2.5 | Cilia and Microvilli

This high-magnification electron micrograph illustrates the ultrastructural differences between cilia (singular, cilium) and microvilli (singular, microvillus). Both **cilia (1)** and **microvilli (2)** project from the apical surfaces of certain cells in the body. The cilia (1) are long, motile structures, with a core of uniformly arranged **microtubules (3)** in longitudinal orientation. The core of each cilium contains a constant number of nine microtubule doublets located peripherally and two single microtubules in the center. Each cilium is attached to and extends from the **basal body (4)** in the apical region of the cell. Instead of nine microtubule doublets, the basal bodies exhibit nine microtubule triplets and no central microtubules.

In contrast to cilia, microvilli (2) are smaller, shorter, closely packed fingerlike extensions that greatly increase the surface area of certain cells. Microvilli (2) are nonmotile and exhibit a core of thin microfilaments called actin. The actin filaments extend from the microvilli (2) into the apical cytoplasm of the cell to form a terminal web, a complex network of actin filaments.

1 Nucleus

2 Nuclear envelope

3 Nuclear pores

4 Mitochondria

5 Basal membrane infoldings

6 Hemidesmosome

7 Basal lamina

8 Nucleolus

9 Nuclear chromatin

10 Mitochondria

11 Basal membrane interdigitations

12 Hemidesmosome

13 Basal lamina

FIGURE 2.4 ■ Basal region of an ion-transporting cell. ×16,600.

1 Cilia

2 Microvilli with microfilaments

3 Microtubules in cilia

4 Basal bodies of cilia

FIGURE 2.5 ■ Cilia and microvilli. ×20,000.

FIGURE 2.6 | Nuclear Envelope and Nuclear Pores

A high-magnification electron micrograph illustrates in detail part of a **nucleus (8)** and the surrounding membrane, the **nuclear envelope (3)**, which consists of an **outer nuclear membrane (3a)** and an **inner nuclear membrane (3b)**. Between the two nuclear membranes (3a, 3b) is a space. The outer nuclear membrane (3a) is in contact with the **cell cytoplasm (4)**, whereas the inner nuclear membrane (3b) is associated with the **nuclear chromatin (7)**. The nuclear envelope is continuous with the **RER (1)**, and the outer nuclear membrane (3a) usually contains ribosomes. At certain intervals around the nucleus, the two membranes of the nuclear envelope (3) fuse and form numerous **nuclear pores (2, 6)**.

FUNCTIONAL CORRELATIONS 2.3 | Cytoplasmic Organelles: Part 1

CILIA

Cilia are highly motile surface modifications in cells that line the respiratory organs, oviducts or uterine tubes, and efferent ducts in the testes. Cilia are inserted into the **basal bodies** beneath the cell membrane. The main function of cilia is to sweep or move fluids, cells, or particulate matter across cell surfaces. In the lungs, the cilia rid the air passages of particulate matter or mucus. In the oviduct, cilia move eggs and sperm along the passageway, and in the testes, cilia move mature sperm into the epididymis.

The motility exhibited by cilia is caused by the sliding of adjacent microtubule doublets in the core of the cilia. Each of the nine doublets in the cilia consists of two subfibers, A and B. Extending from the A subfiber are two armlike filaments containing the **motor protein dynein**, which exhibits ATPase activity. This protein uses the energy of ATP hydrolysis to move cilia. Dynein armlike extensions from one doublet temporarily attach and detach from the subfiber B of the adjacent doublet, producing a sliding force between the doublets. These rapid back-and-forth changes between adjacent doublets produce cilia motility.

MICROVILLI

In contrast to cilia, **microvilli** are nonmotile. Microvilli are highly developed on the apical surfaces of epithelial cells of the small intestine and kidney. Here, the main functions of the microvilli are to absorb nutrients from the digestive tract of the small intestine or the glomerular filtrate in the kidney.

NUCLEUS, NUCLEOLUS, AND NUCLEAR PORES

The **nucleus** is the control center of the cell; it stores and processes most of the cell's genetic information. The nucleus directs all the activities of the cell through the process of protein synthesis and ultimately controls the structural and functional characteristics of each cell. The cell's genetic material, **deoxyribonucleic acid (DNA)**, is visible in the cell in the form of **chromatin**. When the cells are not actively producing protein, the DNA is not condensed and does not stain.

The **nucleolus** is a dense-staining, nonmembrane-bound structure within the nucleus. One or more nucleoli may be visible in a given cell. The nucleolus functions in synthesis, processing, and assembly of **ribosomes**. In nucleoli, the ribosomal **ribonucleic acid (RNA)** is produced and combined with proteins to form ribosomal subunits. These ribosomal subunits are then transported to the cell cytoplasm through the nuclear pores to form complete ribosomes. Consequently, nucleoli are prominent in cells that synthesize large amounts of proteins. **Nuclear pores** control the transport of macromolecules between the nucleus and the cytoplasm. The nuclear pore membrane, like other cell membranes, shows selective permeability. As a result, some of the larger molecules travel through the pores via an active transport mechanism.

FUNCTIONAL CORRELATIONS 2.3 | Cytoplasmic Organelles: Part 1 *(Continued)*

MITOCHONDRIA

These organelles produce most of the high-energy molecule **adenosine triphosphate (ATP)** present in cells and are, therefore, considered the powerhouses of the cells. The numerous cristae in the mitochondria increase the surface area of the inner membrane. The cristae contain most of the respiratory chain enzymes as well as **ATP synthetase**, which is responsible for cell respiration (oxidative phosphorylation) and production of cell ATP, which is the chemical energy responsible for the different metabolic activities of the cells.

The number of mitochondria in the cell is directly related to its energy needs. Thus, such cells as cardiac or skeletal muscle cells with continuous high-energy needs exhibit numerous mitochondria, whereas cells with low-energy needs have few mitochondria. Also, in these high-energy cells, the mitochondria exhibit large numbers of closely packed cristae, whereas in cells with low-energy metabolism, the cristae are less extensively developed. Surrounding the cristae is an amorphous **mitochondrial matrix**, which contains enzymes, ribosomes, and, unlike other cytoplasmic organelles, a small, circular DNA molecule called **mitochondrial DNA**. New mitochondria arise from preexisting mitochondria by growth and division.

FIGURE 2.6 ■ Nuclear envelope and nuclear pores. ×110,000.

FIGURE 2.7 | Mitochondria

A high-magnification electron micrograph illustrates the ultrastructure of **mitochondria (1, 4)** in a **longitudinal section (1)** and in **cross section (4)**. Note that the mitochondria (1, 4) also exhibit two membranes. The **outer mitochondrial membrane (5, 9)** is smooth and surrounds the entire organelle. The inner mitochondrial membrane is highly folded, surrounds the matrix of the mitochondria, and projects inward into the organelle to form the numerous, shelflike **cristae (6)**. Some mitochondrial matrix may contain dense-staining granules. Also visible in the **cytoplasm (8)** of the cell are variously sized, light-staining **vacuoles (7)**, a section of **RER (2)**, and free **ribosomes (3)**. This type of mitochondria with shelflike cristae (6) is normally found in protein-secreting cells and muscle cells.

FIGURE 2.8 | Rough Endoplasmic Reticulum

A high-magnification electron micrograph illustrates the components of the **RER (3)** in the cytoplasm of a cell. It consists of stacked layers of membranous cavities called **cisternae (3)**. In the RER, ribosomes are attached to the outer surface of the membranes. Also present in the cytoplasm are **free ribosomes (4, 13)**, some of which attach to other ribosomes and form ribosome groups called **polyribosomes (4, 13)**. Visible in the cytoplasm are also numerous **mitochondria (2, 10)**, in longitudinal **(10)** and cross section (2), **dense secretory granules (8)**, and very thin strands of **microfilaments (5, 11)**. In the lower right corner of the micrograph, the smooth cisternae and associated vesicles of the **Golgi apparatus (14)** are visible. Note the **cell membranes (1, 9)** of adjacent cells, **nuclear envelope (6)**, and portions of the **nucleus (7)** and nuclear **chromatin (12)**.

1 Mitochondrion (longitudinal section)

2 RER

3 Free ribosomes

4 Mitochondria (cross section)

5 Outer mitochondrial membrane

6 Cristae

7 Vacuoles

8 Cytoplasm

9 Outer mitochondrial membrane

FIGURE 2.7 ■ Mitochondria (longitudinal and cross section). ×49,500.

1 Cell membrane

2 Mitochondria

3 Cisternae of RER

4 Free ribosomes

5 Microfilaments

6 Nuclear envelope

7 Nucleus

8 Dense secretory granules

9 Cell membrane

10 Mitochondria (longitudinal section)

11 Microfilaments

12 Nuclear chromatin

13 Free ribosomes

14 Golgi apparatus

FIGURE 2.8 ■ Rough endoplasmic reticulum. ×32,000.

FIGURE 2.9 | Smooth Endoplasmic Reticulum

This high-magnification electron micrograph illustrates the structure of the **SER (2)** in two adjacent cells. SER (2) is devoid of ribosomes and consists primarily of smooth, anastomosing tubules. In this micrograph, the tubules of the SER (2) are primarily seen in cross section. In other sections, the SER (2) can be seen as flattened vesicles. In some cells, the SER is continuous with **cisternae** of the **RER (7)**, as seen in this micrograph.

Also seen in the micrograph are the **cell membranes (6, 11)** of the two cells, the **cell membrane interdigitations (10)**, and the **extracellular matrix (9)** between the two cell membranes. A section of the **nucleus (4, 5)**, **nuclear envelope (8)**, **nuclear chromatin (3)**, and **mitochondrion (1)** in cross section is also visible in the two cells. The mitochondria (1) in these cells contain tubular cristae, indicating that the cells synthesize products other than proteins.

FIGURE 2.10 | Golgi Apparatus

A high-magnification electron micrograph illustrates the components of the **Golgi apparatus (2)**. This apparatus consists of membrane-bound **Golgi cisternae (2)** with numerous membranous **Golgi vesicles (1)** located near the end of the cisternae. The Golgi apparatus (2) usually exhibits a crescent shape. Its convex side is called the *cis* **face (3)**, and the opposite, concave side is called the *trans* **face** (9) of the Golgi apparatus (2). This micrograph illustrates the Golgi apparatus (2) in the seminiferous tubule of the testis, where a spermatid is undergoing transformation into a sperm. At this stage of the transformation, the Golgi apparatus (2) is packaging and condensing the secretory product into an electron-dense **acrosome granule (7)**. The acrosome granule (7) is located in the **acrosomal vesicle (8)** that adheres to the **nuclear envelope (6)** at the anterior pole of the spermatid. In the left corner of the micrograph, note a short cisterna of the **granular (rough) endoplasmic reticulum (4)** and some **free ribosomes (5)** in the **cytoplasm (11)** of the spermatid. A **cell membrane (10)** surrounds the cell.

1 Mitochondrion

2 Tubules of SER

3 Nuclear chromatin

4 Nucleus

5 Nucleus

6 Cell membrane

7 Cisternae of RER

8 Nuclear envelope

9 Extracellular matrix

10 Cell membrane interdigitations

11 Cell membrane

FIGURE 2.9 ■ Smooth endoplasmic reticulum. ×11,500.

1 Golgi vesicles

2 Cisterna of Golgi apparatus

3 *Cis* face of Golgi apparatus

4 Cisterna of RER

5 Free ribosomes

6 Nuclear envelope of spermatid

7 Acrosome granule

8 Acrosome vesicle

9 *Trans* face of Golgi apparatus

10 Cell membrane

11 Cell cytoplasm

FIGURE 2.10 ■ Golgi apparatus. ×23,000.

A medium-magnification electron micrograph illustrates numerous dense-staining **lysosomes** (3) in the cytoplasm of a tissue macrophage. The lysosomes (3) show great variation in size, appearance, density, and the contents. Also visible in the cell cytoplasm are what appear to be the **residual bodies (1, 4)**, consisting of lipid-like material and dense undigested matter enclosed in a membrane. Distinguishing between material being digested in the lysosomes and the residual bodies is often quite difficult. Located also in the cytoplasm are numerous **mitochondria (2)**, sectioned in different planes. Note also the difference in size between the mitochondria and the variably sized lysosomes. In the left-hand corner is a section of a cytoplasm from an adjacent cell.

FUNCTIONAL CORRELATIONS 2.4 | Cytoplasmic Organelles: Part 2

ROUGH ENDOPLASMIC RETICULUM

Cells that synthesize large amounts of protein for export, such as pancreatic acinar cells or salivary gland cells, exhibit a highly developed and extensive **rough endoplasmic reticulum (RER)** with numerous stacks of flattened cisternae. Thus, the main function of RER is **protein synthesis**. Proteins that will be either transported or exported to the outside of the cell or packaged in organelles such as lysosomes are synthesized by the ribosomes attached to the surface of the RER. In addition, **integral membrane proteins** and **phospholipid molecules** are synthesized by the RER and become part of the cell membrane. In contrast, proteins for the cytoplasm, nucleus, and mitochondria use are synthesized by the **free ribosomes** located within the cell cytoplasm.

SMOOTH ENDOPLASMIC RETICULUM

Although the **smooth endoplasmic reticulum (SER)** is continuous with the RER, its membranes lack ribosomes, and, therefore, its functions are completely different and unrelated to protein synthesis. SER is found in abundance in cells that synthesize **phospholipids** that constitute all cell membranes, **cholesterol**, and **steroid hormones**, such as estrogens, testosterone, and corticosteroids. When liver cells (hepatocytes) are exposed to potentially harmful drugs and chemicals, SER proliferates and inactivates or **detoxifies** the chemicals. Similarly, in hepatocytes, SER is involved in **carbohydrate metabolism** that converts glycogen to glucose. Skeletal and cardiac muscle fibers also exhibit an extensive network of SER, called **sarcoplasmic reticulum**, whose primary functions is **calcium storage** (sequestering) between contractions and calcium release for initiation of muscular contractions.

GOLGI APPARATUS

The **Golgi apparatus** is present in almost all cells. Its size and development vary, depending on the cell function; however, it is most highly developed in **secretory cells**. Most of the new proteins synthesized by the cisternae of the RER are transported in the cell cytoplasm as **transfer vesicles** to the *cis* face of the Golgi apparatus, which faces the RER. Within the Golgi cisternae are different types of enzymes that modify, sort, and package proteins for different destinations in the cell. As the protein molecules move through the different Golgi cisternae, sugars are added to the proteins and lipids to form **glycoproteins** and **glycolipids**. Also, proteins are added to lipids to form **lipoproteins**. As the secretory molecules near the exit or *trans* face of the Golgi cisternae, they are further modified, sorted, and packaged as membrane-bound vesicles, which then separate from the Golgi cisternae. Some secretory vesicles become lysosomes and remain in the cytoplasm. Other proteins migrate to the cell membrane and are incorporated into the cell membrane itself, thus contributing proteins and phospholipids to the membrane. Still other secretory granules become vesicles filled with a secretory product destined for **exocytosis** (export) to the outside of the cell.

1 Residual bodies

2 Mitochondria

4 Lysosomes

5 Residual bodies

FIGURE 2.11 ■ Ultrastructure of lysosomes and residual bodies in the cytoplasm of a tissue macrophage. Courtesy of Dr. Rex A. Hess, Professor Emeritus, Comparative Biosciences, College of Veterinary Medicine, University of Illinois, Urbana, Illinois. ×16,000.

Cell and Cytoplasm

- Cells maintain proper homeostasis of the body
- Certain structural features are common to all cells

The Cell Membrane

- Consists of phospholipid bilayer and integral (transmembrane) membrane proteins
- Peripheral membrane proteins are located on external and internal cell surfaces
- Peripheral proteins are anchored to microfilaments of cytoskeleton
- Transmembrane proteins are located within the lipid bilayer of the cell membrane
- Transmembrane proteins transport molecules across the lipid bilayer
- Cholesterol molecules within the cell membrane stabilize the cell membrane
- Carbohydrate glycocalyx covers cell surfaces
- Glycocalyx is important for cell recognition, cell adhesion, and receptor-binding sites

Molecular Organization of the Cell Membrane

- Lipid bilayer is in a fluid state, hence the fluid mosaic model
- Phospholipids form two layers with polar heads facing inner and outer surfaces
- Nonpolar tails are in the center of membrane

Cell Membrane Permeability and Transport

- Cell membrane shows selective permeability and forms a barrier between internal and external cell environments
- Permeable to oxygen, carbon dioxide, water, steroids, and lipid-soluble chemicals
- Larger molecules enter the cell by specialized transport mechanisms
- Endocytosis is ingestion of extracellular material into the cell
- Exocytosis is the release of material from the cell
- Pinocytosis is the ingestion of extracellular fluid into the cell
- Phagocytosis is the uptake of large, solid particles into the cell
- Receptor-mediated endocytosis involves pinocytosis or phagocytosis via receptors on the cell membrane and the formation of clathrin-coated pits
- Uptake of low-density lipoproteins and insulin as example of receptor-mediated endocytosis

Cellular Organelles

- Membrane bound: nucleus, mitochondria, endoplasmic reticulum, Golgi complex, lysosomes, and peroxisomes
- Nonmembrane bound: ribosomes, basal bodies, and centrosomes

Mitochondria

- Surrounded by cell membrane
- Shelflike cristae in protein-secreting cells and tubular cristae in steroid-secreting cells
- Present in all cells, especially numerous in highly metabolic cells
- Produce high-energy ATP molecules
- Cristae contain respiratory chain enzymes for ATP production
- Matrix contains enzymes, ribosomes, and circular mitochondrial DNA
- Arise from preexisting mitochondria by growth and division

Rough Endoplasmic Reticulum

- Exhibits interconnected cisternae that are covered with ribosomes
- Highly developed in protein-synthesizing cells
- Synthesizes proteins for export or lysosomes
- Synthesizes integral membrane proteins and phospholipids for the cell membrane
- Free ribosomes synthesize proteins for the cell cytoplasm

Smooth Endoplasmic Reticulum

- Devoid of ribosomes and consists of anastomosing tubules
- Found in cells that synthesize phospholipids, cholesterol, and steroid hormones
- In liver cells, proliferates to deactivate or detoxify harmful chemicals; is involved with carbohydrate metabolism and converts glycogen to glucose
- In skeletal and cardiac muscle fibers, stores and releases calcium between contractions

Golgi Apparatus

- Present in all cells, highly developed in secretory cells
- Consists of stacked, curved cisternae with a convex side known as the *cis* face
- Mature concave side is the *trans* face
- New synthesized proteins are transported in transfer vesicles to the Golgi apparatus
- Cisternae modify enzymes, sort, and package proteins
- Adds sugars to proteins and lipids to form glycoproteins, glycolipids, and lipoproteins
- Secretory granules are modified, sorted, and packaged in membranes for export outside of the cell or for lysosomes
- Other proteins and phospholipids are incorporated into the cell membrane

Ribosomes

- Appear as free and attached (as to the endoplasmic reticulum)
- Most abundant in protein-synthesizing cells
- Decode genetic messages from nucleus for amino acid sequence of protein synthesis
- Free ribosomes synthesize proteins for cell use
- Attached ribosomes synthesize proteins that are packaged for export or lysosomes' use
- Ribosomal subunits are synthesized in nucleolus and transported to the cytoplasm via nuclear pores

Lysosomes

- Membrane-bound vesicles filled with hydrolyzing or digesting enzymes called acid hydrolases
- Synthesized in RER and packaged in the Golgi apparatus
- Separated from the cytoplasm by the membrane to prevent damage to the cell
- Functions in intracellular digestion or phagocytosis
- Digest microorganisms, cellular debris, worn-out cells, and cell organelles
- Residual bodies are seen after phagocytosis
- Very abundant in tissue macrophages and the white blood cells of neutrophils

Peroxisomes

- Contain oxidases that form cytotoxic hydrogen peroxide
- Contain enzyme catalase to eliminate excess hydrogen peroxide
- Abundant in liver and kidney cells, which remove much of the toxic material
- Detoxify, degrade alcohol, oxidize fatty acids, and metabolize compounds

Cell Cytoskeleton

Microfilaments

- Thinnest microfilaments in the cytoskeleton
- Composed of the protein actin and contribute to cell and organelle movements
- Distributed throughout the cell and used as anchors at cell junctions
- Form the core of microvilli and the terminal web at cell apices
- Actin–myosin interactions produce muscle contractions

Intermediate Filaments

- Thicker than microfilaments
- Epithelial cells contain keratin filaments
- In skin cells, they terminate at desmosomes and hemidesmosomes

- Vimentin filaments are found in mesenchymal cells
- Desmin filaments are found in smooth and skeletal muscles
- Glial filaments are found in astrocytic cells of the nervous system
- Lamin filaments are found in the nuclear membrane

Microtubules

- Largest filaments in cytoskeleton and found in most cells except red blood cells
- Composed of α and β tubulin
- Originate from the centrosome
- Determine cell shape and function in intracellular transport
- Form spindles and separate duplicated chromosomes during cell mitosis
- Present in cilia, flagella, centrioles, and basal bodies

Centrosome and Centrioles

- Centrosomes are located near the nucleus and contain two centrioles
- Major microtubule forming both the center and mitotic spindles
- Centrioles are perpendicular to one another; contain nine clusters of three microtubules, each arranged in a circle
- Before mitosis, centrioles replicate
- During mitosis, centrioles form mitotic spindles to control the distribution of chromosomes
- Centrioles induce the formation of basal bodies and microtubules in cilia and flagella

Cytoplasmic Inclusions

- Temporary structures, such as lipids, glycogen, crystals, and pigment

Nucleus and Nuclear Envelope

- Nucleus contains chromatin, nucleoli, nuclear matrix, and cellular DNA
- Double membrane called the nuclear envelope surrounds the nucleus
- Nucleolus is not membrane bound
- Outer membrane of the nuclear envelope contains ribosomes and is continuous with RER
- Nuclear pores at intervals in the nuclear envelope
- Nuclear pores control movements of the material between the nucleus and the cytoplasm

Surfaces of Cells

Junctional Complex

- Zonula occludentes or tight junctions form an effective epithelial barrier
- Transmembrane proteins called claudins fuse the outer membranes of adjacent cells to form tight junctions
- In zonula adherens or adhering junctions, transmembrane proteins attach to the cytoskeleton and bind adjacent cells
- Actin filaments attach zonula adherens
- Desmosomes are spotlike structures, very prominent in skin and cardiac cells
- Desmosomes anchor cells through extension of transmembrane proteins into intercellular spaces between adjacent cells
- Desmosomes are bound to intermediate filaments
- Hemidesmosomes are present at the base of epithelial cells
- Gap junctions are spotlike structures with fluid channels called connexons
- Ions and chemicals diffuse through connexons from cell to cell
- Gap junctions allow rapid communications between cells for synchronized action

Basal Regions of Cells

Infolded Basal Regions of the Cell

- Infolded basal and lateral cell membranes function in ionic transport
- Found in kidney and salivary gland cells
- Na^+/K^+-ATPase (sodium pumps) are embedded in infolded membranes
- Numerous and long mitochondria in infoldings supply ATP for ion transport

Cilia

- Motile apical surface modifications that are inserted into basal bodies
- Line cells in the respiratory organs, uterine tubes, and efferent ducts in testes
- Motility caused by sliding microtubule doublets
- Motor protein dynein uses ATP to move cilia

Microvilli

- Nonmotile apical surface modifications
- Well developed in small intestines and kidney
- Main function is the absorption of nutrients from intestines and glomerular filtrate

OVERVIEW FIGURE 3.1 ■ Cell cycle.

CHAPTER 3

Cells and the Cell Cycle ▪

During embryonic development, the cells divide and multiply to form new cells, tissues, and organs. In an adult organism, however, not all cells retain the ability to further divide and reproduce. As a result, different populations of cells are recognized based on their ability or inability to divide and reproduce.

Permanent Cell Population in Adult Organisms

Nerve cells in the nervous system and **muscle cells** (skeletal and cardiac) continue to divide during embryonic development. Once these cells establish the organs in postnatal life, however, their ability to further divide ceases, and they cannot be replaced if they are damaged or destroyed.

Stable Cell Population

In organs such as the **liver**, cells remain stable in postnatal life and do not divide under normal conditions. However, when part of the liver is surgically removed or is damaged, the liver cells can then proliferate and replace lost cells in order to maintain the normal functions of the organ.

Renewing Cell Population

These cells constantly divide to replace lost or worn-out cells in different tissues and organs of the body. **Skin cells** and cells in the **gastrointestinal epithelium (oral cavity, esophagus, stomach**, and **small** and **large intestines)** continually divide. Similarly, numerous **blood cells** have short life spans and are continually produced to replace the worn-out cells. Also, **germ cells** (spermatagonia) in **testes** constantly divide to produce new sperm.

The Cell Cycle—Interphase and Mitosis

The time interval between two successive cell divisions represents the **cell cycle**. It involves cell replication by duplicating the cell's genetic contents and producing two identical daughter cells. The cell cycle is divided into two main phases: **interphase** and **mitosis**. Interphase consists of a prolonged interval comprising different phases during which time the cell size and its contents increase. In addition, DNA, centrioles, and chromosomes replicate, and the cell prepares for division, or mitosis, which exhibits four distinct and histologically recognizable stages or phases.

Prophase

During this first prolonged phase of mitosis, the **chromosomes** condense and become histologically visible. Each chromosome consists of two genetically identical sister **chromatids** that are joined together at a pinched area called the **centromere**. With the condensation of the chromosomes, the nuclear envelope and nucleolus disappear (fragment) with only fragments visible in the cell. The **centrosome** divides, and the **centrioles** migrate to the opposite poles of the cell to form **microtubules** of the **mitotic spindle** (Figure 3.1a). The microtubule spindles continue to grow toward the chromosomes, where some of them attach to a platelike protein complex called the **kinetochore**, which appears on each side of the centromere. These **kinetochore microtubules** eventually align the chromosomes in the middle of the cell. The microtubules that do not attach to the chromosomes at the kinetochore become the **polar microtubules**.

Metaphase

In this short phase, the chromosomes become highly condensed. The chromosomes are aligned along the equator of the cell as a result of their attachment to the **kinetochore microtubules** of the mitotic spindles that radiate from both spindle poles. The kinetochore microtubules direct the movement of chromosomes toward the middle of the cells, forming the **metaphase** or **equatorial plate** (Figure 3.1a, b).

Anaphase

During this phase, the chromatid pairs separate at the centromere due to an enzymatic action, and each chromatid now becomes a separate chromosome. These chromosomes now begin their migration to the opposite poles of the cell, pulled by the shortening of the kinetochore microtubules, which are attached to the centromeres. The migrating or pulled chromosomes exhibit a V shape in the cell. In late anaphase, a **cleavage furrow** in the cell membrane appears at the cell equator, indicating the area where the cell will divide (Figure 3.1c).

Telophase

This is the terminal phase of mitosis. It begins when the chromosomes complete their migration to the opposite side of the mitotic spindle, and the chromosomes decondense into the chromatin of the interphase cell. Also, the **nucleolus** reappears, and the rough endoplasmic reticulum begins to form a new **nuclear envelope**. A constriction of the cytoplasm is formed by the **contractile ring** composed of **actin** filaments, which becomes the site of cleavage for the separation of daughter cells. **Cleavage** of the joined daughter cells now follows. **Cytokinesis** is the process by which the cytoplasm is divided into two genetically identical cells (Figure 3.1d, e).

Interphase

Mitosis is now complete, and the cell is ready for the new interphase to begin. The chromosomes have unraveled to become visible as **chromatin** material in the nucleus. The resulting cell division has produced two new cells that are identical in their genetic content to the parent cell (Figure 3.1e).

Meiosis

Meiosis is a special type of cell division that is restricted to **male** and **female germ cells**. This type of division produces an ova and a spermatozoa whose chromosome numbers have been reduced from **diploid** (46 chromosomes) to **haploid** (23 chromosomes).

The process of meiosis involves two successive cell divisions after one DNA replication. This ensures that haploid cells are produced from every cell that enters meiosis. The recombination of genes and the establishment of a full chromosome count occur at fertilization of the ovum by the sperm, thus ensuring variability of the progeny. Additional information concerning the meiotic process is described in Chapter 20, "Male Reproductive System," and Chapter 21, "Female Reproductive System."

 Supplemental micrographic images are available at **www.thePoint.com/Eroschenko12e** under Cell and Cytoplasm.

FIGURE 3.1 ■ Different phases of mitosis and cytokinesis.

Cell Populations in Adults

- Permanent—nerve and muscle cells are not replaced when damaged
- Stable cell population—liver cells can proliferate to replace removed or damaged cells
- Renewing cell population—skin, gastrointestinal organs, blood cells, and germ cells in testes are constantly replaced

Cell Cycle—Interphase and Mitosis

- Divided into interphase and mitosis
- Interphase is prolonged and consists of different phases that replicate cell contents
- Mitosis consists of four phases—prophase, metaphase, anaphase, and telophase

Prophase

- Condensation of chromosomes to form two identical chromatids
- Chromatids are joined together at the centromere
- Nuclear envelope and nucleolus disappear
- Centrosome divides, and centrioles move to the opposite poles of the cell
- Centrioles form microtubules of the mitotic spindle
- Microtubules attach to kinetochores of chromatids and align chromosomes in the middle of the cell

Metaphase

- Chromosomes highly condensed
- Kinetochore aligns chromosomes along the equator of the cell
- Formation of equatorial plate

Anaphase

- Chromatid pairs separate at the centromere due to enzymatic action and become chromosomes
- Chromosomes migrate to opposite poles of the cell due to shortening of kinetochore microtubules
- Migrating chromosomes form a V shape in the cell
- Cleavage furrow appears at the cell equator

Telophase

- Terminal phase of mitosis
- Chromosomes complete their migration to the opposite side of the mitotic spindle
- Chromosomes condense to form chromatin of the interphase cell
- Nucleolus reappears, and a nuclear envelope is formed
- Contractile ring becomes the site of cleavage for separation of daughter cells
- Cytokinesis is the division of genetically identical cells during mitosis

Meiosis

- Specialized cell division restricted to male and female germ cells
- Produces ova and sperm with haploid number (23) of chromosomes
- Recombination of genes occurs at fertilization of ovum by sperm

PART III

Tissues

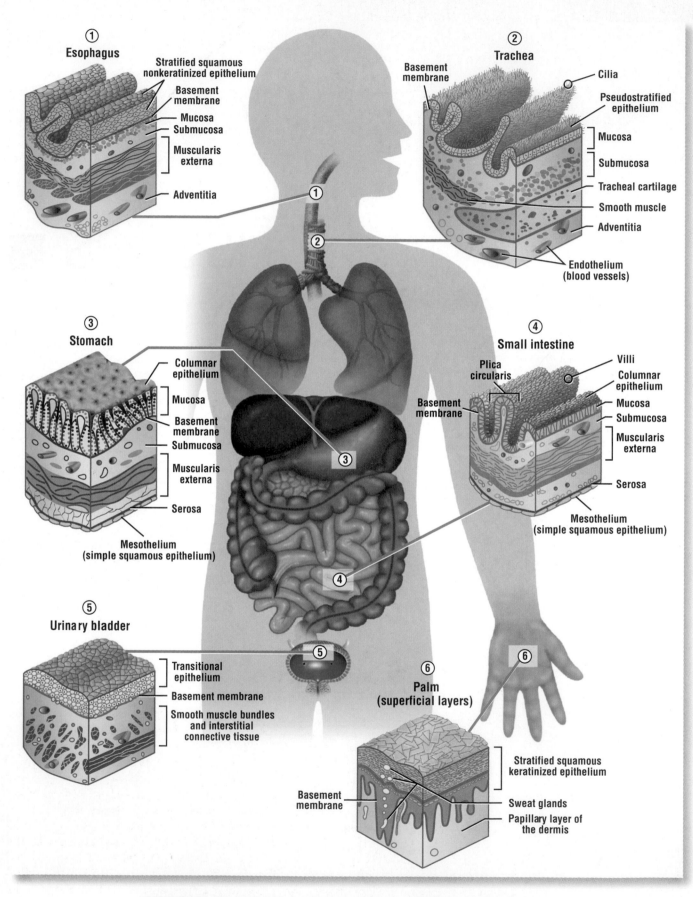

OVERVIEW FIGURE 4.1 ■ Different types of epithelia in selected organs.

Epithelial Tissue ▪

SECTION 1 Classification of Epithelial Tissue

Location of Epithelium

The four basic tissue types in the body are the epithelial, connective, muscular, and nervous tissue. These tissues exist and function in close association with one another.

The **epithelial tissue**, or **epithelium**, consists of sheets of cells that cover the **external surfaces** of the body, line the **internal cavities** and the **organs**, form various **organs** and **glands**, and line their **ducts**. Epithelial cells are in contact with each other, either in a single cell layer or in multiple cell layers. The morphology of any epithelium, however, differs from organ to organ, depending on its location and its function. For example, epithelium that covers the outer surfaces of the body and serves as a protective layer differs from the epithelium that lines the internal organs or their ducts.

Epithelium is not supplied by the blood vessels and is therefore **nonvascular**. Oxygen, nutrients, and metabolites **diffuse** from the blood capillaries located in the underlying connective tissue. In contrast to the other basic tissues, epithelial cells exhibit a high **mitotic rate** with continuous cell renewal and replacement of the worn-out cells.

Overview Figure 4.1 shows different types of epithelia in selected organs.

Classification of Epithelium

Epithelium is classified according to the number of **cell layers** and the **morphology** or structure of the **surface cells**. A **basement membrane** is a thin, noncellular region that separates the epithelium from the underlying **connective tissue** and is easily seen with a light microscope. An epithelium with a single layer of cells is called **simple**, and that with numerous cell layers is called **stratified**. A **pseudostratified** epithelium consists of a single layer of cells that attaches to a **basement membrane**, but not all cells reach the surface. An epithelium that exhibits flat cells is called **squamous**. When the surface cells are round, or as tall as they are wide, the epithelium is **cuboidal**. When the cells are taller than they are wide, the epithelium is called **columnar**.

Special Surface Modifications and Junctional Complexes in Epithelial Cells

Epithelial cells in different organs exhibit special cell membrane modifications on their **apical** (upper) **surfaces**. These modifications are cilia, stereocilia, or microvilli. **Cilia** are motile structures found on certain cells in the **uterine tubes**, **uterus**, **efferent ducts** in the **testes**, and conducting tubes of the **respiratory system**. **Microvilli** are small, nonmotile projections that cover the surfaces of all absorptive cells in the small intestine and the proximal convoluted tubules in the kidney. **Stereocilia** are long, nonmotile, branched microvilli that line the cell surfaces in the **epididymis** and **vas deferens**. The function of microvilli and stereocilia is **absorption**.

Various specialized structures in the epithelium link the individual cells into a functional unit that provides strong adhesion to and rapid communication between neighboring cells. The apical **zonulae occludentes** (tight junctions) form a seal that prevents the entrance of material between the epithelial cells. The **zonulae adherens** (adhering junctions) provide firm adhesion between cells, whereas the strong attachment sites of **desmosomes** provide stability to cells subject to shearing stresses. At the base of epithelial cells, **hemidesmosomes** attach the cells to the basement membrane, whereas the **gap junctions** allow for selective diffusion of molecules between cells as well as rapid cell-to-cell communication.

Types of Epithelia

Simple Epithelium

Simple squamous epithelium that covers the external surfaces of the digestive organs, lungs, and heart is called **mesothelium**. Simple squamous epithelium that lines the lumina of the heart chambers and all blood and lymphatic vessels is called **endothelium.**

Simple cuboidal epithelium lines small excretory ducts in different organs. In the proximal convoluted tubules of the kidney, the apical surfaces of the simple cuboidal epithelium are lined with a **brush border** consisting of **microvilli.**

Simple columnar epithelium covers the **digestive organs** (stomach, small and large intestines, and gallbladder). In the small intestine, simple columnar absorptive cells that cover the **villi** also exhibit **microvilli**. Villi are fingerlike structures that project into the lumen of the small intestine. In uterine tubes and the uterine cavity of the female reproductive tract, the simple columnar epithelium is lined with motile **cilia.**

Pseudostratified Columnar Epithelium

Pseudostratified columnar epithelium lines the **respiratory passages** and lumina of the **epididymis** and **vas deferens**. In the trachea, bronchi, and larger bronchioles, some surface cells are lined with motile **cilia**; in the epididymis and vas deferens, the surface cells exhibit nonmotile **stereocilia**, which are branched or modified microvilli.

Stratified Epithelium

Stratified squamous epithelium contains multiple cell layers. The basal cells are cuboidal to columnar; these cells produce cells that migrate toward the surface and become squamous. There are two types of stratified squamous epithelia: nonkeratinized and keratinized.

Nonkeratinized epithelium exhibits live surface cells and covers moist cavities, such as the mouth, pharynx, esophagus, vagina, and anal canal. **Keratinized epithelium** lines the external surfaces of the body. The surface layers contain nonliving, keratinized cells that are filled with the protein **keratin**. The exposed epithelium that covers the palms and soles exhibits especially thick layers of keratinized cells for added protection against abrasion.

Stratified cuboidal epithelium and **stratified columnar epithelium** have a limited distribution in the body. Both types of epithelia line the larger **excretory ducts** of the pancreas, salivary glands, and sweat glands. In these ducts, the epithelium exhibits two or more layers of cells.

Transitional epithelium lines the minor and major calyces, pelvis, ureters, and the bladder of the **urinary system**. This type of epithelium changes shape and can resemble either stratified squamous or stratified cuboidal epithelium, depending on whether it is stretched or contracted. When transitional epithelium is **contracted**, the surface cells appear **dome shaped**; when **stretched**, the epithelium appears **squamous** and resembles the stratified epithelium of other organs.

 Supplemental micrographic images are available at **www.thePoint.com/Eroschenko12e** under Epithelial Tissue.

FIGURE 4.1 | Simple Squamous Epithelium: Surface View of Peritoneal Mesothelium

To visualize the surface of the simple squamous epithelium, a small piece of mesentery was fixed and treated with silver nitrate and then counterstained with hematoxylin. The cells of the simple squamous epithelium (**mesothelium**) appear flat, adhere tightly to each other, and form a sheet with the thickness of a single cell layer. The irregular **cell boundaries (1)** of the epithelium stain dark and are highly visible owing to silver deposition between the cell boundaries; they form a characteristic mosaic pattern. The blue-gray **cell nuclei (2)** are centrally located in the yellow-to-brown-stained **cytoplasm (3).**

1 Cell boundaries
3 Cytoplasm
2 Nuclei (2)

FIGURE 4.1 ■ Simple squamous epithelium: surface view of peritoneal mesothelium. Stain: silver nitrate with hematoxylin. High magnification.

Simple squamous epithelium is common in the body. It covers the surfaces that allow passive transport of gases or fluids and lines the pleural (thoracic), pericardial (heart), and peritoneal (abdominal) cavities.

FIGURE 4.2 | Simple Squamous Epithelium: Peritoneal Mesothelium Surrounding Small Intestine (Transverse Section)

The simple squamous epithelium that lines different organs in the pleural and peritoneal cavities is called mesothelium. A transverse section of a wall of the small intestine illustrates **mesothelium (1)**, a thin layer of spindle-shaped cells with prominent and oval nuclei. A thin **basement membrane (2)** is located directly under the mesothelium (1). In a surface view, the disposition of these cells would appear similar to those shown in Figure 4.1.

Mesothelium (1) and the underlying irregular **connective tissue (5)** form the serosa of the peritoneal cavity. Serosa is attached to a layer of **smooth muscle fibers (6)** called the muscularis externa **serosa** (see Overview Figure 4.1 parts 3 and 4). In this illustration, the bundles of smooth muscle fibers (6) are cut in the transverse plane. Also present in the connective tissue are small **blood vessels (4)**, lined also by a simple squamous epithelium called the **endothelium (4)**, and numerous **fat (adipose) cells (3)**.

| FUNCTIONAL CORRELATIONS 4.1 | Simple Squamous Epithelium |

In the peritoneal cavity, simple squamous epithelium **reduces friction** between visceral organs by producing lubricating fluids and **transports fluid**. In the cardiovascular system, this epithelium or endothelium allows for passive **transport** of fluids, nutrients, and metabolites across the thin capillary walls to the surrounding cells. In the lungs, the simple squamous epithelium provides for an efficient means of **gas exchange** or **transport** between the thin-walled capillaries and alveoli.

1 Mesothelium
2 Basement membrane
3 Fat cells
4 Endothelium in blood vessels
5 Connective tissue
6 Smooth muscle fibers (cross section)

FIGURE 4.2 ■ Simple squamous epithelium: peritoneal mesothelium surrounding small intestine (transverse section). Stain: hematoxylin and eosin. High magnification.

FIGURE 4.3 | Different Epithelial Types in the Kidney Cortex

This high-power photomicrograph of the kidney illustrates the different types of epithelia that are present in the kidney cortex (peripheral region). **Simple squamous epithelium (1)** lines the outer portion of the double-layered epithelial capsule called the **Bowman capsule (5)**. The inner layer of the capsule surrounds the **capillaries (3)** of the **glomerulus (2)**. The glomerulus (2) is a tuft of capillaries (3) where blood filtration takes place. Simple squamous epithelium called **endothelium (4, 9)** also lines the capillaries (3) and all **blood vessels (8)**. **Simple cuboidal epithelium (6)** lines the lumina of the surrounding **convoluted tubules (7)**. The blue-staining fibers surrounding the Bowman capsule (5), convoluted tubules (7), and blood vessels (8) in the kidney cortex are the collagen fibers of the **connective tissue (10)**.

1 Simple squamous epithelium
2 Glomerulus
3 Capillaries
4 Endothelium
5 Bowman capsule
6 Simple cuboidal epithelium
7 Convoluted tubules
8 Blood vessels
9 Endothelium
10 Connective tissue

FIGURE 4.3 ■ Different epithelial types in the kidney cortex. Stain: Masson trichrome. ×120.

FIGURE 4.4 | Simple Columnar Epithelium: Stomach Surface

The surface of the stomach is covered by a tall, **simple columnar epithelium (1)**. The illustration shows the light-staining **apical cytoplasm (1a)** and the dark-staining **basal nuclei (1b)** of the simple columnar epithelium (1). The epithelial cells are in close contact with each other and are arranged in a single row. A thin, connective tissue **basement membrane (2, 9)** separates the surface epithelium (1) from the underlying collagen fibers and cells of the **connective tissue (3, 10)**, called the **lamina propria**. Small **blood vessels (5)**, lined with endothelium, are present in the connective tissue (3, 10).

In some areas, the surface epithelium has been sectioned in a transverse or oblique plane. When a plane of section passes close to the free surface of the epithelium, the sectioned **apices (6)** of the epithelium resemble a layer of stratified, enucleated polygonal cells. When a plane of section passes through **bases (7)** of the epithelial cells, the nuclei resemble a stratified epithelium.

The surface cells of the stomach secrete a protective coat of mucus. The pale appearance of cytoplasm is caused by the routine histologic preparation of the tissues. The mucigen droplets that filled the apical cytoplasm (1a) were lost during section preparation. The more granular cytoplasm is located basally (1b) and stains more acidophilic.

In an empty stomach, the stomach wall exhibits numerous **temporary folds (8)** that disappear when the stomach is filled with solid or fluid material. Also, the surface epithelium extends downward to form numerous indentations or pits in the surface of the stomach called **gastric pits (11)**, seen in both longitudinal section and transverse section.

1 Simple columnar
surface epithelium
a. Apical cytoplasm
b. Basal nuclei

2 Basement membrane

3 Connective tissue
(lamina propria)

4 Connective tissue cells

5 Blood vessel

6 Apices of epithelium
(cytoplasm, oblique
section)

7 Bases of epithelium
(nuclei, oblique
section)

8 Temporary folds

9 Basement membrane

10 Connective tissue
(lamina propria)

11 Gastric pits
(longitudinal and
transverse sections)

FIGURE 4.4 ■ Simple columnar epithelium: surface of stomach. Stain: hematoxylin and eosin. Medium magnification.

FUNCTIONAL CORRELATIONS 4.2	Simple Cuboidal Epithelium and Simple Columnar Epithelium

Simple cuboidal epithelium lines various ducts of glands and organs, where it covers the surface for sturdiness and protection. In kidneys, this epithelium functions in transport, absorption of filtered substances, and active secretion of substances into the filtrate. Simple columnar epithelium covers the surface of the stomach. These cells are **secretory** and produce **mucus**. The mucus covers the stomach surface and **protects** its surface lining from the corrosive gastric secretions normally found in the stomach during food processing and digestion.

FIGURE 4.5 | Simple Columnar Epithelium on Villi in Small Intestine: Cells with Striated Borders (Microvilli) and Goblet Cells

The intestinal **villi (1)**, illustrated in transverse section and longitudinal section, are covered by simple columnar epithelium. In the small intestine, the epithelium consists of two cell types: columnar cells with **striated borders (5, 7)** and oval-shaped **goblet cells (6, 13)**. The striated border (5, 7) is seen as a reddish outer cell layer with faint vertical striations; these striations represent microvilli on the apices of columnar cells.

Pale-staining goblet cells (6, 13) are interspersed among the columnar cells. During routine histologic preparation, the mucus is lost; hence, the goblet cell cytoplasm appears clear or only lightly stained (6, 13). Normally, the mucigen droplets occupy **cell apices (4)** and the nucleus cell **bases (4)**.

When the epithelium at the tip of a villus is sectioned in an oblique plane, the cell apices (4) of the columnar cells appear as a mosaic of enucleated cells, whereas the cell bases (4) appear as stratified epithelium.

A thin connective tissue **basement membrane (8)** is visible directly under the epithelium. The connective tissue **lamina propria (12)** contains an empty lymphatic vessel with a very thin endothelium called the **central lacteal (2, 9)**. Also present in the lamina propria (12) are numerous **blood vessels (10)** and a **capillary (14)** lined with endothelium. **Smooth muscle fibers (3, 11)** extend into the villi. In this illustration, smooth muscle fibers (3, 11) are cut in transverse section (3) and longitudinal section (11).

1 Villi (longitudinal and transverse sections

2 Central lacteal

3 Smooth muscle fibers (transverse section)

4 Oblique section of epithelium (cell apices and cell bases)

5 Striated border

6 Goblet cells

7 Striated border

8 Basement membrane

9 Central lacteal

10 Blood vessel

11 Smooth muscle fibers (longitudinal section)

12 Connective tissue (lamina propria)

13 Goblet cells

14 Capillary

FIGURE 4.5 ■ Simple columnar epithelium on villi in small intestine: cells with striated borders (microvilli) and goblet cells. Stain: hematoxylin and eosin. Medium magnification.

The connective tissue lamina propria also contains numerous other connective tissue cells, such as plasma cells, lymphocytes, macrophages, and fibroblasts. These cells are normally seen with higher magnification.

FUNCTIONAL CORRELATIONS 4.3	Epithelium with Striated Borders (Small Intestine) and Brush Borders (Kidney)

The main function of the epithelium in the small intestine is **absorption** of nutrients. This function is enhanced by the presence of fingerlike **villi**, which increase the absorptive surface area and are covered by simple columnar epithelium with **striated borders,** or **microvilli**. These microvilli absorb nutrients and fluids from the intestinal contents. The intestinal epithelium also contains numerous **goblet cells**. These cells secrete **mucus**, which **protects** the surface lining from corrosive secretions that enter the small intestine from the stomach during digestion.

Production of urine by the kidney involves filtration, absorption, and excretion. The apical surfaces of the simple cuboidal epithelium in the proximal convoluted tubules of the kidney are also covered with **brush borders** or **microvilli**. The main function of these microvilli is to **absorb** the nutrient material and fluid from the filtrate that passes through the tubules.

FIGURE 4.6 | Pseudostratified Columnar Ciliated Epithelium: Respiratory Passages—Trachea

Pseudostratified columnar ciliated epithelium lines the upper respiratory passages, such as the trachea and bronchi. In this type of epithelium, the cells appear to form several layers. Serial sections show that all cells reach the **basement membrane (4, 13)**; however, because the epithelial cells are of different shapes and heights, not all reach the surface. For this reason, this type of epithelium is called pseudostratified rather than stratified.

Numerous motile and closely spaced **cilia (1, 8)** (cilium, singular) cover all cell apices of the ciliated cells, except those of the light-staining, oval **goblet cells (3, 11)** that are interspersed among the ciliated cells. Each cilium arises from a **basal body (9)**, whose internal morphology is identical to the centriole. The basal bodies (9) are located directly beneath the apical cell membrane and are adjacent to each other; they often give the appearance of a continuous dark, apical membrane (9).

In pseudostratified epithelium, the deeper nuclei belong to the intermediate and short **basal cells (12)**. The more superficial, oval nuclei belong to the columnar ciliated cells (1, 8). The small, round, heavily stained nuclei, without any visible surrounding cytoplasm, are those of **lymphocytes (2, 10)**. These cells migrate from the underlying **connective tissue (5)** through the epithelium.

A clearly visible basement membrane (4, 13) separates the pseudostratified epithelium from the underlying connective tissue (5). Visible in the connective tissue (5) are **fibrocytes (5a)**, dense **collagen fibers (5b)**, scattered lymphocytes, and small **blood vessels (14)**. Deeper in the connective tissue are glands with **mucous acini (6)** and **serous acini (7, 15)**. These provide secretions that moisten the respiratory passages.

| FUNCTIONAL CORRELATIONS 4.4 | Epithelium with Cilia or Stereocilia |

In most **respiratory passages** (trachea and bronchi), **pseudostratified epithelium** contains both **goblet cells** and **ciliated cells**. The motile cilia on the ciliated cells cleanse the inspired air and transport mucus and entrapped **particulate material** across the cell surfaces to the oral cavity for expulsion.

Simple columnar cells with motile cilia in the **uterine tubes** facilitate the conduction of oocyte and sperm across their surfaces. In the **efferent ductules** of the **testes**, ciliated cells assist in **transporting** sperm out of the testis and into the ducts of the epididymis.

The lumina of the **epididymis** and **vas deferens** are lined by pseudostratified epithelium with prominent **stereocilia**. These are nonmotile structures, and their structure is highly different from that of the motile cilia. However, the major function of stereocilia in these organs, like that of microvilli, is to absorb the testicular fluid in the epididymis and vas deferens that was produced by cells in the testes.

1 Cilia
2 Lymphocyte
3 Goblet cells
4 Basement membrane
5 Connective tissue
  a. Fibrocytes
  b. Collagen fibers
6 Mucous acinus
7 Serous acinus

8 Cilia
9 Basal bodies
10 Lymphocyte
11 Goblet cells
12 Basal cells
13 Basement membrane
14 Blood vessels
15 Serous acini

FIGURE 4.6 ■ Pseudostratified columnar ciliated epithelium: respiratory passages—trachea. Stain: hematoxylin and eosin. High magnification.

FIGURE 4.7 | Transitional Epithelium: Bladder (Unstretched, or Relaxed)

Transitional epithelium (1) is found exclusively in the excretory passages of the urinary system. It covers the lumina of renal calyces, pelvis, ureters, and bladder. This stratified epithelium is composed of several layers of similar cells. The epithelium changes its shape in response to either stretching, as a result of fluid accumulation, or contraction during voiding of urine.

In a relaxed, unstretched condition, the **surface cells (7)** are usually cuboidal and bulge out. Frequently, **binucleate (two nuclei) cells (6)** are visible in the superficial layers or surface cells (7) of the bladder.

Transitional epithelium (1) rests on a **connective tissue (3, 8)** layer, composed primarily of **fibroblasts (8a)** and **collagen fibers (8b)**. Between the connective tissue (3, 8) and the transitional epithelium (1) is a thin **basement membrane (2)**. The base of the epithelium is not indented by connective tissue papillae, and it exhibits an even contour.

Small **blood vessels**, **venules (4, 11)**, and **arterioles (9)** of various sizes are present in the connective tissue (3, 8). Deeper in the connective tissue are strands of **smooth muscle fibers (5, 10)**, sectioned in both cross (5) and longitudinal (10) planes. The muscle layers in the bladder are located deep to the connective tissue (3, 8).

FIGURE 4.7 ■ Transitional epithelium: bladder (unstretched, or relaxed). Stain: hematoxylin and eosin. High magnification.

FIGURE 4.8 | Transitional Epithelium: Bladder (Stretched)

When fluid begins to fill the bladder, the **transitional epithelium (1)** changes its shape. Increased volume in the bladder appears to reduce the number of cell layers. This is because the **surface cells (5)** flatten to accommodate increasing surface area. In the stretched condition, the transitional epithelium (1) may resemble stratified squamous epithelium found in other regions of the body. Note also that the folds in the bladder wall disappear, and the **basement membrane (2)** is smoother. As in the empty bladder (see Figure 4.7), the underlying **connective tissue (6)** contains **venules (3)** and **arterioles (7)**. Below the connective tissue (6) are **smooth muscle fibers (4, 8)**, sectioned in cross (4) and longitudinal (8) planes. (Compare transitional epithelium with the stratified squamous epithelium of the esophagus, shown in Figure 4.9.)

FUNCTIONAL CORRELATIONS 4.5 | Transitional Epithelium

Transitional epithelium allows **distension** of the urinary organs (calyces, pelvis, ureters, bladder) during urine accumulation and **contraction** of these organs during the emptying process without breaking the cell contacts in the epithelium. This change in cell shape is owing to the unique feature of the cell membrane in the transitional epithelium. Here are found specialized regions called **plaques**. When the bladder is empty, the plaques are folded into irregular contours. During bladder filling and stretching of the epithelium, the plaques disappear. In addition, because plaques appear impermeable to fluids and salts, transitional epithelium forms a **protective osmotic barrier** against the hypertonic and cytotoxic effect of urine in the bladder and the underlying connective tissue.

FIGURE 4.9 | Stratified Squamous Nonkeratinized Epithelium: Esophagus

Stratified squamous epithelium is characterized by numerous cell layers, with the outermost layer consisting of flat or squamous cells, which contain nuclei and are alive. The thickness of the epithelium varies among different regions of the body, and, as a result, the composition of the epithelium also varies. Illustrated in this figure is an example of the moist, **nonkeratinized stratified squamous epithelium (1)** that lines the esophagus as well as the oral cavity, vagina, and anal canal.

Cuboidal or low columnar **basal cells (5)** are located at the base of the stratified epithelium. The cytoplasm is finely granular, and the oval, chromatin-rich nucleus occupies most of the cell. Cells in the intermediate layers of the epithelium are **polyhedral (4)** with round or oval nuclei and more visible cell cytoplasm and membranes. **Mitoses (6)** are frequently observed in the deeper cell layers and in the basal cells (5). Cells and their nuclei become progressively flatter as the cells migrate toward the free surface of the epithelium. Above the polyhedral cells (4) are several rows of flattened or **squamous cells (3)**.

A fine **basement membrane (7)** separates the epithelium (1) from the underlying **connective tissue**, the **lamina propria (2)**. **Papillae (10)** or extensions of connective tissue indent the lower surface of the epithelium (1), giving it a characteristic wavy appearance. The connective tissue (2) contains **collagen fibers (11)**, **fibrocytes (9)**, **capillaries (12)**, and **arterioles (8)**.

In areas where stratified squamous epithelium is exposed to increased wear and tear, the outermost layer, called the stratum corneum, becomes thick and keratinized, as illustrated in the epidermis of the palm in Figure 4.10.

An example of thin, stratified squamous epithelium without connective tissue papillae indentation is found in the cornea of the eye; the surface underlying the epithelium is smooth. This type of epithelium is only a few cell layers thick, but it has the characteristic arrangement of basal columnar, polyhedral, and superficial squamous cells.

1 Transitional epithelium

2 Basement membrane

3 Venules

4 Smooth muscle (cross section)

5 Surface cells

6 Connective tissue

7 Arterioles

8 Smooth muscle (longitudinal section)

FIGURE 4.8 ■ Transitional epithelium: bladder (stretched). Stain: hematoxylin and eosin. High magnification.

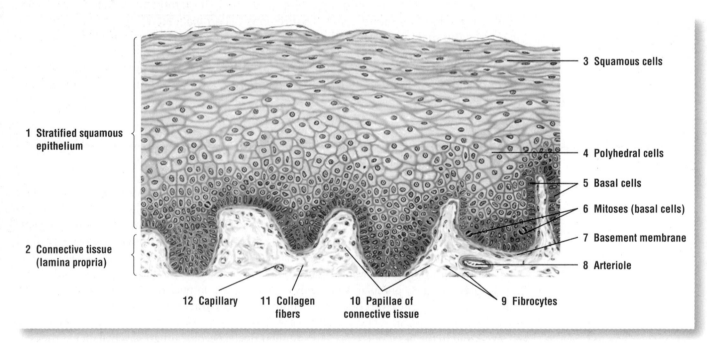

1 Stratified squamous epithelium

2 Connective tissue (lamina propria)

3 Squamous cells

4 Polyhedral cells

5 Basal cells

6 Mitoses (basal cells)

7 Basement membrane

8 Arteriole

9 Fibrocytes

12 Capillary   11 Collagen fibers   10 Papillae of connective tissue

FIGURE 4.9 ■ Stratified squamous nonkeratinized epithelium: esophagus. Stain: hematoxylin and eosin. Medium magnification.

FIGURE 4.10 | Stratified Squamous Keratinized Epithelium: Palm of the Hand

The skin is covered with **stratified squamous keratinized epithelium (1)**. The outermost layer of the skin contains dead cells and is called the **stratum corneum (5)**. In the palms and soles, the stratum corneum (5) is thick, whereas in the rest of the body, it is thinner. Inferior to the stratum corneum (5) are the different cell layers that give rise to the stratum corneum (5).

This medium-power photomicrograph illustrates the stratified squamous keratinized epithelium (1) of the palm and the cell layers **stratum granulosum (6)** and **stratum spinosum (7)** as well as the basal cell layer, **stratum basale (8)**. The epithelium is attached to the underlying **connective tissue (3)** layer composed of dense collagen fibers and fibroblasts. The underlying surface of the epithelium (1) is indented by connective tissue (3) extensions called **papillae (2)** that form the characteristic wavy boundary between the epithelium (1) and the connective tissue (3). Passing through the connective tissue (3) and the epithelium (1) are **excretory ducts of the sweat glands (4)** that are located deep to the epithelium.

FIGURE 4.11 | Stratified Cuboidal Epithelium: An Excretory Duct in the Salivary Gland

The stratified cuboidal epithelium has a limited distribution and is seen in only a few organs. The larger excretory ducts in the salivary glands and in the pancreas are lined with stratified cuboidal epithelium. This figure illustrates a high-power photomicrograph of a large excretory duct of a salivary gland. The luminal lining consists of two layers of cuboidal cells, forming the **stratified cuboidal epithelium (1)**. Surrounding the excretory duct are collagen fibers of the **connective tissue (2, 7)** and **blood vessels (3, 5)** that are lined by simple squamous epithelium called **endothelium (4, 6)**.

FUNCTIONAL CORRELATIONS 4.6 | Stratified Epithelium—Nonkeratinized and Keratinized

Stratified squamous nonkeratinized epithelium is well suited to withstand increased wear and tear in the moist cavities of the esophagus, vagina, and oral cavity. Its multilayered cellular composition protects the surfaces of these organs. In the larger excretory ducts of kidney, salivary glands, and pancreas, another cell layer is added to form either stratified cuboidal or stratified columnar epithelium for even more protection (see Figure 4.11).

For additional protection from abrasion, desiccation, and bacterial invasion, the epithelium on the surfaces of the skin, hands, and feet is **keratinized** and consists of superficial layers of dead cells filled with **keratin protein**.

1 Stratified squamous keratinized epithelium

2 Papillae

3 Connective tissue with collagen fibers

4 Excretory ducts of sweat glands

5 Stratum corneum

6 Stratum granulosum

7 Stratum spinosum

8 Stratum basale

FIGURE 4.10 ■ Stratified squamous keratinized epithelium: palm of the hand. Stain: hematoxylin and eosin. ×40.

1 Stratified cuboidal epithelium

2 Connective tissue

3 Blood vessel

4 Endothelium

5 Blood vessel

6 Endothelium

7 Connective tissue

FIGURE 4.11 ■ Stratified cuboidal epithelium: an excretory duct in the salivary gland. Stain: hematoxylin and eosin. ×100.

CHAPTER 4 SUMMARY

SECTION 1 • Classification of Epithelial Tissue

Epithelial Tissue

Major Features

- Classification is based on number of cell layers and cell morphology
- Basement membrane separates epithelium from connective tissue
- All epithelia are nonvascular; delivery of nutrients to cells and removal of metabolic waste occurs via diffusion from adjacent capillaries
- Surface modifications include motile cilia, microvilli, and stereocilia
- Lateral cell surface modification includes zonulae occludentes, zonulae adherens, desmosomes, gap junctions, and hemidesmosomes basally

Types of Epithelia

Simple Squamous Epithelium

- Single layer of flat or squamous cells; includes mesothelium and endothelium
- Mesothelium lines external surfaces of digestive organs, lung, and heart
- Endothelium lines inside of heart chambers, blood vessels, and lymphatic vessels
- Functions in filtration, diffusion, transport, secretion, and reduction of friction

Simple Cuboidal Epithelium

- Single layer of round cells
- Lines small ducts and kidney tubules
- Protects ducts; transports and absorbs filtered material in kidney tubules

Simple Columnar Epithelium

- All cells are tall, some lined by microvilli
- Lines the lumina of digestive organs
- Secretes protective mucus for stomach lining
- Absorption of nutrients in small intestine

Pseudostratified Columnar Epithelium, Epithelium With Cilia or Stereocilia

- All cells reach basement membrane, but not all reach the surface
- Ciliated cells interspersed among mucus-secreting goblet cells
- In respiratory passages, ciliated and mucus cells clean inspired air and transport particulate matter across cell surfaces
- In uterine tubes and the efferent ducts of testes, ciliated cells transport oocytes and sperm across cell surfaces, respectively
- In the epididymis and vas deferens, the lining stereocilia absorb testicular fluid

Stratified Epithelium

- Formed by multiple layers of cells, the superficial cell layer determining epithelial type
- Nonkeratinized squamous epithelium contains live superficial cell layer
- Nonkeratinized squamous forms moist and protective layer in esophagus, vagina, anal canal, and oral cavity
- Keratinized epithelium contains dead superficial cell layer
- Keratinized epithelium provides protection against abrasion, bacterial invasion, and desiccation
- Cuboidal epithelium lines large excretory ducts in different organs
- Cuboidal epithelium provides protection for the ducts

Transitional Epithelium

- Found exclusively in renal calyces, renal pelvis, ureters, and bladder
- Changes shape in response to distensions caused by fluid accumulation
- During extension or contraction, cell-to-cell contact remains unbroken
- Forms protective osmotic barrier between hypertonic urine and underlying tissue

SECTION 2 Classification of Glandular Tissue

The body contains a variety of glands. They are classified as either **exocrine glands** or **endocrine glands**. These glands develop from epithelial cells that extend from the surface into the underlying connective tissue. Exocrine glands are connected to the surface epithelium by excretory **ducts**, into which they secrete their secretory products that pass to the external surface. In contrast, the endocrine glands have lost their connection to the surface epithelium and their secretory products are delivered directly into the capillaries of the connective tissue that surrounds the **circulatory system**.

Exocrine Glands

Exocrine glands are either **unicellular** or **multicellular**. Unicellular glands consist of single cells. The mucus-secreting **goblet cells** found in the epithelia of the small and large intestines and in the respiratory passages are the best examples of unicellular glands.

Multicellular glands are characterized by a **secretory portion**, an end piece where the epithelial cells secrete a product, and an epithelium-lined excretory **ductal portion**, through which the secretion from the secretory regions is delivered to the exterior of the gland. Larger excretory ducts are usually lined by stratified epithelium, either cuboidal or columnar.

Simple and Compound Exocrine Glands

Multicellular exocrine glands are divided into two major categories depending on the structure of their ductal portion. A **simple exocrine gland** exhibits an unbranched duct, which may be straight or coiled. Also, if the terminal secretory portion of the gland is shaped in the form of a tube, the gland is called a **tubular gland**.

An exocrine gland that shows a repeated branching pattern of the ducts that drain the secretory portions is called a **compound exocrine gland**. Furthermore, if the secretory portions of the gland are shaped like a flask or a tube, the glands are called **acinar (alveolar) glands** or **tubular glands**, respectively. Certain exocrine glands exhibit a mixture of both tubular and acinar secretory portions. Such glands are called **tubuloacinar glands**.

Exocrine glands may also be classified on the basis of the secretory products of their cells. Glands with cells that produce a viscous secretion that lubricates or protects the inner lining of the organs are **mucous glands**. These glands produce the lubricating product **mucus**. Glands with cells that produce watery secretions that are often rich in enzymes are **serous glands**. Certain glands in the body contain a mixture of both mucous and serous secretory cells; these are **mixed (seromucous) glands**.

Merocrine and Holocrine Glands

Exocrine glands may also be classified according to the method by which their secretory product is discharged. **Merocrine glands**, such as pancreas and sweat glands, release their secretion by exocytosis without any loss of cellular components. Most exocrine glands in the body secrete their product in this manner. In **holocrine glands**, such as the sebaceous glands of the skin, the cells themselves become the secretory product that accumulates in the glands. Here, gland cells accumulate lipids, die, and degenerate to become **sebum**, the secretory product. Another type of gland, called **apocrine glands** (mammary glands), discharges part of the secretory cell as the secretory product. However, almost all glands that were once classified as apocrine are now regarded as merocrine glands.

Endocrine Glands

Endocrine glands differ from exocrine glands in that they do not have excretory ducts for their secretory products. Instead, endocrine glands are highly vascularized, and their secretory cells are surrounded by rich **capillary networks**. The close proximity of the secretory cells to the capillaries allows for efficient release of the secretory products into the **bloodstream** and their distribution to different organs via the systemic circulation.

The endocrine glands can be **individual cells** (unicellular glands) as seen in the digestive organs as enteroendocrine cells; **endocrine tissue** in mixed glands (both endocrine and exocrine) as seen in the pancreas and male and female reproductive organs; or separate **endocrine organs** as the pituitary gland, thyroid glands, parathyroid glands, and adrenal glands. Individual endocrine cells, called enteroendocrine cells, are found in the digestive organs. Endocrine tissues are seen in such mixed glands as the pancreas and the reproductive organs of both sexes.

 Supplemental micrographic images are available at **www.thePoint.com/Eroschenko12e** under Cell and Cytoplasm.

FIGURE 4.12 | Unbranched Simple Tubular Exocrine Glands: Intestinal Glands

Unbranched simple tubular glands without excretory ducts are best represented by the **intestinal glands** (crypts of Lieberkühn) in the **large intestine (A and B)** and **rectum**. The **surface epithelium** and the **secretory cells** of the glands in the intestines are lined with numerous goblet cells; these are unicellular exocrine glands. Similar but shorter intestinal glands with goblet cells are also found in the small intestine.

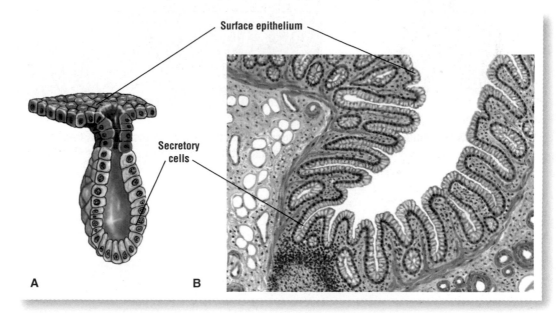

FIGURE 4.12 ■ Unbranched simple tubular exocrine glands: intestinal glands. (A) Diagram of gland. (B) Transverse section of large intestine. Stain: hematoxylin and eosin. Medium magnification.

FIGURE 4.13 | Simple Branched Tubular Exocrine Glands: Gastric Glands

Simple or slightly branched tubular glands without excretory ducts are found in the stomach. These are the **gastric glands** (**A** and **B**). In the fundus and body of the stomach, they are lined with modified columnar cells that are highly specialized for secreting hydrochloric acid and the precursor for the proteolytic enzyme pepsin.

FIGURE 4.13 ■ Simple branched tubular exocrine gland: gastric glands. (A) Diagram of gland. (B) Transverse section of stomach. Stain: hematoxylin and eosin. Low magnification.

FIGURE 4.14 | Coiled Tubular Exocrine Glands: Sweat Glands

Sebaceous glands in the skin are coiled tubular glands with long, unbranched ducts (**A** and **B**). Note the **secretory cells** of the gland and the **excretory duct**, which delivers the secretory product to the surface. Note also the transition from single layer of cells in the secretory portion of the gland and the stratified cuboidal epithelium in the excretory duct.

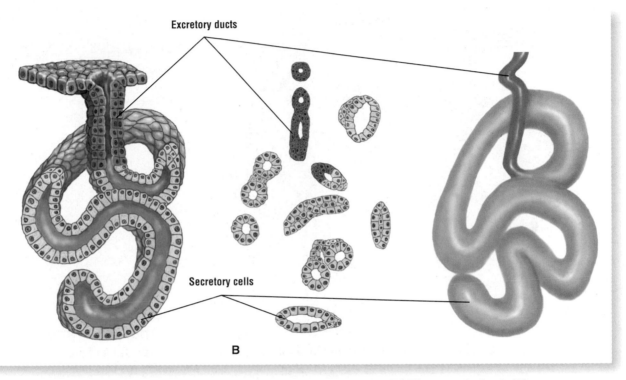

Excretory ducts

Secretory cells

A

B

FIGURE 4.14 ■ Coiled tubular exocrine glands: sweat glands. (A) Diagram of gland. (B) Transverse and three-dimensional view of coiled sweat gland. Stain: hematoxylin and eosin. Medium magnification.

FIGURE 4.15 | Compound Acinar (Exocrine) Gland: Mammary Glands

The mammary gland is an example of a **compound acinar (alveolar) gland** (**A** and **B**). The lactating mammary gland contains enlarged **secretory acini (alveoli)** with large lumina that are filled with milk. Draining these acini (alveoli) are **excretory ducts**, some of which contain secretory material and are lined by stratified epithelium.

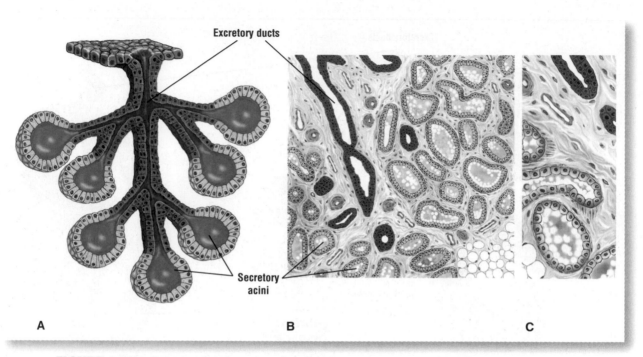

Excretory ducts

Secretory
acini

A B C

FIGURE 4.15 ■ Compound acinar exocrine gland: mammary gland. **(A)** Diagram of gland.
(B and C) Mammary gland during lactation. Stain: hematoxylin and eosin. **(B)** Low magnification. **(C)** Medium magnification.

FIGURE 4.16 | Compound Tubuloacinar (Exocrine) Gland: Salivary Glands

The salivary glands (parotid, submandibular, and sublingual) best illustrate **compound tubuloacinar glands** (**A** and **B**). The glands contain **secretory acinar elements** and **secretory tubular elements**. In addition, the submandibular and sublingual salivary glands contain both serous and mucous acini. Details and comparisons of these acini are described in Chapter 13, "Digestive System Part I: Oral Cavity and Major Salivary Glands." The **excretory ducts** are lined with cuboidal, columnar, or stratified epithelium and are named according to their location in the gland.

FIGURE 4.16 ■ Compound tubuloacinar (exocrine) gland: salivary gland. (A) Diagram of gland. (B) Submandibular salivary gland. Stain: hematoxylin and eosin. Low magnification.

FIGURE 4.17 | Compound Tubuloacinar (Exocrine) Gland: Submaxillary Salivary Gland

A photomicrograph of a submaxillary salivary gland shows the secretory units of a compound tubuloacinar gland. The grapelike **secretory acinar elements (1)** are circular in transverse section and are distinguished from the longer **secretory tubular elements (7)** of the gland. Empty lumina can be seen in some sections of both types of secretory elements. This salivary gland is a mixed gland and contains both the **mucous cells (4)**, which stain light, and **serous cells (5)**, which stain dark. Draining the secretory elements of the gland are **excretory ducts (3, 6, 8)**. The small excretory ducts are lined by simple cuboidal epithelium and surrounded by **connective tissue (2)**, which also surrounds all of the secretory elements.

1 Secretory acinar elements

2 Connective tissue

3 Excretory duct

4 Mucous cells

5 Serous cells

6 Excretory duct

7 Secretory tubular elements

8 Excretory ducts

FIGURE 4.17 ■ Compound tubuloacinar (exocrine) gland: submaxillary salivary gland. Stain: hematoxylin and eosin. ×64.

FIGURE 4.18 | Endocrine Gland: Pancreatic Islet

An example of an endocrine gland is illustrated as a pancreatic islet from the pancreas. The pancreas is a mixed gland, containing both an **exocrine portion** and **endocrine portion**. In the pancreas, the exocrine acini surround the endocrine pancreatic islets (**A** and **B**).

The structure and function of other endocrine organs (glands) are presented in greater detail in Chapter 19, "Endocrine System."

A

B

FIGURE 4.18 ■ Endocrine gland: pancreatic islet. (A) Diagram of pancreatic islet. (B) High magnification of endocrine and exocrine pancreas. Stain: hematoxylin and eosin. High magnification.

FIGURE 4.19 | Endocrine and Exocrine Pancreas

A photomicrograph of the pancreas shows a mixed gland with both endocrine and exocrine portions. The **exocrine pancreas (3)** consists of numerous secretory acini that deliver their secretory material into the **excretory duct (1)**, which is lined by simple cuboidal epithelium and surrounded by a layer of connective tissue. The **endocrine pancreas (5)** is called the pancreatic islet (5) because it is separated from the cells of the exocrine pancreas (3) by a thin **connective tissue capsule (4)**. The endocrine pancreatic islet (5) does not contain excretory ducts. Instead, it is highly vascularized, and all of the secretory products leave the pancreatic islet via numerous **blood vessels (capillaries) (2)**.

1 Excretory duct

2 Blood vessels

3 Exocrine pancreas

4 Connective tissue capsule

5 Endocrine pancreas

FIGURE 4.19 ■ Endocrine and exocrine pancreas. Stain: Mallory-Azan. ×100.

SECTION 2 • Glandular Tissue

Glandular Tissue

Exocrine Glands

- Can be unicellular or multicellular
- Multicellular glands contain secretory portion and ductal portion
- Secretions enter the ductal system
- Simple tubular glands exhibit unbranched duct; found in intestinal glands
- Coiled tubular glands seen in sweat glands
- Compound glands exhibit repeated ductal branching with either acinar (alveolar) or tubular secretory portions
- Compound acinar glands seen in mammary glands
- Compound tubuloacinar glands seen in salivary glands
- Mucous glands lubricate and protect inner linings of organs
- Serous glands produce watery secretions that contain enzymes

- Mixed glands contain both serous and mucous cells
- Merocrine glands, like pancreas, release secretion without cell loss
- Holocrine glands, like sebaceous skin glands, release secretion with cell components

Endocrine Glands

- Are individual cells as enteroendocrine cells in digestive organs
- Are endocrine portions in organs such as pancreatic islets in pancreas
- Are endocrine glands such as pituitary, thyroid, or adrenal glands
- Do not have ducts and are highly vascularized
- Secretory products enter bloodstream (capillaries) for systemic distribution

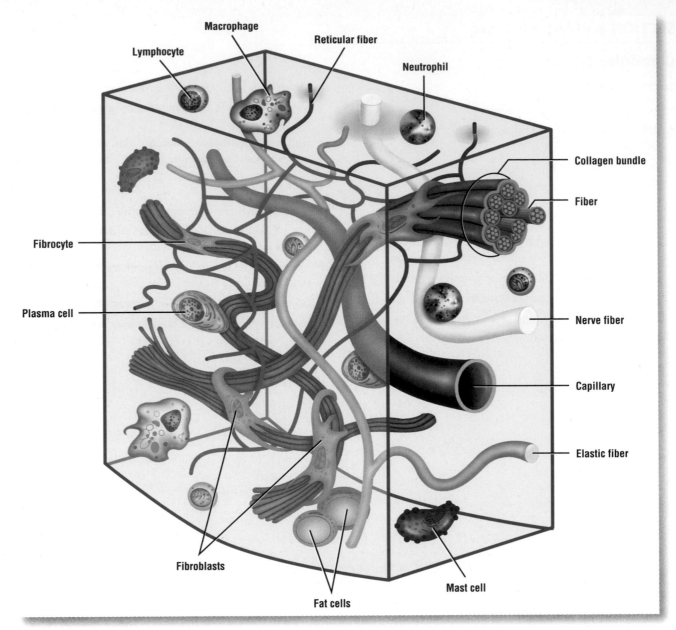

OVERVIEW FIGURE 5.1 ■ Composite illustration of loose connective tissue with its predominant cells and fibers.

CHAPTER 5

Connective Tissue ■

The connective tissue develops from **mesenchyme cells,** an embryonic type of tissue. The embryonic connective tissue is present in the umbilical cord and in the pulp of the developing teeth. During embryonic development, mesenchyme cells also give rise to other connective tissues such as cartilage, bone, and blood. With the exceptions of blood and lymph, the **connective tissue** consists of **cells** and **extracellular material** called **matrix.** The extracellular matrix consists of connective **tissue fluid,** the **ground substance** within which are embedded the different protein **fibers** (collagen, reticular, and elastic). The connective tissue binds, anchors, and supports various cells, tissues, and organs of the body. It also provides a gel-like medium of the ground substance for exchange of nutrients, oxygen, and metabolic waste. In addition, the connective tissue matrix contains numerous cell types that provide **protection** and **defense** against bacterial invasion and foreign bodies. The connective tissue is classified as either loose connective tissue or dense connective tissue, depending on the amount, type, arrangement, and abundance of cells, fibers, and ground substance.

Classification of Connective Tissue

Loose Connective Tissue

Loose connective tissue is more prevalent in the body than dense connective tissue. It is characterized by a loose, irregular arrangement of connective tissue fibers and abundant ground substance. Numerous connective tissue cells and fibers are found in the matrix. **Collagen fibers, fibroblasts, adipose cells, mast cells, plasma cells,** and **macrophages** predominate in the loose connective tissue, with fibroblasts being the most common cell types. Overview Figure 5.1 shows the various types of cells and fibers that are present in loose connective tissue.

Dense Connective Tissue

In contrast, **dense connective tissue** contains thicker and more densely packed collagen fibers, with fewer cell types and less ground substance. The collagen fibers in the **dense irregular connective tissue** exhibit a random and irregular orientation. The dense irregular connective tissue is present in the dermis of skin, in capsules of different organs, and in areas that need strong binding and support. In contrast, the **dense regular connective tissue** contains densely packed collagen fibers that exhibit a regular and parallel arrangement. This type of tissue is primarily found in the **tendons** and **ligaments.** In both dense connective tissue types, **fibroblasts** are the most abundant cells, which are located between the dense collagen bundles.

Cells of the Connective Tissue

The two most common cell types in the connective tissue are the active **fibroblasts** and the inactive or resting fibroblasts, the **fibrocytes.** Fusiform fibroblasts synthesize all the connective tissue fibers (collagen, elastic, and reticular) and the extracellular ground substance, including proteoglycans, glycosaminoglycans, and adhesive glycoproteins.

Adipose (fat) cells, which may occur singly or in groups, are seen frequently in the connective tissue; these cells store fat. There are two types of adipose cells. Cells with a large, single, or unilocular lipid droplet are **white adipose tissue.** Cells with numerous or multilocular lipid droplets are **brown adipose tissue**. White adipose tissue is more abundant than brown adipose tissue, and when adipose cells predominate, the connective tissue is called **adipose tissue**.

Macrophages or **histiocytes** are phagocytic cells that ingest foreign material or dead cells and are most numerous in loose connective tissue, after fibroblasts. They are difficult to distinguish from fibroblasts, unless they are performing phagocytic activity and contain ingested material in their cytoplasm. The macrophages, however, are called by different names in different tissues/organs. Their location and names are listed in Functional Correlations 5.1.

Mast cells are normal elements of the connective tissue, usually closely associated with blood vessels. They are widely distributed in the connective tissue of the skin and in the digestive and respiratory organs. Mast cells are spherical cells filled with fine, regular, dark-staining, basophilic granules. However, the cells exhibit variation in size and granule content.

Plasma cells arise from the lymphocytes that migrate into the connective tissue. These cells have a wide distribution in the body. They are especially found in great abundance in the loose connective tissue and lymphatic tissue of the respiratory and digestive tracts, respectively.

Leukocytes (white blood cells), neutrophils, and eosinophils, migrate from the blood vessels and capillaries into the connective tissue. Their main function is to defend the organism against bacterial invasion or foreign matter.

Fibroblasts and adipose cells are permanent or resident connective tissue cells. Neutrophils, eosinophils, plasma cells, mast cells, and macrophages migrate from the blood vessels and take up residence in the connective tissue of different regions of the body.

Fibrous Components of the Connective Tissue

There are three distinctive types of connective tissue fibers: **collagen**, **elastic**, and **reticular**. The amount and arrangement of these fibers depend on the function of the tissues or organs in which they are found. **Fibroblasts** synthesize all the collagen, elastic, and reticular fibers. The primary function of the fibrous components within the connective tissue is to provide strength and resistance to stretching and deformation. Thus, the mechanical and physical properties of the fibrous components of the connective tissue primarily depend on the mixture of the fibers in the extracellular matrix and the predominance of any single fiber type.

Types of Collagen Fibers

Collagen fibers are tough, thick, fibrous proteins that do not branch. They are the most abundant fibers and are found in almost all the connective tissues of all organs. The most frequently recognized fibers in histologic slides are the following:

- **Type I** collagen fibers: These are the most common fibers and are found in the dermis of the skin, tendons, ligaments, fasciae, fibrocartilage, the capsules of organs, and bones. They are very strong and offer great resistance to tensile stresses.

- **Type II** collagen fibers: These are present in hyaline cartilage, in elastic cartilage, and in the vitreous body of the eye. The fibers provide resistance to pressure.

- **Type III** collagen fibers: These are the thin, branching reticular fibers that form the delicate supporting meshwork in such organs as the lymph nodes, spleen, and bone marrow, where they form the main extracellular matrix support for the cells of these organs.

- **Type IV** collagen fibers: These are present as meshwork in the basal lamina of the basement membrane, to which the basal regions of the cells attach with the hemisdesmosomes.

Reticular Fibers

Reticular fibers consist mainly of type III collagen, are thin, and form a delicate netlike support framework in the liver, lymph nodes, spleen, hemopoietic organs, and other locations where blood and lymph are filtered. Reticular fibers also support capillaries, nerves, and muscle cells. These fibers become visible only when the tissue or organ is stained with silver stain.

Elastic Fibers

Elastic fibers are thin, small, branching fibers that are capable of stretching and returning to their original length. They have less tensile strength than collagen fibers and are composed of microfibrils and the protein **elastin**. When stretched, elastic fibers return to their original size (recoil) without deformation. Elastic fibers are found in abundance in the lungs, bladder wall, and skin. In the walls of the aorta and pulmonary trunk, the presence of elastic fibers allows for stretching and recoiling of these vessels during powerful blood ejections from the heart ventricles. In the walls of the large vessels, the **smooth muscle cells** synthesize the elastic fibers; in other organs, fibroblasts synthesize elastic fibers.

 Supplemental micrographic images are available at **www.thePoint.com/Eroschenko12e** under Connective Tissue.

FIGURE 5.1 | Loose Connective Tissue (Spread)

The plate illustrates a composite image of mesentery that was stained to show different fibers and cells. Mesentery is a thin sheet composed of loose connective tissue.

The pink **collagen fibers (3)** are the thickest, largest, and most numerous fibers. In this connective tissue preparation, the collagen fibers (3) course in all directions.

The elastic **fibers (5, 10)** are thin, fine, single fibers that are usually straight; however, after tissue preparation, the fibers may become wavy as a result of the release of tension. Elastic fibers (5, 10) form branching and anastomosing networks. Fine reticular fibers are also present in loose connective tissue, but these are not included in this illustration.

The fixed permanent cells of connective tissues are the **fibroblasts (2)**. The fibroblasts (2) are flattened cells with an oval nucleus, sparse chromatin, and one or two nucleoli. Fixed **macrophages**, or **histiocytes (12)**, are always present in the connective tissue. When inactive, they appear similar to fibroblasts, although their processes may be more irregular and their nuclei smaller. Phagocytic inclusions, however, alter the cytoplasm of the macrophages. In this illustration, the cytoplasm of different macrophages (12) is filled with dense-staining particles that were ingested by these cells.

Mast cells (1, 9) are also present in the loose connective tissue and are seen as single or grouped cells along small blood vessels (**capillary, 7**). The mast cells (1, 9) are usually ovoid, with a small, centrally placed nucleus and cytoplasm filled with fine, closely packed granules that stain dense or deep red with neutral red stain.

Numerous different blood cells are also seen in the loose connective tissue. **Small lymphocytes (6)** exhibit a dense-staining nucleus that occupies most of the cell cytoplasm. **Large lymphocytes (8)** also exhibit a dense nucleus with more cytoplasm. Loose connective tissue also contains blood cells, such as eosinophils and neutrophils, and adipose cells. These are illustrated in greater detail in Figure 5.2, in the loose connective tissue in Figure 5.4, and in the mesentery of an intestine in Figure 5.12.

The faint background around the fibers and cells is the ground substance.

1 Mast cell

2 Fibroblasts

3 Collagen fibers

4 Plasma cell

5 Elastic fibers

6 Small lymphocyte

7 Capillary with erythrocytes

8 Large lymphocyte

9 Mast cell

10 Elastic fibers

11 Plasma cells

12 Macrophage with ingested particles

FIGURE 5.1 ■ Loose connective tissue (spread). Stained for cells and fibers. High magnification.

FIGURE 5.2 | Individual Cells of Connective Tissue

The main cells of the connective tissue are the fibroblasts and fibrocytes. The **fibroblast (1)** is an elongated cell with cytoplasmic projections, an ovoid nucleus with sparse chromatin, and one or two nucleoli. The **fibrocyte (6)** is a more mature, smaller spindle-shaped cell without cytoplasmic projections; the nucleus is similar but smaller than that in the fibroblast.

The **plasma cell (2)** exhibits a smaller, eccentrically placed nucleus with condensed, coarse chromatin clumps distributed peripherally in a characteristic radial (cartwheel) pattern and one central mass. A prominent, clear area in the cytoplasm is adjacent to the nucleus.

The large **adipose cell (3)** exhibits a narrow rim of cytoplasm and a flattened, eccentric nucleus. In histologic sections, the large fat globules of adipose cells have been dissolved by different chemicals, leaving a large, highly characteristic empty space.

The **large lymphocyte (4)** and **small lymphocyte (10)** are spherical cells that differ primarily in the greater amount of cytoplasm that is present in the large lymphocyte (4). The dense-staining nuclei of all lymphocytes have condensed chromatin but no nucleoli.

The free **macrophage (5)** usually appears round with irregular cell outlines but exhibits a variable appearance. In the illustration, the macrophage exhibits a small nucleus rich in chromatin and cytoplasm filled with dense, ingested particles.

An **eosinophil (7)** is a large blood cell with a bilobed nucleus and large, eosinophilic cytoplasmic granules that fill the cytoplasm.

A **neutrophil (8)** is also a large blood cell, characterized by a multilobed nucleus and a lack of stained granules in the cytoplasm.

Cells with **pigment granules (9)** may be seen in the connective tissue. Also, the basal epithelial cells of the skin contain brown-staining pigment or melanin granules.

A **mast cell (11)** is usually ovoid, with a small, centrally placed nucleus. The cytoplasm is normally filled with fine, closely packed, dense-staining granules.

FUNCTIONAL CORRELATIONS 5.1 | Individual Cells in Connective Tissue

Fibroblasts are the dominant cells in the connective tissue. These highly active cells with irregularly branched cytoplasm synthesize **collagen**, **reticular**, and **elastic fibers** as well as carbohydrates, such as glycosaminoglycans, proteoglycans, and adhesive glycoproteins of the **extracellular matrix**. The spindle-shaped **fibrocytes** are smaller than the fibroblasts and are mature and less active cells of the fibroblast line.

Macrophages or histiocytes are **phagocytes** that are attracted to the sites of inflammation. They ingest bacteria, dead cells, cell debris, and other foreign matter that enters the connective tissue. These cells also enhance immunologic activities of the lymphocytes. Macrophages are **antigen-presenting cells** to lymphocytes that perform important functions in the immune response. The cells are part of the **mononuclear phagocyte system**, derived from circulating blood **monocytes** that take up residence in the connective tissue. Although present throughout the body, macrophages have specific names in different organs. **Dusts cells** are found in the alveoli of the lungs, **Kupffer cells** line the sinusoids in the liver, **Langerhans cells** are in the epidermis of the skin, **microglia** in the tissues of the brain, **monocytes** in the circulating blood, and **osteoclasts** are found in the bone.

Lymphocytes are the most numerous cells in the loose connective tissue of the respiratory and gastrointestinal tracts. They do not have any function in the bloodstream but leave the circulatory system and enter the connective tissue through the capillaries. They mediate immune responses to antigens that enter these organs and, once activated, produce antibodies and kill virus-infected cells by inducing cell death (apoptosis).

Plasma cells are derived from lymphocytes that have been exposed to antigens and become activated. They synthesize and secrete **antibodies** that destroy specific antigens and defend the body against infections.

FUNCTIONAL CORRELATIONS 5.1 | Individual Cells in Connective Tissue *(Continued)*

Adipose cells store fat (lipid) and provide protective packing material and insulation in and around numerous vital organs. In addition, adipose cells provide energy for metabolic functions.

Neutrophils are active and powerful phagocytes; they leave the bloodstream to engulf and destroy bacteria at sites of infections.

Eosinophils become active and increase in number after parasitic infections or allergic reactions. They phagocytize antigen–antibody complexes formed during allergic reactions.

Mast cells synthesize and release **histamine** and **heparin**. Their location near small blood vessels and capillaries allows them to perform numerous defensive functions. Exposure of mast cells to allergens causes rapid release of histamine and other vasoactive chemicals. Histamine is a potent inflammatory mediator. It causes dilation of blood vessels and increases the permeability of capillaries and venules, thereby causing local edema and the migration of white blood cells from circulation. Histamine also induces signs and symptoms of immediate hypersensitive (allergic) reactions. In contrast, heparin acts locally as a weak anticoagulant.

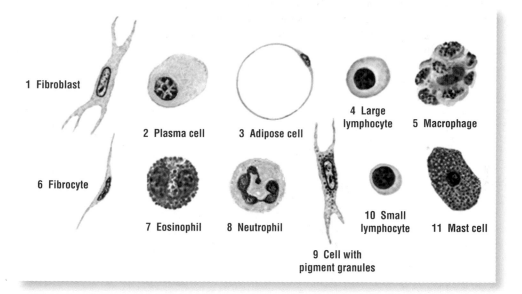

FIGURE 5.2 ■ Cells of the connective tissue. Stain: hematoxylin and eosin. High magnification or oil immersion.

FIGURE 5.3 | Connective Tissue, a Capillary, and a Mast Cell in the Mesentery of a Small Intestine

This micrograph illustrates the contents of the connective tissue from the mesentery of a small intestine. Closely associated with the **capillary (3)** and sectioned in a longitudinal plane is a **mast cell** with dense **granules (5)** in its cytoplasm and a red-staining nucleus. The capillary (3) is packed with **red blood cells (6)**. Because the lumen of the capillary is about the size of a red blood cell (RBC), the RBCs in its lumen are lined up in a row. Located above the capillary (3) is a larger vessel, a **venule (2)**, sectioned in a transverse plane and also packed with RBCs. Surrounding the blood vessels (2, 3) are numerous **adipose cells (1)** with their lipid contents washed out during slide preparation. Also present are the dense layers of blue-staining **collagen fibers (4)** and **fibrocytes (7)** that are closely associated with the blood vessels and the capillaries.

FIGURE 5.4 | Embryonic Connective Tissue

The embryonic connective tissue resembles the mesenchyme or mucous connective tissue; this is loose and irregular connective tissue. The difference in ground substance (semifluid vs. jellylike) is not apparent in these sections.

The **fibroblasts (4)** are numerous, and fine **collagen fibers (1)** are found between them, some coming in close contact with fibroblasts. The embryonic connective tissue is vascular. **Capillaries (3)** lined with endothelium and filled with **RBCs (2)** are visible in the ground substance.

At higher magnification, primitive **fibroblasts (5)** are seen as large, branching cells with cytoplasm, prominent cytoplasmic processes, an ovoid nucleus with fine chromatin, and one or more nucleoli. The widely separated **collagen fibers (6)** are more apparent at this magnification.

1 Adipose cells

2 Venule

3 Capillary

4 Collagen fibers

5 Mast cell with dense granules

6 Red blood cells

7 Fibrocytes

FIGURE 5.3 ■ Connective a tissue, a capillary, and a mast cell in the mesentery of a small intestine. Stain: Mallory-Azan. ×205.

1 Collagen fibers

2 RBCs in capillary

3 Capillaries lined with endothelium

4 Nuclei of fibroblasts

5 Nuclei and cytoplasm of fibroblasts

6 Collagen fibers

FIGURE 5.4 ■ Embryonic connective tissue. Stain: hematoxylin and eosin. *Left*, low magnification; *right*, high magnification.

FIGURE 5.5 | Loose Connective Tissue

Collagen fibers (9) predominate in loose connective tissue, course in different directions, and form a loose fiber meshwork. In the illustration, collagen fibers (9) are sectioned in various planes, and transverse ends may be seen. The fibers are acidophilic and stain pink with eosin. Thin elastic fibers are also present in loose connective tissue but are difficult to distinguish with this stain and at this magnification.

The **fibroblasts (2)** are the most numerous cells in the loose connective tissue and may be sectioned in various planes, so that only parts of the cells may be seen. Also, during section preparation, the cytoplasm of these cells may shrink. A typical fibroblast (2) shows an oval nucleus with sparse chromatin and lightly acidophilic cytoplasm, with a few short processes.

Also present in loose connective tissue are various blood cells such as the **neutrophils (6)** with lobulated nuclei, **eosinophils (3)** with red-staining granules, and small **lymphocytes (7)** with dense-staining nuclei and sparse cytoplasm. The **fat (adipose) cells (5)** appear characteristically empty with a thin rim of cytoplasm and peripherally displaced flat **nuclei (4)**.

The connective tissue is highly vascular; **capillaries (8)** sectioned in different planes (t.s., transverse section; l.s., longitudinal section) are visible. Larger blood vessels, such as an **arteriole (1) with RBCs**, are also seen in the loose connective tissue.

FIGURE 5.6 | Dense Irregular and Loose Irregular Connective Tissue (Elastin Stain)

This figure illustrates a section of connective tissue that shows a transition zone between loose irregular connective tissue in the upper region and more dense irregular connective tissue in the lower region of the illustration. In addition, the tissue section has been specially prepared to show the presence and distribution of elastic fibers in the connective tissue.

The **elastic fibers (1, 7)** have been selectively stained a deep blue using the Verhoeff method. Using Van Gieson stain as a counterstain, acid fuchsin stains **collagen fibers** red **(2, 6)**. Cellular details of fibroblasts are not obvious, but the **fibroblast nuclei (3, 5)** stain deep blue. **Blood vessels (4)** are also present.

The characteristic features of dense irregular and loose connective tissues become apparent with this staining technique. In dense irregular connective tissue, the collagen fibers (6) are larger, more numerous, and more concentrated. Elastic fibers are also larger and more numerous (7). In contrast, in the loose connective tissue, both fiber types are smaller (1, 2) and more loosely arranged. Fine elastic networks are seen in both types of connective tissue.

1 Arteriole with RBCs

2 Nuclei of fibroblasts

3 Eosinophil

4 Nuclei of adipose cells

5 Adipose cells

6 Neutrophils

7 Lymphocytes

8 Capillaries (t.s. and l.s.)

9 Collagen fibers

FIGURE 5.5 ■ Loose connective tissue with blood vessels and adipose cells. Stain: hematoxylin and eosin. High magnification.

1 Thin elastic fibers

2 Collagen fibers

3 Nuclei of fibrocytes

4 Blood vessel

5 Nuclei of fibrocytes

6 Collagen fibers

7 Elastic fibers

FIGURE 5.6 ■ Dense irregular and loose irregular connective tissue. Stains: Verhoeff and Van Gieson. Medium magnification.

FIGURE 5.7 | Loose Irregular and Dense Irregular Connective Tissue

This figure illustrates a gradual transition from **loose irregular connective tissue (5)** to **dense irregular connective tissue (1)**. Where firmer support and more strength are required, dense irregular connective tissue replaces the loose type.

The **collagen fibers (2, 9)** in both types of tissues are large, typically found in bundles, and sectioned in several planes because they course in various directions. Also present here are thin, wavy elastic fibers that form fine networks. However, these fibers are not obvious in routine histologic preparations.

In the **dense connective tissue (1)**, the **fibroblasts (3)** are often found compressed among the collagen fibers (2). In the loose connective tissue (5), the collagen fibers (9) are less compressed and the fibroblasts **(10)** are more visible. Also illustrated in the connective tissue are **capillaries (4)**, a small **venule (11)**, an **eosinophil (6)** with lobulated nucleus, **lymphocytes (7)** with large round nuclei without visible cytoplasm, a **plasma cell (8)**, and numerous **adipose cells (12)**.

FIGURE 5.8 | Dense Irregular Connective Tissue and Adipose Tissue

Illustrated in this photomicrograph is a deep section of the skin called the dermis. This region contains **dense irregular connective tissue (1)** and the collagen-producing **fibroblasts (3)**. In this type of connective tissue, the **collagen fibers (2)** show a very random and irregular orientation. Adjacent to the dense irregular connective tissue (1) is a region of **adipose tissue (4)** with its numerous **adipose cells (5)**. Because of the tissue preparation with different chemicals, the individual adipose cells appear empty, and only their flattened, dense-staining nuclei are visible. Deep in the skin are also found numerous sweat glands. The light-staining regions are the **secretory cells of the sweat gland (7)**. The dark-staining cells form a **stratified cuboidal epithelium** of the **excretory duct of the sweat gland (6, 8)**. The excretory duct (6, 8) continues through the connective tissue and the stratified squamous epithelium of the skin and exits on the surface of the skin (see Figure 4.10).

FUNCTIONAL CORRELATIONS 5.2 | Ground Substance and Connective Tissue

The **ground substance** in connective tissue consists primarily of amorphous, transparent, and colorless **extracellular matrix**, which has the properties of a semifluid gel and high water content. The matrix supports, surrounds, and binds all the connective tissue cells and fibers. The ground substance contains different types of mixed, unbranched polysaccharide chains of **glycosaminoglycans**, **proteoglycans**, and **adhesive glycoproteins**. **Hyaluronic acid** constitutes the principal glycosaminoglycan of connective tissue. Except for hyaluronic acid, the various glycosaminoglycans are bound to a core protein to form much larger molecules called **proteoglycan aggregates**. These proteoglycans attract increased amounts of water, which forms the hydrated gel of the ground substance.

The semifluid consistency of the ground substance in the connective tissue facilitates **diffusion** of oxygen, electrolytes, nutrients, fluids, metabolites, and other water-soluble molecules between the cells and the blood vessels. Similarly, waste products from the cells diffuse through the ground substance back into the blood vessels. Also, because of its viscosity, the ground substance serves as an efficient **barrier**. It prevents movement of large molecules and the spread of pathogens from the connective tissue into the bloodstream. However, certain bacteria can produce hyaluronidase, an enzyme that hydrolyzes hyaluronic acid and reduces the viscosity of the gel-like ground substance, allowing pathogens to invade the surrounding tissues.

The density of ground substance depends on the amount of extracellular tissue fluid or water that it contains. Mineralization of ground substance, as a result of increased calcium deposition, changes its density, rigidity, and permeability to diffusion, as seen in normal developing cartilage models and bones.

In addition to proteoglycans, connective tissue also contains several cell **adhesive glycoproteins**, which bind cells to the fibers. One glycoprotein, the **fibronectin**, is the adhesion protein. It binds connective tissue cells, collagen fibers, and proteoglycans, thereby interconnecting all three components of the connective tissue. Integral proteins of the plasma membrane, called **integrins**, bind to extracellular collagen fibers and to actin filaments in the cytoskeleton, thus establishing a structural continuity between the cytoskeleton and the extracellular matrix. **Laminin** is a large glycoprotein and a major component of the cell basement membrane. This protein binds epithelial cells to the basal lamina.

FIGURE 5.7 ■ Dense irregular and loose irregular connective tissue. Stain: hematoxylin and eosin. High magnification.

FIGURE 5.8 ■ Dense irregular connective tissue and adipose tissue. Stain: hematoxylin and eosin. ×64.

FIGURE 5.9 | Dense Regular Connective Tissue: Tendon (Longitudinal Section)

Dense regular connective tissue is present in ligaments and tendons. Shown here is a section of a tendon in the longitudinal plane in which some of the collagen fibers are stretched, and some are relaxed.

The **collagen fibers (2, 5, 8)** are arranged in compact, parallel bundles. Between collagen bundles (2, 5, 8) are thin partitions of looser connective tissue that contain parallel rows of **fibroblasts (1, 3)**. The fibroblasts (1, 3) have short processes (not visible here) and nuclei that appear ovoid when seen in **surface view (3)** or flat and rodlike in **lateral view (1)**. When the tendon is stretched, the bundles of collagen fibers (2) are straight. When the tendon is relaxed, the bundles of collagen fibers (8) become wavy.

Dense irregular connective tissue with less regular fiber arrangement than in the tendon also surrounds and partitions the collagen bundles as the **interfascicular connective tissue (4)**. Here are also found **fibroblasts (6)** and numerous blood vessels, such as this **arteriole (7)**, that supply the connective tissue cells.

FIGURE 5.10 | Dense Regular Connective Tissue: Tendon (Longitudinal Section)

A photomicrograph of dense regular connective tissue of a tendon shows that it has a compact, regular, and parallel arrangement of **collagen fibers (1)**. Between the densely packed collagen fibers are seen flattened nuclei of the **fibroblasts (2)**. A small **blood vessel (3)** with blood cells courses between the dense bundles of collagen fibers to supply the connective tissue cells of the tendon.

FUNCTIONAL CORRELATIONS 5.3 | Dense Connective Tissue

DENSE IRREGULAR CONNECTIVE TISSUE

Dense irregular connective tissue consists primarily of **collagen fibers (type I collagen)** with minimal amounts of surrounding ground substance. Except for the **fibroblasts** and/or **fibrocytes**, cells in this type of connective tissue are sparse. Collagen fibers exhibit great **tensile strength**, and their main function is **support**. In dense irregular connective tissue, collagen fibers exhibit **random orientation** and are most highly concentrated in those areas of the body where strong support is needed to resist pulling forces from different directions.

DENSE REGULAR CONNECTIVE TISSUE

Dense regular connective tissue exhibits a predominance of **collagen fibers (type I collagen)** and is present where **great tensile strength** is required, such as in **ligaments** and **tendons**. The parallel and dense arrangements of collagen fibers offer strong resistance to forces pulling along a **single axis or direction**.

Tendons and ligaments are attached to bones and are constantly subjected to strong pulling forces. Because of the dense arrangement of collagen fibers, little ground substance is present, and the predominant cell types that synthesize the collagen fibers are the **fibroblasts** that are located between rows of parallel collagen fibers.

1 Nuclei of fibroblasts (lateral view)

2 Bundle of collagen fibers (stretched condition)

3 Nuclei of fibroblasts (surface view)

4 Interfascicular connective tissue

5 Collagen fibers (in bundle)

6 Fibroblasts

7 Arteriole

8 Bundle of collagen fibers (relaxed condition)

FIGURE 5.9 ■ Dense regular connective tissue: tendon (longitudinal section). Stain: hematoxylin and eosin. Medium magnification.

1 Collagen fibers

2 Fibroblasts

3 Blood vessel

FIGURE 5.10 ■ Dense regular connective tissue: tendon (longitudinal section). Stain: hematoxylin and eosin. ×64.

FIGURE 5.11 | Dense Regular Connective Tissue: Tendon (Transverse Section)

A transverse section of a tendon is illustrated at a lower magnification (*left side*) and a higher magnification (*right side*). Within each large bundle of **collagen fibers (3, 7)** are **fibroblasts (nuclei) (1, 8)** sectioned transversely. The fibroblasts are located between the bundles of collagen fibers (3, 7). These fibroblasts (8) are better distinguished at the higher magnification on the right side, which shows bundles of collagen fibers (7) and the branched shape of fibroblasts (8) in transverse section.

Between the large collagen bundles are the **interfascicular connective tissue (2)** partitions. These partitions contain blood vessels, an **arteriole** and **venules (6)**, nerves, and, occasionally, the sensitive pressure receptors **Pacinian corpuscles (9)**.

Also illustrated on the left side of the figure is a transverse section of several **skeletal muscle fibers (4)**. These are adjacent to the tendon but are separated from it by a connective tissue partition. Note that the **nuclei (5)** of skeletal muscle fibers (4) are located on the periphery of the fibers, whereas the fibroblasts (1, 8) are located between bundles of collagen fibers (3, 7).

FIGURE 5.12 | Adipose Tissue: Intestine

A small section of intestinal mesentery is illustrated, in which large accumulations of **adipose (fat) cells (4, 8)** are organized into adipose tissue. The **connective tissue (9)** that surrounds the adipose tissue is covered by a simple squamous epithelium called **mesothelium (10)**.

Adipose cells (4, 8) are closely packed and separated by thin strips of **connective tissue septa (3)**, in which are found compressed **fibroblasts (7)**, **arterioles (1)**, **venules (2, 6)**, nerves, and **capillaries (5)**.

Individual adipose cells (4) appear as empty cells because the fat was dissolved by chemicals used during routine histologic preparation of the tissue. The **adipose cell nuclei (8)** are compressed to the peripheral rim of the cytoplasm, and, in certain sections, it is difficult to distinguish between fibroblast nuclei (7) and adipose cell nuclei (8).

FUNCTIONAL CORRELATIONS 5.4 | Adipose Tissue

The two distinct types of adipose tissues in the body are **white adipose tissue** and **brown adipose tissue**. These adipose tissues represent the main sites of **lipid storage** and **metabolism** in the body.

WHITE ADIPOSE TISSUE

White adipose tissue is the more common type. Cells of white adipose tissue, the **adipocytes**, are large and store lipids as a single, large droplet. The lipids stored in adipose cells are primarily **triglycerides** (fatty acids and glycerol) derived from the intestinal lipoproteins and the very-low-density lipoproteins from the liver. This adipose tissue also exhibits a wider distribution than brown adipose tissue. White adipose tissue is distributed throughout the body, with the distribution pattern showing variations that are highly dependent on the gender and age of the individual. In addition to serving as an important energy source, white adipose tissue provides **insulation** under the skin and forms cushioning **fat pads** around different organs. This tissue is also highly vascularized as a result of its high metabolic activity. The white adipose cells also have receptors for insulin, glucocorticoids, growth hormone, and other factors that influence adipose tissue to accumulate and release lipids. Furthermore, white adipose tissue also functions as an important endocrine organ. These cells are the sole source of a hormone called **leptin**, which increases carbohydrate and lipid metabolism in cells. This hormone also influences the cells in the **hypothalamus** that inhibit or suppress appetite and food intake.

BROWN ADIPOSE TISSUE

In contrast to the white adipose tissue, which is present throughout the body, brown adipose tissue has a more limited distribution. The cells of brown adipose tissue are

FUNCTIONAL CORRELATIONS 5.4 | Adipose Tissue *(Continued)*

smaller than white adipose tissue cells and store lipids as multiple small droplets. Brown adipose tissue is found in all mammals, but is best developed in animals that **hibernate**. The main function of brown adipose tissue is to supply the body with **heat** through nonshivering thermogenesis. In newborn humans exposed to cold and in fur-bearing animals emerging from hibernation, brown adipose tissue is especially useful to generate and increase body heat during these critical periods. The production of heat by brown adipose tissue is regulated by the sympathetic nervous system, which releases **norepinephrine** to promote hydrolysis of lipids to fatty acids and glycerol. The amount of brown adipose tissue gradually decreases in older individuals and is mainly found around the adrenal glands, great vessels, and in the neck region. However, as an adaptation, the cold environment activates the development of brown adipose cells and tissue.

1 Fibroblasts

2 Interfascicular connective tissue

3 Bundles of collagen fibers

4 Skeletal muscle fibers

5 Nuclei of skeletal muscles

6 Arteriole and venules

7 Collagen fibers

8 Nuclei of fibroblasts

9 Pacinian corpuscle

FIGURE 5.11 ■ Dense regular connective tissue: tendon (transverse section). Stain: hematoxylin and eosin. *Left*, low magnification; *right*, high magnification.

1 Arteriole

2 Venule

3 Connective tissue septa

4 Adipose cells

5 Capillary

6 Venule

7 Fibroblasts

8 Nuclei of adipose cells

9 Connective tissue

10 Mesothelium

FIGURE 5.12 ■ Adipose tissue in the intestine. Stain: hematoxylin and eosin. Medium magnification.

Connective Tissue

- Develops from mesenchyme and consists of cells and extracellular matrix
- Matrix consists of tissue fluid, the ground substance
- Embryonic connective tissue is present in the umbilical cord and developing teeth
- Ground substance is a medium for exchange of nutrients, oxygen, and waste
- Contains cells that protect and defend body against bacteria and foreign bodies
- Classified as loose or dense connective tissue

Classification

Loose Connective Tissue

- More prevalent in body and exhibits a loose, irregular arrangement of cells and fibers
- Abundant ground substance
- Collagen fibers, fibroblasts, adipose cells, mast cells, plasma cells, and macrophages predominate

Dense Irregular Connective Tissue

- Consists primarily of fibroblasts and thick, densely packed collagen fibers
- Fewer other cell types and minimal ground substance
- Collagen fibers exhibit random orientation and provide strong tissue support
- Concentrated in areas where resistance to forces from different directions is needed

Dense Regular Connective Tissue

- Fibers densely packed with regular, parallel orientation
- Present in tendons and ligaments that are attached to bones
- Great resistance to forces pulling along single axis or direction
- Minimal ground substance; predominant cell type is fibroblast

Cells of Connective Tissue

Fibroblasts

- Are active permanent cells that synthesize all collagen, reticular, and elastic connective tissue fibers
- Synthesize glycosaminoglycans, proteoglycans, and adhesive glycoproteins of ground substance

Fibrocytes

- Smaller than fibroblasts
- Inactive or resting connective tissue cells

White Adipose (Fat) Cells

- Most common type of adipose tissue with wider distribution
- Occur singly or in groups and contain single or unilocular lipid droplets
- When adipose cells predominate, the connective tissue is adipose tissue
- Store fat (lipid) as a single large droplet, primarily as tryglycerides
- Lipids derived from intestinal lipoproteins and low lipid lipoproteins from liver
- Appear as empty cells because lipid is dissolved during tissue preparation
- Distributed throughout the body, serves as insulation, and forms fat pads for organ protection
- Highly vascularized owing to high metabolic activity
- Exhibit numerous receptors for different hormones that influence accumulation and release of lipid
- Sole source of hormone leptin that increases lipid metabolism and regulates appetite

Brown Adipose Cells

- Exhibits more limited distribution
- Cells smaller than white adipose cells; store fat as multiple lipid droplets
- Best developed in hibernating animals
- In newborns or animals emerging from hibernation, generates body heat
- Norepinephrine from sympathetic nervous system promotes hydrolysis of lipids
- As an adaptation to cold environment, cell numbers and tissue increase

Macrophages

- Most numerous in loose connective tissue
- Ingest bacteria, dead cells, cell debris, and foreign matter
- Are antigen-presenting cells to lymphocytes for immunologic response
- Derived from circulating blood monocytes
- Called Kupffer cells in liver, osteoclasts in bone, microglia in central nervous system, Langerhans cells in skin, monocytes in blood, and osteoclasts in bone

Lymphocytes

- Most numerous in loose connective tissue of respiratory and gastrointestinal tracts
- Produce antibodies and kill virus-infected cells

Plasma Cells

- Characterized by chromatin distributed in radial pattern
- Derived from lymphocytes exposed to antigens
- Produce antibodies to destroy specific antigens

Mast Cells

- Closely associated with blood vessels
- Found in skin, respiratory, and digestive system connective tissue

- Spherical cells with fine, regular basophilic granules
- Release histamine and vasoactive chemicals when exposed to allergens, causing adamant allergic reactions
- Heparin is a weak anticoagulant

Neutrophils

- Active phagocytes; engulf and destroy bacteria

Eosinophils

- Increase after parasitic infestation
- Phagocytize antigen–antibody complexes during allergic reactions

Collagen Fibers

- Type I most common and very strong; found in skin, tendons, ligaments, and bone
- Type II found in hyaline and elastic cartilage and the vitreous body of the eye; provide resistance to pressure
- Type III forms meshwork in liver, lymph node, spleen, and hemopoietic organs
- Type IV found in basal lamina of basement membrane; associated with hemidesmosomes

Reticular Fibers

- Consist mainly of type III collagen; form delicate netlike framework in different organs
- Visible only when stained with silver stain

Elastic Fibers

- Thin, branching fibers that allow stretch
- Composed of microfibrils and the protein elastin
- After stretching, return (recoil) to original size without deformation
- Found in lungs, bladder, skin, and walls of large blood vessels
- In large blood vessel walls, smooth muscle synthesizes elastic fibers

Ground Substance and Connective Tissue

- Consists of extracellular matrix, a semifluid gel with high water content
- Matrix binds, supports, and surrounds cells and fibers
- Contains polysaccharide chains of glycosaminoglycans, proteoglycans, and adhesive glycoproteins
- Hyaluronic acid is the main glycosaminoglycan
- Other glycosaminoglycans form proteoglycan aggregates, which attract water
- Facilitates diffusion of different substances between cells and blood vessels
- Acts as an efficient barrier to the spread of pathogens
- Bacteria can hydrolyze hyaluronic acid and reduce barrier viscosity
- Contains several adhesive glycoproteins, such as fibronectin, that bind cells to fibers
- Integrin protein binds collagen fibers to actin
- Laminin is a component of basement membrane and binds epithelial cells to basal lamina

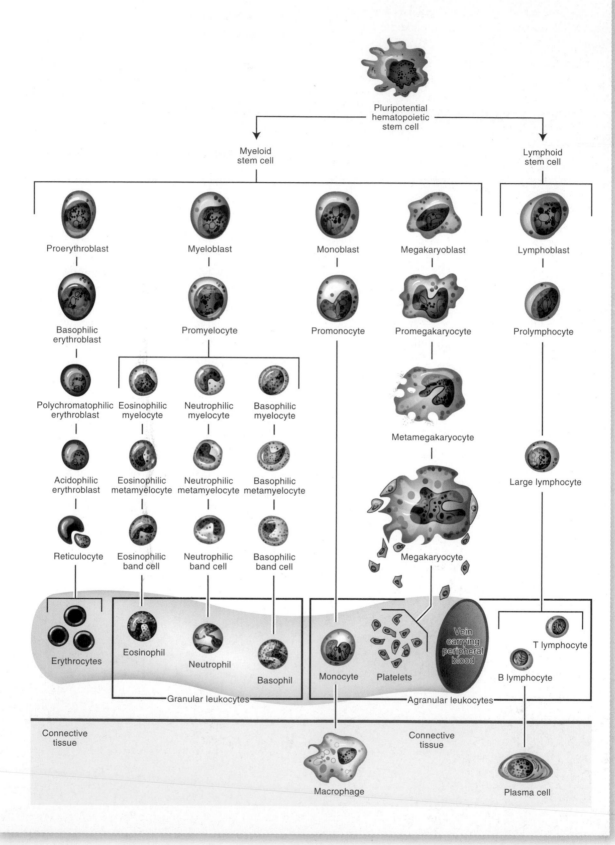

OVERVIEW FIGURE 6.1 ■ Differentiation of myeloid and lymphoid stem cells into their mature forms and their distribution in the blood and connective tissue.

CHAPTER 6

Hematopoietic Tissue ■

SECTION 1 Blood

Blood is a unique form of **connective tissue** in which its cells are suspended in a circulating fluid. The three major cell types that are found in this fluid are the erythrocytes (red blood cells [RBCs]), leukocytes (white blood cells [WBCs]), and platelets (thrombocytes). These cells, also called the **formed elements** of blood, are suspended in a liquid medium called **plasma**. Blood cells transport gases, nutrients, waste products, hormones, antibodies, various chemicals, ions, and other substances in plasma to and from different cells, tissues, and organs in the body. Blood cells have a limited life span, and, as a result, they wear out and need to be continuously replaced in the body. The process of blood cell production is called **hemopoiesis**.

Sites of Hemopoiesis

Hemopoiesis occurs in different organs of the body, depending on the stage of development of the individual. In a developing **embryo**, hemopoiesis initially occurs in the **yolk sac** and later in the development in liver, spleen, lymph nodes, and bone marrow. After birth, hemopoiesis continues almost exclusively in the **red marrow** of different bones. In the newborn, all bone marrow is red and functions in hemopoiesis.

The red bone marrow is a highly cellular structure and consists of hemopoietic **stem cells** and the precursors of different blood cells. Red marrow also contains a loose arrangement of fine reticular fibers that form an intricate network. As the individual ages and becomes an adult, the red marrow is found primarily in the flat bones of the skull, sternum and ribs, vertebrae, and pelvic bones. The remaining bones, primarily the long bones in the limbs of the body, gradually accumulate fat, and their marrow becomes yellow. Consequently, they lose the hemopoietic functions.

Hemopoiesis

In this process, all blood cells originate from a common stem cell in the **red bone marrow** that is self-renewing. Because this stem cell type can produce all blood cell types, it is called the **pluripotential hemopoietic stem cell**. Pluripotential stem cells, in turn, produce two major cell lineages that form the **pluripotential myeloid stem cells** and **pluripotential lymphoid stem cells**. Before maturation and release into the bloodstream, the stem cells from each lineage undergo numerous divisions and intermediate stages of differentiation before maturation (Overview Figure 6.1).

Myeloid stem cells develop in the red bone marrow and eventually give rise to **erythrocytes, eosinophils, neutrophils, basophils, monocytes,** and **megakaryocytes. Lymphoid stem cells** also develop in the red bone marrow. Some lymphoid cells remain in the bone marrow, proliferate, mature, and become **B lymphocytes**. Others leave the bone marrow and migrate via the bloodstream to **lymph nodes** and the **spleen**, where they proliferate and differentiate into B lymphocytes, after which they colonize peripheral lymploid tissues (connective tissues, lymphoid tissues, and lymphoid organs).

Other undifferentiated lymphoid cells migrate to the **thymus gland**, where they proliferate and differentiate into immunocompetent **T lymphocytes**. Afterward, T lymphocytes enter the bloodstream and migrate to reside in the connective tissues and specific regions of peripheral lymphoid organs of the body. Both B and T lymphocytes reside in numerous peripheral lymphoid tissues, lymph nodes, and spleen. Here, they initiate immune responses when exposed to antigens. Both the

B and T lymphocytes are morphologically indistinguishable. Only the different protein markers on their cell surfaces allow these cells to be distinguished by immunohistochemical means.

Because all blood cells have a limited life span, the pluripotential hemopoietic stem cells continually divide and differentiate to produce new progeny of cells. When the blood cells become worn out and die, they are destroyed by macrophages in different lymphoid organs such as the spleen.

Formed Elements: Major Blood Cell Types

Microscopic examination of a stained blood smear reveals the major blood cell types. **Erythrocytes,** or RBCs, are nonnucleated cells and are the most numerous blood cells. During their maturation process, the erythrocytes extrude their nuclei, and the mature blood cells enter the bloodstream, without their nuclei. Erythrocytes remain in the blood and perform their major functions within the blood vessels.

In contrast, **leukocytes**, or WBCs, are nucleated and subdivided into **granulocytes** and **agranulocytes**, depending on the presence or absence of granules in their cytoplasm. Granulocytes are the neutrophils, eosinophils, and basophils. Agranulocytes are the monocytes and lymphocytes. Leukocytes perform their major functions outside the blood vessels. They migrate out of the blood vessels through capillary walls and enter the connective tissue, lymphatic tissue, and bone marrow.

The primary function of leukocytes is to defend the body against bacterial invasion or the presence of foreign material. Consequently, most leukocytes are concentrated in the connective tissue of different organs.

Platelets

Platelets or **thrombocytes** are not blood cells. Instead, they are the smallest, nonnucleated formed elements that appear in the blood of all mammals. Platelets are membrane-bound cytoplasmic fragments or remnants of **megakaryocytes**, the largest cells in the bone marrow. Platelets are produced when small, uneven portions of the cytoplasm separate or fragment from the peripheries of the megakaryocytes and are extruded into the bloodstream. Like the erythrocytes, platelets perform their major functions within the blood vessels. Their main function is to continually monitor the vascular system and detect any damage to the endothelial lining of the vessels. If the endothelial lining breaks, the platelets adhere to the damaged site and initiate a highly complex chemical process that produces a blood clot.

 Supplemental micrographic images are available at **www.thePoint.com/Eroschenko12e** under Blood Cells.

FIGURE 6.1 | Human Blood Smear

A smear of human blood examined under lower magnification illustrates the formed elements. **Erythrocytes (1)** are the most abundant elements and the easiest to identify. Erythrocytes (RBCs) are enucleated (without a nucleus) and stain pink with eosin. They are uniform in size and measure approximately 7.5 µm in diameter, which is the approximate size of capillaries. Erythrocytes can be used as a size reference for other cell types.

Several leukocytes (WBCs) are visible in the blood smear. Leukocytes are subdivided into categories according to the shape of their nuclei, the absence or presence of cytoplasmic granules, and the staining affinities of the granules. Two **neutrophils (2, 4)**, one **eosinophil (7)** filled with red-pink granules, and one small **lymphocyte (5)** with a thin, bluish cytoplasm are visible. Scattered among the blood cells are small, blue-staining fragments called **platelets (3, 6)**.

FIGURE 6.2 | Human Blood Smear: RBCs, Neutrophils, Large Lymphocyte, and Platelets

A photomicrograph of a human blood smear shows different blood cell types. The most numerous blood cells are the **erythrocytes** (RBCs) **(1)**. Also visible are two **neutrophils (2, 4)**, a **large lymphocyte (5)**, and numerous **platelets (3)**.

1 Erythrocytes

2 Neutrophil

3 Platelets

4 Neutrophil

5 Lymphocyte

6 Platelets

7 Eosinophil

FIGURE 6.1 ■ Human blood smear: erythrocytes, neutrophils, eosinophils, lymphocyte, and platelets. Stain: Wright stain. High magnification.

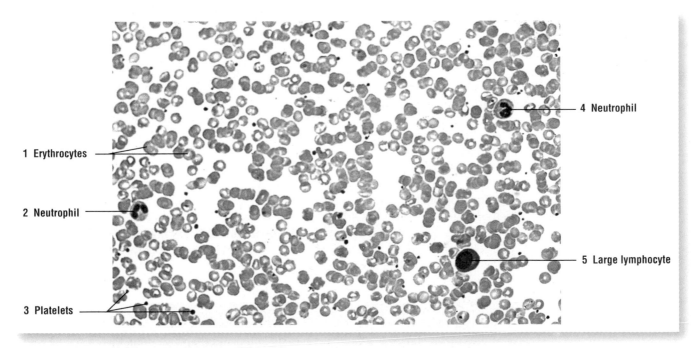

1 Erythrocytes

2 Neutrophil

3 Platelets

4 Neutrophil

5 Large lymphocyte

FIGURE 6.2 ■ Human blood smear: RBCs, neutrophils, large lymphocytes, and platelets. Stain: Wright stain. ×205.

FIGURE 6.3 | Erythrocytes and Platelets

This illustration shows numerous **erythrocytes (1)** and **platelets (2)** that are usually seen in a blood smear. Blood platelets (2) are the smallest of the formed elements; they are nonnucleated cytoplasmic remnants of large-cell megakaryocytes, which are found only in the red bone marrow. Platelets (2) appear as irregular masses of the basophilic (blue) cytoplasm, and they tend to form clumps in blood smears. Each platelet exhibits a light blue peripheral zone and a dense central zone containing purple granules.

FIGURE 6.4 | Neutrophils

The leukocytes that contain cytoplasmic granules and lobulated nuclei are the polymorphonuclear granulocytes, of which the **neutrophils (1)** are the most abundant. The neutrophil cytoplasm (1) contains fine violet or pink granules that are difficult to see with a light microscope. As a result, the cytoplasm (1) appears clear or neutral. The nucleus (1) consists of several lobes connected by narrow chromatin strands. Immature neutrophils (1) contain fewer nuclear lobes.

Neutrophils (1) constitute approximately 60% to 70% of blood leukocytes.

FUNCTIONAL CORRELATIONS 6.1 | Erythrocytes

Mature erythrocytes are specialized to transport **oxygen** and **carbon dioxide**. This specialization is attributable to the presence of the protein **hemoglobin** in their cytoplasm. Iron molecules in hemoglobin bind with oxygen molecules. As a result, most of the oxygen in the blood is carried in the combined form of **oxyhemoglobin**, which is responsible for the bright red color of arterial blood. Carbon dioxide diffuses from the cells and tissues into the blood vessels. It is carried to the lungs partly dissolved in the blood and partly in combination with hemoglobin in the erythrocytes as **carbaminohemoglobin**, which gives venous blood its bluish color.

During differentiation and maturation in the bone marrow, erythrocytes synthesize large amounts of hemoglobin. Before an erythrocyte is released into the systemic circulation, the nucleus is extruded from the cytoplasm, and the mature erythrocyte assumes a biconcave shape. This shape provides more surface area for carrying respiratory gases. Thus, mature mammalian erythrocytes in the circulation are **nonnucleated** biconcave disks surrounded by a cell membrane and filled with hemoglobin and some enzymes.

The life span of erythrocytes is approximately 120 days, after which the worn-out cells are removed from the blood and phagocytosed by macrophages in the **spleen**, **liver**, and **bone marrow**.

FUNCTIONAL CORRELATIONS 6.2 | Platelets

The main function of platelets is to repair minor tears in the walls of the blood vessels and promote **blood clotting**, thus preventing blood loss. When the wall and the endothelium of the blood vessel are damaged, platelets aggregate at the site and **adhere** to the damaged wall. The platelets are activated and form a plug to occlude the site of damage. The platelets in the plug release adhesive glycoproteins that increase the plug size by adhesion of other platelets, which is then reinforced by a polymer **fibrin** formed from numerous plasma proteins. Fibrin forms a mesh around the plug, trapping other platelets and blood cells to form a blood clot. After blood clot formation and cessation of bleeding, the aggregated platelets contribute to **clot retraction**, which pulls the damaged edges of the blood vessels closer together. Following the vessel repair, the clot is removed through the action of a proteolytic enzyme, **plasmin**, formed from the circulating plasminogen.

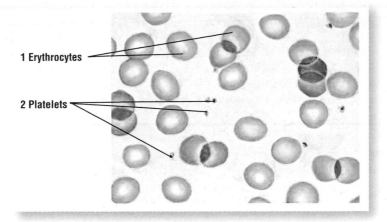

1 Erythrocytes

2 Platelets

FIGURE 6.3 ■ Erythrocytes and platelets in a blood smear. Stain: Wright stain. Oil immersion.

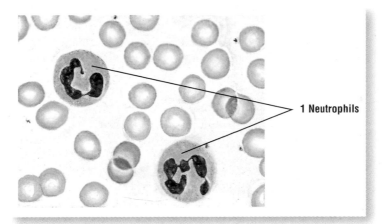

1 Neutrophils

FIGURE 6.4 ■ Neutrophils and erythrocytes. Stain: Wright stain. Oil immersion.

FIGURE 6.5 | Eosinophils

Eosinophils (1) are identified in a blood smear by their cytoplasm, which is filled with distinct, large, eosinophilic (bright pink) granules. The nucleus in eosinophils (1) typically is bilobed, but a small third lobe may be present.

Eosinophils (1) constitute approximately 2% to 4% of blood leukocytes.

FIGURE 6.6 | Lymphocytes

Agranular leukocytes have few or no cytoplasmic granules and exhibit round to horseshoe-shaped nuclei. **Lymphocytes (1, 2)** vary in size from cells smaller than erythrocytes to cells almost twice as large. For a size comparison between lymphocytes and erythrocytes, this illustration of a human blood smear depicts a **large lymphocyte (1)** and a **small lymphocyte (2)** surrounded by the red-staining erythrocytes. In small lymphocytes (2), the densely stained nucleus occupies most of the cytoplasm, which appears as a thin basophilic rim around the nucleus. The cytoplasm in lymphocytes is usually agranular but may sometimes contain a few granules. In large lymphocytes (1), the basophilic cytoplasm is more abundant, and the larger and paler nucleus may contain one or two nucleoli.

Lymphocytes (1, 2) constitute approximately 20% to 30% of blood leukocytes. Most of the lymphocytes in the blood, about 90%, are the small lymphocytes.

1 Eosinophil

FIGURE 6.5 ■ Eosinophil. Stain: Wright stain. Oil immersion.

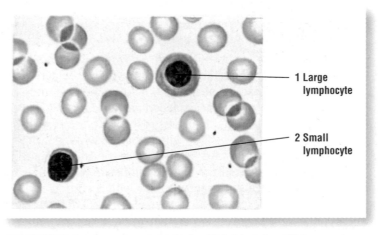

1 Large
lymphocyte

2 Small
lymphocyte

FIGURE 6.6 ■ Lymphocytes. Stain: Wright stain. Oil immersion.

FIGURE 6.7 | Monocytes

Monocytes (1) are the largest agranular leukocytes. The nucleus (1) varies from round or oval to indented or horseshoe shaped and stains lighter than the lymphocyte nucleus. The nuclear chromatin is finely dispersed in monocytes (1), and the abundant cytoplasm is lightly basophilic with few fine granules.

Monocytes (1) constitute approximately 3% to 8% of blood leukocytes.

FIGURE 6.8 | Basophils

The granules in **basophils (1)** are not as numerous as in eosinophils (see Figure 6.5); however, they are more variable in size, less densely packed, and stain dark blue or brown. Although the nucleus is not lobulated and stains palely basophilic, it is usually obscured by the density and number of granules.

The basophils (1) constitute less than 1% of blood leukocytes and are, therefore, the most difficult to find and identify in a blood smear.

FUNCTIONAL CORRELATIONS 6.3	Leukocytes

Neutrophils have a short life span. They circulate in blood for about 10 hours and then enter the connective tissue, where they survive for another 2 or 3 days. Neutrophils are active **phagocytes**, and they concentrate at the sites of infection. They are attracted by **chemotactic factors** (chemicals) released by damaged or dead cells, tissues, or microorganisms, especially bacterial, which they phagocytose (ingest) and quickly destroy with their lysosomal enzymes.

Eosinophils also have a short life span. They remain in blood for up to 10 hours and then migrate into the connective tissue, where they remain for up to 10 days. Eosinophils are also **phagocytic** cells with a particular affinity for **antigen–antibody complexes** that are formed in tissues after allergic responses. The cells also release chemicals that neutralize histamine and other mediators related to inflammatory allergic reactions. Eosinophils also increase in number during **parasitic infestation** and defend the organism against helminthic parasites by destroying them.

Lymphocytes have a variable life span, from days to months, and show size variability. The difference between small and large lymphocytes has a functional significance. Large lymphocytes represent the cells that were activated by specific antigens. Lymphocytes are essential for **immunologic defense** of the organism. Some lymphocytes (B lymphocytes), when stimulated by specific antigens, differentiate into **plasma cells** in the connective tissue and produce **antibodies** to counteract or destroy the invading organisms.

Monocytes can live in the blood for 2 to 3 days, after which they move into the connective tissue, where they may remain for a few months or longer. Blood monocytes are precursors of the mononuclear phagocyte system. After entering the connective tissue, monocytes become powerful **phagocytes**. At the site of infection, monocytes differentiate into **tissue macrophages** and then destroy bacteria, foreign matter, and cellular debris.

Basophils have a short life span, and their function is similar to that of mast cells. Their granules contain **histamine** and **heparin**. Exposure to allergens results in release of histamine and other chemicals that mediate and intensify inflammatory responses. These reactions cause severe allergic reactions, vascular changes that lead to increased fluid leakage from blood vessels (tissue edema), and hypersensitivity responses and anaphylaxis.

1 Monocyte

FIGURE 6.7 ■ Monocyte. Stain: Wright stain. Oil immersion.

1 Basophil

FIGURE 6.8 ■ Basophil. Stain: Wright stain. Oil immersion.

FIGURE 6.9 | Human Blood Smear: Basophil, Neutrophil, Erythrocytes, and Platelets

A high-magnification photomicrograph of a human blood smear shows **erythrocytes (3)**, a **basophil (1)**, a **neutrophil (5)**, and **platelets (4)**. The basophil (1) cytoplasm is filled with dense **basophilic granules (2)** that obscure the nucleus. In contrast, the neutrophil (5) cytoplasm does not show granules, and its **nucleus** is **multilobed (6)**.

FIGURE 6.10 | Human Blood Smear: Monocyte, Erythrocytes, and Platelets

A high-magnification photomicrograph shows numerous **erythrocytes (1)**, **platelets (2)**, and a large **monocyte (3)** with a characteristic kidney-shaped nucleus and nongranular cytoplasm.

1 Basophil

2 Basophilic granules

3 Erythrocytes

4 Platelets

5 Neutrophil

6 Multilobed nucleus

FIGURE 6.9 ■ Human blood smear: basophil, neutrophil, erythrocytes, and platelets. Stain: Wright stain. ×320.

1 Erythrocytes

2 Platelets

3 Monocyte

FIGURE 6.10 ■ Human blood smear: monocyte, erythrocytes, and platelets. Stain: Wright stain. ×320.

SECTION 1 • Blood

- Unique form of connective tissue in which cells are suspended in circulating fluid
- Consists of formed elements, erythrocytes, leukocytes, and platelets suspended in plasma
- Blood cells have limited life span and are continually replaced in the red bone marrow

Sites of Hemopoiesis

- Depend on the stage of development of the organism
- In embryo, the initial hemopoietic site is the yolk sac
- Later in development, liver, spleen, lymph nodes, and bone marrow form blood
- In adults, red marrow is limited to the skull, sternum, vertebrae, and pelvic bones
- Long bones contain yellow marrow and lose hemopoietic functions

Hemopoiesis

- Common pluripotential stem cell forms pluripotential myeloid and lymphoid stem cells
- Myeloid stem cells give rise to erythrocytes, eosinophils, neutrophils, basophils, monocytes, and megakaryocytes
- Lymphoid stem cells give rise to B lymphocytes and T lymphocytes
- B and T lymphocytes reside in peripheral lymphoid tissue, lymph nodes, and spleen

Formed Elements: Major Blood Cell Types

Erythrocytes

- Most numerous cells in blood
- Erythrocytes are nonnucleated cells that remain in blood
- Contain hemoglobin with iron molecules in the cytoplasm
- Carry oxygen as oxyhemoglobin and carbon dioxide as carbaminohemoglobin
- Biconcave shape increases the surface area to carry respiratory gases
- Life span is about 120 days, after which cells are phagocytosed in the spleen, liver, and bone marrow

Platelets

- Membrane-bound fragments of bone marrow megakaryocytes, not blood cells
- Function in blood vessels to promote blood clotting when the blood vessel wall is damaged
- In damaged vessels form a plug; increase plug size through adhesive glycoproteins and fibrin

- Fibrin traps more platelets and blood cells and forms a blood clot
- Cause clot retraction and pull damaged edges of the blood vessel together
- Following vessel repair, the clot is removed by the proteolytic enzyme plasmin

Leukocytes

- Contain nuclei and are subdivided into granulocytes and agranulocytes
- Granulocytes contain cytoplasmic granules; they are neutrophils, eosinophils, and basophils
- Agranulocytes are without cytoplasmic granules; they are monocytes and lymphocytes

Granulocytes

Neutrophils

- Cytoplasm appears clear under microscope
- Nucleus contains several lobes connected by thin chromatin strands
- Short life span in blood or connective tissue, ranging from hours to days
- Very active phagocytes that are attracted to foreign material by chemotactic factors
- Destroy phagocytosed (ingested) material with lysosomal enzymes
- Constitute about 60% to 70% of blood leukocytes

Eosinophils

- Cytoplasm filled with large pink or eosinophilic granules
- Nucleus typically bilobed
- Short life span, in blood or connective tissue
- Phagocytic with affinity for antigen–antibody complexes
- Release a chemical that neutralizes histamine and other mediators of inflammatory reactions
- Increase during parasitic infestation to destroy helminthic parasites
- Constitute about 2% to 4% of blood leukocytes

Basophils

- Cytoplasm contains dark blue or brown granules
- Short life span
- Nucleus stains palely basophilic, but is normally obscured by dense cytoplasmic granules
- Granules contain histamine and heparin

- Exposure to allergens releases histamine that causes intense inflammatory response in severe allergic reactions
- Constitute less than 1% of blood leukocytes

Agranulocytes

Lymphocytes

- No granules in cytoplasm and vary in size from small to large
- Dense-staining nucleus surrounded by a narrow cytoplasmic rim
- Life span is from days to months
- Essential in immunologic defense of organism

- When exposed to specific antigens, B lymphocytes form plasma cells in the connective tissue
- Plasma cells release antibodies to counteract or destroy invading organisms
- Constitute about 20% to 30% of blood leukocytes

Monocytes

- Largest agranular leukocyte characterized primarily by a horseshoe-shaped nucleus
- Live in connective tissue for months where they become powerful phagocytes
- Are part of the mononuclear phagocyte system
- Constitute about 3% to 8% of blood leukocytes

SECTION 2 Bone Marrow

Although bones provide important structural support for the body, they also serve as important sites for blood cell formation. Bone marrow is a highly cellular tissue that is located in the medullary cavities of the bone. **Red bone marrow** is the principal site of blood cell formation, or **hemopoiesis**, which is located between the bony trabeculae of the bone. Red bone marrow consists of densely packed cords and islands of blood-forming (hemopoietic) stem cells. They are surrounded by numerous macrophages and an abundant blood supply that form extensive and branching sinusoidal capillaries opening into the thin venous sinuses. These sinuses provide the main exit route through the openings in their endothelial lining for the newly differentiated blood cells to enter the systemic circulation. A connective tissue stroma of reticular cells and reticular fibers also form a delicate **meshwork** that surrounds the islands of hematopoietic cells and provides support for the bone marrow.

The active red bone marrow in selected bones provides a steady rate of blood cell renewal to replace those that are worn out or lost. Also, the red bone marrow is the site where tissue macrophages engulf and phagocytose worn-out erythrocytes and store the iron recovered from the hemoglobin breakdown for the next generation of blood cells.

 Supplemental micrographic images are available at **www.thePoint.com/Eroschenko12e** under Blood Cells

---

FIGURE 6.11 | Development of Different Blood Cells in the Red Bone Marrow (Decalcified Section)

In a section of the red bone marrow, all types of developing blood cells are difficult to distinguish. The cells are densely packed, and different cell types are intermixed. During the maturation process, hemopoietic cells become smaller and their nuclear chromatin more condensed. As the blood cells pass through a series of developmental stages, they exhibit morphologic changes and become microscopically identifiable.

This section of bone marrow is stained with hematoxylin and eosin stain. At this magnification, little differentiation of cytoplasm is visible. In the erythrocytic line, early **basophilic erythroblasts (7, 21)** are recognized by a large but not very dense nucleus and basophilic cytoplasm. These cells give rise to the smaller **polychromatophilic erythroblasts (8, 22)** with a more condensed nuclear chromatin and a more variable color of the cytoplasm, with the cytoplasm becoming more eosinophilic. The most recognizable cells of the erythrocytic line are **normoblasts (2, 23)**. They are characterized by small, dark-staining pyknotic nuclei and a reddish, or eosinophilic, cytoplasm. Early normoblasts (2, 23) exhibit **mitotic activity (6)** in the bone marrow. As normoblasts (2, 23) mature, the cells lose the ability to divide and extrude their densely staining nuclei to become **erythrocytes (3)**. Cells of the erythrocytic lineage do not display any granules in their cytoplasm. Erythrocytes (3) are abundant in red bone marrow and are seen in the numerous **sinusoids (1, 12)**, **venule (14)**, and **arteriole (15)** as they are released into systemic circulation.

The early granulocytes initially exhibit numerous primary, or azurophilic, granules in their cytoplasm. As a result, the immature forms of neutrophils, eosinophils, and basophils are morphologically indistinguishable and become recognizable only in the myelocyte stage, when specific granules appear in quantity in their cytoplasm. In neutrophilic cells, the specific granules are only faintly stained, and the cytoplasm appears clear. In the eosinophilic line, the specific granules stain deep red, or eosinophilic. Basophilic granulocytes are rarely observed in the bone marrow because of their small numbers. The cytoplasm of mature basophils exhibits a bilobed nucleus and dense blue, or basophilic, granules.

The granulocytic **myelocytes (13, 19)** exhibit a large spherical nucleus and a cytoplasm with many azurophilic granules. The myelocytes (13, 19) give rise to **metamyelocytes (4, 11, 20)**, whose nuclei are bean or horseshoe shaped. The **neutrophilic metamyelocytes (17)** exhibit a deeply indented nuclei and cytoplasm with azurophilic granules and faintly stained specific granules. In contrast, a cell with bright-staining red (eosinophilic) granules in the cytoplasm is an **eosinophilic myelocyte (18)**.

The stroma of the reticular connective tissue in the bone marrow is almost obscured by hemopoietic cells. In less dense areas, the reticular connective tissue with the elongated **reticular cells (16)** is visible. Also, numerous thin-walled sinusoids (1, 12) and different types of blood vessels (14, 15) containing erythrocytes and leukocytes are present in the bone marrow. Conspicuous in the bone marrow are the large **adipose cells (5)**, each exhibiting a large vacuole (because of fat removal during section preparation) and a small, peripheral cytoplasm that surrounds the **nucleus (5)**. Other identifiable cells in the bone marrow are the very large **megakaryocytes (9, 10)** with varied nuclear lobulation. One of these megakaryocytes (10) is situated adjacent to a blood sinusoid, into which the fragments from its cytoplasmic extension can be discharged as platelets.

Selected blood cells from the red bone marrow are illustrated below at a higher magnification.

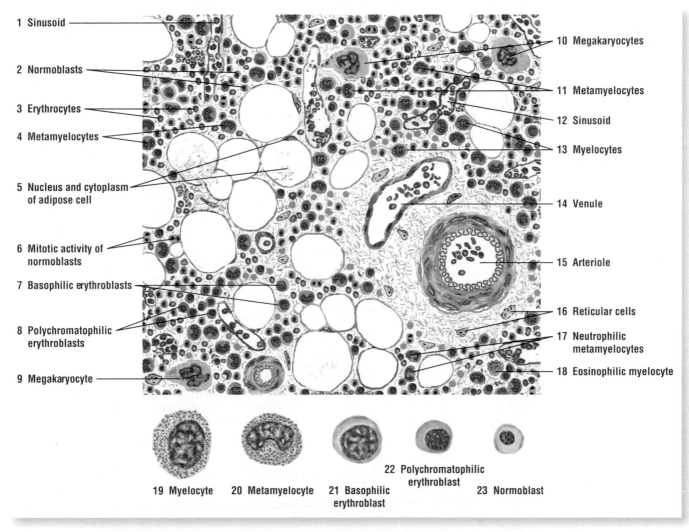

1 Sinusoid

2 Normoblasts

3 Erythrocytes

4 Metamyelocytes

5 Nucleus and cytoplasm of adipose cell

6 Mitotic activity of normoblasts

7 Basophilic erythroblasts

8 Polychromatophilic erythroblasts

9 Megakaryocyte

10 Megakaryocytes

11 Metamyelocytes

12 Sinusoid

13 Myelocytes

14 Venule

15 Arteriole

16 Reticular cells

17 Neutrophilic metamyelocytes

18 Eosinophilic myelocyte

19 Myelocyte 20 Metamyelocyte 21 Basophilic erythroblast 22 Polychromatophilic erythroblast 23 Normoblast

FIGURE 6.11 ■ Development of different blood cells in the red bone marrow (decalcified). Stain: hematoxylin and eosin. Upper image: high magnification; lower image: oil immersion.

FIGURE 6.12 | Bone Marrow Smear: Development of Different Cell Types

A bone marrow smear shows a few typical blood cells in different stages of development. In the erythrocytic series, the precursor cell **proerythroblast (3)** exhibits a thin rim of basophilic cytoplasm and a large, oval nucleus that occupies most of the cell. The chromatin is dispersed uniformly, and two or more nuclei may be present. Azurophilic granules are absent from the cytoplasm in all cells of the erythrocytic series. The proerythroblasts (3) divide to form the smaller **basophilic erythroblasts (8, 16)**.

Basophilic erythroblasts (8, 16) are characterized by a rim of basophilic cytoplasm and a decreased cell and nuclear size. The nuclear chromatin is coarse and exhibits the characteristic "checkerboard" pattern. Nucleoli are either inconspicuous or absent. Basophilic erythroblasts (8, 16) give rise to the **polychromatophilic erythroblasts (12)**, which are similar in size to basophilic erythroblasts (8, 16). The cytoplasm of the polychromatophilic erythroblast (12) becomes progressively less basophilic and more acidophilic as a result of increased hemoglobin accumulation. The nuclei of polychromatophilic erythroblasts (12) are smaller and exhibit a coarse checkerboard pattern.

When the polychromatophilic cells (12) acquire a more eosinophilic (pink) cytoplasm as a result of increased hemoglobin accumulation, their size decreases and they become **orthochromatophilic erythroblasts (late normoblasts) (1)**. These cells are capable of **mitosis (2)**. Initially, the nucleus of orthochromatophilic erythroblasts (1) exhibits a concentrated checkerboard chromatin pattern. Eventually the nucleus decreases in size, becomes pyknotic, and is extruded from the cytoplasm, forming a biconcave-shaped cell with a bluish pink cytoplasm called a reticulocyte or young erythrocyte. With special supravital staining, a delicate reticulum is seen in the reticulocyte cytoplasm because of the remaining polyribosomes (see Figure 6.13). After polyribosomes are lost from the cytoplasm, the cells become mature **erythrocytes (9)**, which then enter the systemic circulation via the numerous blood channels. Erythrocytes (9) are small cells with a homogeneous eosinophilic, or pink, cytoplasm.

Also visible in the bone marrow smear are different types of myelocytes and metamyelocytes of the granulocytic cell line. Myelocytes exhibit an eccentric nucleus with condensed chromatin and a less basophilic cytoplasm with few azurophilic granules. Different types of myelocytes exhibit varying number of granules. More mature myelocytes, such as **neutrophilic myelocytes (14)**, an **eosinophilic myelocyte (15)**, and a rare **basophilic myelocyte (11)**, show an abundance of specific granules in their slightly acidophilic cytoplasm. The myelocyte is the last cell of the granulocytic line capable of mitosis, after which they mature into metamyelocytes.

The shape of the nucleus in the neutrophilic line changes from oval to one with indentation, as seen in **neutrophilic metamyelocytes (4)**. Before complete maturation and segmentation of the nucleus into distinct lobes, the neutrophils pass through a **band cell (10)** stage, in which the nucleus assumes a nearly uniform curved rod or band shape.

Mature neutrophils (13) with segmented nuclei are also present in the bone marrow smear, as well as a **mature eosinophil (7)** with specific pink granules filling its cytoplasm.

A section of a giant cell **megakaryocyte (17)** is visible. These cells measure approximately 80 to 100 μm in diameter and have a large, slightly acidophilic cytoplasm filled with fine azurophilic granules. Cytoplasmic fragments derived from megakaryocytes are shed as **platelets (18)**.

1 Orthochromatophilic erythroblasts (normoblasts)

2 Mitosis of orthochromatophilic erythroblast (normoblast)

3 Proerythroblast

4 Neutrophilic metamyelocyte

5 Eosinophilic metamyelocyte

6 Platelets

7 Mature eosinophil

8 Basophilic erythroblast

9 Mature erythrocytes

10 Neutrophil (band cell)

11 Basophilic myelocyte

12 Polychromatophilic erythroblast

13 Mature neutrophils

14 Neutrophilic myelocytes

15 Eosinophilic myelocyte

16 Basophilic erythroblast

17 Megakaryocyte

18 Platelets derived from megakaryocyte

FIGURE 6.12 ■ Bone marrow smear: development of different blood cell types. Stain: Giemsa stain. High magnification.

FIGURE 6.13 | Bone Marrow Smear: Selected Precursors of Different Blood Cells

This figure shows at a higher magnification the selected precursor cells of different blood cells that develop and mature in the red bone marrow.

A common stem cell gives rise to different hemopoietic cell lines, from which arise erythrocytes, granulocytes, lymphocytes, and megakaryocytes. Because of its ability to differentiate into all blood cells, this cell is called the pluripotential hemopoietic stem cell. Although this cell cannot be recognized microscopically, it resembles a large lymphocyte. In adults, the greatest concentration of pluripotential stem cells is found in the red bone marrow.

Development of Erythrocytes

In the erythrocytic cell line, the **pluripotential stem cell** differentiates into a **proerythroblast (1)**, a large cell with loose chromatin, one or two nucleoli, and a basophilic cytoplasm. The proerythroblast (1) divides to produce a smaller cell called a **basophilic erythroblast (2)** with a rim of basophilic cytoplasm and a more condensed nucleus without visible nucleoli. In the next stage, a smaller cell called the **polychromatophilic erythroblast (3)** is produced. These cells show a decrease in basophilic ribosomes and an increase in the acidophilic hemoglobin content of their cytoplasm. As a result, staining these cells produces several colors in their cytoplasm. As differentiation continues, there is a further reduction of the cell size, condensation of nuclear material, and a more uniform eosinophilic cytoplasm. At this stage, the cell is called an **orthochromatophilic erythroblast (normoblast) (4)**. After extruding its nucleus, the orthochromatophilic erythroblast (4) becomes a **reticulocyte (5)** because a small number of ribosomes can be stained in its cytoplasm. After losing the ribosomes, the reticulocyte becomes a **mature erythrocyte (6)**.

Development of Granulocytes

The **myeloblast (7)** is the first recognizable precursor in the granulocytic cell line. The myeloblast (7) is a small cell with a large nucleus, dispersed chromatin, three or more nucleoli, and a basophilic cytoplasm rim that lacks specific granules. As development progresses, the cell enlarges, acquires azurophilic granules, and becomes a **promyelocyte (8, 9)**. The chromatin in the oval nucleus is dispersed, and multiple nucleoli are evident. In more advanced promyelocytes, the cells become smaller, the nucleoli become inconspicuous, the number of azurophilic granules increases, and specific granules with different staining properties begin to appear in the perinuclear region. Promyelocytes (8, 9) divide to form smaller **myelocytes (10, 13, 14)**. The cytoplasm of myelocytes (10, 13, 14) is less basophilic and contains many azurophilic granules. Myelocytes differentiate into three kinds of granulocytes, which can be recognized only by the increased accumulation and staining of the specific granules in their cytoplasm, as seen in the **eosinophilic myelocyte (13)** with red or eosinophilic granules and the rare **basophilic myelocyte (14)** with blue or basophilic granules. Myelocytes develop into metamyelocytes.

The cytoplasm of **neutrophilic metamyelocyte (11)** contains deep-staining azurophilic granules, lightly stained specific granules, and an indented, kidney-shaped nucleus. The **eosinophilic metamyelocytes (15)** are larger cells, and their specific cytoplasmic granules stain eosinophilic.

Megakaryoblasts (12) are large cells with a basophilic, homogeneous cytoplasm largely free of specific granules. The voluminous nucleus is ovoid or kidney shaped, contains numerous nucleoli, and exhibits a loose chromatin pattern. Platelets are not formed at this stage.

During differentiation, megakaryoblasts (12) become very large. Their nucleus becomes convoluted, with multiple, irregular lobes interconnected by constricted regions. The chromatin becomes condensed and coarse, and nucleoli are not visible. In mature **megakaryocytes (17)**, the plasma membrane invaginates the cytoplasm and forms demarcation membranes. This delimits the areas of the megakaryocyte cytoplasm that is then shed into the blood as small cell fragments in the form of **platelets (16)**.

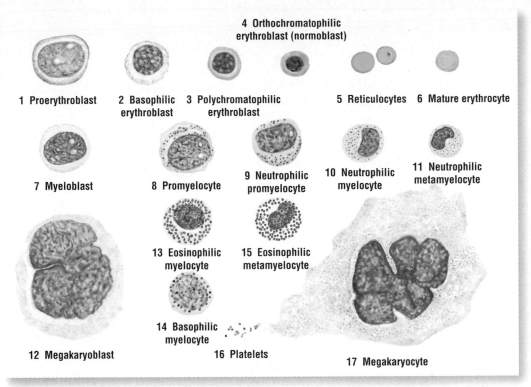

FIGURE 6.13 ■ Bone marrow smear: selected precursors of different blood cells. Stain: Giemsa stain. High magnification or oil immersion.

SECTION 2 • Bone Marrow

- Located in medullary cavities between bony trabeculae
- Red marrow is the principal site of hemopoiesis
- Consists of cords and islands of hemopoeitic stem cells that replace lost cells
- A branching capillary network surrounds hemopoeitic stem cells
- The site of macrophage breakdown of worn-out erythrocytes and storage of iron

Developing Blood cells

Development of Erythrocytes

- Precursor proerythroblast shows a rim of basophilic cytoplasm and a large nucleus
- Early basophilic erythroblasts are smaller and exhibit large nuclei and basophilic cytoplasm
- Polychomatophilic erythroblasts exhibit more condensed nuclei and more eosinophilic cytoplasm
- Increased hemoglobin accumulation, eosinophilic cytoplasm, and decreased size produce orthochromatophilic erythroblasts (late normoblasts)
- Most recognizable erythrocytic line are normoblasts with early stages exhibiting mitosis
- Mature normoblasts lose the ability to divide, extrude their highly condensed pyknotic nuclei, and become eosinophilic erythrocytes

- Erythrocytes do not exhibit cytoplasmic granules and enter systemic circulation

Development of Granulocytes

- Myeloblast, first recognizable granulocytic cell line, gives rise to promyelocyte
- Early granulocytes exhibit numerous azurophilic granules in the cytoplasm
- Promyelocytes divide and form myelocytes, which differentiate into three different kinds of granulocytes
- Myelocyte is the last stage of the granulocyte line that can divide
- Granulocyte cell lines are recognized in myelocytes as specific granules appear in the cytoplasm
- Myelocytes develop into metamyelocytes whose nuclei appear bean or kidney shaped
- Neutrophilic metamyelocytes show indented nuclei and faintly staining specific granules
- At maturation, neutrophils exhibit segmented nucleus into three lobes
- Eosinophilic metamyelocytes exhibit red or eosinophilic-specific granules in the cytoplasm
- Basophilic metamyelocytes exhibit dark or basophilic-specific granules in the cytoplasm

OVERVIEW FIGURE 7.1 ■ Endochondral ossification illustrating the progressive stages of bone formation, from a cartilage model to bone, including the histology of a section of formed compact bone.

CHAPTER 7

Skeletal Tissue: Cartilage and Bone

SECTION 1 Cartilage

Characteristics of Cartilage

Cartilage is a special form of connective tissue that also develops from **mesenchymal cells**. Similar to other types of connective tissue in the body, cartilage consists of cells and an **extracellular matrix** composed of connective tissue fibers and ground substance. In contrast to other connective tissue, however, cartilage does not have a direct blood supply, or is **nonvascular** (avascular). Cartilage receives its nutrition and eliminates its metabolic waste via diffusion through the extracellular matrix.

Cartilage exhibits tensile strength, provides firm structural support for soft tissues, allows flexibility without distortion, and is resilient to compression. Cartilage consists mainly of cells called **chondrocytes** and **chondroblasts** that synthesize the extensive extracellular matrix. There are three main types of cartilage in the body: hyaline, elastic, and fibrocartilage. Their classification is based on the amount and types of connective tissue fibers that are present in the extracellular matrix.

Cartilage Types

Hyaline Cartilage

Hyaline cartilage is the most common type. In embryos, hyaline cartilage serves as a skeletal model for most bones. As the individual grows, the cartilage model is gradually replaced with bone by a process called **endochondral ossification**. In developing bones of young individuals, hyaline cartilage persists in the **epiphyseal plates**, where its presence allows the bones to grow in length. In adults, most of the hyaline cartilage model is replaced with bone, except on the articular surfaces of bones, ends of ribs (costal cartilage), the nose, larynx, trachea, and in bronchi. Here, the hyaline cartilage persists throughout life and does not calcify to become bone.

Elastic Cartilage

Elastic cartilage is similar in appearance to hyaline cartilage, except for the presence of numerous branching elastic fibers within its matrix. Elastic cartilage is highly flexible and occurs in the external ear, walls of the auditory tube, epiglottis, and larynx.

Fibrocartilage

Fibrocartilage is characterized by large amounts of irregular and dense bundles of coarse collagen fibers in its matrix. In contrast to hyaline and elastic cartilage, fibrocartilage consists of alternating layers of cartilage matrix and thick, strong, and dense layers of **type I collagen** fibers. The collagen fibers normally orient themselves in the direction of functional stress. Fibrocartilage has a limited distribution in the body and is primarily found in the intervertebral disks, symphysis pubis, and certain joints.

Perichondrium

Most of the hyaline and elastic cartilage is surrounded by a peripheral layer of vascularized, dense, irregular connective tissue called the **perichondrium**. Its outer fibrous layer contains type I collagen fibers and fibroblasts. The inner layer of perichondrium is cellular and contains **chondrogenic cells**, which differentiate to form the chondroblasts that secrete the cartilage matrix. Hyaline cartilage on the articulating surfaces of bones, however, has a free surface and is not lined or covered by perichondrium. Similarly, because fibrocartilage is always associated with dense connective tissue collagen fibers, it does not exhibit the identifiable perichondrium seen in other types of cartilage.

Cartilage Matrix

Cartilage matrix is produced and maintained by chondrocytes and chondroblasts. The collagen or elastic fibers give cartilage matrix its firmness and resilience. Similar to loose connective tissue, the extracellular **ground substance** of cartilage contains sulfated **glycosaminoglycans** and **hyaluronic acid** that are closely associated with the elastic and collagen fibers within the ground substance. Also, cartilage matrix is highly hydrated because of its high **water** content, which allows for diffusion of molecules to and from the chondrocytes and also allows cartilage to resist compression. Cartilage is also a semirigid tissue and can act as a shock absorber. Embedded within its matrix are varying proportions of collagen and elastic fibers. The proportion of these fibers characterizes the cartilage type as hyaline cartilage, elastic cartilage, or fibrocartilage.

Hyaline cartilage matrix consists of the fine **type II collagen fibrils** embedded in a firm amorphous hydrated matrix rich in proteoglycans and structural glycoproteins. Most of the proteoglycans in the cartilage matrix exist as large **proteoglycan aggregates**, which contain sulfated glycosaminoglycans linked to core proteins and molecules of nonsulfated glycosaminoglycan hyaluronic acid. The proteoglycan aggregates bind to the thin fibrils of the collagen matrix. Numerous negatively charged ions are associated with the large proteoglycan molecules that attract hundreds of Na^+ ions, resulting in increased attraction of water molecules and hydration of the cartilage matrix.

In addition to type II collagen fibrils and proteoglycans, cartilage matrix also contains an adhesive glycoprotein called **chondronectin**. These macromolecules bind to glycosaminoglycans and collagen fibers, providing adherence of chondroblasts and chondrocytes to collagen fibers of surrounding matrix.

Although hyaline cartilage contains type II collagen fibers in its matrix, in routine histologic preparations, these collagen fibers are not seen because their reflective index is similar to that of the surrounding ground substance.

 Supplemental micrographic images are available at **www.thePoint.com/Eroschenko12e** under Cartilage.

FIGURE 7.1 | Fetal Hyaline Cartilage

This figure illustrates hyaline cartilage in an early stage of development. Superficial **mesenchyme (1)** with cells and **blood vessels (5)** surrounds the nonvascular fetal cartilage. At this stage, lacunae around the **fetal chondroblasts (4, 7)** are not visible, and the chondroblasts (4, 7) resemble superficial mesenchymal cells (1). Fetal chondroblasts (4, 7) are randomly distributed without forming isogenous groups and secrete the **intercellular cartilage matrix (8)**.

During fetal development, mesenchymal cells (1) concentrate on the periphery of the cartilage, and their nuclei become elongated. This region develops into the **perichondrium (2, 6)**, a sheath of dense irregular connective tissue with fibroblasts (2, 6) that surrounds hyaline and elastic cartilage. The inner layer of the perichondrium (2, 6) becomes the **chondrogenic layer (3)** that gives rise to chondroblasts (4, 7).

1 Superficial mesenchyme with cells

2 Perichondrium with fibroblasts

3 Chondrogenic layer

4 Fetal chondroblasts

5 Blood vessels

6 Perichondrium with fibroblasts

7 Fetal chondroblasts

8 Intercellular cartilage matrix

FIGURE 7.1 ■ Developing fetal hyaline cartilage. Stain: hematoxylin and eosin. Medium magnification.

FIGURE 7.2 | Hyaline Cartilage and Surrounding Structures: Trachea

This illustration depicts a section of a hyaline cartilage plate from the trachea. The **perichondrium (5)** with **fibroblasts (7)** surrounds the cartilage. The inner **chondrogenic layer (4)** produces **chondroblasts (8)** that differentiate into chondrocytes. **Chondrocytes** in lacunae appear either singly or in **isogenous groups (3)**. Lacunae and chondrocytes (3) in the middle of the cartilage plate are large and spherical but become progressively flatter toward the periphery, where these cells are differentiating chondroblasts (8). The **interterritorial** (intercellular) **matrix (1)** stains lighter, whereas the **territorial matrix (2)** around the lacunae stains darker.

Vascular **(9) connective tissue (10)** and tracheal glands with grapelike secretory units called acini are visible near the cartilage. **Serous acini (11)** produce watery secretions, whereas **mucous acini (12)** secrete a lubricating mucus. An **excretory duct (6)** delivers these secretions to the tracheal lumen.

FUNCTIONAL CORRELATIONS 7.1	Cartilage Cells

Cartilage develops from primitive **mesenchymal cells** that differentiate into **chondroblasts**. These cells divide mitotically and synthesize the cartilage **matrix** and **extracellular material** around them. As the cartilage model grows, the individual chondroblasts become surrounded by the extracellular matrix and trapped in matrix compartments called **lacunae** (singular, lacuna). In the lacunae are found mature cartilage cells called **chondrocytes**. The main function of chondrocytes is to maintain the cartilage matrix. Some lacunae may contain more than one chondrocyte; these groups of chondrocytes are called **isogenous groups**.

Mesenchymal cells can also differentiate into fibroblasts that form the **perichondrium**, a dense, irregular connective tissue layer that invests the cartilage. The inner cellular layer of the perichondrium contains chondrogenic cells, which can differentiate into chondroblasts, secrete the cartilage matrix, and become trapped in lacunae as chondrocytes.

FIGURE 7.3 | Cells and Matrix of Mature Hyaline Cartilage

Higher magnification illustrates an interior or central region of mature hyaline cartilage. Distributed throughout the homogeneous ground substance, the **matrix (4, 5)**, are ovoid spaces called **lacunae (3)** containing mature cartilage cells, the **chondrocytes (1, 2)**. In intact cartilage, chondrocytes fill the lacunae. Each chondrocyte has a granular cytoplasm and a **nucleus (1)**. During histologic preparations, chondrocytes (1, 2) shrink, and the lacunae (3) appear as clear spaces. Cartilage cells in the matrix are seen either singly or in isogenous groups.

Hyaline cartilage matrix (4, 5) appears homogeneous and usually basophilic. The lighter-staining matrix between chondrocytes (2) is called **interterritorial matrix (5)**. The more basophilic or darker matrix adjacent to the chondrocytes is the **territorial matrix (4)**.

1 Interterritorial matrix

2 Territorial matrix

3 Isogenous chondrocytes in lacunae

4 Inner chondrogenic layer

5 Perichondrium

6 Excretory duct of tracheal gland

7 Fibroblasts of perichondrium

8 Differentiating chondroblasts

9 Blood vessel

10 Connective tissue

11 Serous acini

12 Mucous acini

FIGURE 7.2 ■ Hyaline cartilage and surrounding structures: trachea. Stain: hematoxylin and eosin. Medium magnification.

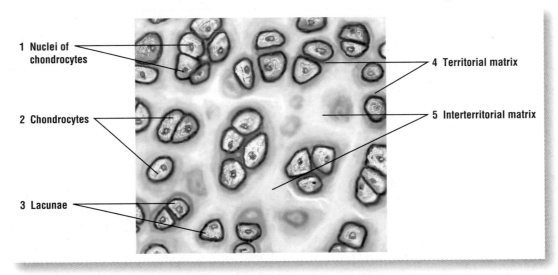

1 Nuclei of chondrocytes

2 Chondrocytes

3 Lacunae

4 Territorial matrix

5 Interterritorial matrix

FIGURE 7.3 ■ Cells and matrix of mature hyaline cartilage. Stain: hematoxylin and eosin. High magnification.

FIGURE 7.4 | Hyaline Cartilage: Developing Bone

A photomicrograph of a section through a developing bone shows a portion of the hyaline cartilage and its characteristic homogenous **matrix (1)**. Located within the matrix (1) are the mature hyaline cartilage cells, the **chondrocytes (3)** in their **lacunae (2)**. Surrounding the hyaline cartilage is the dense, irregular connective tissue, the **perichondrium (5)**. On the inner surface of the perichondrium (5) is the **chondrogenic layer (4)**. Note that the more central cells in the cartilage appear as rounded chondrocytes, whereas the peripheral cells are more flattened and appear as typical chondroblasts.

FUNCTIONAL CORRELATIONS 7.2 | Cartilage (Hyaline, Elastic, and Fibrocartilage)

Cartilage is nonvascular, but it is surrounded by vascular connective tissue, the **perichondrium**. Because of the high water content in the cartilage, all nutrients enter and metabolites leave the cartilage by diffusing through the matrix. Also, the cartilage matrix is soft and pliable, not as hard as bone. As a result, cartilage can simultaneously grow by two different processes: interstitial growth and appositional growth.

Interstitial growth of cartilage involves mitosis of chondroblasts within the matrix and deposition of new matrix between and around the newly formed cells. This growth process increases cartilage growth and size from within. In contrast, **appositional growth** occurs on the periphery of the cartilage. Here, chondroblasts differentiate from the inner cellular layer of the perichondrium and deposit a layer of cartilage matrix that is apposed to the existing cartilage layer. This growth process increases cartilage width.

Hyaline cartilage provides a firm structural and flexible support. Elastic cartilage, owing to the numerous branching elastic fibers in its matrix, confers structural support as well as increased flexibility. In contrast to hyaline cartilage, which can calcify with aging, the matrix of elastic cartilage does not calcify, and the cartilage maintains its high flexibility.

The main function of dense fibrocartilage is to provide tensile strength, bear weight, and resist stretch or compression. This cartilage type is always associated with dense type I collagen fibers.

FIGURE 7.5 | Elastic Cartilage: Epiglottis

Elastic cartilage differs from hyaline cartilage principally by the presence of numerous **elastic fibers (4)** in its **matrix (7)**. Staining the cartilage of the epiglottis with silver reveals thin elastic fibers (4). Elastic fibers (4, 7) enter the cartilage matrix from the surrounding connective tissue **perichondrium (1)** and become distributed as branching and anastomosing fibers of various sizes. The density of the fibers varies among elastic cartilages as well as among different areas of the same cartilage.

As in hyaline cartilage, larger **chondrocytes** in the **lacunae (3, 8)** are more prevalent in the interior of the plate. The smaller and flatter chondrocytes are located peripherally in the inner **chondrogenic layer** of the **perichondrium (2)**, from which chondroblasts develop to synthesize the cartilage matrix. Also visible in the perichondrium (1) are the connective tissue **fibrocytes (5)** and a **venule (6)**.

1 Matrix

2 Lacunae

3 Chondrocytes

4 Chondrogenic layer

5 Perichondrium

FIGURE 7.4 ■ Hyaline cartilage: developing bone. Stain: hematoxylin and eosin. ×80.

1 Perichondrium

2 Chondrogenic layer of perichondrium

3 Lacunae with chondrocytes

4 Elastic fibers

5 Fibrocytes of perichondrium

6 Venule

7 Cartilage matrix with elastic fibers

8 Nuclei of chondrocytes

FIGURE 7.5 ■ Elastic cartilage: epiglottis. Stain: silver. High magnification.

FIGURE 7.6 | Elastic Cartilage: Epiglottis

A photomicrograph of a section of an epiglottis shows that this type of structure is characterized by the presence of a cartilage with fine, branching **elastic fibers (2)** in its **matrix (5)**, in addition to distinct **chondrocytes (3)** and **lacunae (4)**. The presence of elastic fibers (2) gives this cartilage flexibility, in addition to support. Surrounding the elastic cartilage is a layer of dense, irregular connective tissue, the **perichondrium (1)**.

FIGURE 7.7 | Fibrocartilage: Intervertebral Disk

In fibrous cartilage, the **matrix (5)** is filled with dense **collagen fibers (2, 6)**, which frequently exhibit parallel arrangement, as seen in tendons. Small **chondrocytes (1, 4)** in **lacunae (3)** are usually distributed in **rows (4)** within the fibrous cartilage matrix (5), rather than at random or in isogenous groups, as is seen in hyaline or elastic cartilage. All chondrocytes and lacunae (1, 3, 4) are of similar size; there is no gradation from larger central chondrocytes to smaller and flatter peripheral cells.

A perichondrium, normally present around hyaline cartilage and elastic cartilage, is absent because fibrous cartilage usually forms a transitional area between hyaline cartilage and tendon or ligament.

The proportion of collagen fibers (2, 6) to cartilage matrix (5), the number of chondrocytes, and their arrangement in the matrix (5) may vary. Collagen fibers (2, 6) may be so dense that the matrix (5) is invisible. In such case, chondrocytes and lacunae will appear flattened. Collagen fibers within a bundle are normally parallel, but collagen bundles may course in different directions.

1 Perichondrium

2 Elastic fibers

3 Chondrocytes

4 Lacunae

5 Matrix

FIGURE 7.6 ■ Elastic cartilage: epiglottis. Stain: silver. ×80.

1 Nuclei of chondrocytes

2 Collagen fibers

3 Lacunae

4 Row of chondrocytes

5 Cartilage matrix

6 Collagen fibers

FIGURE 7.7 ■ Fibrous cartilage: intervertebral disk. Stain: hematoxylin and eosin. High magnification.

FIGURE 7.8 | Fibrocartilage: Intervertebral Disk

This high-power photomicrograph from a section of an intervertebral disk illustrates the dense composition of the fibrocartilage. Numerous **chondrocytes** in **lacunae (1, 4, 5, 7)**, some dispersed individually (1, 4) or in rows (7), are visible between the layers of **dense collagen fibers (3, 6)** that course throughout the fibrous portion of the disk. The lighter-staining area between the collagen fibers (3, 6) and the chondrocytes (1, 4, 7, 7) is the **cartilage matrix (2)**

1 Condrocyte
in lacuna

2 Cartilage matrix

3 Collagen fibers

4 Nuclei of
chondrocytes

5 Nuclei of
chondrocytes
in lacunae

6 Collagen fibers

7 Row of
chondrocytes
in lacunae

FIGURE 7.8 ■ Fibrocartilage—intervertebral disk. Stain: hematoxylin and eosin. ×205.

SECTION 1 • Cartilage

Characteristics of Cartilage

- Develops from mesenchyme and consists of cells, connective tissue fibers, and ground substance
- Nonvascular, gets nutrients via diffusion through ground substance
- Performs numerous supportive functions
- Cells include chondrocytes and chondroblasts
- Three types of cartilage are hyaline, elastic, and fibrocartilage

Hyaline Cartilage

- Most common in the body and serves as a skeletal model for most bones
- In developing bones, cartilage present in epiphyseal plates for bone growth in length
- Replaced by bone during endochondral ossification
- Contains type II collagen fibrils, which are not seen in histologic sections due to reflective index that is similar to that of ground substance
- In adults, present on articular surfaces of bones, ends of ribs, nose, larynx, trachea, and bronchi

Elastic Cartilage

- Contains branching elastic fibers in matrix and is highly flexible
- Found in external ear, auditory tube, epiglottis, and larynx

Fibrocartilage

- Filled with dense bundles of type I collagen fibers that alternate with cartilage matrix
- Provides tensile strength, bears weight, and resists compression
- Found in intervertebral disks, symphysis pubis, and certain joints

Perichondrium

- Found on peripheries of hyaline and elastic cartilage
- Peripheral layer is dense vascular connective tissue with type I collagen
- Inner layer is chondrogenic and gives rise to chondroblasts that secrete cartilage matrix
- Articular hyaline cartilage of bones and fibrocartilage not lined by perichondrium

Cartilage Matrix

- Produced and maintained by chondrocytes and chondroblasts
- Contains large proteoglycan aggregates and is highly hydrated (high water content)
- Allows diffusion and is semirigid shock absorber
- Adhesive glycoprotein chondronectin binds cells and fibrils to the surrounding matrix
- Elastic cartilage provides structural support and increased flexibility

Cartilage Cells

- Primitive mesenchymal cells differentiate into chondroblasts that synthesize the matrix
- Mesenchyme also differentiates into fibroblasts of the perichondrium
- Mature cartilage cells, chondrocytes, become enclosed in lacunae
- Main function of chondrocytes is to maintain the cartilage matrix
- Inner layer of surrounding connective tissue perichondrium is chondrogenic
- Cartilage grows by both interstitial and appositional growth

SECTION 2 Bone

Characteristics of Bone

Similar to cartilage, **bone** is also a special form of connective tissue that consists of **cells**, **connective tissue fibers**, and **extracellular matrix**. In contrast to cartilage, as the bone develops, minerals are deposited in the matrix and the bones become calcified. As a result, bones become hard and can bear more weight, serve as a rigid skeleton for the body, and provide attachment sites for muscles and organs.

Because of their strength, bones also protect the brain in the skull, the heart and lungs in the thorax, and the urinary and reproductive organs between the pelvic bones. In addition, bones in adults that contain red marrow serve an essential function in **hemopoiesis** (blood cell formation). Bones also serve as crucial **reservoirs** for calcium, phosphate, and other essential minerals. Almost all (99%) of the calcium in the body is stored in bones, from which the body draws its daily calcium needs.

Bone Microarchitecture

All adult bones exhibit similar histology, which consists of cells, bony matrix, and the neurovascular supply. Examination of bone in cross section shows two types: **compact bone** and **cancellous (spongy) bone** (see Overview Figure 7.1). In long bones, the outer cylindrical part represents the dense compact bone. The inner surface of compact bone adjacent to the marrow cavity is the cancellous (spongy) bone. Cancellous bone contains numerous interconnecting areas and is not dense; however, both types of bone have a similar microscopic appearance. In newborns, the marrow cavities of long bones are red and produce blood cells. In adults, the marrow cavities of long bones are normally yellow and filled with adipose (fat) cells.

In compact bone, the collagen fibers are arranged in thin layers of bone called **lamellae** that are parallel to each other in the periphery of the bone or concentrically arranged around the blood vessels. In a long bone, the **outer circumferential lamellae** are deep to the surrounding connective tissue **periosteum**. **Inner circumferential lamellae** are located around the bone marrow cavity. **Concentric lamellae** surround the canals that contain an artery, vein, nerve, and loose connective tissue. Each concentric lamellar complex is called the **osteon (Haversian system)**. The space in the osteon that contains blood vessels and nerves is the **central (Haversian) canal**. Most of the compact bone consists of **osteons**, which are usually oriented in the long axis of the bone (see Overview Figure 7.1).

Bone Types

Distribution and orientation of the collagen fibers in the bone matrix indicates the bone type. The compact and cancellous bones of an adult exhibit a consistent structural pattern that is seen following the maturation and mineralization of bone. In contrast, **woven (immature** or **primary) bone** shows a random arrangement of collagen fibers that are oriented in different directions. This type of arrangement is nonlamellar. The woven bone is encountered in the fetus during initial skeletal development and in repair of bone fractures. Also, the woven bone is **temporary**, and, as the individual ages, it is replaced by lamellar or mature bone in postnatal life.

The **lamellar (secondary** or **mature) bone** exhibits highly organized lamellae and is found in adults. This bone exhibits either multiple parallel or concentric layers of calcified matrix called **lamellae** arranged in an orderly manner around the central canals that contain the neurovascular bundle, or the osteons. Each lamella exhibits a parallel arrangement of the collagen fibers that follow a helical course. Also, the bone cells, called osteocytes, are found in lacunae at regular intervals between the concentric layers of lamellae and are arranged circumferentially around the central canal. The matrix is more calcified in the lamellar bone than in the woven bone, and, as a result, the lamellar bone is stronger than the woven or immature bone.

FUNCTIONAL CORRELATIONS 7.3 | Bone Cells and Their Function

Developing and adult bones contain four cell types: osteoprogenitor cells, osteoblasts, osteocytes, and osteoclasts.

Osteoprogenitor cells are undifferentiated, pluripotent stem cells derived from the connective tissue **mesenchyme**. These cells are located on the inner layer of the connective tissue, the periosteum, and in the single layer of the internal endosteum that lines the marrow cavities, the osteons (Haversian system), and the perforating canals in the bone (see Overview Figure 7.1). The main functions of the periosteum and the endosteum are to provide nutrition for the bone as well as a continuous supply of new osteoblasts for growth, remodeling, and bone repair. During bone development, osteoprogenitor cells proliferate by mitosis and differentiate into osteoblasts, which then begin to secrete collagen fibers and the bony matrix.

Osteoblasts, derived from osteoprogenitor cells, are present on the surfaces of bone. They synthesize, secrete, and deposit **osteoid**, the organic components of new bone matrix, which includes type I collagen fibers, several glycoproteins, and proteoglycans. Osteoid is uncalcified and does not contain any minerals; however, shortly after its deposition, it is rapidly mineralized and becomes hard bone. Osteoblasts regulate the mineralization process of osteoid by releasing **matrix vesicles**, which serve as centers for formation of **hydroxyapatite** crystals and the first steps of calcification. Further calcification surrounds and embeds the collagen fibers and the various glycoproteins.

Osteocytes are the mature forms of osteoblasts that become surrounded by the mineralized bone matrix. They are also smaller than osteoblasts and become the principal cells of the bone. Like the chondrocytes in cartilage, osteocytes are trapped by the surrounding bone matrix that was produced by osteoblasts. Osteocytes are also located in the cavelike **lacunae** and are very close to a blood vessel. In contrast to cartilage, only one osteocyte is found in each bony lacuna. Also, because mineralized bone matrix is much harder than cartilage, nutrients and metabolites cannot freely diffuse through it to the osteocytes. Consequently, bone is highly vascular and possesses a unique system of channels or tiny canals called **canaliculi**, which open into the osteons.

Osteocytes exhibit numerous branches. Their cytoplasmic extensions enter the canaliculi, radiate in all directions from each lacuna, and make contact with neighboring osteocytes through **gap junctions**. These connections allow the passage of ions and small molecules from cell to cell. The canaliculi contain extracellular fluid, and the gap junctions in the cytoplasmic extensions allow individual osteocytes to communicate with adjacent osteocytes and with materials in the nearby blood vessels of the central canal. In this manner, the canaliculi form complex connections around the blood vessels in the osteons and constitute an efficient exchange mechanism: nutrients are brought to the osteocytes, gaseous exchange takes place between the blood and cells, and metabolic wastes are removed from the osteocytes. The canaliculi system keeps the osteocytes alive, and the osteocytes, in turn, maintain the homeostasis of the surrounding bone matrix and blood concentrations of calcium and phosphates. When an osteocyte dies, the surrounding bone matrix is reabsorbed by another type of bone cell, the osteoclasts.

Osteoclasts are large, multinucleated cells found along bone surfaces where resorption (removal of bone), remodeling, and repair of bone take place. They do not belong to the osteoprogenitor cell line. Instead, the osteoclasts originate from the fusion of blood or hemopoietic progenitor cells that belong to the mononuclear macrophage–monocyte cell line of the red bone marrow. The main function of osteoclasts is bone resorption during bone remodeling (renewal or restructuring). Osteoclasts are often located on the resorbed surfaces or in shallow depressions in the bone matrix called **Howship lacunae.** Lysosomal enzymes released by osteoclasts erode these depressions. During bone development, bone deposition by osteoblasts is coordinated with bone remodeling by the osteoclasts. This coordinated activity between these two cell types maintains the bone development and the same bone mass.

Bone Matrix

The bone matrix consists of **inorganic** (minerals) and **organic** (collagen fibers) components. The bone matrix also consists of living cells and extracellular material. Because the bone matrix is calcified or mineralized, it is harder than cartilage. As a result, diffusion is not possible through the calcified matrix; therefore, bone matrix is highly vascularized. Bones are surrounded by dense connective tissue, the **periosteum**. Blood vessels from the periosteum penetrate and enter the bone matrix via the **perforating (Volkmann) canals**. These canals run perpendicular to and join the vessels in the central canals of the osteon, which then supply the cellular components of the bone matrix.

The organic components enable bones to resist tension, whereas the mineral components resist compression. The major organic components of bone matrix are the coarse **type I collagen fibers**, which are the predominant proteins. The other organic components are sulfated glycosaminoglycans and hyaluronic acid that form larger proteoglycan aggregates. The glycoproteins **osteocalcin** and **osteopontin** bind tightly to calcium crystals and promote mineralization and calcification of the bone matrix. Another matrix protein, sialoprotein, binds osteoblasts to the extracellular matrix through the integrins of the plasma membrane proteins.

The inorganic component of bone matrix consists of the minerals calcium and phosphate in the form of hydroxyapatite crystals. The association of coarse collagen fibers with hydroxyapatite crystals provides the bone with its hardness, durability, and strength. In addition, as the need arises, actions of hormones such as the **parathyroid** hormone from the parathyroid gland and **calcitonin** from the thyroid gland on the bone adjust and maintain a proper mineral content in the blood.

The Process of Bone Formation (Ossification)

Bone development begins in the embryo by two distinct processes: endochondral ossification and intramembranous ossification. Although the resulting bones are produced by two different methods, they exhibit the same histologic structure or morphology (see Overview Figure 7.1).

Endochondral Ossification

Most bones in the body develop by the process of **endochondral ossification**, in which a temporary hyaline cartilage model precedes bone formation. This method of ossification allows the model to grow in length and width. Mesenchymal cells proliferate and differentiate into chondroblasts, which form the cartilage model for the future bone. This cartilage model, surrounded by the connective tissue **perichondrium**, continues to grow by both interstitial and appositional means and is primarily used to form the short and long bones of the body. As development progresses, the chondroblasts divide, hypertrophy (enlarge), and mature, and the hyaline cartilage model begins to calcify. As calcification of the cartilage model progresses, diffusion of nutrients and gases through the calcified cartilage matrix decreases. Consequently, chondrocytes begin to degenerate and die, leaving a fragmented calcified matrix as scaffolding that serves as a structural framework on which the deposition of bony material will take place.

As soon as a layer of bony material is deposited around the calcifying cartilage, the inner perichondrial cells exhibit their osteogenic potential, and a thin periosteal collar of bone forms around the midpoint of the shaft of the bone. This external surrounding connective tissue around the newly formed bone is now called the **periosteum**. Mesenchymal cells differentiate into **osteoprogenitor cells** from the inner layer of periosteum, and blood vessels from the vascular periosteum invade the calcified and degenerating cartilage model, bringing with them mesenchymal and osteoprogenitor cells. The osteoblasts attach to the calcified cartilage remnants and begin to synthesize the bone matrix. Osteoprogenitor cells continue to proliferate and differentiate into **osteoblasts** that continue to secrete the osteoid matrix, initially a soft collagenous tissue that lacks minerals but is quickly mineralized into bone. The osteoblasts become eventually surrounded by bone in the cavelike **lacunae** and are now called **osteocytes**; there is one osteocyte per lacuna. Osteocytes establish a complex cell-to-cell connection through tiny canals in the bone called **canaliculi**; these eventually open into channels that house the blood vessels. Osteoprogenitor cells also arise from the inner surface of bone called **endosteum**. Endosteum lines all internal cavities in the bone and consists of a single layer of osteoprogenitor cells.

Mesenchymal tissue, osteoblasts, and blood vessels form the **primary ossification center** in the developing bone that first appears in the **diaphysis** or the shaft of the long bone, followed somewhat later by a **secondary ossification center** in the **epiphysis** or the articular surface of the expanded end of the bone. In all developing long bones, cartilage in the diaphysis and epiphysis is gradually replaced by bone, except in the **epiphyseal plate** region, which is located between the diaphysis and epiphysis. Growth of cartilage in this region continues and is responsible for lengthening the bone until bone growth stops. Expansion of the two ossification centers eventually replaces all cartilage with bone, including the epiphyseal plate. At this time, bone lengthening ceases. The only exceptions in which the hyaline cartilage is not replaced by bone are the free or articulating ends of long bones. Here, a layer of permanent hyaline cartilage covers the bone and is called the **articular cartilage**.

Intramembranous Ossification

In **intramembranous ossification**, bone development is not preceded by a hyaline cartilage model. Instead, bone develops from the condensation of the connective tissue **mesenchyme** that forms an **ossification center**. Most flat bones develop by this method. The mesenchymal cells differentiate directly into osteoblasts that produce the surrounding **osteoid matrix**, which quickly calcifies. Numerous ossification centers are formed, anastomose, and produce a network of **spongy bone** that consists of thin rods, plates, and spines called **trabeculae**. Located between the trabeculae is the hemopoietic tissue. The osteoblasts then become surrounded by bone in the **lacunae** and become **osteocytes**. As in endochondral ossification, once osteocytes are trapped in the lacunae, they establish a complex cell-to-cell connection through the **canaliculi**.

The **mandible**, **maxilla**, **clavicles**, and most of the **flat bones of the skull** are formed by the intramembranous method. In the developing skull, the centers of bone development grow radially, replace the connective tissue, and then fuse. In newborns, the **fontanelles** in the skull represent the soft membranous regions where intramembranous ossification of skull bones is in the process of ossification. The surrounding mesenchymal connective tissue that does not ossify becomes the periosteum and endosteum of the new bone.

 Supplemental micrographic images are available at **www.thePoint.com/Eroschenko12e** under Bone Development.

FIGURE 7.9 | Endochondral Ossification: Development of a Long Bone (Panoramic View, Longitudinal Section)

During endochondral ossification, the bone is first formed as a model of embryonic hyaline cartilage. As bone development progresses, the cartilage model is replaced by bone. The process of endochondral ossification can be followed by examining the upper part of the illustration and proceeding downward.

In the upper part, the hyaline cartilage is surrounded by the connective tissue **perichondrium (13)**. The **zone of reserve cartilage (1)** shows chondrocytes in their lacunae distributed singly or in small groups. Below this region is the **zone of proliferating chondrocytes (2)** where the chondrocytes divide and become arranged in vertical columns. **Chondrocytes in lacunae (14)** increase in size in the **zone of chondrocyte hypertrophy (3)** as a result of swelling of the nucleus and cytoplasm. The hypertrophied chondrocytes degenerate, forming thin **plates of calcified cartilage matrix (15)**. Below this region is the **zone of ossification (4)**, where a bony material is deposited on the plates of calcified cartilage matrix (15).

Blood sinusoids (20) or capillaries invade the calcifying cartilage. Lacunar walls and the calcified cartilage (15) are eroded, and the **red bone marrow cavity (16)** is formed. The connective tissue around the newly formed bone is called **periosteum (5, 6, 17)**, and this region is now the zone of ossification (4). In this illustration, bone is stained dark red. Osteoprogenitor cells from the **inner periosteum (6)** continue to differentiate into osteoblasts, deposit **osteoid and bone (8)** around the remaining plates of calcified cartilage (15), and form the **periosteal bone collar (7)**.

Formation of new periosteal bone (7) keeps pace with the formation of new endochondral bone. The bone collar (7) increases in thickness and compactness as development of bone proceeds. The thickest portion of the bone collar (7) is seen in the central part of the developing bone called the diaphysis. The primary center of ossification is located in the diaphysis, where the initial periosteal bone collar (7) is formed.

Red bone marrow (16) fills the cavity of newly formed bone with hemopoietic (blood forming) cells. Fine reticular connective tissue fibers in the bone marrow (16) are obscured by masses of developing erythrocytes, granulocytes, **megakaryocytes (12)**, **bony spicules (11, 22)**, numerous blood sinusoids (20), capillaries, and blood vessels.

Surrounding the shaft of the developing bone are the soft tissues. The **epidermis (18)** of skin is lined by stratified squamous epithelium. Below the epidermis (18) is the subcutaneous **connective tissue of the dermis (19)**, in which are seen **hair follicles (9)**, **blood vessels (10)**, **adipose cells (21)**, and **sweat glands (23)**.

1 Zone of reserve cartilage

2 Zone of proliferating chondrocytes

3 Zone of chondrocyte hypertrophy and calcification of cartilage

4 Zone of ossification

5 Outer periosteum

6 Inner periosteum

7 Periosteal bone collar

8 Osteoid and bone

9 Hair follicles

10 Blood vessels

11 Bony spicules

12 Megakaryocytes

13 Perichondrium

14 Chondrocytes in lacunae

15 Plates of calcified cartilage matrix

16 Red bone marrow cavity

17 Periosteum

18 Epidermis

19 Connective tissue of dermis

20 Blood sinusoids

21 Adipose cells

22 Bony spicules

23 Sweat glands in dermis

FIGURE 7.9 ■ Endochondral ossification: development of a long bone (panoramic view, longitudinal section). Stain: hematoxylin and eosin. Low magnification.

FIGURE 7.10 | Endochondral Ossification: Zone of Ossification

This figure shows endochondral ossification at higher magnification and in greater detail and corresponds to the upper region of Figure 7.9.

Proliferating chondrocytes (1, 14) are arranged in distinct vertical columns. Below is the zone of **hypertrophied chondrocytes (2, 15)**. Chondrocytes and lacunae undergo hypertrophy as a result of increased glycogen and lipid accumulations in their cytoplasm and nuclear swelling. The cytoplasm of hypertrophied chondrocytes (2, 15) becomes **vacuolized (16)**, the nuclei become pyknotic, and the thin cartilage plates become surrounded by **calcified matrix (5, 17)**.

Osteoblasts (6, 20) line up along remaining plates of calcified cartilage (5, 17) and lay down a layer of **osteoid (19)** and bone. Osteoblasts trapped in the osteoid or bone become **osteocytes (9, 21)**. **Capillaries (8, 18)** from the **marrow cavity (10)** invade the newly ossified area.

The developing marrow cavity (10) contains numerous **megakaryocytes (13, 24)** and pluripotent stem cells that give rise to erythrocytic and granulocytic **blood cells (23)**. Multinucleated **osteoclasts (11, 22)** lie in shallow depressions called **Howship lacunae (11, 22)** and are adjacent to the bone that is being resorbed.

The left side of the illustration shows an area of **periosteal bone (7)** with osteocytes (9) in their lacunae. The new bone is added peripherally by osteoblasts (6), which develop from osteoprogenitor cells of the **inner periosteum (12)**. The outer layer of periosteum continues as the connective tissue **perichondrium (3)**.

FIGURE 7.11 | Endochondral Ossification: Zone of Ossification

This photomicrograph illustrates the transformation of hyaline cartilage into bone through the process of endochondral ossification. The **hyaline cartilage matrix (6)** contains **proliferating chondrocytes (7)** and **hypertrophied chondrocytes (1)** with **vacuolated cytoplasm (2)**. Below these cells are plates or **spicules** of **calcified cartilage (3)** surrounded by **osteoblasts (4)**. As the cartilage calcifies, a **marrow cavity (5)** is formed with blood vessels, **hemopoietic tissue (10)**, osteoprogenitor cells, and osteoblasts (4). The hyaline cartilage is surrounded by the connective tissue **perichondrium (8)**. The marrow cavity in the new bone is surrounded by the connective tissue **periosteum (9)**.

1 Proliferating chondrocytes
2 Hypertrophied chondrocytes
3 Perichondrium
4 Degenerating chondrocytes
5 Calcified matrix
6 Osteoblasts
7 Periosteal bone
8 Capillary
9 Osteocyte
10 Marrow cavity
11 Osteoclast
12 Inner periosteum
13 Megakaryocyte

14 Proliferating chondrocytes
15 Hypertrophied chondrocyte
16 Vacuolized cytoplasm
17 Calcified matrix
18 Capillary
19 Osteoid
20 Osteoblasts
21 Osteocyte
22 Osteoclast (in a Howship lacuna)
23 Developing blood cells
24 Megakaryocyte

FIGURE 7.10 ■ Endochondral ossification: zone of ossification. Stain: hematoxylin and eosin. Medium magnification.

1 Hypertrophied chondrocytes
2 Vacuolated cytoplasm
3 Spicules of calcified cartilage
4 Osteoblasts
5 Marrow cavity

6 Hyaline cartilage matrix
7 Proliferating chondrocytes
8 Perichondrium
9 Periosteum
10 Hemopoietic tissue

FIGURE 7.11 ■ Endochondral ossification: zone of ossification. Stain: hematoxylin and eosin. ×50.

FIGURE 7.12 | Endochondral Ossification: Formation of Secondary (Epiphyseal) Centers of Ossification and Epiphyseal Plate in Long Bones (Longitudinal Section, Decalcified Bone)

The hyaline cartilage in the epiphyseal ends of two developing bones is illustrated. Both bones exhibit **secondary centers of ossification (5, 11)**. Although cartilage is nonvascular, numerous **blood vessels (1, 6)**, sectioned in a different plane, pass through the cartilage matrix to supply the osteoblasts and osteocytes in the secondary centers of ossification (5, 11). **Articular cartilage (4, 12)** covers both articulating ends of the future bone. A **synovial** or **joint cavity (3)** separates the two cartilage models. The inner synovial membrane of squamous cells lines the synovial cavity (3), except over the articular cartilages (4, 12). A synovial membrane, together with the connective tissue, may extend into the joint cavity as **synovial folds (2, 13)**. The synovial cavity (3) is covered by a connective tissue capsule.

In the lower bone, an active **epiphyseal plate (16)** is seen between the secondary ossification center (5) and the developing shaft of the bone. A **zone** of **proliferating chondrocytes (7)** and a **zone of chondrocyte hypertrophy** and **calcification** of **cartilage (8)** are clearly visible in the epiphyseal plate (16). Small **spicules of calcified cartilage (9, 15)** surrounded by red-stained bony material and **primitive bone marrow cavities** with **hemopoiesis (14, 17)** are seen in the shaft of the bone and the secondary center of ossification (5). A **megakaryocyte (18)** is also visible in the lower bone marrow cavity (17). A connective tissue, **periosteum (19)**, surrounds the compact **bone (10)**.

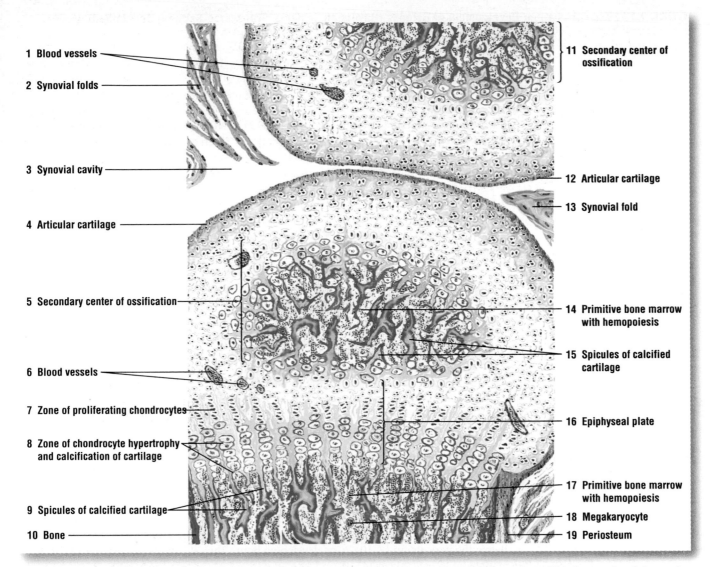

1 Blood vessels

2 Synovial folds

3 Synovial cavity

4 Articular cartilage

5 Secondary center of ossification

6 Blood vessels

7 Zone of proliferating chondrocytes

8 Zone of chondrocyte hypertrophy and calcification of cartilage

9 Spicules of calcified cartilage

10 Bone

11 Secondary center of ossification

12 Articular cartilage

13 Synovial fold

14 Primitive bone marrow with hemopoiesis

15 Spicules of calcified cartilage

16 Epiphyseal plate

17 Primitive bone marrow with hemopoiesis

18 Megakaryocyte

19 Periosteum

FIGURE 7.12 ■ Endochondral ossification: formation of secondary (epiphyseal) centers of ossification and epiphyseal plate in long bone (decalcified bone, longitudinal section). Stain: hematoxylin and eosin. Low magnification.

FIGURE 7.13 | Bone Formation: Development of Osteons (Haversian Systems; Transverse Section, Decalcified)

This illustration shows the **primitive bone marrow (15)** and developing osteons in a compact bone. Vascular tufts of connective tissue from the periosteum or endosteum invade and erode the bone and form primitive osteons. Bone reconstruction or remodeling will continue as the initial osteons, and then later ones, are broken down or eroded, followed by the formation of new osteons.

The new **bone matrix (11)** and **bone spicule (12)** of an immature compact bone are stained deep red with eosin owing to the presence of collagen fibers in the matrix. Numerous primitive osteons are visible in the transverse section, with large **central (Haversian) canals (2, 9)** surrounded by a few concentric **lamellae (9)** of bone and **osteocytes in lacunae (10)**. The central (Haversian) canals (2, 9) contain **primitive osteogenic connective tissue (13)** and **blood vessels (2)**. Bone deposition is continuing in some of the primitive osteons (2, 9), as indicated by the presence of **osteoblasts (1, 14)** around the central (Haversian) canals (2, 9) and the margin of the innermost bone lamella. In some osteons, the multinucleated **osteoclasts (6)** have formed and eroded shallow depressions called **Howship lacunae (5)** in the bone. Osteoclasts (6) continue to resorb and remodel the bone as it forms.

Primitive osteogenic connective tissue (13) passes through the bone, from which arise tufts of vascular connective tissue that give rise to new central (Haversian) canals (2, 9). Osteoblasts (1, 14) are located along the periphery of the developing central canals.

In the lower left corner of the figure is the primitive bone marrow (15), in which hemopoiesis (blood cell formation) is in progress; this is the red marrow. Also present in the bone marrow cavity (15) are developing erythrocytes and granulocytes, **megakaryocytes (4, 8)**, **blood sinusoids (vessels) (3, 7)**, and osteoclasts (6) in the eroded Howship lacunae (5). Some megakaryocytes (4, 8) are adjacent to the blood sinusoids. Their cytoplasmic processes protrude into these blood sinusoids, where they eventually fragment and enter the bloodstream as platelets.

FIGURE 7.14 | Intramembranous Ossification: Developing Mandible (Decalcified Bone, Transverse Section)

This illustration depicts a section of mandible in the process of intramembranous ossification. External to the developing bone is the stratified squamous keratinized epithelium of the **skin (1)**. Inferior to the skin (1), the embryonic mesenchyme has differentiated into the highly vascular primitive **connective tissue (2)** with **nerves** and **blood vessels (9)**, and a denser connective tissue, the **periosteum (3, 10)**.

Below the periosteum (3, 10) is the developing bone. The cells in the periosteum (3, 10) have differentiated into **osteoblasts (6, 10)** and formed numerous anastomosing **trabeculae of bone (7, 11)** that surround the primitive **marrow cavities (8, 15)**. In the marrow cavities (8, 15) are embryonic connective tissue cells and fibers, **blood vessels (4)**, **arterioles (12)**, and nerves. Peripherally, collagen fibers of the periosteum (3, 10) are in continuity with the fibers of the embryonic connective tissue of adjacent marrow cavities (3) and with collagen fibers within the trabeculae of bone (7, 11).

Osteoblasts (6, 10) actively deposit the bony matrix and are seen in linear arrangement along the developing trabeculae of bone (7, 11). **Osteoid (14)**, the newly synthesized bony matrix, is seen on the margins of certain bony trabeculae. The **osteocytes (5)** are located in lacunae of the trabeculae (7, 11). **Osteoclasts (13)** are multinucleated large cells that are associated with bone resorption and remodeling during bone formation.

Although collagen fibers embedded in the bony matrix are obscured, the continuity with embryonic connective tissue fibers in the marrow cavities may be seen at the margins of numerous trabeculae (3).

Formation of new bone is not a continuous process. Inactive areas appear where ossification has temporarily ceased. Osteoid and osteoblasts are not present in these areas. In some primitive marrow cavities, fibroblasts differentiate into osteoblasts (3, 10).

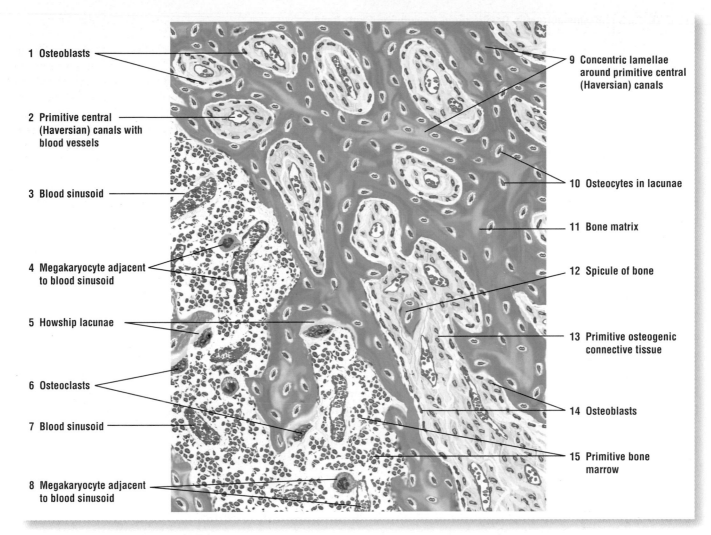

1 Osteoblasts

2 Primitive central (Haversian) canals with blood vessels

3 Blood sinusoid

4 Megakaryocyte adjacent to blood sinusoid

5 Howship lacunae

6 Osteoclasts

7 Blood sinusoid

8 Megakaryocyte adjacent to blood sinusoid

9 Concentric lamellae around primitive central (Haversian) canals

10 Osteocytes in lacunae

11 Bone matrix

12 Spicule of bone

13 Primitive osteogenic connective tissue

14 Osteoblasts

15 Primitive bone marrow

FIGURE 7.13 ■ Bone formation: primitive bone marrow and development of osteons (Haversian systems; decalcified bone, transverse section). Stain: hematoxylin and eosin. Medium magnification.

1 Skin

2 Connective tissue

3 Continuity of periosteum with marrow cavity

4 Blood vessels

5 Osteocytes

6 Osteoblasts

7 Trabeculae of bone

8 Marrow cavity

9 Nerves and venule

10 Developing osteoblasts from periosteum

11 Trabeculae of bone

12 Arteriole

13 Osteoclasts

14 Osteoid

15 Marrow cavity

FIGURE 7.14 ■ Intramembranous ossification: developing mandible (decalcified bone, transverse section). Stain: Mallory-Azan. Low magnification.

FIGURE 7.15 | Intramembranous Ossification: Developing Skull Bone

A higher-power photomicrograph illustrates the development of skull bone by the process of intramembranous ossification. The connective tissue **periosteum (5)** surrounds the developing bone and gives rise to the **osteoblasts (1, 6)** that form the **bone (7)**. Osteoblasts (1, 6) are located along the developing **bony trabeculae (3)**. Trapped within the formed bone (7) and the bony trabeculae (3) are the **osteocytes (2)** in their lacunae. Also associated with the bony trabeculae (3) are the multinuclear **osteoclasts (8)** that remodel the developing bone. A primitive **marrow cavity (4)** with **blood vessels (9)**, **blood cells (9)**, and hemopoietic tissue is located between the formed bony trabeculae (3).

FIGURE 7.16 | Cancellous Bone With Trabeculae and Marrow Cavities: Sternum (Transverse Section, Decalcified)

Cancellous bone consists primarily of slender **bony trabeculae (5)** that ramify, anastomose, and enclose irregular **marrow cavities with blood vessels (4)**. The **periosteum (2, 7)** that surrounds the trabeculae (5) of cancellous bone merges with adjacent dense irregular **connective tissue with blood vessels (1)**. Inferior to the periosteum (2, 7), the bony trabeculae (5) merge with a thin layer of **compact bone (9)** that contains a forming or **primitive osteon (6)** and a mature **osteon (Haversian system) (8)** with concentric lamellae.

Except for concentric lamellae in the primitive osteon (6) and the mature osteon (8), the bone inferior to the periosteum (2, 7) and the bony trabeculae (5) exhibit parallel lamellae. **Osteocytes (3)** in lacunae are visible in trabeculae (5) and compact bone (9).

Between bony trabeculae (5) are the marrow cavities with blood vessels (4) and **hemopoietic tissue (11)** that gives rise to new blood cells. Because of the low magnification, individual red and white blood cells are not recognizable. Lining the bony trabeculae (5) in the marrow cavities (4) is a thin inner layer of cells called **endosteum (10)**. Cells in the periosteum (2, 7) and in the endosteum (10) give rise to bone-forming osteoblasts.

1 Osteoblasts
2 Osteocytes
3 Bony trabeculae
4 Marrow cavity
5 Periosteum
6 Osteoblasts
7 Bone
8 Osteoclast
9 Blood vessels with blood cells

FIGURE 7.15 ■ Intramembranous ossification: developing skull bone. Stain: Mallory-Azan. ×64.

1 Connective tissue with blood vessels
2 Periosteum
3 Osteocytes in lacunae
4 Marrow cavities with blood vessels
5 Bony trabeculae
6 Primitive osteon
7 Periosteum
8 Osteon
9 Compact bone
10 Endosteum
11 Hemopoietic tissue

FIGURE 7.16 ■ Cancellous bone with trabeculae and bone marrow cavities: sternum (decalcified bone, transverse section). Stain: hematoxylin and eosin. Low magnification.

FIGURE 7.17 | Cancellous Bone: Sternum (Transverse Section, Decalcified)

This photomicrograph shows a section of cancellous bone from the sternum. Cancellous bone is composed of numerous **bony trabeculae (1)** separated by the **marrow cavity (5)** that contains **blood vessels (7)** and different types of **blood cells (8)**. Bony trabeculae (1) are lined by a thin inner layer of cells called the **endosteum (4, 6)**. Osteoprogenitor cells in the endosteum (4, 6) give rise to osteoblasts. Formed bone matrix contains numerous **osteocytes** in **lacunae (2)**. The large, multinuclear **osteoclasts (3)** are eroding or remodeling the formed bone matrix. Osteoclasts (3) erode part of the bone through enzymatic action and lie in the eroded depressions called Howship lacunae.

FUNCTIONAL CORRELATIONS 7.4 | Bone

Bones are dynamic structures. They are continually renewed, or remodeled, in response to the mineral needs of the body, mechanical stress, thinning as a result of age or disease, and fracture healing. Calcium and phosphate are either stored in the bone matrix or released into the blood to maintain proper levels. Maintenance of normal blood calcium levels is critical to life, because calcium is essential for muscle contraction, blood coagulation, cell membrane permeability, transmission of nerve impulses, and numerous other functions.

Hormones regulate both the calcium release into the bloodstream and its deposition in the bones. When the calcium level falls below normal, **parathyroid hormone**, released from the parathyroid glands, indirectly promotes an increase in **osteoclast** numbers and osteoclast activity by stimulating **osteoblasts** to produce osteoclast-stimulating (differentiating) factors. This action induces increased breakdown of bone matrix by the osteoclasts and release of calcium. In addition, parathyroid hormone also increases calcium reabsorption in the kidneys and small intestine. These hormonal effects increase the calcium levels in the blood to normal range. When the calcium level is above normal, a hormone called **calcitonin**, released by parafollicular cells in the thyroid gland, inhibits osteoclast activity, decreases bone reabsorption, and decreases blood calcium levels. In addition, the kidneys increase their excretion of both calcium and phosphate. These effects lower the circulating calcium levels in the body. The actions of both thyroid and parathyroid glands and their hormones are discussed in more detail in Chapter 19, "Endocrine System."

FIGURE 7.18 | Compact Bone, Dried (Transverse Section)

This illustration depicts a transverse section of a dried compact bone. The bone was ground to a thin section to show empty canals for blood vessels, lacunae for osteocytes, and the connecting canaliculi.

The structural units of a compact bone matrix are the **osteons (Haversian systems) (3, 10)**. Each osteon (3, 10) consists of layers of concentric **lamellae (3b)** arranged around a **central (Haversian) canal (3a)**. Central canals are shown in cross section (3a) and in oblique section (10, middle leader). Lamellae are thin plates of bone that contain osteocytes in almond-shaped spaces called **lacunae (3c, 9)**. Radiating from each lacuna in all directions are tiny canals, the **canaliculi (2)**. Canaliculi (2) penetrate the lamellae (3b, 8), anastomose with canaliculi (2) from other lacunae (3c, 9), and form a network of communicating channels with other osteocytes. Some of the canaliculi (2) open directly into central (Haversian) canals (3a) of the osteon (3) and the marrow cavities of the bone. The small irregular areas of bone between osteons (3, 10) are the **interstitial lamellae (5, 12)** that represent the remnants of eroded or remodeled osteons.

External circumferential lamellae (7) form the external wall of a compact bone (beneath the connective tissue periosteum) and run parallel to each other and to the long axis of the bone. The internal wall of the bone (the endosteum along the marrow cavity) is lined by **internal circumferential lamellae (1)**. Osteons (3, 10) are located between the internal circumferential lamellae (1) and the external circumferential lamellae (7).

In a living bone, the lacunae of each osteon (3c, 9) house osteocytes. The central canals (3a) contain reticular connective tissue, blood vessels, and nerves. The boundary between each osteon (3, 10) is outlined by a refractile line of modified bone matrix called the **cement line (4, 11)**. Anastomoses between central canals (3a) are called **perforating (Volkmann) canals (6)**.

1 Bony trabeculae

2 Osteocytes in lacunae

3 Osteoclasts

4 Endosteum

5 Marrow cavity

6 Endosteum

7 Blood vessel

8 Blood cells

FIGURE 7.17 ■ Cancellous bone: sternum (decalcified bone, transverse section). Stain: hematoxylin and eosin. ×64.

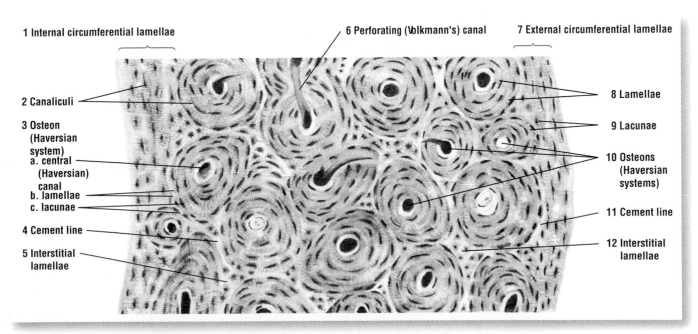

1 Internal circumferential lamellae

2 Canaliculi

3 Osteon (Haversian system)
  a. central (Haversian) canal
  b. lamellae
  c. lacunae

4 Cement line

5 Interstitial lamellae

6 Perforating (Volkmann's) canal

7 External circumferential lamellae

8 Lamellae

9 Lacunae

10 Osteons (Haversian systems)

11 Cement line

12 Interstitial lamellae

FIGURE 7.18 ■ Dry, compact bone: ground, transverse section. Low magnification.

FIGURE 7.19 | Compact Bone, Dried (Longitudinal Section)

This figure represents a small area of a dried compact bone, ground in a longitudinal plane. Because **central canals (1, 9)** course longitudinally, each central canal is seen as a vertical tube that shows branching. Central canals (1, 9) are surrounded by **lamellae (2, 6)** with **lacunae (4)** and radiating **canaliculi (5)**. The lamellae (2, 6), lacunae (4), and the osteon boundaries, the **cement lines (3, 8)**, course parallel to the central canals (1, 9).

Other canals that extend in either a transverse or oblique direction are called **perforating (Volkmann) canals (7)**. Perforating canals (7) join the central canals (1, 9) of osteons with the marrow cavity. The perforating canals (7) do not have concentric lamellae. Instead, they penetrate directly through the lamellae (2, 6).

FIGURE 7.20 | Compact Bone, Dried: Osteon (Transverse Section)

A higher magnification illustrates the details of one osteon and portions of adjacent osteons. Located in the center of the osteon is the dark-staining **central (Haversian) canal (3)** surrounded by the concentric **lamellae (4)**. Between adjacent osteons are the **interstitial lamellae (5)**. The dark, almond-shaped structures between the lamellae (4) are the **lacunae (1, 7)** that house osteocytes in living bone.

Tiny **canaliculi (2)** radiate from individual lacuna (1, 7) to adjacent lacunae and form a system of communicating canaliculi (2) throughout the bony matrix and within the central canal (3). The canaliculi (2) contain tiny cytoplasmic extensions of the osteocytes. In this manner, osteocytes around the osteon communicate with each other and blood vessels in the central canals. The outer boundary of the osteon is separated by a **cement line (6)**.

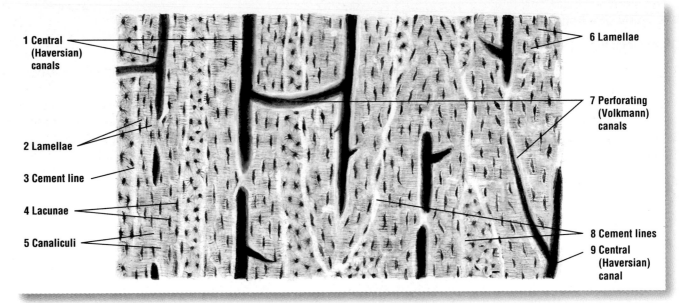

1 Central (Haversian) canals

2 Lamellae

3 Cement line

4 Lacunae

5 Canaliculi

6 Lamellae

7 Perforating (Volkmann) canals

8 Cement lines

9 Central (Haversian) canal

FIGURE 7.19 ■ Dry, compact bone: ground, longitudinal section. Low magnification.

1 Lacunae

2 Canaliculi

3 Central (Haversian) canal

4 Lamellae

5 Interstitial lamellae

6 Cement line

7 Lacunae

FIGURE 7.20 ■ Dry, compact bone: an osteon, transverse section. High magnification.

SECTION 2 • Bone

Characteristics of Bone

- Consists of cells, connective tissue fibers, and extracellular material
- Mineral deposits in the bone matrix produce a hard structure for protecting various organs
- Functions in hemopoiesis and as reservoir for calcium and minerals

Bone Microarchitecture

- All bones exhibit similar histology; there are two types of bones
- Compact bone is the outer cylindrical part of long bone
- Inner bone adjacent to bone marrow is the cancellous (spongy) bone
- In newborn bones, marrow is red and hemopoietic; in adults, the marrow of long bone is yellow
- Outer circumferential lamellae are located deep to the periosteum
- Inner circumferential lamellae are located around the bone marrow
- Concentric lamellae form osteons in compact bone and surround the central canal
- Most osteons are oriented in the long axis of the bone

Bone Types

- Orientation of collagen fibers indicates bone type
- Compact and cancellous bones show similar microscopic structure
- Woven (immature) bone has a random orientation of collagen fibers and is nonlamellar
- Woven bone is seen during fetal bone development and bone repair
- Lamellar (mature) bone with concentric lamellae around the central canal is found in adults
- In lamellar bone, collagen fibers exhibit parallel arrangements that follow a helical course
- Osteocytes in lamellar bone are arranged around the central canal

Bone Cells and Their Function

- Osteoprogenitor cells are derived from mesenchyme and are located in the inner layer of periosteum, endosteum, osteons, and perforating canals that differentiate into osteoblasts
- Osteoblasts are on the bone surfaces and synthesize the osteoid matrix with collagen fibers and different glycoproteins

- Osteoblasts release matrix vesicles that form hydroxyapatite and calcification of osteoid
- Osteocytes are mature osteoblasts, are branched, are located in lacunae, and use canaliculi for communication and exchange of metabolic products and nutrients
- Osteocytes maintain homeostasis of bone and blood concentrations of calcium and phosphate
- Osteoclasts are multinucleated cells responsible for resorption, remodeling, and bone repair
- Osteoclasts belong to the mononuclear macrophage–monocyte cell line and are found in enzyme-eroded depressions (Howship lacunae)

Bone Matrix

- Highly vascularized with blood vessels from periosteum to aid diffusion through calcified matrix
- Organic components of bone resist tension, whereas mineral components resist compression
- Major organic component is coarse type I collagen fibers
- Glycoprotein components bind to calcium crystals during mineralization
- Inorganic components are calcium and phosphate in the form of hydroxyapatite crystals
- Hormones from the parathyroid gland (parathyroid hormone) and the thyroid gland (calcitonin) are responsible for maintaining the proper mineral content of blood

Process of Bone Formation (Ossification)

Endochondral Ossification

- Most bones develop by this process, with a hyaline cartilage model preceding bone
- Hyaline cartilage model grows in length and width, then calcifies, and chondrocytes die
- Mesenchymal cells in the periosteum differentiate into osteoprogenitor cells and form osteoblasts
- Osteoblasts synthesize the osteoid matrix, which calcifies and traps osteoblasts in lacunae as osteocytes
- Osteocytes establish cell-to-cell communication via canaliculi that open into blood channels
- Primary ossification center forms in the diaphysis and secondary center of ossification in the epiphysis
- Epiphyseal plate between the diaphysis and epiphysis allows for growth in bone length
- Eventually all cartilage is replaced by bone except the articular cartilage

Intramembranous Ossification

- Mesenchymal cells differentiate directly into osteoblasts
- Osteoblasts produce the osteoid matrix that quickly calcifies
- Osteoblasts initially form spongy bone that consists of trabeculae and trap osteocytes
- Mandible, maxilla, clavicle, and flat skull bones are formed by this process
- Fontanelles in newborn skulls represent intramembranous ossification in progress

Bone Types

- In long bones, the outer part is compact bone, and the inner surface is cancellous bone
- Both bone types have the same microscopic appearance
- In compact bones, collagen fibers arranged in lamellae
- Lamellae deep to the periosteum are outer circumferential lamellae
- Lamellae surrounding the bone marrow are inner circumferential lamellae
- Lamellae surrounding the blood vessels, nerves, and loose connective tissue are osteons
- Within an osteon is the central canal, which is found in most compact bone

Functional Correlations of Bone

- Continually remodeled in response to mineral needs, mechanical stress, thinning, or disease
- Maintain normal calcium levels in blood; critical to functions of numerous organs and life
- Parathyroid hormone increases calcium levels by indirectly stimulating osteoclasts to resorb bone as well as reabsorb calcium in the kidney and small intestine
- Hormones from the thyroid gland parafollicular cells counteract parathyroid hormone
- Calcitonin inhibits osteoclasts, decreases calcium reabsoption, and increases calcium excretion in kidneys

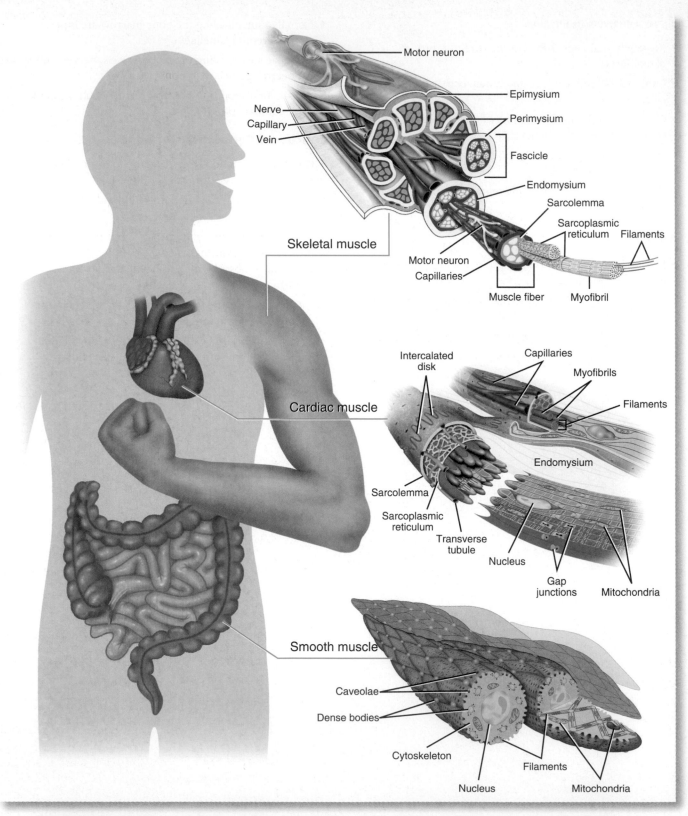

Motor neuron
Epimysium
Perimysium
Nerve
Capillary
Vein
Fascicle
Endomysium
Sarcolemma
Sarcoplasmic reticulum
Filaments
Skeletal muscle
Motor neuron
Capillaries
Muscle fiber
Myofibril

Intercalated disk
Capillaries
Myofibrils
Filaments
Cardiac muscle
Endomysium
Sarcolemma
Sarcoplasmic reticulum
Transverse tubule
Nucleus
Gap junctions
Mitochondria

Smooth muscle
Caveolae
Dense bodies
Cytoskeleton
Filaments
Nucleus
Mitochondria

OVERVIEW FIGURE 8.1 ■ Diagrammatic representation of the microscopic appearance of muscle tissue.

CHAPTER 8

Muscle Tissue

SECTION 1   Skeletal Muscle

There are three types of muscle tissues in the body: **skeletal muscle**, **cardiac muscle**, and **smooth muscle**. These muscles can be identified by their structure and function, with each muscle type showing morphologic and functional similarities as well as differences. All muscle tissues consist of elongated cells called **fibers**. The cytoplasm of muscle cells is called **sarcoplasm**, and the surrounding cell membrane or plasmalemma is called **sarcolemma**.

Skeletal muscle fibers are long, cylindrical, **multinucleated cells**, with peripheral nuclei. The multiple nuclei in skeletal muscle fibers are due to the fusion of numerous mesenchymal cells **myoblasts** during the embryonic development. The elongated and flattened nuclei of the muscle fibers are normally seen under the cell membrane sarcolemma. Each muscle fiber is composed of subunits called **myofibrils** that extend the entire length of the fiber. The myofibrils, in turn, are composed of smaller **myofilaments** formed by the contractile thin protein **actin** and the thick protein **myosin**.

In the sarcoplasm of the skeletal muscle, the arrangement of actin and myosin filaments is very regular, forming the distinct **cross-striation** patterns, which are seen under a light microscope as lighter-staining **I bands** and dark-staining **A bands** in each muscle fiber. Because of these cross-striations, skeletal muscle is also called **striated muscle**. Transmission electron microscopy illustrates the internal organization of the contractile proteins in each myofibril. These high-resolution images show that each light I band is bisected by a dense transverse **Z line** (disk or band). Between the two adjacent Z lines is found the smallest structural and functional contractile unit of the muscle, the **sarcomere**. Sarcomeres are the repeating contractile units seen along the entire length of each myofibril and are highly characteristic features of the sarcoplasm of skeletal and cardiac muscle fibers.

The center and the dark-staining part of each sarcomere contains the thick (myosin) filaments, which form the A band. The peripheries and the light-staining portion of the sarcomere contain the light-staining, thin actin filaments. Actin and myosin filaments are precisely aligned and stabilized within individual myofibrils and sarcomeres by accessory proteins. The thin actin filaments are bound to the protein α-**actinin**, which binds them to the dense Z line (band). The thick myosin filament are anchored to the Z line by the very large protein called **titin**. Titin positions and centers the myosin filaments on the Z line and acts like a spring between the end of the myosin filament and the Z line.

Entire skeletal muscles are surrounded by a dense, irregular connective tissue layer called **epimysium**. From the epimysium, a less dense and thinner irregular connective tissue layer, called **perimysium**, extends inward and divides the interior of the muscle into smaller bundles of muscle fibers called **fascicles**; each fascicle is thus surrounded by perimysium. A thin layer of reticular connective tissue fibers, called **endomysium**, invests individual muscle fibers. Located in all the different connective tissue sheaths are blood vessels, nerves, and lymphatics, with a rich capillary plexus seen in the endomysium (Overview Figure 8.2).

 Supplemental micrographic images are available at **www.thePoint.com/Eroschenko12e** under Muscle Tissue.

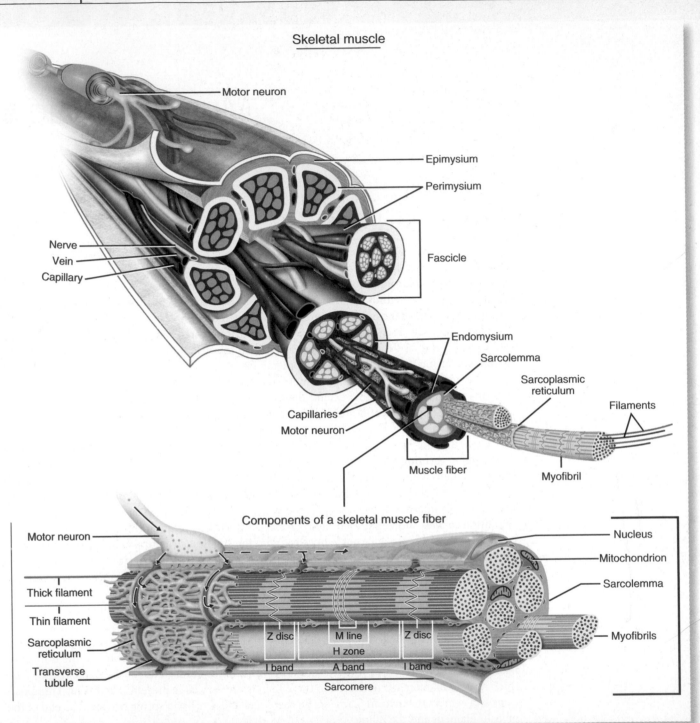

Skeletal muscle

Motor neuron

Epimysium

Perimysium

Fascicle

Nerve
Vein
Capillary

Endomysium

Sarcolemma

Sarcoplasmic reticulum

Filaments

Capillaries
Motor neuron

Muscle fiber

Myofibril

Components of a skeletal muscle fiber

Motor neuron

Nucleus

Mitochondrion

Sarcolemma

Thick filament

Thin filament

Sarcoplasmic reticulum

Transverse tubule

Myofibrils

Z disc   M line   Z disc
H zone

I band   A band   I band
Sarcomere

OVERVIEW FIGURE 8.2 ■ Diagrammatic representation of the microscopic appearance of skeletal muscle.

FIGURE 8.1 | Longitudinal and Transverse Sections of Skeletal (Striated) Muscles: Tongue

In the tongue, skeletal muscle fibers are arranged in bundles and course in different directions. This image illustrates the tongue muscle fibers in both the longitudinal (*upper region*) and transverse (*lower region*) sections.

Each skeletal **muscle fiber (9, transverse section; 11, longitudinal section)** is multinucleated. The **nuclei (1, 6)** are situated peripherally and immediately below the sarcolemma of each muscle fiber. (The sarcolemma is not visible in the figure.) Also, each skeletal muscle fiber shows **cross-striations (3)**, which are visible as alternating dark **A bands (3a)** and light **I bands (3b)**. With higher magnification and transmission electron microscopy, additional details of the cross-striations are visible (Figures 8.4 and 8.5).

Skeletal muscle fibers are aggregated into bundles or **fascicles (15)**, surrounded by fibers of **connective tissue (5)**. The connective tissue (5) sheath around each muscle fascicle (15) is called the **perimysium (12)**. From each perimysium (12), thin partitions of connective tissue extend into each muscle fascicle (15) and invest individual muscle fibers (9, 11) with a connective tissue layer called the **endomysium (4, 7)**. Small **blood vessels (8)** and **capillaries (2, 14)** are present in the connective tissue (5) around each muscle fiber (9, 11).

The skeletal muscle fibers that were sectioned longitudinally (11) show light and dark cross-striations (3a, 3b). The muscle fibers that were sectioned transversely (9) exhibit cross sections of **myofibrils (13)** and peripheral nuclei (6).

1 Nucleus
2 Capillary
3 Cross-striations
 a. A band
 b. I band
 (light)
4 Endomysium
5 Connective tissue
6 Nuclei of muscle fibers
7 Endomysium
8 Blood vessel

10 Fibroblast in endomysium
11 Muscle fiber
12 Perimysium
13 Myofibrils
14 Capillary

9 Muscle fiber
15 Muscle fascicle

FIGURE 8.1 ■ Longitudinal and transverse sections of skeletal (striated) muscles of the tongue. Stain: hematoxylin and eosin. High magnification.

FIGURE 8.2 | Skeletal (Striated) Muscles: Tongue (Longitudinal Section and Cross Section)

A higher-magnification photomicrograph of the tongue illustrates individual **skeletal muscle fibers (3, 9)** in both cross section (3) and longitudinal section (9). In each, the muscle fibers are visible as tiny **myofibrils (4)**. In the longitudinal section of the muscle fiber (9), the multiple **cross-striations (10)** are visible. Note that in the skeletal muscle fibers, the **nuclei (5, 9)** are located on the peripheries. Surrounding each skeletal muscle fiber (3, 9) is a thin layer of connective tissue called **endomysium (2, 6)**, seen both in cross section (2) and in longitudinal section (6). The thicker connective tissue layer called **perimysium (1, 7)** surrounds a group of individual muscle fibers called fascicles. Visible in the surrounding connective tissue perimysium (7) are tiny **capillaries** with flattened **erythrocytes (8)**.

1 Perimysium

2 Endomysium

3 Muscle fibers

4 Myofibrils

5 Peripheral nuclei
in muscle fibers

6 Endomysium

7 Perimysium

8 Capillaries with
erythrocytes

9 Peripheral nuclei
in muscle fibers

10 Cross-striations

FIGURE 8.2 ■ Skeletal (striated) muscles of the tongue (longitudinal and transverse section). Stain: Masson trichrome. ×130.

FIGURE 8.3 | Skeletal Muscle Fibers (Longitudinal Section)

A higher-magnification illustration shows greater detail of individual skeletal muscle fibers and the cross-striations. A cell membrane, or **sarcolemma (4)**, surrounds each skeletal **muscle fiber (2)**. Note the peripheral location of the flattened muscle fiber **nuclei (1, 10)**. Adjacent to the nuclei (1, 10) is the thin cytoplasm or **sarcoplasm (5)** with its organelles. Each muscle fiber (2) consists of **individual myofibrils (8)** that are arranged longitudinally. Myofibrils (8) are best seen in cross sections of the skeletal muscle fibers in Figure 8.2. Surrounding each skeletal muscle fiber (2) is a thin connective tissue **endomysium (9)**, containing the connective tissue cells, **fibrocytes (3, 6)**, and **capillaries (7)** with blood cells.

With higher magnification, the cross-striations of skeletal muscle fibers are recognized as the light-staining **I bands** and dark-staining **A bands**. Each A band is bisected by the lighter H band and the darker **M band**. Crossing the central region of each I band is a distinct, narrow **Z line**. The filamentous and cellular segments between the Z lines represent a **sarcomere**, the structural and functional unit of striated muscles (skeletal and cardiac). When the myofibrils (8) are separated from the muscle fiber (2), the A, I, and Z lines remain visible. The close longitudinal arrangement of parallel myofibrils gives the skeletal muscle fibers their characteristic striated appearance. For a better understanding of the cross-striations and internal composition of the myofibrils, a direct comparison with the ultrastructural image of the myofibrils is presented in the next figure.

FIGURE 8.4 | Ultrastructure of Myofibrils in Skeletal Muscle

For comparison with the light microscope illustration of Figure 8.3, a small section of the skeletal muscle is illustrated with a much higher magnification and higher resolution. This transmission electron micrograph illustrates the organization of the myofibrils and myofilaments in a partially contracted skeletal muscle. Each myofibril consists of repeating units called sarcomeres, the contractile elements in striated muscles. A **sarcomere (5)** is located between two electron-dense **Z lines**. Located in each sarcomere (5) are the light-staining thin actin and the dark-staining thick myosin myofilaments. The thin actin filaments extend from the Z lines and form the light-staining **I bands**. In the center of each sarcomere (5) is the dark-staining **A band**, which consists mainly of the thick myosin filaments overlapping the thin actin filaments. Each A band is bisected by a denser **M band** where the adjacent myosin filaments are linked. On each side of the M band are smaller lighter **H bands (2, 3)** that consist only of myosin filaments. Surrounding each sarcomere in a repeating fashion are the tubules of **sarcoplasmic reticulum (4)** and **mitochondria (1)**. During muscle contraction, the length of the thick and thin filaments remains unchanged, whereas the size of each sarcomere (5) decreases (see Figure 8.5).

1 Nucleus of muscle fiber
2 Muscle fiber
3 Fibrocyte in endomysium
4 Sarcolemma
5 Sarcoplasm

6 Fibrocyte
7 Erythrocyte in capillary
8 Myofibrils
9 Endomysium
10 Nucleus of muscle fiber

Sarcomere   I band   A band   Z line   M band

1 Mitochondria

3 H bands

2 H bands

4 Sarcoplasmic reticulum

5 Sarcomere

FIGURE 8.3 ■ Skeletal muscle fibers (longitudinal section). Stain: hematoxylin and eosin. Plastic section. High magnification.

FIGURE 8.4 ■ Ultrastructure of myofibrils in skeletal muscle. Courtesy of Carter Rowley, Ft. Collins, CO. ×33,500.

FIGURE 8.5 | Ultrastructure of Sarcomeres, Tubules, and Triads in Skeletal Muscle

A higher magnification with the transmission electron micrograph illustrates the sarcomeres in a contracted skeletal muscle. Note that as the muscle contracts and the sarcomere shortens, the **Z lines (2, 6)** are drawn closer together, and the thick and thin filaments slide past each other. This action narrows the **I bands (7)** and **H bands (8)**, whereas the **A band (1)** remains unchanged. Also visible in the middle of the sarcomere is the dense-staining **M band (4)**. The tubules or the cisternae of the sarcoplasmic reticulum surround every sarcomere of every myofibril (see Figure 8.4). At the A band (1) and I band (7) junction (A–I junctions), the sarcoplasmic reticulum tubules expand into terminal cisternae. To allow synchronous stimulation and contraction of all sarcomeres, tiny tubular invaginations of the sarcolemma, called the **T tubules (3)**, penetrate every myofibril, and are located at the A–I junctions (1, 7). Here, one T tubule (3) is surrounded on each side by the expanded terminal cisternae of the sarcoplasmic reticulum and forms a **triad (5)**. In mammalian skeletal muscles, the triads (5) are located at the A–I junctions. The stimulus for muscle contraction, delivered via a nerve, is then disseminated to each sarcomere of each myofibril through the T tubules (3) in the triads (5).

1 A band

2 Z line

3 T tubule

4 M band

5 Triads

6 Z line

7 I bands

8 H bands

FIGURE 8.5 ■ Ultrastructure of sarcomeres, T tubules, and triads in skeletal muscle. Courtesy of Carter Rowley, Ft. Collins, CO. ×50,000.

FIGURE 8.6 | Skeletal Muscles, Nerves, and Motor Endplates

A group of **skeletal muscle fibers (6, 7)** have been teased apart and stained to illustrate nerve terminations or myoneural junctions on individual muscle fibers. Note the characteristic **cross-striations (2, 8)** that are visible in the individual skeletal muscle fibers (6, 7). The dark-stained, string like structures between the separated muscle fibers (6, 7) are the **myelinated motor nerves (3)** and their branches, the **axons (1, 5, 10)**. The motor nerve (3) courses within the muscle, branches, and distributes its axons (1, 5, 10) to the individual muscle fibers (6, 7). The axons (1, 5, 10) terminate on individual muscle fibers as specialized junctional regions called **motor endplates (4, 9)**. The small, dark, round structures seen in each motor endplate (4, 9) are the terminal expansion of the axons (1, 5, 10). Some axons (1) are also seen without motor endplates as a result of tissue preparation.

FUNCTIONAL CORRELATIONS 8.1 | Skeletal Muscles

SKELETAL MUSCLE AND MOTOR ENDPLATES

Skeletal muscles are **voluntary** because the stimulation for their contraction and relaxation is under conscious control. Large motor nerves or axons innervate skeletal muscles. Near the skeletal muscle, the motor nerve branches, and a smaller axon branch individually innervates a single muscle fiber. As a result, skeletal muscle fibers contract only when stimulated by an axon. Also, each skeletal muscle fiber exhibits a specialized site where the axon terminates. This **neuromuscular junction,** or **motor endplate,** is the site where the impulse from the axon is transmitted to the skeletal muscle fiber.

The terminal end of each efferent (motor) axon contains numerous small **vesicles** that contain the neurotransmitter **acetylcholine**. Arrival of a nerve impulse, or **action potential,** at the axon terminal causes the synaptic vesicles to fuse with the plasma membrane of the axon and release the acetylcholine into the **synaptic cleft**, a small gap between the axon terminal and cell membrane of the muscle fiber. The neurotransmitter then diffuses across the synaptic cleft, combines with **acetylcholine receptors** on the cell membrane of the muscle fiber, and stimulates the muscle to contract. An enzyme called **acetylcholinesterase**, located in the basal lamina of the synaptic cleft, inactivates or neutralizes the released and excess acetylcholine. Inactivation of acetylcholine is necessary in order to prevent further muscle stimulation and muscle contraction until the next impulse arrives at the axon terminal.

CONTRACTION OF SKELETAL MUSCLES

Before the arrival of the nerve stimulus to the muscle, the muscle is relaxed, and **calcium ions** are stored in the cisternae of the **sarcoplasmic reticulum**. Muscle contractions depend on the availability of calcium ions. After the arrival of the nerve stimulus and the release of the neurotransmitter at the motor endplates, the sarcolemma is depolarized, or activated. The stimulus signal (action potential) is propagated along the entire length of the sarcolemma and rapidly transmitted deep to every myofiber by the network of the **T tubules**, which are located at the **A–I junctions** in mammalian skeleton muscles. Expanded terminal cisternae of the sarcoplasmic reticulum and T tubules form **triads**. At each triad, the action potential is transmitted from the T tubules to every myofiber and myofibril as well as the sarcoplasmic reticulum membrane. After stimulation, cisternae of the sarcoplasmic reticulum

FUNCTIONAL CORRELATIONS 8.1 | Skeletal Muscles *(Continued)*

in each myofibril release calcium ions into the individual sarcomeres and the over-lapping thick and thin myofilaments of the myofibril. Calcium ions activate binding between actin and myosin, which results in their sliding past each other, causing muscle contraction and muscle shortening. When the stimulus subsides and the membrane is no longer stimulated, calcium ions are actively transported back into and stored in the cisternae of the sarcoplasmic reticulum, causing muscle relaxation.

Nearly all skeletal muscles contain sensitive stretch receptors called **neuromuscular spindles**. These spindles consist of a connective tissue **capsule**, in which are found modified muscle fibers called **intrafusal fibers** and numerous **nerve endings**, surrounded by a fluid-filled space. The muscles that surround the neuromuscular spindles are called the **extrafusal fibers**. The neuromuscular spindles monitor the changes (distension) in muscle length and activate complex reflexes to regulate muscle activity. When skeletal muscles are stretched, the neuromuscular spindles initiate a reflex contraction and shortening of the muscle.

1 Axon terminals

2 Cross-striations

3 Myelinated nerve

4 Motor endplates

5 Axons

6 Skeletal muscle fibers

7 Skeletal muscle fibers

8 Cross-striations

9 Motor endplates

10 Axons

FIGURE 8.6 ■ Skeletal muscles, nerves, axons, and motor endplates. Stain: silver. High magnification.

FIGURE 8.7 | Skeletal Muscle With Muscle Spindle (Transverse Section)

Skeletal muscles contain sensory stretch receptors called muscle spindles that are surrounded by connective tissue capsules. A transverse section of an extraocular skeletal muscle shows individual **muscle fibers (2)** surrounded by connective tissue, the **endomysium (6)**. The muscle fibers (2), in turn, are grouped into **fascicles (1)** and surrounded by interfascicular connective tissue called **perimysium (4)**. Located within the muscle fascicles (1) is a cross section of a **muscle spindle (3)**. Surrounding the muscle spindle (3) and the skeletal muscle fibers (2) are **arterioles (5)** in the perimysium (4).

The connective tissue **capsule (8)** surrounding the muscle spindle (3) extends from the adjacent **perimysium (11)** and encloses several components of the spindle. The specialized muscle fibers located in the spindle and surrounded by the capsule (8) are called **intrafusal fibers (10)**, in contrast to the extrafusal **skeletal muscle fibers (7)** located outside of the spindle capsule (8). Small nerve fibers associated with the muscle spindles (3) are the myelinated and terminal unmyelinated **nerve fibers (axons) (9)** surrounded by the supportive Schwann cells. Small blood vessels and an **arteriole (12)** from the perimysium (11) are found in and around the capsule of the muscle spindle (3).

FUNCTIONAL CORRELATIONS 8.2 | Muscle Spindles

Muscle spindles are highly specialized **stretch receptors** located parallel to muscle fibers in nearly all skeletal muscles. Their main function is to detect changes in the length of the muscle fibers. An increase in the length of muscle fibers stimulates the muscle spindle and sends **impulses** via the afferent (sensory) axons into the spinal cord. These impulses result in a **stretch reflex** that immediately causes **contraction** of the **extrafusal muscle fibers**, thereby shortening the stretched muscle and producing movement. A decrease in skeletal muscle length stops the stimulation of the muscle spindle fibers and the conduction of its impulses to the spinal cord.

The simple **stretch reflex arc** illustrates the function of these receptors. Gently tapping the patellar tendon on the knee with a rubber mallet stretches the skeletal muscle and stimulates the muscle spindle. This action results in rapid muscle contraction of the stretched muscle and produces an involuntary response, or stretch reflex.

1 Fascicles

2 Skeletal muscle fibers

3 Muscle spindle

4 Perimysium

5 Arterioles

6 Endomysium

7 Extrafusal fibers

8 Capsule of muscle spindle

9 Nerve fibers with Schwann cells

10 Intrafusal fibers

11 Perimysium

12 Arteriole

FIGURE 8.7 ■ Skeletal muscle with muscle spindle (transverse section). Frozen section stained with modified Van Gieson method (hematoxylin, picric acid–ponceau stain). Left, medium magnification; right, high magnification. Courtesy of Dr. Mark DeSantis, Professor Emeritus, WWAMI Medical Program, University of Idaho, Moscow, ID.

OVERVIEW FIGURE 8.3 ■ Diagrammatic representation of the microscopic appearance of cardiac muscle.

SECTION 2   Cardiac Muscle

Cardiac muscle fibers are also cylindrical. They are primarily located in the walls and septa of the **heart** and in the walls of the large vessels attached to the heart (the aorta and pulmonary trunk). Similar to skeletal muscle, cardiac muscle fibers exhibit distinct **cross-striations** as a result of the regular arrangements of actin and myosin filaments in the sarcomeres. Transmission electron microscopy reveals similar A bands, I bands, Z lines, and the repeating sarcomere units. In contrast to skeletal muscles, however, the cardiac muscle fibers exhibit some important differences. The cardiac muscles develop by joining the cells end to end through anchoring cell junctions called the

intercalated disks that form the distinguishing characteristic features of cardiac muscles. These dense-staining disks are special attachment sites that cross the cardiac cells in a stepwise fashion at irregular intervals. Cardiac muscle cells also exhibit only one or two **central nuclei**, are likewise shorter than the skeletal muscle, and exhibit **branching** (see Overview Figure 8.2).

 Supplemental micrographic images are available at **www.thePoint.com/Eroschenko12e** under Muscle Tissue.

FIGURE 8.8 | Longitudinal and Transverse Sections of Cardiac Muscle

Cardiac muscle fibers exhibit some of the features that are seen in skeletal muscle fibers. This figure illustrates a section of a cardiac muscle cut in both longitudinal (*upper portion*) and transverse (*lower portion*) planes. The **cross-striations (2)** in the cardiac muscle fibers closely resemble those seen in skeletal muscles. In contrast, the cardiac muscle fibers show **branching (5, 10)** without much change in their diameters. Also, each cardiac muscle fiber is shorter than a skeletal muscle fiber and contains a single, centrally located **nucleus (3, 7)**. **Binucleate** (two nuclei) **muscle fibers (8)** are also occasionally seen. The nuclei (7) are clearly visible in the center of each muscle fiber when they are cut in a transverse section. Around these nuclei (3, 7, 8) are the clear zones of nonfibrillar **perinuclear sarcoplasm (1, 13)**. In transverse sections, the perinuclear sarcoplasm (13) appears as a clear space if the section is not through the nucleus. Also visible in transverse sections are the **myofibrils (14)** of individual cardiac muscle fibers.

Highly distinguishing and characteristic features of cardiac muscle fibers are the **intercalated disks (4, 9)**. These dark-staining structures are found in the cardiac muscle at irregular intervals and represent the specialized junctional complexes between cardiac muscle fibers.

Cardiac muscle has a vast blood supply. Numerous small blood vessels and **capillaries (6)** are found in the **connective tissue (11)** septa and the delicate **endomysium (12)** between individual muscle fibers.

Other examples of cardiac muscles are seen in Chapter 10, "Circulatory System."

1 Perinuclear sarcoplasm
2 Cross striations
3 Central nucleus
4 Intercalated disk
5 Branching cardiac fiber
6 Capillary
7 Central nucleus
8 Binucleate fiber
9 Intercalated disks
10 Branching cardiac fiber
11 Connective tissue
12 Endomysium
13 Perinuclear sarcoplasm
14 Myofibrils

FIGURE 8.8 ■ Longitudinal and transverse sections of cardiac muscle. Stain: hematoxylin and eosin. High magnification.

FIGURE 8.9 | Cardiac Muscle (Longitudinal Section)

A high-magnification photomicrograph illustrates a section of the cardiac muscle cut in a longitudinal plane. **Cardiac muscle fibers (1)** exhibit **cross-striations (3), branching fibers (8)**, and a single central **nucleus (6)**. The dark-staining **intercalated disks (2)** connect individual cardiac muscle fibers (1). Small **myofibrils (4)** are visible within each cardiac muscle fiber (1). The flattened and fusiform cells surrounding the cardiac muscle fibers (1) represent the **fibrocytes** of the **endomysium (5)**. Although not visible in this illustration, delicate strands of connective tissue endomysium surround the individual cardiac muscle fibers.

FIGURE 8.10 | Cardiac Muscle in Longitudinal Section

Comparison of the cardiac muscle fibers with skeletal muscles at higher magnification and with the same stain (Figure 8.3) illustrates the similarities and differences between the two types of muscle tissue.

The cross-striations **(1)** are similar in both the skeletal and cardiac muscle types but are less prominent in cardiac muscle fibers. The branching **cardiac fibers (9)** are in contrast to the individual, elongated fibers of the skeletal muscle. The characteristic **intercalated disks (5, 7)** of cardiac muscle fibers and their irregular structure are more prominent at higher magnification. The intercalated disks (5, 7) appear as either straight bands (5) or staggered (7) across individual fibers.

The large, oval **nuclei (3)**, usually one per cell, occupy the central position of the cardiac fibers, in contrast to the numerous flattened and peripheral nuclei in each skeletal muscle fiber. Surrounding the nucleus of a cardiac muscle fiber is a prominent **perinuclear sarcoplasm (2, 10)** that is devoid of cross-striations and myofibrils.

The connective tissue **fibrocytes (6, 8)** and the fine connective tissue fibers of **endomysium (4)** surround the cardiac muscle fibers. **Capillaries** with **erythrocytes (11)** are normally seen in the endomysium (4, 6, 8).

1 Cardiac muscle fibers

2 Intercalated disks

3 Striations

4 Myofibrils

5 Fibrocytes of endomysium

6 Nuclei

7 Intercalated disks

8 Branching cardiac muscle fiber

FIGURE 8.9 ■ Cardiac muscle (longitudinal section). Stain: Masson trichrome. ×130.

1 Cross-striations

2 Perinuclear sarcoplasm

3 Central nuclei

4 Endomysium

5 Intercalated disk

6 Fibrocyte in endomysium

7 Intercalated disks

8 Fibrocyte in endomysium

9 Branching cardiac fiber

10 Perinuclear sarcoplasm

11 Erythrocytes in capillary

FIGURE 8.10 ■ Cardiac muscle in longitudinal section. Stain: hematoxylin and eosin. High magnification.

FIGURE 8.11 | Ultrastructure of Cardiac Muscle in Longitudinal Section

This ultrastructure image illustrates the internal structures of cardiac muscle fiber. A distinct **sarcomere (1)** with regular arrangements of thin actin and thick myosin filaments is located between the dense-staining **Z lines (3)**. Visible in the sarcomere (1) is the denser **A band (2)** containing both actin and myosin filaments and the light-staining **I band (8)** with actin filaments that are bisected by the Z lines (3). Located between the myofibrils are the large **mitochondria (4)** that are highly characteristic of cardiac muscle. In contrast to skeletal muscle, however, the **sarcoplasmic reticulum (5)** in the cardiac muscle is not as well organized and exhibits only small terminal cisternae. In addition, cardiac muscles exhibit only one **T tubule (9)** per sarcomere, which is seen at the level of the Z line (3). In the middle of the sarcomere (1) are visible **M bands (7)**, darker bands that represent the linkages of the thick myosin filaments. A highly characteristic feature of the cardiac muscle is the dense-staining **intercalated disk (6)** with its irregular, zigzag pattern that crosses the cardiac muscle fibers. These disks represent important attachment sites between individual cardiac muscle fibers. The clear spaces between the myofibrils represent the branching features of different cardiac muscle fibers.

FUNCTIONAL CORRELATIONS 8.3 | Cardiac Muscle

Although the organization of the contractile proteins (actin and myosin) in cardiac myofibers and their arrangement in sarcomeres is essentially the same as in skeletal muscles, there are important differences. The **T tubules** are located at the Z lines and are much larger than those in skeletal muscles. Furthermore, the sarcoplasmic reticulum is less well developed. Also, the mitochondria are larger and more abundant in the cardiac cells, which reflects the increased metabolic demands on the cardiac muscle fibers for continuous function.

Cardiac cells are joined end to end by specialized, interdigitating junctional complexes called **intercalated disks**, which consist of fascia adherens, desmosomes, and **gap junctions**. The gap junctions functionally couple all cardiac muscle fibers and allow a rapid spread of stimuli throughout the entire muscle mass. Conduction of excitatory impulses to the cardiac sarcomeres is through the T tubules and the sarcoplasmic reticulum. Diffusion of ions through the pores in gap junctions between individual cardiac muscle fibers coordinates heart function and allows the cardiac muscle to act as a **functional syncytium**, allowing the stimuli for contraction to pass through the entire cardiac musculature mass.

As in the skeletal muscle, calcium is essential for cardiac muscle contractions. In cardiac muscles, however, the sarcoplasmic reticulum is less well developed and does not store sufficient amounts of calcium for uninterrupted contractions. As a result, during muscle stimulation and contraction, calcium is imported from outside the cardiac muscle cells into the sarcoplasm as well as from the sparse sarcoplasmic reticulum. At the end of the stimulus, this calcium movement is reversed.

Cardiac muscle fibers exhibit **autorhythmicity**, an ability to spontaneously generate stimuli. Both the **parasympathetic** and **sympathetic divisions** of the autonomic nervous system innervate the heart. Nerve fibers from the parasympathetic division, by way of the vagus nerve, slow the heart and decrease blood pressure. Nerve fibers from the sympathetic division produce the opposite effect and increase heart rate and blood pressure.

Additional information on cardiac muscle histology, the heart pacemaker, Purkinje fibers, and heart hormones is presented in more detail in Chapter 10, "Circulatory System."

1 Sarcomere

2 A band

3 Z lines

4 Mitochondria

5 Sarcoplasmic reticulum

6 Intercalated disk

7 M bands

8 I band

9 T tubules

FIGURE 8.11 ■ Ultrastructure of cardiac muscle in longitudinal section. Used with permission from D. Cui. Atlas of Histology with Functional and Clinical Correlations. Wolters Kluwer/Lippincott Williams and Wilkins, Baltimore: 2011. ×24,800.

Smooth muscle

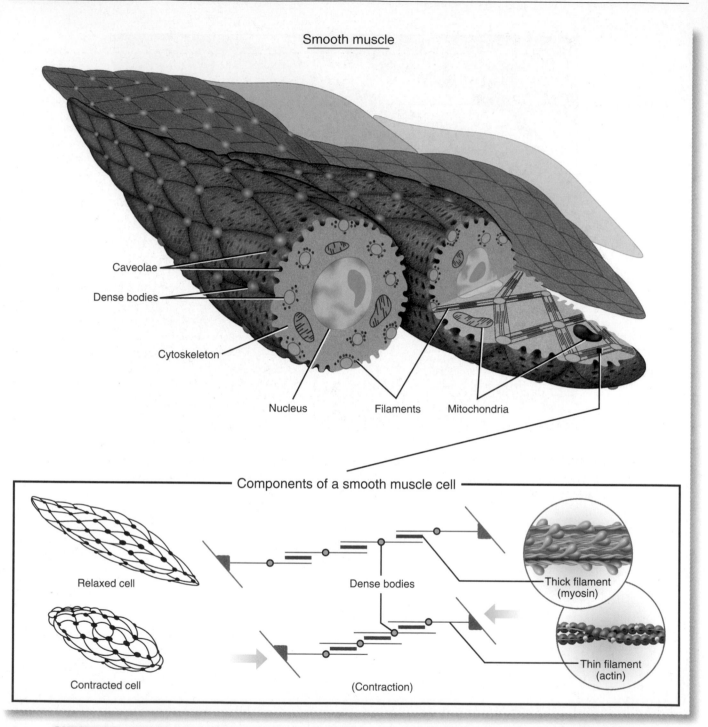

Caveolae

Dense bodies

Cytoskeleton

Nucleus

Filaments

Mitochondria

Components of a smooth muscle cell

Relaxed cell

Contracted cell

Dense bodies

(Contraction)

Thick filament (myosin)

Thin filament (actin)

OVERVIEW FIGURE 8.4 ■ Diagrammatic representation of the microscopic appearance of smooth muscle.

SECTION 3   Smooth Muscle

Smooth muscles have a wide distribution in the body and are predominantly found in the linings of **visceral hollow organs** and **blood vessels**. In digestive tract organs, the uterus, ureters, and other hollow organs, smooth muscles occur in large sheets or layers. In the dermis of the skin, smooth muscles are seen as small strips associated with hair follicles. Zonula adherens bind the cells, whereas the numerous **gap junctions** provide functional coupling between individual smooth muscle cells.

Under a light microscope, smooth muscle appears as elongated individual fibers with fusiform shapes of slender bundles called fascicles. The muscle fibers are also small and contain a single central **nucleus**. Connective tissue surrounds individual muscle fibers as well as muscle layers. In the blood vessels, smooth muscle fibers are arranged in a circular pattern, where they control blood pressure by altering luminal diameters. In intestines, smooth muscles are also arranged in concentric layers around the organs.

Individual smooth muscle fibers contain contractile **actin** and **myosin** filaments; however, they are not arranged in the regular, cross-striated patterns that are visible in both the skeletal and cardiac muscle fibers. Instead, actin and myosin course obliquely throughout the cell in the form of a lattice network that crisscrosses the sarcoplasm. As a result of the irregular distribution of contractile elements, these muscle fibers appear **smooth,** or **nonstriated**. The actin filaments attach to **dense bodies**, structures that are unique to smooth muscles. The dense bodies are either scattered throughout the cytoplasm or attached to the cytoplasmic side of the cell membrane. The intermediate and actin filaments attach to the dense bodies in the cytoplasm and the dense bodies in the cell membrane. The dense bodies also contain **α-actinin** and other accessory Z disk proteins and are similar to the Z disks of the striated muscles. Another characteristic feature of smooth muscle fibers is the presence of numerous vesicular invaginations of the cell membrane that look like the endocytotic or pinocytotic vesicles in other cells. These are the caveolae and are believed to function like the T tubules of skeletal muscles.

 Supplemental micrographic images are available at **www.thePoint.com/Eroschenko12e** under Muscle Tissue.

FIGURE 8.12 | Longitudinal and Transverse Sections of Smooth Muscle: Wall of Small Intestine

In the muscular region of the small intestine, smooth muscle fibers are arranged in two concentric layers: an inner circular layer and an outer longitudinal layer. Here, the muscle fibers are tightly packed, and the muscle fibers of one layer are arranged at right angles to the fibers of the adjacent layer.

The upper region of the illustration shows the smooth muscle fibers of the inner circular layer cut in longitudinal section. **Smooth muscle fibers (1)** are spindle-shaped cells with tapered ends. The cytoplasm (sarcoplasm) of each muscle fiber stains dark. An elongated or ovoid single **nucleus (7)** is present in the center of each smooth muscle fiber.

The lower region of the figure shows the muscles of the adjacent longitudinal layer cut in transverse section. Because the spindle-shaped cells are sectioned at different places along their length, the cells with their central nuclei exhibit different shapes and sizes. Large **nuclei (5)** are seen only in those **smooth muscle fibers (5)** that have been sectioned through their center. Muscle fibers that were not sectioned through the center appear only as deeply stained areas of clear **cytoplasm (sarcoplasm) (3**, upper leader; **9**, lower leader) or exhibit only a small portion of their cytoplasm with a section of their nuclei (3, lower leader; 9 upper leader).

In the small intestine, the smooth muscle layers are close to each other with only a minimal amount of **connective tissue fibers** and **fibrocytes (4, 8, 10)** present between the two layers. Smooth muscle also has a rich blood supply, evidenced by the numerous **capillaries (6, 11)** between individual fibers and layers. Note that between the inner circular muscle layer and the outer longitudinal muscle layer are found numerous **neurons** of the **myenteric nerve plexus (2)**.

FIGURE 8.13 | Smooth Muscle: Wall of the Small Intestine (Transverse and Longitudinal Sections)

A photomicrograph of the small intestine illustrates its muscular outer wall. The smooth muscle fibers are arranged in two layers: an **inner circular layer (7)** and an **outer longitudinal layer (8)**. In the inner circular layer (7), a single **nucleus (1)** is visible in the center of the **cytoplasm (2)** of different fibers. In the outer longitudinal layer (8), cut in transverse section, the **cytoplasm (5)** appears empty, and single **nuclei (6)** of individual muscle fibers are visible if the plane of section passes through them. Located between the two smooth muscle layers is a group of autonomic **neurons** of the **myenteric nerve plexus (3)**. Small **blood vessels (4)** are seen between individual muscle fibers and muscle layers.

1 Smooth muscle fibers

2 Neurons of myenteric nerve plexus

3 Smooth muscle fibers

4 Fibrocyte

5 Nucleus of smooth muscle fiber

6 Capillary

7 Nucleus of smooth muscle fiber

8 Connective tissue and fibrocyte

9 Nucleus and cytoplasm of smooth muscle fiber

10 Connective tissue

11 Capillary

FIGURE 8.12 ■ Longitudinal and transverse sections of smooth muscle in the wall of the small intestine. Stain: hematoxylin and eosin. High magnification.

1 Nuclei

2 Cytoplasm

3 Neurons of myenteric nerve plexus

4 Blood vessels

5 Cytoplasm

6 Nuclei

7 Inner circular layer

8 Outer longitudinal layer

FIGURE 8.13 ■ Smooth muscle: wall of the small intestine (transverse and longitudinal section). Stain: hematoxylin and eosin. ×80.

FIGURE 8.14 | Ultrastructure of Smooth Muscle Fibers From a Section of an Intestinal Wall

In comparing the ultrastructure of the skeletal (see Figures 8.4 and 8.5) and cardiac (see Figure 8.11) muscle fibers with smooth muscle fibers, there is a significant difference in their morphology. The orderly arrangement of actin and myosin that gave skeletal and cardiac muscles a striated appearance is absent. Although individual fibers are visible in the **cell cytoplasm (4)** of smooth muscle fibers, their overall arrangement is highly random. The thin actin filaments attach to the **dense bodies (1, 5)** at the **cell membrane (1, 5)** or to **dense bodies (6, 9)** that are found scattered in the cytoplasm (4) of each smooth muscle cell (4). The dense bodies (1, 5, 6, 9) are functionally similar to the Z disks of the skeletal and cardiac muscles. Note also the numerous invaginations along muscle cell membranes. These invaginations are the **caveolae** (arrows). Within the cell cytoplasm (4) are also seen a **mitochondrion (8)** and remnants of **sarcoplasmic reticulum (7)**. Smooth muscle cytoplasm (4) is surrounded by **basal lamina (3)**, and, between individual smooth muscle fibers, there are numerous collagen fibers of the **connective tissue (2, 10)**.

FUNCTIONAL CORRELATIONS 8.4 | Smooth Muscle

There are no T tubules in the smooth muscles, and the sarcoplasmic reticulum is not well developed for storing much calcium. In addition, smooth muscles exhibit numerous vesicular invaginations of the cell membrane called **caveolae**. These caveolae may have the same function as the T tubules of striated muscles by controlling the influx of calcium into the cells following stimulation. During stimulation and contraction of the smooth muscle, calcium enters the sarcoplasm from the sarcoplasmic reticulum and from the cell membrane caveolae. After the calcium ions enter the cell, it binds to a protein called **calmodulin**, a calcium-binding protein that stimulates the interaction of actin and myosin, which then slide past each other. Both actin and myosin contract by a sliding filament mechanism that is similar to that in skeletal muscles. This action causes the **dense bodies** to be pulled closer together, producing contraction and shortening of the smooth muscle. Because the dense bodies of the neighboring smooth muscle cells are connected, the force of contraction is transmitted to all smooth muscle cells, allowing the smooth muscles to function as a unit.

Smooth muscle usually exhibits spontaneous wavelike activity that passes in a slow, sustained contraction throughout the entire muscle. In this manner, smooth muscle produces a continuous contraction of low force and maintains **tonus** in hollow structures. In ureters, the uterus, and digestive organs, contraction of smooth muscle produces **peristaltic contractions**, which propel the contents along the lengths of these organs. In arteries and other blood vessels, smooth muscles regulate the luminal diameters.

Smooth muscle fibers also make close contacts with each other via specialized **gap junctions**. These gap junctions allow for rapid ionic communications between the smooth muscle fibers, resulting in coordinated activity in smooth muscle sheets or layers. Smooth muscles are also **involuntary** muscles. They are innervated and regulated by nerves from postganglionic neurons whose cell bodies are located in the **sympathetic** and **parasympathetic divisions** of the **autonomic nervous system**. These innervations influence the rate and force of contractility. In addition, smooth muscle fibers contract and relax in response to nonneural stimulation, such as **stretching** or exposure to different **hormones**.

1 Dense body (cell membrane)

2 Connective tissue

3 Basal lamina

4 Cell cytoplasm

5 Dense body (cell membrane)

6 Dense bodies (cytoplasm)

7 Sarcoplasmic reticulum

8 Mitochondrion

9 Dense body (cytoplasm)

10 Connective tissue

FIGURE 8.14 ■ Ultrastructure of smooth muscle fibers from a section of an intestinal wall. Courtesy of Dr. Rex A. Hess, Professor Emeritus Comparative Biosciences, College of Veterinary Medicine, Univrsity of Illinois, Urbana, Illinois. Approximately ×10,500.

Muscle Tissue

- Three muscle types are skeletal muscle, cardiac muscle, and smooth muscle
- All muscles show similarities and differences
- All muscles are composed of elongated cells called fibers
- Muscle cytoplasm is sarcoplasm, and muscle cell membrane is sarcolemma
- Muscle fibers contain myofibrils made of contractile proteins actin and myosin

Skeletal Muscle

- Fibers are multinucleated with peripheral nuclei
- Multiple nuclei due to fusion of mesenchyme myoblasts during embryonic development
- Each muscle fiber is composed of myofibrils and myofilaments
- Actin and myosin filaments form distinct cross-striation patterns
- Light I bands contain thin actin, and dark A bands contain thick myosin filaments
- Dense Z line bisects I bands; between Z lines is the contractile unit, the sarcomere
- Accessory proteins align and stabilize actin and myosin filaments
- Titin protein anchors myosin filaments, and α-actinin binds actin filaments to Z lines
- Titin centers, positions, and acts like a spring between myosin and Z lines
- Muscle is surrounded by connective tissue epimysium
- Muscle fascicles are surrounded by connective tissue perimysium
- Each muscle fiber is surrounded by connective tissue endomysium
- Voluntary muscles are under conscious control
- Neuromuscular spindles are specialized stretch receptors in almost all skeletal muscles
- Intrafusal fibers and nerve endings are found in spindle capsules
- Stretching of muscle produces a stretch reflex and movement to shorten muscle

Transmission Electron Microscopy of Skeletal Muscle

- Light bands are I bands and are formed by thin actin filaments
- I bands are crossed by dense Z lines
- Between Z lines is the smallest contractile unit of muscle, the sarcomere
- Dark bands are A bands and are located in the middle of sarcomere
- A bands are formed by overlapping actin and myosin filaments
- M bands in the middle of A bands represent linkage of myosin filaments
- H bands on each side of M bands contain only myosin filaments
- Sarcoplasmic reticulum and mitochondria surround each sarcomere

Functional Correlations of Skeletal Muscles

- Skeletal muscles are voluntary, are under conscious control, and contract only when stimulated
- Motor endplates are the sites of nerve innervations and transmission of stimuli to muscle
- Axon terminals of motor endplates contain vesicles with the neurotransmitter acetylcholine
- Action potential releases acetylcholine into synaptic cleft
- Acetylcholine combines with its receptors on muscle membrane
- Acetylcholinesterase neutralizes acetylcholine and prevents further contraction
- Before arrival of impulse, calcium is stored in sarcoplasmic reticulum
- Sarcolemma invaginations into each myofiber form T tubules
- Expanded terminal cisternae of sarcoplasmic reticulum and T tubules form triads
- Triads are located at A–I junctions in mammalian skeletal muscles
- Stimulus for muscle contraction carried by T tubules to every myofiber, myofibril, and sarcoplasmic reticulum membrane
- After stimulation, sarcoplasmic reticulum releases calcium ions into sarcomeres
- Calcium activates the binding of actin and myosin, causing muscle contraction and shortening
- After the end of stimulus, calcium is actively transported and stored in sarcoplasmic reticulum
- When muscle contracts, I and H bands shorten, whereas A bands stay the same
- Muscle contraction and shortening draw Z lines closer together and shorten sarcomere

Cardiac Muscle

- Located in heart and large vessels attached to heart
- Cross-striations of actin and myosin form similar I bands, A bands, and Z lines as in skeletal muscle
- Characterized by dense junctional complexes called intercalated disks that contain gap junctions

- Contain one or two central nuclei, fibers are shorter and show branching
- T tubules are located at Z lines and are larger than in skeletal muscle
- Sarcoplasmic reticulum is less well developed than in skeletal muscles
- Mitochondria are larger and more abundant in cardiac fibers
- Gap junctions couple all fibers for rhythmic contraction and form functional syncytium
- For contraction, calcium is imported from outside cell and from sarcoplasmic reticulum
- Exhibit autorhythmicity and spontaneously generate stimuli
- Autonomic nervous system innervates heart and influences heart rate and blood pressure

Smooth Muscle

- Found in hollow organs and blood vessels
- Zonula adherens binds muscle cells, whereas gap junctions provide functional coupling
- Contain actin and myosin filaments without cross-striation patterns
- Fibers are fusiform in shape and contain single central nuclei
- In intestines, muscles are arranged in concentric layers, and in blood vessels in a circular pattern
- Actin and myosin filaments are present, but they do not show regular arrangement or striations

- Actin and myosin form lattice network, and they insert into dense bodies in sarcoplasm and cytoplasm
- Dense bodies contain α-actinin and other Z disk proteins
- Sarcoplasmic reticulum is not well developed for calcium storage
- Sarcolemma contains invaginations called caveolae
- Caveolae may control influx of calcium into cell after stimulation
- Following stimulation, calcium enters sarcoplasm from caveolae and sarcoplasmic reticulum
- Calmodulin, a calcium-binding protein, stimulates actin and myosin interaction
- Actin and myosin contract muscle by a sliding mechanism similar to skeletal muscle
- Connection of dense bodies with adjacent cells transmits force of contraction to all cells
- Exhibit spontaneous activity and maintain tonus in hollow organs
- Peristaltic contractions propel contents in the organs
- Gap junctions couple muscles and allow ionic communication between all fibers
- Innervated by postganglionic neurons of sympathetic and parasympathetic divisions
- Involuntary muscles regulated by autonomic nervous system, hormones, and stretching

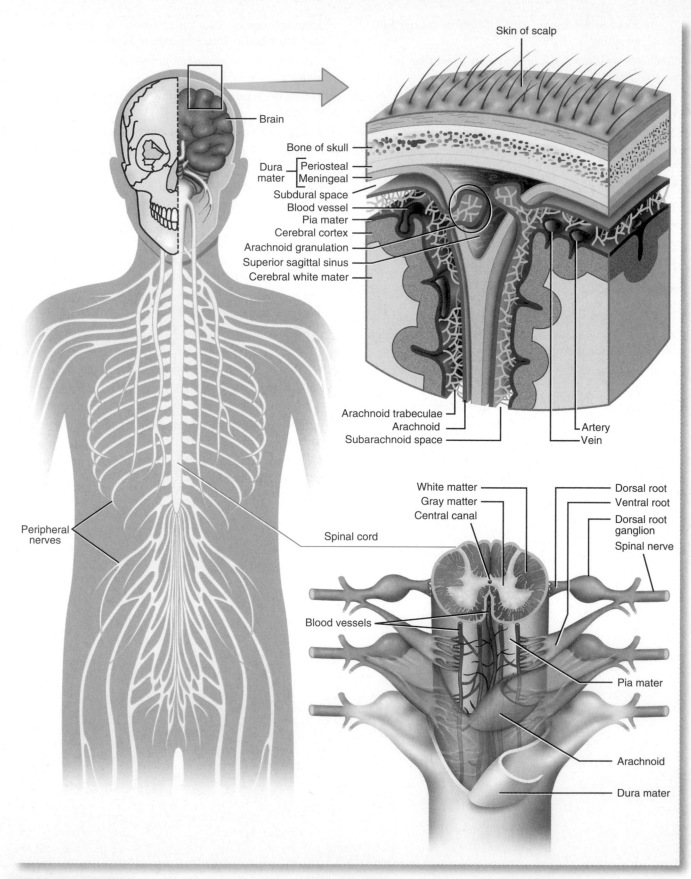

OVERVIEW FIGURE 9.1 ■ Central nervous system (CNS). The CNS is composed of the brain and spinal cord. A section of the brain and spinal cord is illustrated with their protective connective tissue layers called meninges (dura mater, arachnoid mater, and pia mater).

Nervous Tissue ■

SECTION 1 Central Nervous System: Brain and Spinal Cord

Introduction

The mammalian nervous system is the most complex system in the body. It is divided into two major parts: the **central nervous system (CNS)**, which consists of the **brain** and **spinal cord**, which are surrounded and protected by the cranium and vertebral bones, respectively, and the **peripheral nervous system (PNS)**, which is located outside of the CNS and consists of cranial, spinal, and peripheral nerves that conduct information to (afferent or sensory) and from (efferent or motor) the CNS.

Protective Layers of the Central Nervous System

Because the nervous tissue is very delicate, bones, connective tissue layers, and a watery cerebrospinal fluid (CSF) surround and protect the brain and the spinal cord. Deep to the cranial bones in the skull and the vertebral foramen are the meninges, a connective tissue that consists of three distinct layers: the dura mater, arachnoid mater, and pia mater (Overview Figure 9.1).

The outermost meningeal layer is the **dura mater**, a tough, strong, and thick layer of dense connective tissue fibers. Deep to the dura mater is a more delicate connective tissue, the **arachnoid mater**. The dura mater and arachnoid mater surround the brain and spinal cord on their external surfaces. The innermost meningeal layer is the delicate connective tissue **pia mater**. This layer contains numerous blood vessels and adheres directly to the surfaces of the brain and spinal cord.

Between the arachnoid mater and the pia mater is the **subarachnoid space**. Delicate, web-like strands of collagen and elastic fibers attach the arachnoid mater to the pia mater. Filling and circulating in the subarachnoid space is the CSF that bathes and protects both the brain and spinal cord from shock and injury.

Cerebrospinal Fluid

The **CSF** is a clear, colorless fluid that cushions the brain and spinal cord and gives them buoyancy as a means of protection from physical injuries. CSF is continually produced by the **choroid plexuses** in the lateral, third, and fourth ventricles or cavities of the brain, with the majority of the fluid produced in the lateral ventricles. Choroid plexuses are small, vascular extensions of dilated and fenestrated capillaries that penetrate the interior of brain ventricles. Blood is selectively filtered through the cells of the choroids plexus, which results in the production of the CSF. The CSF then circulates through the ventricles and around the outer surfaces of the brain and spinal cord in the subarachnoid space. It also fills the central canal of the spinal cord.

CSF is important for homeostasis and brain metabolism. It brings nutrients to nourish brain cells, removes metabolites that enter the CSF from the brain cells, and provides an optimal chemical environment for neuronal functions and impulse conduction. After circulation, CSF is reabsorbed from the arachnoid space via the **arachnoid villi** into venous blood, mainly at the superior sagittal sinus—a major vein that drains the brain. Arachnoid villi are small, thin-walled arachnoid extensions that penetrate the dura mater and project into the blood-filled venous sinuses located between the periosteal and meningeal layers of dura mater.

Morphology of a Typical Neuron

The nervous system is composed of highly complex intercommunicating networks of nerve cells that receive and conduct **impulses** along their neural pathways or axons to the CNS for analysis, integration, interpretation, and response. Ultimately, the appropriate response to a given stimulus from the neurons of the CNS is the activation of muscle (skeletal, smooth, or cardiac) functions or glandular secretions (endocrine or exocrine).

The structural and functional cells of the nervous tissue are the **neurons**. (The general structure of a neuron and examples of different types of neurons are shown in Overview Figure 9.2.) Although neurons vary in size and shape, the general structure of these cells can be described. Each neuron consists of **soma** or **cell body**, numerous **dendrites**, and a single **axon**. The cell body, or soma, contains the nucleus, nucleolus, numerous different organelles, and the surrounding cytoplasm, or perikaryon. Projecting from the cell body are numerous cytoplasmic extensions called dendrites that form a dendritic tree.

Surrounding the neurons are the smaller and more numerous supportive cells collectively called **neuroglia**. These cells form the nonneural components of the CNS.

Types of Neurons in the Central Nervous System

The three major types of neurons in the nervous system are multipolar, bipolar, and unipolar. This anatomic classification is based on the number of dendrites and axons that originate from the cell body.

- **Multipolar neurons.** These are the most common type in the CNS and include all **motor neurons** and **interneurons** of the brain, cerebellum, and spinal cord. Projecting from the cell body of a multipolar neuron are numerous branched dendrites. On the opposite side of the multipolar neuron is a single axon.
- **Bipolar neurons.** These are not as common and are purely **sensory neurons**. In bipolar neurons, a single dendrite and a single axon are associated with the cell body. Bipolar neurons are found in the retina of the eye, in the organs of hearing and equilibrium in the inner ear, and in the olfactory epithelium in the upper region of the nose (the latter two are found in the PNS).
- **Unipolar neurons.** Most neurons in the adult organism that exhibit only one process leaving the cell body were initially bipolar during embryonic development. The two neuronal processes fuse during later development and form one axon process. This process then divides close to the cell body into two long axonal branches. One of these branches continues to the CNS, whereas the other branch extends to the peripheral organ. The unipolar neurons (formerly called pseudounipolar neurons) are also **sensory**. The cell bodies of unipolar neurons are found in numerous dorsal root ganglia of spinal nerves and cranial nerve ganglia.

Myelin Sheath and Myelination of Axons

Highly specialized cells present in both the CNS and the PNS surround and wrap around the axon multiple times. This process builds up successive layers of modified cell membrane and forms a lipid-rich, insulating sheath around the axon called the **myelin sheath**. As the wrapping around the axon by these cells continues, the cytoplasm is gradually forced or squeezed out from between the membranes of the concentric layers. The myelin sheath extends from the initial segments of the axon to the terminal branches. Interspersed along the length of a myelinated axon are small gaps or spaces in the myelin sheath because the myelin sheath is formed by numerous cells. Where the myelinating cells meet is devoid of myelin. These gaps in myelin sheath between the myelinating cells are called **nodes of Ranvier**. Axons in both the CNS and the PNS can be either myelinated or remain unmyelinated.

In the PNS, all axons are surrounded by specialized **Schwann cells** that either myelinate the axons or envelope the unmyelinated axons with their cytoplasm. Schwann cells myelinate individual peripheral axons and extend along their length, from their origin to their termination in the muscle or gland. In contrast, each Schwann cell cytoplasm can envelope numerous unmyelinated axons. Unmyelinated axons enveloped by Schwann cells do not show nodes of Ranvier. Smaller axons in the peripheral nerves, such as those in the autonomic nervous system (ANS), are unmyelinated and surrounded only by the Schwann cell cytoplasm.

There are no Schwann cells in the CNS. Instead, neuroglial cells called **oligodendrocytes** myelinate the axons in the CNS. Oligodendrocytes differ from Schwann cells in that the cytoplasmic branching processes extend radially from one oligodendrocyte to envelope and myelinate numerous axons.

Gray and White Matter

The brain and the spinal cord contain gray matter and white matter. The **gray matter** of the CNS consists of neurons, their dendrites, and the supportive cells called **neuroglia**. This region also represents the site of connections or **synapses** between a multitude of neurons and dendrites. Gray matter forms the outer surface of the brain (cerebrum) and cerebellum. The size, shape, and mode of branching of these neurons are highly variable and depend on which region of the CNS is examined.

The gray matter also contains a meshwork of neural tissues such as axonal, dendritic, and glial processes that are packed very tightly together and that fill the interneural spaces. This associated meshwork of processes in the gray matter is called the **neuropil**.

White matter in the CNS is devoid of neuronal cell bodies and consists primarily of myelinated axons, some unmyelinated axons, the supportive neuroglial oligodendrocytes, and blood vessels. The myelin sheaths around the axons impart a white color to this region of the CNS.

Synapses

Synapses are specialized sites for chemical or electrical transmission for communication between neurons, interneurons, and effector cells, such as the muscle fibers or glands. Synapses are too small to be visible with routine histologic preparations but can be seen ultrastructurally with transmission electron microscopy. The transmission of an impulse at the synapse is from one **presynaptic** cell to a **postsynaptic** cell and is always unidirectional. Synapses that occur between axons and dendrites are classified as **axodendritic**, between an axon and the neuron cell body as **axosomatic**, and between axons as **axoaxonic**. A typical synapse in the CNS consists of a presynaptic component with a **presynaptic membrane**, a **synaptic cleft**, and a **postsynaptic membrane**. The synaptic cleft separates the presynaptic and postsynaptic membranes.

Supporting Cells in the Central Nervous System: Neuroglia

Neuroglia are the highly branched, supportive, nonneuronal cells in the CNS that surround the neurons, their axons, and dendrites. These cells do not become stimulated or conduct impulses and are morphologically and functionally different from the neurons. Neuroglial cells can be distinguished by their much smaller size and dark-staining nuclei. The CNS contains approximately 10-fold more neuroglial cells than neurons. The four types of neuroglial cells are **astrocytes**, **oligodendrocytes**, **microglia**, and **ependymal cells**.

 Supplemental micrographic images are available at **www.thePoint.com/Eroschenko12e** under Nervous Tissue.

FIGURE 9.1 | Spinal Cord: Midthoracic Region (Transverse Section)

The transverse section of a spinal cord cut in the midthoracic region and stained with hematoxylin and eosin is illustrated. Although a basic structural pattern is seen throughout the spinal cord, the shape and structure of the cord vary at different levels (cervical, thoracic, lumbar, and sacral).

The thoracic region of the spinal cord differs from the cervical region illustrated in Figure 9.3. The thoracic spinal cord exhibits slender **posterior gray horns (6)** and smaller **anterior gray horns (10, 20)** with fewer **motor neurons (10, 20)**. The **lateral gray horns (8, 19)**, on the other hand, are well developed in the thoracic region of the spinal cord. These contain the **motor neurons (8, 19)** of the sympathetic division of the ANS.

The remaining structures in the midthoracic region of the spinal cord closely correspond to the structures illustrated in the cervical cord region in Figure 9.3. These are the **posterior median sulcus (15)**, **anterior median fissure (22)**, **fasciculus gracilis (16)** and **fasciculus cuneatus (17)** (seen in the mid-to-upper-thoracic region of the spinal cord) of the **posterior white column (16, 17)**, **lateral white column (7)**, **central canal (9)**, and the **gray commissure (18)**. Associated with the posterior gray horns (6) are axons of the **posterior roots (5)**, and leaving the anterior gray horns (10, 20) are the **axons (11, 21)** of the **anterior roots (11)**.

Surrounding the spinal cord are the connective tissue layers of the meninges. These are the thick and fibrous outer **dura mater (2)**, the thinner and middle **arachnoid mater (3)**, and the delicate inner **pia mater (4)**, which closely adheres to the surface of the spinal cord. Located in the pia mater (4) are numerous anterior and posterior **spinal blood vessels (1, 12)** of various sizes. Between the arachnoid (3) and the pia mater (4) is the **subarachnoid space (14)**. Fine trabeculae located in the subarachnoid space (14) connect the pia mater (4) with the arachnoid mater (3). In life, the subarachnoid space (14) is filled with circulating CSF. Between the arachnoid mater (3) and the dura mater (2) is the **subdural space (13)**. In this preparation, the subdural space (13) appears unusually large because of the artifactual retraction of the arachnoid during the specimen preparation.

FIGURE 9.2 | Spinal Cord: Anterior Gray Horn, Motor Neurons, and Adjacent Anterior White Matter

A higher magnification of a small section of the spinal cord illustrates the appearance of **white matter**, **gray matter**, neurons, **neuroglia**, and axons stained with hematoxylin and eosin. The cells in the anterior gray horn of the thoracic region of the spinal cord are **multipolar motor neurons (2, 7, 10)**. The cytoplasm is characterized by a prominent vesicular **nucleus (10)**, a distinct **nucleolus (10)**, and coarse clumps of basophilic material called the **Nissl substance (3)**. The Nissl substance extends into the **dendrites** but not into the axons. Two of the neurons exhibit the axons and their **axon hillocks (4, 9)**, which is devoid of the Nissl substance; this feature characterizes the axon hillock. In certain **multipolar neurons (7)**, the plane of section did not pass through the nucleus, and, as a result, the cytoplasm appears enucleated (without a nucleus) and exhibits only the Nissl substance in the cytoplasm.

The nonneural supportive neuroglia (8), seen here only as basophilic nuclei, are small in comparison to the prominent multipolar neurons (2, 7, 10). The neuroglia (8) occupy the spaces between the neurons. The anterior white matter of the spinal cord contains myelinated axons of various sizes. Because of the chemicals used in the histologic preparation of this section, the myelin sheaths were dissolved and appear only as clear spaces around the dark-staining **axons (5)**. Also visible in the image are capillaries, venules, and an **arteriole (6)**.

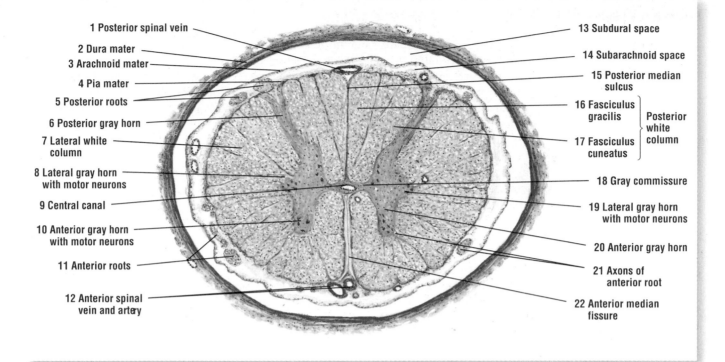

FIGURE 9.1 ■ Spinal cord: midthoracic region (transverse section). Stain: hematoxylin and eosin. Low magnification.

FIGURE 9.2 ■ Spinal cord: anterior gray horn, motor neuron, and adjacent white matter. Stain: hematoxylin and eosin. Medium magnification.

FIGURE 9.3 | Spinal Cord: Midcervical Region (Transverse Section)

To illustrate the **white matter** and the **gray matter** of the spinal cord, a cross section of the cord was prepared with the silver impregnation technique. After staining, the dark brown, outer white matter (3) and the light-staining, inner gray matter (4, 14) are clearly visible. The white matter (3) consists primarily of ascending and descending myelinated nerve fibers, or axons. By contrast, the gray matter contains the cell bodies of neurons and interneurons. The gray matter also exhibits a symmetrical H-shape, with the two sides connected across the midline of the spinal cord by the **gray commissure (15)**. The center of the gray commissure is located at the **central canal (16)** of the spinal cord.

The anterior **horns (6)** of the gray matter extend toward the front of the cord and are more prominent than the **posterior horns (2, 13)**. The anterior horns contain the cell bodies of the large **motor neurons (7, 17)**. Some **axons (8, 20)** from the motor neurons of the anterior horns cross the white matter and exit from the spinal cord as components of the **anterior roots (9, 21)** of the peripheral nerves. The posterior horns (2, 13) are the sensory areas and contain cell bodies of smaller neurons.

The spinal cord is surrounded by connective tissue meninges, consisting of an outer dura mater, a middle **arachnoid mater (5)**, and an inner **pia mater (18)**. The spinal cord is also partially divided into right and left halves by a narrow, posterior (dorsal) groove—the **posterior median sulcus (10)**—and a deep, anterior (ventral) cleft—the **anterior median fissure (19)**. In this illustration, pia mater (18) is best seen in the **anterior median fissure (19)**.

Between the posterior median sulcus (10) and the posterior horns (2, 13) of the gray matter are the prominent posterior columns of the white matter. In this midcervical region of the spinal cord, each dorsal column is subdivided into two fascicles, the posteromedial column—the **fasciculus gracilis (11)**—and the posterolateral column—the **fasciculus cuneatus (1, 12)**.

FIGURE 9.4 | Spinal Cord: Anterior Gray Horn, Motor Neurons, and Adjacent Anterior White Matter

A small section of the white matter and the gray matter of the anterior horn of the spinal cord are illustrated at a higher magnification. The gray matter of the anterior horn contains large, **multipolar motor neurons (2, 3)**. These are characterized by numerous **dendrites (5, 6)** that extend in different directions from the perikaryon (cell bodies). In some sections of the neurons, the **nucleus (8)** is visible with its prominent **nucleolus (8)**. In other neurons, the plane of section has missed the nucleus and the perikaryon appears empty (2). Located in the vicinity of the motor neurons are the small, light-staining, supportive cells, the **neuroglia (7)**.

The white matter contains closely packed groups of myelinated axons. In cross sections, the **axons (1)** appear dark-stained and surrounded by clear spaces, which are the remnants of the myelin sheaths. The axons of the white matter represent the ascending and descending tracts of the spinal cord. On the other hand, the **axons (4)** of the anterior horn motor neurons aggregate into groups, pass through the white matter, and exit from the spinal cord as the anterior (ventral) root fibers (see Figure 9.3).

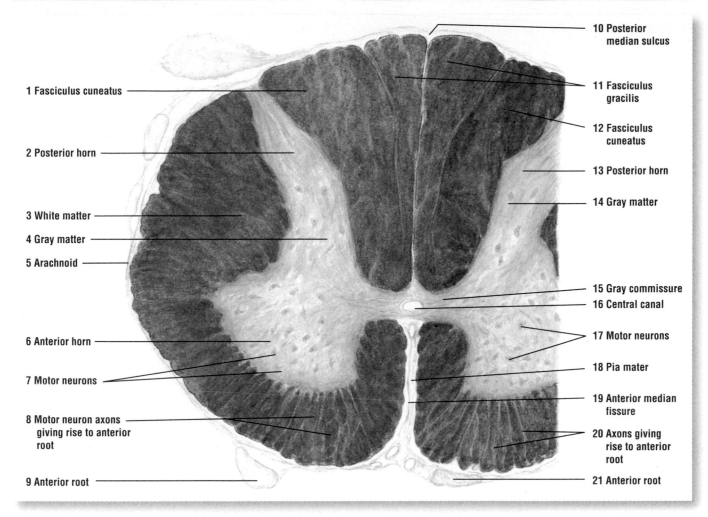

1 Fasciculus cuneatus

2 Posterior horn

3 White matter

4 Gray matter

5 Arachnoid

6 Anterior horn

7 Motor neurons

8 Motor neuron axons giving rise to anterior root

9 Anterior root

10 Posterior median sulcus

11 Fasciculus gracilis

12 Fasciculus cuneatus

13 Posterior horn

14 Gray matter

15 Gray commissure

16 Central canal

17 Motor neurons

18 Pia mater

19 Anterior median fissure

20 Axons giving rise to anterior root

21 Anterior root

FIGURE 9.3 ■ Spinal cord: midcervical region (transverse section). Stain: silver impregnation (Cajal method). Low magnification.

White matter

Gray matter of anterior horn

1 Axons

2 Multipolar motor neuron (plane of section missed nucleus)

3 Multipolar motor neurons

4 Axons of motor neurons entering white matter

5 Dendrites

6 Dendrite

7 Neuroglia

8 Nucleolus and nucleus of anterior horn cell

FIGURE 9.4 ■ Spinal cord: anterior gray horn, motor neurons, and adjacent anterior white matter. Stain: silver impregnation (Cajal method). Medium magnification.

FIGURE 9.5 | Ultrastructure of Typical Axodendritic Synapses in the CNS

It is not possible to see synapses in the CNS with routine hematoxylin and eosin preparations. This high magnification transmission electron micrograph shows two typical **axodendritic synapses (2, 4)** in the CNS. The terminal end of the **presynaptic component (1, 3)** is somewhat expanded and contains numerous small **neurotransmitter vesicles (1, 3)**. A small intercellular space, called the **synaptic cleft (2, 4)**, is located between and separates the **presynaptic membrane (2, 4)** from the **postsynaptic membranes (8)**. The postsynaptic membranes (8) appear thicker and denser than the presynaptic membrane (2, 4). In the center of the image is a section of a **dendrite (7)** with **neurofilaments**, **microtubules**, and large **mitochondria (7)**. Located peripherally around the dendrite (7) are numerous smaller **myelinated axons (5)** surrounded by a dense, thick **myelin sheath (9)**. In the upper region of the figure are numerous **unmyelinated axons (6)**. Also visible in both the myelinated axons (5) and the unmyelinated axons (6, 7) are dark-staining, oval **mitochondria (6)** with shelflike cristae.

FUNCTIONAL CORRELATIONS 9.1 | Synapses

Synapses are specialized membrane junctions where transmissions of nerve impulses are conveyed unidirectionally from a **presynaptic** neuron to a **postsynaptic** membrane of a neuron; effector cells, such as muscle fibers; or gland cells. The major function of the synapse is to process and convert an impulse from the presynaptic cell into a signal that affects the postsynaptic cell membranes and initiates neuronal activities. Most synapses in mammals release chemical **neurotransmitters** from the presynaptic portion of one axon or dendrite to the postsynaptic membrane of another cell. Neurotransmitter chemicals must first cross the **synaptic cleft** and bind to specific **neurotransmitter receptors** on the postsynaptic membrane to produce an effect. The release of neurotransmitters from the presynaptic portion can produce either an **excitatory** response or an **inhibitory** response at the postsynaptic membrane. The final generation of nerve impulse in a postsynaptic cell depends on the summation of excitatory or inhibitory effects of many synapses on the target cell, which allows for a more precise regulation of responses from postsynaptic neurons, muscles, or glands. Thus, the synapses regulate neuronal activity in the nervous system by inducing either excitatory or inhibitory effects on the target cells. Once the neurotransmitters induce their effects on the target cell, the neurotransmitter chemicals are rapidly removed from the synaptic cleft by enzymes, diffusion, or endocytosis.

1 Neurotransmitter vesicles in presynaptic component

2 Presynaptic membrane and synaptic cleft of a synapse

3 Neurotransmitter vesicles in presynaptic component

4 Presynaptic membrane and synaptic cleft of a synapse

5 Myelinated axons

6 Mitochondria in unmyelinated axons

7 Dendrite with neurofilaments, microtubules, and mitochondria

8 Postsynaptic membranes

9 Myelin sheath

FIGURE 9.5 ■ Ultrastructure of typical axodendritic synapses in the CNS. Transmission electron micrograph. Courtesy of Dr. Mark DeSantis, Professor Emeritus, WWAMI Medical Program, University of Idaho, Moscow, Idaho. ×75,000.

FIGURE 9.6 | Motor Neurons: Anterior Horn of the Spinal Cord

The large, multipolar **motor neurons (7)** of the CNS have a large central **nucleus (11)**, a prominent **nucleolus (12)**, and several radiating cell processes—the **dendrites (10, 16)**. A single, thin **axon (5, 14)** arises from a cone-shaped, clear area of the neuron; this is the **axon hillock (6, 13)**. The axons (5, 14) that leave the motor neurons (7) are thinner and much longer than the thicker but have shorter dendrites (10, 16).

The cytoplasm, or perikaryon, of the neuron is characterized by numerous clumps of coarse granules (basophilic masses). These are the **Nissl bodies (4, 8)**, and they represent the granular endoplasmic reticulum of the neuron. When the plane of section misses the nucleus (4), only the dark-staining Nissl bodies (4) are seen in the perikaryon of the neuron. The Nissl bodies (4, 8) extend into the dendrites (10, 16) but not into the axon hillock (6, 13) or into the axon (5, 14). This feature distinguishes the axons (5, 14) from the dendrites (10, 16). The nucleus of the neuron is outlined distinctly and stains light because of the uniform dispersion of the chromatin. The nucleolus (12), on the other hand, is prominent, dense, and stains dark. The **nuclei (2, 9)** of the surrounding **neuroglia (2, 9)** are stained prominently, whereas their small cytoplasm remains unstained. The neuroglia (2, 9) are nonneural cells of the CNS; they provide the structural and metabolic support for the neurons (7).

Surrounding the neurons (7) and the neuroglia (2, 9) are numerous **blood vessels (1, 3, 15)** of various sizes.

FUNCTIONAL CORRELATIONS 9.2 | Neurons, Interneurons, Axons, and Dendrites

Functionally, neurons are classified as **afferent** (sensory), **efferent** (motor), or **interneurons**. Sensory or afferent neurons conduct impulses from receptors in the internal organs or from the external environment to the CNS. **Somatic afferent** fibers conduct impulses from the body surface and body organs, such as muscles, tendons, and joints. **Visceral afferent** fibers conduct impulses from internal organs, glands, and blood vessels. Motor, or efferent, fibers convey impulses from the CNS to the effector muscles or glands in the peripheries. Interneurons constitute the majority of the neurons in the CNS. They serve as intermediaries or integrators of nerve impulses and connect neuronal circuits between sensory neurons, motor neurons, and other interneurons in the CNS.

Neurons are highly specialized for **irritability**, **conductivity**, and **synthesis** of neuroactive substances, such as **neurotransmitters** and **neurohormones**. After a mechanical or chemical stimulus, these neurons react (irritability) to the stimulus and transmit (conductivity) the information via axons to other neurons or interneurons in different regions of the nervous system. Strong stimuli create a wave of excitation, or nerve impulse (action potential), which is then propagated along the entire length of the axon (nerve fiber).

Extending from the neurons are numerous dendrites that divide in a treelike fashion, which allows the dendrites to connect with and receive stimuli from many axon terminals of other neurons. The surface of the dendrites is covered by **dendritic spines** that connect (synapse) with axon terminals from other neurons. The surface membrane of the neuron and the dendrites are specialized to receive and to integrate information from other dendrites, neurons, or axons. The axons, in turn, conduct the received information away from the neuron to an interneuron; another neuron; or to an effector organ, such as a muscle or gland.

Axons arise from the funnel-shaped region of the cell body called the **axon hillock**. The **initial segment** of the axon is located between the axon hillock and where myelination starts. It is at the initial segment that the stimuli, whether inhibitory or stimulatory, are summated and the resulting nerve stimuli are generated. The rate

FUNCTIONAL CORRELATIONS 9.2	Neurons, Interneurons, Axons, and Dendrites *(Continued)*

of conduction of the stimulus is dependent on the size of the axon and myelination. Myelinated axons conduct impulses at a much faster rate (velocity) than the unmyelinated axons of the same size. To initiate a nerve impulse, neurotransmitters are released at different synapses.

In addition to conducting impulses, axons also exhibit a **bidirectional transport** of chemical substances, organelles, or membrane-bound neurotransmitters between the neuron and the axon terminals. Materials that are first synthesized in the neurons are then transported in tiny tubules called **microtubules** to the region where the axon terminates or **synapses** with other dendrites, a cell body, or other axons. This method of movement in axons is called **anterograde transport**. Similar material carried away from the axon terminals and dendrites toward the nerve cells body is called **retrograde transport**. Transport by microtubules in either direction requires the expenditure of energy, which is used by microtubule-associated motor proteins. The mechanism for anterograde transport involves **kinesin**, a microtubule-associated motor protein that directs substances along the microtubules in axons away from the neuron. The retrograde transport in axons toward the neurons is mediated by another microtubule-associated motor protein called **dynein**.

In addition, microtubules and microfilaments serve an important role in the growth of axons during development and in their regeneration following an injury.

1 Arteriole

2 Nuclei of neuroglia

3 Capillary

4 Nissl bodies

5 Axon

6 Axon hillock

7 Motor neuron

8 Nissl bodies

9 Nuclei of neuroglia

10 Dendrites

11 Nucleus

12 Nucleolus

13 Axon hillock

14 Axon

15 Venule

16 Dendrites

FIGURE 9.6 ■ Motor neurons: anterior horn of the spinal cord. Stain: hematoxylin and eosin. High magnification.

FIGURE 9.7 | Neurofibrils and Motor Neurons in the Gray Matter of the Anterior Horn of the Spinal Cord

This section of the anterior horn of the spinal cord was prepared by silver impregnation (the Cajal method) to demonstrate the distribution of **neurofibrils** in both the **gray matter** and **motor neurons**. Fine neurofibrils (2, 4) are distributed throughout the **cytoplasm (perikaryon) (4)** and **dendrites (2, 9)** of the motor neurons (1, 10, 11).

Because of the silver impregnation technique, axons and additional details of the motor neurons are not visible. The nuclei of the **motor neurons (1, 11)** appear yellow stained and their **nucleoli (5, 10)** appear dark stained. Not all motor neurons were sectioned through the middle. As a result, some motor neurons show only a **nucleus (1)** without a nucleolus, whereas others show only the **peripheral cytoplasm (8)** without a nucleus.

There are also many neurofibrils in the gray matter (3). Some of these neurofibrils (3) belong to the axons of anterior horn neurons (1, 11) or the adjacent **neuroglia (7)**, whose **nuclei (7)** are visible throughout the gray matter (3) (see also Figure 9.8).

The clear spaces around the neurons and their processes are artifacts that were caused by the chemical preparations of the nervous tissue.

FIGURE 9.8 | Anterior Gray Horn of Spinal Cord: Multipolar Motor Neurons, Axons, and Neuroglial Cells

This medium-magnification photomicrograph of the anterior horn of the spinal cord was prepared with silver stain to show the morphology of neurons and **axons** of the CNS. The large multipolar **motor neurons (1)** of the gray horn exhibit numerous **dendrites (4)**. Each motor neuron (1) contains a distinct **nucleus (5)** and a prominent **nucleolus (6)**. Within the cytoplasm of the motor neurons (1) is the cytoskeleton, which consists of numerous **neurofibrils (3)** that course through the cell body and extend into the dendrites (4) and axons (8). Coursing past the motor neurons (1) are numerous axons of a size different from that of the other nerve cells in the spinal cord. Surrounding the motor neurons (1) are numerous **nuclei** of **neuroglial cells (2)** and a **blood vessel (7)** with blood cells.

Similar to what is seen in Figure 9.6, the clear spaces around the neurons and their processes are artifacts caused by tissue shrinkage during the preparation of the spinal cord.

1 Nucleus of motor neuron

2 Neurofibrils in dendrites

3 Gray matter

4 Neurofibrils in cytoplasm

5 Nucleolus

6 Neurofibrils in gray matter

7 Nuclei of neuroglia

8 Peripheral section of motor neuron

9 Dendrites

10 Nucleolus of motor neuron

11 Nucleus of motor neuron

FIGURE 9.7 ■ Neurofibrils and motor neurons in the gray matter of the anterior horn of the spinal cord. Stain: silver impregnation (Cajal method). High magnification.

1 Motor neurons

2 Nuclei of neuroglial cells

3 Neurofibrils

4 Dendrites

5 Nucleus

6 Nucleolus

7 Blood vessel

8 Axons

FIGURE 9.8 ■ Anterior gray horn of the spinal cord: multipolar neurons, axons, and neuroglial cells. Stain: silver impregnation (Cajal method). ×80.

FIGURE 9.9 | Cerebral Cortex: Gray Matter

The different cell types that constitute the gray matter of the cerebral cortex are distributed in six layers, with one or more cell types predominant in each layer. Although there are variations in the arrangement of cells in different parts of the cerebral cortex, distinct layers are recognized in most regions. Horizontal and radial axons associated with neuronal cells in different layers give the cerebral cortex a laminated appearance. The different layers are labeled with Roman numerals on the right side of the figure.

The most superficial is the **molecular layer (I)**. Overlying and covering the molecular cell layer (I) is the delicate connective tissue of the brain, the **pia mater (1)**. The peripheral portion of molecular layer (I) is composed predominantly of **neuroglial cells (2)** and horizontal cells of Cajal. Their axons contribute to the horizontal fibers that are seen in the molecular layer (I).

The external **granular layer (II)** contains mainly different types of neuroglial cells and **small pyramidal cells (3)**. Note that the pyramidal cells get progressively larger in successively deeper layers of the cortex. The **apical dendrites** of the **pyramidal cells (4, 7)** are directed toward the periphery of the cortex, whereas their axons extend from the cell bases (see Figure 9.10 [4, 10]). In the **external pyramidal layer (III)**, **medium-sized pyramidal cells (5)** predominate. The **internal granular layer (IV)** is a thin layer and contains mainly small **granule cells (6)**, some pyramidal cells, and different neuroglia that form numerous complex connections with the pyramidal cells. The **internal pyramidal layer (V)** contains numerous neuroglial cells and the largest **pyramidal cells (8)**, especially in the motor area of the cerebral cortex. The deepest layer is the **multiform layer (VI)**. This layer is adjacent to the **white matter (10)** of the cerebral cortex. The multiform layer (VI) contains intermixed cells of varying shapes and sizes, such as the fusiform cells, granule cells, stellate cells, and cells of Martinotti. **Bundles of axons (9)** enter and leave the white matter (10).

1 Pia mater with blood vessel

2 Neuroglial cells

3 Small pyramidal cells

4 Apical dendrites of pyramidal cells

5 Medium-sized pyramidal cells

6 Granule cells

7 Dendrites of pyramidal cells

8 Large pyramidal cells

9 Bundles of axons

10 White matter

I. Molecular layer

II. External granular layer

III. External pyramidal layer

IV. Internal granular layer

V. Internal pyramidal layer

VI. Multiform layer

FIGURE 9.9 ■ Cerebral cortex: gray matter: Stain: silver impregnation (Cajal method). Low magnification.

FIGURE 9.10 | Layer V of the Cerebral Cortex

A higher magnification of layer V of the cerebral cortex illustrates the large **pyramidal cells (3)**. Note the typical large vesicular **nucleus (3)** with its prominent **nucleolus (3)**. The silver stain also shows the presence of numerous **neurofibrils (9)** in the pyramidal cells (3). The most prominent cell processes are the **apical dendrites (1, 7)** of the pyramidal cells (3), which are directed toward the surface of the cortex. The **axons (4, 10)** of the pyramidal cells (3) arise from the base of the cell body and pass into the white matter (see Figure 9.9 [10]).

The intercellular area is occupied by **neuroglial cells (2, 8)** in the cortex, small astrocytes, and blood vessels—**venule (5)** and **capillary (6)**.

FIGURE 9.11 | Cerebellum (Transverse Section)

The **cerebellar cortex (1, 10)** exhibits numerous deeply convoluted folds called **cerebellar folia (6)** (singular: folium) separated by **sulci (9)**. The cerebellar folia (6) are covered by the thin connective tissue, the **pia mater (7)**, which follows the surface of each folium (6) into the adjacent sulci (9). The detachment of the pia mater (7) from the cerebellar cortex (1, 10) is an artifact caused by tissue fixation and preparation.

The cerebellum (1, 10) consists of an outer **gray matter or cortex (1, 10)** and an inner **white matter (5, 8)**. Three distinct cell layers can be distinguished in the cerebellar cortex (1, 10): an outer **molecular layer (2)** with relatively fewer and smaller neuronal cell bodies and many fibers that extend parallel to the length of the folium; a central or middle **Purkinje cell layer (3)**; and an inner **granular layer (4)** with numerous small neurons that exhibit intensely stained nuclei. The Purkinje cells (3) are pyriform, or pyramidal, in shape with ramified dendrites that extend into the molecular layer (2).

The white matter (5, 8) forms the core of each cerebellar folium (6) and consists of myelinated nerve fibers, or axons. The nerve axons are the afferent and efferent fibers of the cerebellar cortex.

1 Apical dendrite of pyramidal cell

2 Neuroglial cells

3 Pyramidal cells with nucleus and nucleolus

4 Axon of pyramidal cell

5 Venule

6 Capillary

7 Apical dendrites of pyramidal cells

8 Neuroglial cells

9 Neurofibrils

10 Axon of pyramidal cell

FIGURE 9.10 ■ Layer V of the cerebral cortex. Stain: silver impregnation (Cajal method). High magnification.

1 Cerebellar cortex: gray matter

2 Cerebellar cortex: molecular layer

3 Purkinje cell layer

4 Cerebellar cortex: granular layer

5 White matter

6 Cerebellar folium

7 Pia matter

8 White matter

9 Sulci

10 Cerebellar cortex: gray matter

FIGURE 9.11 ■ Cerebellum (transverse section). Stain: silver impregnation (Cajal method). Low magnification.

FIGURE 9.12 | Cerebellar Cortex: Molecular Layer, Purkinje Cell Layer, and Granular Cell Layer

This illustration shows a small section of the cerebellar cortex above the white matter at a higher magnification. The **Purkinje cells (3)** comprising the **Purkinje cell layer (7)**, with their prominent nuclei and nucleoli, are arranged in a single row between the **molecular cell layer (6)** and the **granular cell layer (4)**. The large "flask-shaped" bodies of the Purkinje cells (3, 7) give off thick **dendrites (2)** that branch extensively throughout the molecular cell layer (6) to the cerebellar surface. Thin axons (not shown) leave the base of the Purkinje cells, pass through the granular cell layer (4), become myelinated, and enter the **white matter (5, 11)**.

The molecular cell layer (6) contains scattered **basket cells (1)** with unmyelinated axons that normally course horizontally. Descending collaterals of more deeply placed basket cells (1) arborize around the Purkinje cells (3, 7). Axons of the **granule cells (9)** in the granular cell layer (4) extend into the molecular layer (6) and also course horizontally as unmyelinated axons.

In the granular cell layer (4) are numerous small granule cells (9) with dark-staining nuclei and a small amount of cytoplasm. Also scattered in the granular cell layer (4) are larger **Golgi type II cells (8)** with typical vesicular nuclei and more cytoplasm. Throughout the granular layer are small, irregularly dispersed, clear spaces called the **glomeruli (10)**. These regions contain only synaptic complexes.

1 Basket cells

2 Dendrite of Purkinje cells

3 Purkinje cells with nucleus and nucleolus

4 Granular cell layer

5 White matter

6 Molecular cell layer

7 Purkinje cell layer

8 Golgi type II cells

9 Granule cells

10 Glomeruli

11 Axons

FIGURE 9.12 ■ Cerebellar cortex: molecular, Purkinje cell, and granular cell layers. Stain: silver impregnation (Cajal method). High magnification.

FIGURE 9.13 | Fibrous Astrocytes of the Brain

A section of the brain was prepared by the Cajal method to demonstrate the supportive **neuroglial** cells called astrocytes. The **fibrous astrocytes (2, 5)** exhibit a small **cell body (5)**, a large oval **nucleus (5)**, and a **dark-stained nucleolus (5)**. Extending from the cell body are long, thin, and smooth radiating **processes (4, 6)** that are found between the neurons and blood vessels. A **perivascular fibrous astrocyte (2)** surrounds a **capillary (8)** with red blood cells (erythrocytes). From other fibrous astrocytes (2, 5), the long processes (4, 6) extend to and terminate on the capillary (8) as **perivascular endfeet (3, 7)**.

Also seen in the illustration are nuclei of different neuroglial (1) cells of the brain.

FIGURE 9.14 | Ultrastructure of a Capillary in the Central Nervous System and the Perivascular Endfeet of Astrocytes

This transmission electron micrograph shows a cross section of a continuous type of capillary in the CNS. Lining the **capillary lumen** is a thin endothelial layer and the nucleus of an **endothelial cell (2)**. Attached externally to the **capillary wall (5)** are numerous **perivascular endfeet of astrocytes (3, 4)** that completely envelop the capillary wall (5) to form part of the blood–brain barrier. Surrounding the capillary wall (5) and the endfeet of astrocytes (3, 4) is the **CNS neuropil (1)**, a dense meshwork of fibers from axons, dendrites, and various glial cells that fills the spaces in the CNS. Located below the capillary are a few **myelinated axons (6)** that were myelinated in the CNS by oligodendrocytes (not illustrated).

1 Nuclei of neuroglia

2 Perivascular fibrous astrocyte

3 Perivascular endfeet of fibrous astrocyte

4 Processes of fibrous astrocyte

5 Fibrous astrocyte: cell body, nucleus, and nucleolus

6 Processes of fibrous astrocyte

7 Perivascular endfeet of fibrous astrocyte

8 Capillary with red blood cells

FIGURE 9.13 ■ Fibrous astrocytes and capillary in the brain. Stain: silver impregnation (Cajal method). Medium magnification.

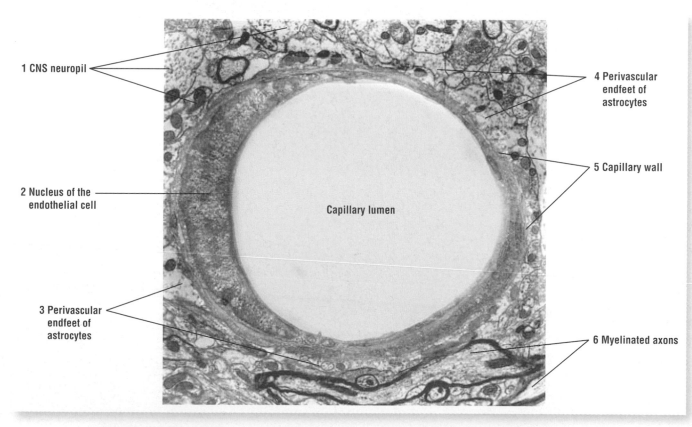

1 CNS neuropil

2 Nucleus of the endothelial cell

3 Perivascular endfeet of astrocytes

4 Perivascular endfeet of astrocytes

5 Capillary wall

6 Myelinated axons

Capillary lumen

FIGURE 9.14 ■ Ultrastructure of a capillary in the CNS and the perivascular endfeet of astrocytes. Transmission electron micrograph. Courtesy of Dr. Mark DeSantis, Professor Emeritus, WWAMI. Medical Program, University of Idaho, Moscow, Idaho. ×20,000.

FIGURE 9.15 | Oligodendrocytes of the Brain

This section of the brain was also prepared with the Cajal method to show the supportive neuroglial cells called **oligodendrocytes (1, 4, 7)**. In comparison to a **fibrous astrocyte (3)**, the oligodendrocytes (1, 4, 7) are smaller and exhibit few, thin, short processes without excessive branching.

The oligodendrocytes (1, 4, 7) are found in both the gray and white matter of the CNS. In the white matter, the oligodendrocytes form myelin sheaths around numerous axons and are analogous to the Schwann cells that myelinate individual axons in the nerves of the PNS.

Two **neurons (2, 6)** are also illustrated to contrast their size with those of a fibrous astrocyte (3) and the oligodendrocytes (1, 4, 7). A **capillary (5)** passes between the different cells.

FIGURE 9.16 | Ultrastructure of an Oligodendrocyte in the Central Nervous System with Myelinated Axons

This transmission electron micrograph illustrates in greater detail the internal morphology of the **oligodendrocyte (2)**, which is the myelin-producing cell of the CNS. The cytoplasm of the cell exhibits a well-developed **granular endoplasmic reticulum (3, 5)**, a **Golgi apparatus (6)**, and numerous free ribosomes scattered around the organelles. Numerous **myelinated axons (1, 4, 8)**, cut in cross section and longitudinal section, are surrounded with dense **myelin sheaths (7)** that are also closely associated with the cytoplasm of the oligodendrocyte. Located in the myelinated axons (1, 4) are oval, dark-staining **mitochondria (4)** and numerous **neurofilaments (8)**.

1 Oligodendrocyte
2 Neuron
3 Fibrous astrocyte
4 Oligodendrocyte
5 Capillary
6 Neuron
7 Oligodendrocyte

FIGURE 9.15 ■ Oligodendrocytes of the brain. Stain: silver impregnation (Cajal method). Medium magnification.

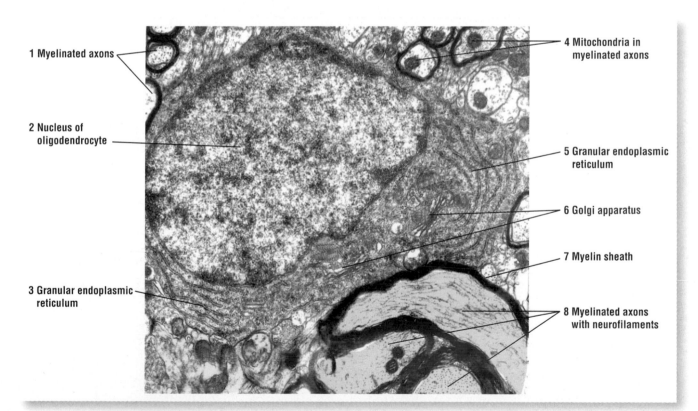

1 Myelinated axons
2 Nucleus of oligodendrocyte
3 Granular endoplasmic reticulum
4 Mitochondria in myelinated axons
5 Granular endoplasmic reticulum
6 Golgi apparatus
7 Myelin sheath
8 Myelinated axons with neurofilaments

FIGURE 9.16 ■ Ultrastructure of an oligodendrocyte in the CNS with myelinated axons. Transmission electron micrograph. Courtesy of Dr. Mark DeSantis, Professor Emeritus, WWAMI Medical Program, University of Idaho, Mascow, Idaho. ×25,000.

FIGURE 9.17 | Ultrastructure of Myelinated axons in the CNS with a Node of Ranvier

A transmission electron micrograph shows in more detail a **myelinated axon** (7) sectioned in a longitudinal plane and a cross section of a **myelinated axon** (2) in close association with the cytoplasm and the organelles of the myelinating cell, the oligodendrocyte. Because the **myelin sheath** is not continuous along the entire length of an axon, there is a small nodal gap called the **node of Ranvier** (4). This region is located where myelin sheaths (5, 6) are absent, and the axon is surrounded by the processes or loops containing the **cellular cytoplasm** (3, 8) of the oligodendrocyte that covers and contacts the axon. At the node of Ranvier (4), the oligodendrocyte cell cytoplasm (3, 8) was not completely displaced to the cell body during the wrapping of the cell around the axon and formation of the myelin sheath (5, 6). Located in the myelinated axons (2) are numerous **neurofilaments** (2, 7) and dark-staining **mitochondria** (1). Located near the myelinated axon (7) are cross sections of **unmyelinated axons** (9) and the **cytoplasm** (10) of an adjacent cell.

1 Mitochondria

2 Myelinated axon
   with neurofilaments

3 Celluar cytoplasm

4 Node of Ranvier

5 Myelin sheath

6 Myelin sheath

7 Myelinated axon
   with neurofilaments

8 Cellular cytoplasm

9 Unmyelinated axons

10 Cytoplasm of
   adjacent cell

FIGURE 9.17 ■ Ultrastructure of myelinated axons in the CNS with a node of Ranvier.
Transmission electron micrograph. Courtesy of Dr. Mark DeSantis, Professor Emeritus, WWAMI
Medical Program, University of Idaho, Mascow, Idaho. Approximately ×55,000.

FIGURE 9.18 | Microglia of the Brain

This section of the brain was prepared with the Hortega method to show the smallest neuroglial cells called **microglia (2, 3)**. The microglia (2, 3) vary in shape and often exhibit irregular contours, and the small, deeply stained nucleus almost fills the entire cell. The cell processes of the microglia (2, 3) are few, short, and slender. Both the cell body and the processes of microglia (2, 3) are covered with small spines. Two **neurons (1)** and a **capillary** with **red blood cells (erythrocytes) (4)** provide a size comparison with the microglia (2, 3).

Microglia are found in both the white and gray matter of the CNS and are the main phagocytes of the CNS.

FUNCTIONAL CORRELATIONS 9.3 | Neuroglia

There are four types of neuroglial cells recognized in the CNS: astrocytes, oligodendrocytes, microglia, and ependymal cells.

Astrocytes are the largest and most abundant neuroglia cells in the gray matter and consist of two types: fibrous astrocytes and protoplasmic astrocytes. In the CNS, both types of astrocytes abut on the surfaces of **capillaries** and **neurons**. Their perivascular endfeet cover the capillary basement membrane, form the tight junctions around the capillaries, and produce part of the **blood–brain barrier.** The blood–brain barrier is a physiologic barrier that regulates the passage of various substances from blood to brain. This allows for a more stable and balanced ionic composition in the interstitial neuronal environment and protects the cells from any potentially harmful substances. The branched processes of astrocytes also extend to the basal lamina of the pia mater to form an impermeable barrier, the **glia limitans,** or glial limiting membrane, which surrounds the brain and spinal cord. They support **metabolic exchange** between the neurons and capillaries of the CNS. In addition, the astrocytes control the **chemical environment** around neurons by clearing intercellular spaces of increased **potassium ions** and released **neurotransmitters,** such as **glutamate,** at active synaptic sites to maintain a proper ionic environment for their function. If these metabolic chemicals are not quickly removed from these sites, they can interfere with proper neuronal functions. Astrocytes remove glutamate and convert it to glutamine, which is then returned to the neurons. Astrocytes also contain reserves of glycogen that they release as glucose and, in this manner, contribute to the energy metabolism of the CNS. Also, the presence of gap junctions allows the astrocytes to form a structural syncytium in the CNS and form a communicating network in the brain. In response to brain injury, the astrocytes exhibit mitosis, proliferate, and form a scar.

Oligodendrocytes are smaller than astrocytes with fewer cytoplasmic processes. Oligodendrocytes produce and **myelinate** the axons in the CNS to provide for their insulation. Because oligodendrocytes have several cytoplasmic processes, a single oligodendrocyte can surround and myelinate several axons. As a result, oligodendrocytes do not surround multiple unmyelinated axons. During myelination, the plasma membrane of the oligodendrocyte is wrapped around the adjacent axons. In intervals between the adjacent oligodendrocytes are the **nodes of Ranvier.** In the PNS, a different type of supporting cell, called the **Schwann cell,** myelinates the axons. In contrast to oligodendrocytes, a Schwann cell forms only a myelin sheath around a single axon.

Microglia are the smallest neuroglial cells. The dark-staining microglia are considered to be part of the **mononuclear phagocyte system** of the CNS, which originates from precursor cells in the bone marrow. Microglia enter the CNS through the vascular system and become scattered throughout it. Their main function is similar

FUNCTIONAL CORRELATIONS 9.3 | Neuroglia *(Continued)*

to that of the **macrophages** of the connective tissue. When nervous tissue is injured or damaged, microglia migrate to the region, proliferate, become phagocytic, and remove dead or foreign tissue. Microglia constitute the brain's major immune system, and, when activated, they function as antigen-presenting cells and secrete immunoregulatory cytokines.

Ependymal cells are simple cuboidal or low columnar epithelial cells that line the ventricles of the brain and the central canal in the spinal cord. Their apices contain cilia and microvilli. Cilia facilitate the movement of the CSF through the central canal of the spinal cord, whereas microvilli may have some absorptive functions.

FIGURE 9.18 ■ Microglia of the brain. Stain: Hortega method. Medium magnification.

CHAPTER 9 SUMMARY

SECTION 1 • Central Nervous System: Brain and Spinal Cord

The Mammalian Nervous System

- CNS consists of the brain and spinal cord
- PNS consists of cranial, spinal, and peripheral nerves
- Afferent nerves conduct to and efferent nerves conduct from the CNS

Protective Layers of the Central Nervous System

- Surrounded by bones, connective tissue, and cerebrospinal fluid (CSF)
- Dura mater is the tough outermost connective tissue layer around the CNS
- Delicate arachnoid mater is located below the dura mater
- Innermost pia mater adheres directly to the surface of the brain and spinal cord
- Between pia mater and arachnoid mater is subarachnoid space that is filled with CSF

Cerebrospinal Fluid

- Clear, colorless fluid that cushions and protects the brain and spinal cord
- Continually produced by choroid plexuses in brain ventricles, with most in the lateral ventricles
- CSF is important for homeostasis, brain metabolism, and optimal neuronal environment
- CSF is reabsorbed into venous blood (superior sagittal sinus) via the arachnoid villi

Morphology and Types of Neurons in the Central Nervous System

- Neurons are structural and functional units of the CNS that receive and conduct impulses
- Consist of soma (cell body), dendrites, and axons
- Three main neuron types are multipolar, bipolar, and unipolar
- Multipolar are most common and include all motor neurons and interneurons of the CNS
- Multipolar neurons contain numerous dendrites and a single axon
- Bipolar neurons are sensory and found in the eyes, nose, and ears
- Bipolar neurons contain a single dendrite and a single axon
- Unipolar neurons are found in sensory ganglia and dorsal root ganglia of spinal and cranial nerves
- Unipolar neurons exhibit one process from the cell body that divides into two axonal branches
- One unipolar branch continues to the CNS, the other to the peripheries
- Interneurons found in the CNS integrate and coordinate stimuli between sensory, motor, and other interneurons

Myelin Sheath and Myelination of Axons

- Specialized cells wrap around axons to form lipid-rich, insulating myelin sheath
- Myelin sheath extends along the length of the axon to its terminal branches
- Gaps between myelin sheaths are nodes of Ranvier
- In the PNS, Schwann cells myelinate individual axons and envelope unmyelinated axons
- Unmyelinated axons do not show nodes of Ranvier
- In the CNS, processes from single neuroglial oligodendrocyte cells extend and myelinate numerous axons

Gray and White Matter

- Gray matter contains neurons, dendrites, and neuroglia
- Gray matter is the site of connections or synapses between neurons and dendrites
- Posterior horns of the spinal cord are associated with axons of posterior roots
- Anterior horns of the spinal cord are associated with axons of anterior roots
- White matter contains only myelinated axons, unmyelinated axons, and neuroglia

Synapses

- Specialized sites for the transmission of chemical/electrical communication
- Transmission is unidirectional from presynaptic to postsynaptic neurons
- The three main synapses are axodendritic, axosomatic, and axoaxonic
- Consist of presynaptic component, synaptic cleft, and postsynaptic membrane
- Transmit nerve impulses from presynaptic to postsynaptic cells
- Convert impulses into signals to affect postsynaptic cell activities
- Most synapses contain chemical neurotransmitters in presynaptic regions
- Neurotransmitters cross synaptic cleft and bind with receptors on the postsynaptic membrane
- Neurotransmitters produce either excitatory or inhibitory responses
- Summation of excitatory or inhibitory effects on the target regulates the effects of stimulus
- After release, the neurotransmitters are quickly removed from synaptic clefts

Spinal Cord

- Thoracic region of spinal cord contains anterior, posterior, and lateral gray horns
- Lateral horns contain motor neurons of sympathetic division of autonomic nervous system
- Anterior horns of gray matter contain motor neurons
- Axons from anterior horns form anterior roots of spinal nerves
- White matter contains closely packed ascending and descending axons
- Posterior columns of white matter contain fasciculus gracilis and fasciculus cuneatus
- Gray matter inside the spinal cord is H shaped and contains neurons and interneurons
- Gray commissure connects two sides of the gray matter and contains the central canal

Neurons, Axons, and Dendrites

- Classified as afferent (sensory), efferent (motor), or interneurons
- Somatic afferent fibers conduct impulses from body surface and body organs to the CNS
- Visceral afferent fibers conduct impulses from internal organs, glands, and blood vessels to the CNS
- Efferent fibers conduct from the CNS to the effector organs in the peripheries
- Interneurons act as intermediaries between different neuron types
- Neuron cell body and dendrites contain Nissl substance (granular endoplasmic reticulum)
- Neurofibrils in the neuron cell body extend into dendrites and axons
- Axons arise from a funnel-shaped region called an axon hillock
- Axons and axon hillocks are devoid of Nissl substance
- Neurons show irritability and conductivity and synthesize various products
- Neurons synthesize neurotransmitters and neurohormones in the cell body
- Axons transport neurotransmitters in microtubules to synapses
- Stimuli cause conduction of nerve impulse (action potential) along the axons
- Initial segment of an axon is the site where stimuli are summated and nerve impulse is generated
- Rate of impulse conduction dependent on axon size and myelination
- Dendrites are covered with dendritic spines for connections (synapses) with other neurons

- Dendrites receive and integrate information from dendrites, neurons, or axons
- Axons also exhibit bidirectional transport of chemicals, organelles, and neurotransmitters
- Anterograde transport in axons is via microtubules in axons to axon terminals or synapses
- Retrograde transport in axons is via microtubules from axon terminals and dendrites to neurons
- Axonal transport requires microtubule-associated motor proteins kinesin and dynein

Supportive Cells in the CNS: Neuroglia

- Supportive, nonneural cells that surround neurons, axons, and dendrites
- Small cells that do not conduct impulses
- Ten times more numerous than neurons
- Four types: astrocytes, oligodendrocytes, microglia, and ependymal cells

Astrocytes

- Are the largest and most numerous in gray matter
- Consist of two types: fibrous astrocytes and protoplasmic astrocytes
- Both types abut on capillaries and form tight junctions and blood–brain barrier
- Form glial limiting membrane that surrounds the brain and the spinal cord
- Support metabolic exchange and contribute to the energy metabolism of the CNS
- Control the chemical environment around neurons by clearing increased potassium ions and neurotransmitters such as glutamate
- Gap junctions form structural syncytia in the CNS and the communication network in the brain
- In response to injury, cells divide and form scar tissue

Oligodendrocytes

- Surround and myelinate numerous axons at one time, in contrast to Schwann cells
- Do not surround multiple and unmyelinated axons

Microglia

- Part of the mononuclear phagocyte system and found throughout the CNS
- Phagocytic cells in the CNS, function similar to that of connective tissue macrophages
- In response to injury, proliferate and become phagocytic
- Are brain's major immune system and function as antigen-presenting cells

Ependymal Cells

- Line the ventricles in the brain and central canal of the spinal cord
- Ciliated cells move the CSF through the central canal of the spinal cord

Cerebral Cortex: Gray Matter (Layers I to IV)

- Molecular layer (I): most superficial and covered by pia mater; contains neuroglial cells and horizontal cells of Cajal
- External granular layer (II): contains neuroglial cells and small pyramidal cells
- External pyramidal layer (III): medium-sized pyramidal cells predominant type
- Internal granular layer (IV): thin layer with small granule, pyramidal cells, and neuroglia

- Internal pyramidal layer (V): contains neuroglial cells and largest pyramidal cells
- Multiform layer (VI): deepest layer, adjacent to white matter with various cell types

Cerebellar Cortex

- Deep folds in the cortex called cerebellar folia separated by sulci
- Outer molecular layer contains small neurons and fibers
- Middle Purkinje layer contains large Purkinje cells whose dendrites branch in molecular layer
- Granule cell layer contains small granule cells, Golgi type II cells, and empty spaces called glomeruli

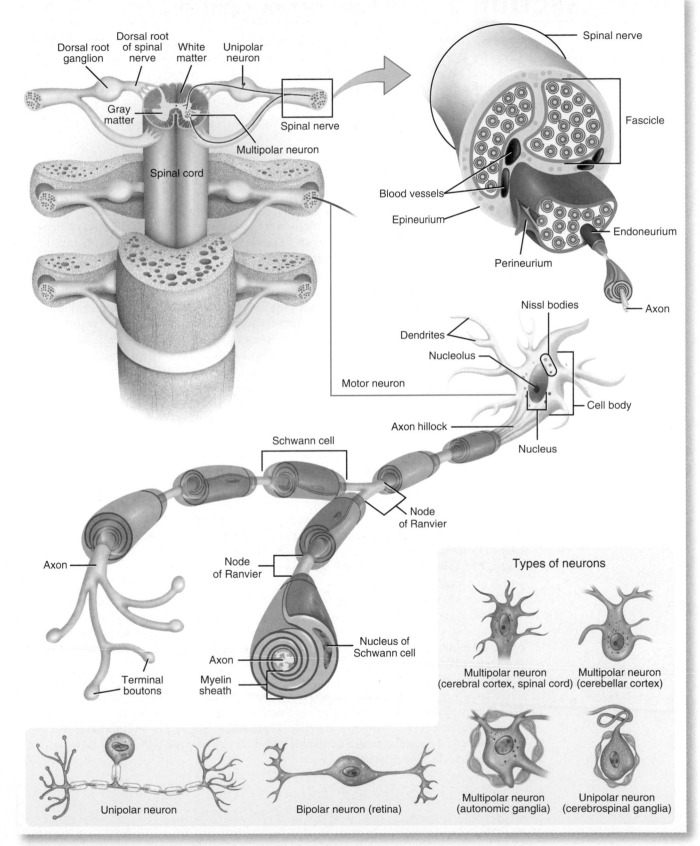

Dorsal root ganglion

Dorsal root of spinal nerve

White matter

Unipolar neuron

Gray matter

Multipolar neuron

Spinal nerve

Spinal cord

Spinal nerve

Fascicle

Blood vessels

Epineurium

Endoneurium

Perineurium

Axon

Nissl bodies

Dendrites

Nucleolus

Motor neuron

Cell body

Axon hillock

Nucleus

Schwann cell

Node of Ranvier

Axon

Node of Ranvier

Nucleus of Schwann cell

Axon

Myelin sheath

Terminal boutons

Types of neurons

Multipolar neuron (cerebral cortex, spinal cord)

Multipolar neuron (cerebellar cortex)

Multipolar neuron (autonomic ganglia)

Unipolar neuron (cerebrospinal ganglia)

Unipolar neuron

Bipolar neuron (retina)

OVERVIEW FIGURE 9.2 ■ **Peripheral nervous system (PNS). The PNS is composed of the cranial and spinal nerves. A cross section of the spinal cord is illustrated with the characteristic features of the motor neuron and a cross section of a peripheral nerve. Also illustrated are types of neurons located in different ganglia and organs outside the CNS.**

SECTION 2 Peripheral Nervous System

The **PNS** consists of neurons, supportive cells, nerves, and axons that are located outside of the CNS. These include **cranial nerves** from the brain and **spinal nerves** from the spinal cord along with their associated **ganglia**. Ganglia (singular, ganglion) are small accumulations of neurons and supportive glial cells surrounded by a connective tissue capsule. The nerves of the PNS contain both sensory and motor axons. These axons transmit information between the peripheral organs and the CNS. The neurons of the peripheral nerves are located either within the CNS or outside of the CNS in different ganglia.

Connective Tissue Layers in the Peripheral Nervous System

A peripheral nerve is composed of numerous axons of various sizes that are surrounded by several layers of connective tissue, which partition the nerve into several nerve (axon) bundles, or **fascicles**. The outermost connective tissue layer is the strong fibrous sheath, the **epineurium,** that binds all fascicles together. It consists of dense irregular connective tissue that completely surrounds the peripheral nerve. A thinner connective tissue layer consists of specialized cells called the **perineurium** that extends into the nerve, subdivides, and surrounds one or more individual nerve fascicles. The cells in the perineum are joined together by **tight junctions,** and the perineum serves as a selective metabolically active diffusion barrier that forms the **blood–nerve barrier**. This barrier restricts passage to many macromolecules and functions in maintaining the proper internal microenvironment and protection of the axons. Within each fascicle are individual axons and their supporting cells, the **Schwann cells**. Each myelinated axon or a cluster of unmyelinated axons associated with a Schwann cell is surrounded by a loose vascular connective tissue layer of thin reticular fibers, called the **endoneurium**.

 Supplemental micrographic images are available at **www.thePoint.com/Eroschenko12e** under Nervous Tissue.

FIGURE 9.19 | Peripheral Nerves and Blood Vessels (Transverse Section)

Several bundles of nerve **axons** (fibers) or **nerve fascicles (1)** and accompanying blood vessels have been sectioned in the transverse plane. Each nerve fascicle (1) is surrounded by a sheath of connective tissue **perineurium (5)** that merges with surrounding **interfascicular connective tissue (9)**. Delicate connective tissue strands from the perineurium (5) surround individual nerve axons (fibers) in a fascicle and form the innermost layer endoneurium (not visible in this figure and at this magnification).

Numerous nuclei are seen between individual nerve axons (fibers) in the nerve fascicles (1). Most of these are the **nuclei** of **Schwann cells (2)**. Schwann cells (2) surround and myelinate the axons. The myelin sheaths that surrounded the tiny axons (3) are seen as empty spaces because of the chemicals used in preparation of the tissue. Other nuclei in the nerve fascicles (1) are the **fibrocytes (4)** of the endoneurium (see Figure 9.22).

The arterial blood vessels in the interfascicular connective tissue (9) send branches into each nerve fascicle (1) where they branch into capillaries in the endoneurium. Different size **arterioles (7, 12)** and **venules (11)** are found in the interfascicular connective tissue (9) that surrounds the nerve fascicles (1). In the larger arteriole (7) are visible blood cells, an **internal elastic membrane (8)**, and a muscular **tunica media (6)**. Different size **adipose cells (10)** are also present in the interfascicular connective tissue (9).

1 Nerve fascicles

2 Nuclei of Schwann cells

3 Myelinated axons

4 Fibrocytes

5 Perineurium with
   fibrocytes

6 Tunica media
   of arteriole

7 Arteriole

8 Internal elastic
   membrane

9 Interfascicular
   connective tissue

10 Adipose cells

11 Venules

12 Arteriole

FIGURE 9.19 ■ Peripheral nerves and blood vessels (transverse section). Stain: hematoxylin and eosin. Medium magnification.

FIGURE 9.20 | Myelinated Nerve Fibers in Longitudinal and Transverse Sections

Schwann cells surround the axons in peripheral nerves and form a myelin sheath. To illustrate the myelin sheath, nerve fibers are fixed in osmic acid; this preparation stains the lipid in the myelin sheath black. In this illustration, a portion of the peripheral nerve has been prepared in a longitudinal section (*upper figure*) and in a cross section (*lower figure*).

In the longitudinal section, the **myelin sheath (1)** appears as a thick, black band surrounding a lighter, central **axon (2)**. The length of an axon myelinated by one Schwann cell is the nodal or internodal segment. Between the internodal segments, which can be a few millimeters in length, the myelin sheath exhibits discontinuity. These regions of discontinuity represent the **nodes of Ranvier (4)**, which can span approximately 1 or 2 micrometers (μm).

A group of nerve fibers or fascicle is also illustrated. Each fascicle is surrounded by a light-appearing connective tissue layer, called the **perineurium (3, 5, 8)**. In turn, each individual nerve fiber or axon is surrounded by a thin layer of connective tissue, called the **endoneurium (7, 10)**. In the transverse plane (*lower figure*), different diameters of myelinated axons are seen. The **myelin sheath (9)** appears as a thick, black ring around the light, unstained **axon (12)**, which, in most fibers, is seen in the center.

The connective tissue surrounding individual nerve fibers, or the fascicle, exhibits a rich supply of **blood vessels (6, 11)** of different sizes.

FUNCTIONAL CORRELATIONS 9.4	Axon Myelination and Supporting Cells in the Peripheral Nervous System

The supportive cells in the PNS are the **Schwann cells**. Their main function is to surround and form the insulating, lipid-rich **myelin sheaths** around the larger axons. The myelin sheaths protect axons and maintain proper ionic environment for impulse conduction and propagation. Each Schwann cell can form a myelin sheath around a portion of a single axon. However, a single Schwann cell can enclose numerous unmyelinated axons. The function of Schwann cells in the PNS is similar to that of the **oligodendrocytes** in the **CNS**, except that processes from a single oligodendrocyte can form myelin sheaths around numerous axons. Myelin sheaths are not continuous, solid sheets along the axon; rather, they are punctuated by small nodal gaps called **nodes of Ranvier** that are located between the myelin sheaths produced by the myelinating cells. The length of the axon covered by the myelin sheath of one Schwann cell is called the internode, or **internodal segment**. The size of the internode varies with the size of the axon. The size of the node of Ranvier is between 1 and 2 μm, whereas the internodes can be a few millimeters, depending on the size of the axon. At the nodes of Ranvier, the axons are not insulated by myelin sheaths. As a result, these nodes significantly accelerate the conduction of **nerve impulses** (action potentials) along the axons. In large, myelinated axons, the nerve impulse, or action potential, jumps from node to node, resulting in a more efficient and faster conduction of the impulse. This type of fast impulse propagation along the myelinated axons is called **saltatory conduction**.

Small unmyelinated axons conduct nerve impulses at a much slower rate than larger, myelinated axons. In unmyelinated axons, even though they are surrounded by the cytoplasm of the Schwann cell, the impulse travels along the entire length of the axon; as a result, conduction efficiency of the impulse and velocity are reduced. Thus, the larger, myelinated axons have the highest velocity of impulse conduction. Also, the rate of impulse conduction depends directly on the axon size and the myelin sheath.

The **satellite cells** are small, flat cells that surround the neurons of PNS ganglia. Ganglia are collections of neurons that are located outside the CNS. Peripheral ganglia are located parallel to the vertebral column near the junction of the dorsal and ventral roots of the spinal nerves and near various visceral organs. Satellite cells provide **structural support** for the neuronal bodies, insulate them, and regulate the exchange of different metabolic substances between the neurons and the interstitial fluid.

1 Myelin sheath

2 Axons

3 Perineurium

8 Perineurium

9 Myelin sheath

4 Nodes of Ranvier

5 Perineurium

6 Blood vessels

7 Endoneurium

10 Endoneurium

11 Blood vessel

12 Axons

FIGURE 9.20 ■ Myelinated nerve fibers (longitudinal and transverse sections). Stain: osmic acid. High magnification.

FIGURE 9.21 | Sciatic Nerve (Longitudinal Section)

A longitudinal section of a sciatic nerve is illustrated at a low magnification. A small portion of the outer layer of dense connective tissue **epineurium (1)** that surrounds the entire nerve is visible. The deeper layer of the epineurium (1) contains numerous **blood vessels (5)** and **adipose cells (6)**.

The connective tissue sheath directly inferior to the epineurium (1) that surrounds bundles of nerve fibers or **nerve fascicles (3)** is the **perineurium (2)**. Extensions of the epineurium (1) with **blood vessels (4)** between the nerve fascicles (3) form the **interfascicular connective tissue (7)**.

In a longitudinal section, the individual axons usually follow a characteristic wavy pattern. Located among the wavy axons in the nerve fascicle (3) are numerous **nuclei (8)** of the Schwann cells and fibrocytes of the endoneurium connective tissue. Schwann cells and fibrocytes cannot be differentiated at this magnification.

FIGURE 9.22 | Sciatic Nerve (Longitudinal Section)

A small portion of the sciatic nerve, illustrated in Figure 9.21, is presented at a higher magnification. The central **axons (1)** appear as slender threads stained lightly with hematoxylin and eosin. The surrounding myelin sheath has been dissolved by chemicals during histologic preparation, leaving a **neurokeratin network (6)** of protein. The sheath or cell membrane of the **Schwann cells (4)** is not always distinguishable from the connective tissue **endoneurium (5)** that surrounds each axon. At the **node** of **Ranvier (2)**, the Schwann cell membrane (4) is seen as a thin, peripheral boundary that descends toward the axon.

Two **Schwann cell nuclei (4)**, cut in different planes, are shown around the periphery of the myelinated axons (1). The **fibrocytes** of the connective tissue **endoneurium (3a)** and **perineurium (3b)** are also seen in the illustration. The fibrocyte of the endoneurium (3a) is outside of the myelin sheath, in contrast to the Schwann cells (4) that myelinate or surround the axons (1). However, it is often difficult to distinguish between the nuclei of Schwann cells (4) and the fibrocytes (3) of the endoneurium.

FIGURE 9.23 | Sciatic Nerve (Transverse Section)

A higher magnification of a transverse section of the sciatic nerve illustrated in Figure 9.21 shows the myelinated nerve fibers. The **axons (5)** appear as thin, dark central structures, surrounded by the dissolved remnants of myelin, the **neurokeratin network (2)** of protein with peripheral radial lines. The nuclei and cell membranes of the **Schwann cells (1)** are peripheral to the myelinated axon (5). The crescent shape of the Schwann cells (1), as they appear to encircle the axons, allows their identification.

The collagen fibers of the connective tissue endoneurium are faintly distinguishable, whereas the **fibrocytes (3a)** in the connective tissue of endoneurium and **perineurium (3b, 6)** are clearly seen. Located in the **interfascicular connective tissue (4)** and draining the nerve fascicles is a small **venule (7)**.

1 Epineurium

2 Perineurium

3 Fascicle

4 Blood vessel

5 Blood vessels

6 Adipose cells

7 Interfascicular connective tissue

8 Nuclei of Schwann cells or fibrocytes

FIGURE 9.21 ■ Sciatic nerve (longitudinal section). Stain: hematoxylin and eosin. Low magnification.

1 Axons

2 Nodes of Ranvier

3 Fibrocytes in:
   a. Endoneurium
   b. Perineurium

4 Nuclei of Schwann cells

5 Endoneurium

6 Neurokeratin network of dissolved myelin

FIGURE 9.22 ■ Sciatic nerve (longitudinal section). Stain: hematoxylin and eosin. High magnification (oil immersion).

1 Schwann cells

2 Neurokeratin network of dissolved myelin

3 Fibrocytes in:
   a. Endoneurium
   b. Perineurium

4 Interfascicular connective tissue

5 Axons

6 Fibrocyte in perineurium

7 Venule

FIGURE 9.23 ■ Sciatic nerve (transverse section). Stain: hematoxylin and eosin. High magnification (oil immersion).

FIGURE 9.24 | Peripheral Nerve: Nodes of Ranvier and Axons

A medium magnification photomicrograph of a peripheral nerve sectioned in a longitudinal plane is shown. The myelin sheaths that normally surround the **axons (2, 8)** have been washed out in this preparation and only **myelin spaces (7)** are seen. A centrally located axon (2, 8) can be seen in some of the nerve fibers that exhibited myelin sheaths. At regular intervals along the axon are seen indentations in the myelin sheaths. These represent the **nodes of Ranvier (1, 9)**, which indicate the edges of two different myelin sheaths that enclose the axon. A possible **Schwann cell nucleus (3)** is seen associated with one of the axons (2, 8) and a thin, blue connective tissue layer **endoneurium (6)** that surrounds some of the axons (2, 8). Outside of the axons (2, 8) are seen a **capillary (4)** with blood cells and **fibrocytes (5)** of the surrounding connective tissue layers.

FIGURE 9.25 | Ultrastructure of Peripheral Nerve Fascicle in the PNS Cut in Transverse Plane

A transmission electron micrograph of a nerve fascicle sectioned in a transverse plane shows in greater detail the two large **myelinated axons (3)** on the left side and numerous small **unmyelinated axons (7)** on the right side. In contrast to the CNS, the Schwann cells only form **myelin sheaths (2)** around a section of one axon. A thin rim of **Schwann cell cytoplasm (5)** surrounds the myelinated axon, which is invested by an outer thin layer of **basal lamina (6)**. Located within the axons are numerous oval-shaped, dense-staining structures; these are the **mitochondria (4)**. On the right side of the image are Schwann cells that are associated with numerous unmyelinated axons (7), which are embedded in the **Schwann cell cytoplasm (8)**. A thin **basal lamina (10)** also surrounds the Schwann cell cytoplasm (8) that encloses the unmyelinated axons (7). Similar oval-shaped **mitochondria (9)** and neurofilaments are found in the unmyelinated axons (7). Enclosing the entire nerve fascicle is a thin layer of connective tissue **perineurium (12)**. Visible on the peripheries of the fascicle are cells with highly developed rough endoplasmic reticulum, which are most likely the **fibroblasts (1, 11)**.

To see the image of the node of Ranvier with a transmission electron micrograph, examine Figure 9.17, which represents the node of Ranvier from the CNS. Except for a few ultrastructural differences, the structures of the nodes of Ranvier in the PNS and the CNS are quite similar. The nodes in the PNS are covered by the **basal lamina**, whereas the nodes in the CNS lack an overlying basal lamina.

1 Node of Ranvier

2 Axon

3 Schwann cell nucleus

4 Capillary

5 Fibrocytes

6 Endoneurium

7 Myelin spaces

8 Axon

9 Node of Ranvier

FIGURE 9.24 ■ Peripheral nerve: nodes of Ranvier and axons. Stain: Masson trichrome. ×100.

1 Fibroblast

2 Myelin sheaths

3 Myelinated axons

4 Mitochondria

5 Schwann cell cytoplasm

6 Basal lamina

7 Unmyelinated axons

8 Schwann cell cytoplasm

9 Mitochondria

10 Basal lamina

11 Fibroblast

12 Perineurium

FIGURE 9.25 ■ Ultrastructure of peripheral nerve fascicle in the PNS cut in transverse plane. Courtesy of Dr. Mark DeSantis, Professor Emeritus, WWAMI Medical Program, University of Idaho, Moscow, Idaho. Approximately ×25,000.

FIGURE 9.26 | Dorsal Root Ganglion with Dorsal and Ventral Roots, and Spinal Nerve (Longitudinal Section)

The dorsal root ganglia are aggregations of neuron cell bodies that are located outside the CNS. The **dorsal (posterior) root ganglion (7)** is situated on the **dorsal (posterior) nerve root (9)**, which joins the spinal cord. Numerous round (pseudo-) **unipolar neurons (2),** or sensory neurons, constitute the majority of the ganglion. Numerous fascicles of **nerve fibers (3)** pass between the unipolar neurons (2) and course either in the dorsal nerve root (9) or the **spinal nerve (5)**. The nerve fibers (3) represent the peripheral processes that are formed by the bifurcation of a single axon that emerges from each unipolar neuron (2).

Each dorsal root ganglion (7) is enclosed by an irregular **connective tissue layer (1)** that contains adipose cells, **nerves (6)**, and **blood vessels (6)**. The connective tissue (1, 6) around the ganglion (7) merges with the connective tissue **epineurium (4)** of the peripheral spinal nerve (5). The nerve fibers in the **ventral (anterior) root (11)** join the nerve fibers that emerge from the ganglion (7) to form the spinal nerve (5). The spinal nerve (5) is formed when the dorsal nerve root (9) and the ventral (anterior) root (11) unite.

On emerging from the spinal cord, the dorsal (9) and ventral roots (11) are surrounded by pia mater and an **arachnoid sheath (8, 10)**. These become continuous with the epineurium (4) of the spinal nerve (5). The connective tissue perineurium around the nerve fascicles (3) and the endoneurium around individual nerve fibers in the spinal nerve (5) or in the ganglion (7) are not distinguishable at this magnification.

FIGURE 9.27 | Cells and Unipolar Neurons of a Dorsal Root Ganglion

The unipolar **neurons (1, 6)** of a dorsal (posterior) root ganglion are illustrated at higher magnification. When the plane of section passes through the middle of a neuron (1, 6), a pink-staining **cytoplasm (1b, 4)** and a round **nucleus (1a)** is visible with its characteristic, dark-staining **nucleolus (1a)**. Some of the unipolar neurons (1, 6) contain small clumps of brownish **lipofuscin pigment (9)** in their cytoplasm (see also Overview Figure 9.2).

The cell body of each unipolar neuron (1, 6) is surrounded by two cellular capsules. The inner cell layer is within the perineuronal space and closely surrounds the unipolar neurons (1, 6). These are the smaller, flat epitheliumlike **satellite cells (3, 8)**. The satellite cells (3, 8) have spherical nuclei, are of neuroectodermal origin, and are continuous with similar **Schwann cells (11)** that surround the unmyelinated and **myelinated axons (5, 10)**. The satellite cells (3, 8) are surrounded by an outer layer of **capsule cells (7)** of the connective tissue. Between the unipolar neurons (1, 6) are numerous **fibrocytes (2)** that are randomly arranged in the surrounding connective tissue and continue into the endoneurium between the axons (5).

With hematoxylin and eosin stain, small axons and individual connective tissue fibers are not clearly defined. Large myelinated axons (5) are recognizable when sectioned longitudinally.

1 Connective tissue layer with blood vessels

2 Unipolar neurons of dorsal root ganglion

3 Nerve fascicles

4 Epineurium of spinal nerve

5 Spinal nerve

6 Nerves and blood vessel in connective tissue layer

7 Dorsal (posterior) root ganglion

8 Arachnoid sheath of dorsal root

9 Dorsal (posterior) nerve root

10 Arachnoid sheath of ventral root

11 Ventral (anterior) nerve root

FIGURE 9.26 ■ Dorsal root ganglion, with dorsal and ventral roots, spinal nerve (longitudinal section). Stain: hematoxylin and eosin. Low magnification.

1 Unipolar neuron
 a. Nucleus and nucleolus
 b. Cytoplasm

2 Fibrocytes

3 Satellite cells

4 Cytoplasm of neurons

5 Myelinated axons

6 Unipolar neuron

7 Capsule cells

8 Satellite cells

9 Lipofuscin pigment

10 Myelinated axon

11 Schwann cells

FIGURE 9.27 ■ Cells and unipolar neurons of a dorsal root ganglion. Stain: hematoxylin and eosin. High magnification.

FIGURE 9.28 | Multipolar Neurons, Surrounding Cells, and Nerve Fibers of a Sympathetic Ganglion

---

In contrast to the neurons of the dorsal root ganglion (Figure 9.27), the **neurons (3, 9)** of the sympathetic trunk are multipolar, smaller, and more uniform in size. As a result, the outlines of the neurons (3, 9) and their **dendritic processes (2, 11)** often appear irregular. Also, if the plane of section does not pass through the middle of the cell, only the **cytoplasm** of the **neuron (1, 10)** is visible. The sympathetic neurons (3, 9) also often exhibit **eccentric nuclei (9)**, and binucleated cells are not uncommon. In older individuals, a brownish **lipofuscin pigment (12)** accumulates in the cytoplasm of numerous neurons (1, 10, 12).

The **satellite cells (8)** surround the multipolar neurons (3, 9) but are usually less numerous than around the cells in the dorsal root ganglion. Also, the connective tissue capsule with its capsule cells may not be well defined. Surrounding the neurons (3, 9) are **fibrocytes (5)** of the intercellular connective tissue and different sizes of blood vessels such as a **venule** with **blood cells (6)**. Unmyelinated and myelinated nerve **axons (4, 7)** aggregate into bundles and course through the sympathetic ganglion. The flattened nuclei on the peripheries of the myelinated axons (4, 7) are the **Schwann cells (4, 7)**. These nerve fibers represent the preganglionic axons, postganglionic visceral efferent axons, and visceral afferent axons.

FIGURE 9.29 | Dorsal Root Ganglion: Unipolar Neurons and Surrounding Cells

---

A medium-magnification photomicrograph of the dorsal root ganglion illustrates the spherical shape of the sensory **unipolar neurons (2)**. The cytoplasm of these neurons contains a central **nucleus (6)** and a prominent dense **nucleolus (5)**. Surrounding the unipolar neurons (2) are the smaller **satellite cells (1)**. Other cells outside the satellite cells are the connective tissue **fibrocytes (3)**. Coursing through the dorsal root ganglion between the unipolar neurons (2) are numerous **bundles of sensory axons (4)** from the periphery.

The clear space around the neurons and the surrounding cells is an artifact caused by the tissue shrinkage during the chemical preparation of the dorsal root ganglion.

1 Cytoplasm of neuron

2 Dendritic process of neuron

3 Nucleus and nucleolus of neuron

4 Axons and Schwann cells

5 Fibrocytes of connective tissue

6 Venule with red blood cells

7 Axons and Schwann cells

8 Satellite cells

9 Eccentric nucleus of neuron

10 Cytoplasm of neuron

11 Dendritic process of neuron

12 Lipofuscin pigment

FIGURE 9.28 ■ Multipolar neurons, surrounding cells, and nerve fibers of the sympathetic ganglion. Stain: hematoxylin and eosin. High magnification.

1 Satellite cells

2 Unipolar neurons

3 Fibrocytes

4 Bundle of sensory axons

5 Nucleolus

6 Nucleus

FIGURE 9.29 ■ Dorsal root ganglion: unipolar neurons and surrounding cells. Stain: hematoxylin and eosin. ×100.

SECTION 2 • Peripheral Nervous System

- Consists of neurons, neuroglia, nerves, and axons outside the CNS
- Cranial nerves arise from the brain and spinal nerves from the spinal cord
- Ganglia are accumulations of neurons and are covered by connective tissue
- Contains both sensory and motor nerves
- Neurons of peripheral nerves can be located in the CNS or in ganglia

Connective Tissue Layers in Peripheral Nerves

- Peripheral nerves are partitioned by layers of connective tissue into fascicles
- Outermost connective tissue around the nerve is the epineurium
- Connective tissue perineurium surrounds one or more nerve fascicles
- Vascular connective tissue layer endoneurium surrounds individual axons

Peripheral Nerves

- Nuclei seen between individual axons are Schwann cells and fibrocytes

- Schwann cells myelinate and surround individual axons or enclose unmyelinated axons
- Between individual Schwann cells in myelinated axons are the nodes of Ranvier
- Conduction along a myelinated axon is called saltatory conduction
- Small satellite cells surround the neurons of PNS ganglia
- Satellite cells provide structural support, insulate, and regulate metabolic exchanges

Dorsal Root Ganglia and Unipolar Neurons of the PNS

- Situated on dorsal nerve roots that join the spinal cord
- Sensory (round) unipolar neurons constitute the ganglia
- Bundles of sensory nerve fibers or axons pass between the unipolar neurons
- Connective tissue capsule encloses the ganglia and merges with the epineurium of the peripheral nerve
- Unipolar neurons are surrounded by satellite cells, which are enclosed by connective tissue capsule cells

PART IV

Systems

Large vein

Valve

Endothelium

Subendothelial layer

Tunica intima

Tunica media

Tunica adventitia

Nerve   Vasa vasorum

Muscular artery

Endothelium

Subendothelial layer

Internal elastic lamina

Tunica intima

Smooth muscle

Elastic fibers

External elastic lamina

Tunica media

Tunica adventitia

Nerve   Vasa vasorum

Sinusoidal (discontinous) capillary

Incomplete basement membrane

Fenestrated capillary

Fenestrae

Lumen

Continuous capillary

Nucleus of endothelial cell

OVERVIEW FIGURE 10.1 ■ Comparison of a muscular artery, a large vein, and the three types of capillaries (transverse sections).

CHAPTER 10

Circulatory System ■

The mammalian circulatory system comprises two major systems: the cardiovascular system and the lymphatic vascular system.

Cardiovascular System

The **cardiovascular system** consists of the heart, major arteries, arterioles, capillaries, venules, and veins that form a closed system of blood vessels that carry blood. Within this system are two major circuits that distribute blood to the body. These are the **systemic circulation** and the **pulmonary circulation**. Both of these circuits depend on the pumping action of the heart to distribute the blood throughout the body. The systemic circulation carries the blood from the heart to all organs, tissues, and cells via arterial vessels and then back to the heart via the venous vessels. The pulmonary system carries blood from the heart to the lungs for gaseous exchange and the oxygenated blood back to the heart for distribution via the systemic circulation.

The main functions of the blood vascular system are gaseous exchange; temperature control; and transport of oxygen, carbon dioxide, nutrients, hormones, metabolic products, cells of immune defense system, and many other essential products. The histology of the heart muscle has been described in detail in Chapter 8, "Muscle Tissue," as one of the four main tissues. In this chapter, heart histology is illustrated only as part of the cardiovascular system.

Types of Arteries

There are three types of arteries in the body: elastic arteries, muscular arteries, and arterioles. Arteries that leave the heart to distribute the oxygenated blood become smaller as they exhibit progressive branching. With each branching, the luminal diameters of the arteries gradually decrease until the smallest vessel, the capillary, is formed.

Elastic arteries are the largest blood vessels in the body and include the **pulmonary trunk** and **aorta** with their major branches, the brachiocephalic, common carotid, subclavian, vertebral, pulmonary, and common iliac arteries. The walls of these vessels are primarily composed of elastic connective tissue fibers interspersed with circularly arranged **smooth muscle cells**. The elastic fibers provide great resilience and flexibility during blood flow.

The large elastic arteries branch and become medium-sized **muscular arteries**, the most numerous vessels in the body. In contrast to the walls of elastic arteries, those of muscular arteries contain greater amounts of **smooth muscle fibers**.

Arterioles are the smallest branches of the arterial system. Their walls consist of one to five layers of smooth muscle fibers. Arterioles deliver blood to the smallest blood vessels, the capillaries. Capillaries connect arterioles with the smallest veins or venules.

Structural Plan of Arteries

The wall of a typical artery contains three concentric layers, or **tunics**. The innermost layer that faces the lumen is the **tunica intima**. This layer consists of a simple squamous epithelium, called **endothelium** in the vascular system, and a thin underlying layer of **subendothelial connective tissue**. The middle layer is the **tunica media**, composed primarily of smooth muscle fibers. Interspersed among the smooth muscle cells are variable amounts of elastic and reticular fibers. In the muscular and elastic arteries, smooth muscles produce the **elastic fibers**, some **collagen fibers**, and other extracellular elements. The collagen fibers provide tensile strength to the arterial walls, whereas the elastic fibers allow for the distention and recoil of the vessel walls during heart contraction and blood ejection. The outermost layer is the **tunica adventitia**, composed primarily of longitudinally oriented collagen fibers and elastic connective tissue fibers; adventitia consists primarily of **collagen type I fibers**.

The walls of some muscular arteries also exhibit two thin, wavy bands of elastic fibers. The **internal elastic lamina (IEL)** is located between the tunica intima and the tunica media and represents the most external layer of tunica intima. This lamina exhibits layers of elastin sheets that contain numerous openings or **fenestrations**. These fenestrations allow for rapid diffusion of nutritive substances through the lamina to reach cells that are deep within the vessel walls. IEL is not seen in smaller arteries.

The **external elastic lamina (EEL)** is located on the periphery of the muscular tunica media and is primarily seen in large muscular arteries. This lamina is a layer of elastin that separates the tunica media from the collagenous tunica adventitia.

Structural Plan of Veins

Capillaries unite to form larger blood vessels called **venules;** venules usually accompany arterioles. Venous blood initially flows into smaller **postcapillary venules** and then into veins of increasing size. The veins are arbitrarily classified as small, medium, and large. Compared with arteries, veins typically are more numerous and have thinner walls, larger diameters, and greater structural variation. Blood that enters the veins is under low pressure. Small-sized and medium-sized veins, particularly veins in the extremities (arms and legs) and those that convey blood against gravity, have **valves**. Because of the low blood pressure in the veins, blood flow to the heart in the veins is slow and can even back up. The presence of valves in veins assists venous blood flow toward the heart by preventing backflow. When blood flows toward the heart, pressure in the veins forces the valves to open. As the blood begins to flow backward, the valve flaps close the lumen and prevent backflow of blood. Venous blood between the valves in the extremities flows toward the heart because of the contraction of surrounding muscles, contractions between muscles, or contractions of organs that have some muscle such as the spleen. However, valves are absent in veins of the central nervous system (CNS), the inferior and superior venae cavae, and the viscera.

The walls of the veins, like the arteries, also exhibit three layers or tunics. However, the muscular layer is much thinner and less prominent. The **tunica intima** in veins exhibits an endothelium and subendothelial connective tissue. In contrast to arteries, the muscular **tunica media** is thin in the veins, and the smooth muscles intermix with connective tissue fibers. The **tunica adventitia** is the thickest and best-developed layer of the three tunics. Longitudinal bundles of smooth muscle fibers are common in the connective tissue of this layer (see Overview Figure 10.1). The structure of the venous walls allows flexibility and the accommodation of a large blood volume. As a result, veins contain most of the blood in the body.

Vasa Vasorum

The walls of medium and large arteries and veins are too thick to provide nourishment to the cells by direct diffusion from their lumina. As a result, these walls are supplied by their own small blood vessels from adjacent small arteries called the **vasa vasorum** (blood vessels of the larger blood vessel). The vasa vasorum allows for the exchange of nutrients and metabolites with cells in the tunica adventitia and the deeper tunica media. The vessels of vasa vasorum are much more extensive in the wall of the veins than in the arteries because of the poor oxygen content of venous blood.

Types of Capillaries

Capillaries are the smallest blood vessels. Their average diameter is about **8 μm**, which is about the size of an **erythrocyte** (red blood cell [RBC]). Each capillary consists of a thin endothelium, an underlying basal lamina, and a few randomly scattered **pericytes**. These cells surround the capillaries with branching cytoplasm and are enclosed by a basal lamina that also encloses the capillary endothelium. There are three types of capillaries: continuous capillaries, fenestrated capillaries, and sinusoids. These structural variations in capillaries allow for different types of metabolic exchange between blood and the surrounding tissues.

Continuous capillaries are the most common. They are found in muscle, connective tissue, nervous tissue, skin, respiratory organs, and exocrine glands. In these capillaries, the **endothelial cells** are joined and form an uninterrupted, solid endothelial lining. Tight junctions, desmosomes, and gap junctions are seen in these capillaries.

Fenestrated capillaries are characterized by openings or **fenestrations** (pores) in the cytoplasm of endothelial cells designed for rapid exchange of molecules between blood and tissues. Fenestrated capillaries are found in those organs/tissues where enhanced exchange of substances occurs between tissues and blood. Endocrine tissues and glands, the small intestine, the kidney glomeruli, and the choroid plexus in the brain ventricles are organs that exhibit fenestrated capillaries.

Sinusoidal (discontinuous) capillaries are blood vessels that exhibit irregular, tortuous paths. Their much wider diameters slow down the flow of blood. Endothelial cell junctions are rare in sinusoidal capillaries, and wide gaps exist between individual endothelial cells. Also, because a **basement membrane** underlying the endothelium is either incomplete or absent, direct exchange of molecules occurs between blood contents and cells. Sinusoidal capillaries are found in the liver, spleen, and bone marrow (see Overview Figure 10.1).

The Lymphatic Vascular System

The lymphatic vascular system is closely associated with the circulatory system. It is composed of vascular channels that drain extracellular fluid called **lymph** from the tissues. The **lymphatic system** consists of lymph capillaries and lymph vessels that originate as blind-ending tubules or lymphatic capillaries in the connective tissue of different organs. The lymph capillaries lie close to the blood capillaries and collect the excess **interstitial fluid (lymph)** from the tissues. The collected lymph is returned to the venous blood via the large **lymph vessels**, the thoracic duct, and the right lymphatic duct after it is filtered through numerous lymph nodes that are located throughout the body. Also, the walls of lymph vessels show more permeability than the walls of blood capillaries because the **endothelium** in lymph capillaries is extremely thin. The structure of larger lymph vessels is similar to that of veins except that their walls are much thinner.

Lymph movement in the lymphatic vessels is similar to that of venous blood movement; that is, the contractions of surrounding skeletal muscles force the lymph to move forward. Also, the lymph vessels contain more **valves** to prevent a backflow of collected lymph. Lymph vessels are found in all tissues except in the CNS, cartilage, bone and bone marrow, thymus, placenta, and teeth. Lymph capillaries also take up and deliver the absorbed lipids from the intestines into the bloodstream.

 Supplemental micrographic images are available at **www.thePoint.com/Eroschenko12e** under Blood Vessels.

FIGURE 10.1 | Different Blood and Lymphatic Vessels in the Connective Tissue

---

This composite figure illustrates a section of irregular connective tissue with nerve fibers, blood and lymphatic vessels, and adipose tissue. To illustrate structural differences, the vessels have been sectioned in transverse, longitudinal, or oblique planes.

A **small artery (3)** with its wall structure is shown in the lower left corner of the illustration. In contrast to **veins (11)**, an artery has a relatively thick wall and a small lumen. In cross section, the wall of a small artery (3) exhibits the following layers:

- **Tunica intima (4)** is the innermost layer. It is composed of **endothelium (4a)**, a **subendo-thelial (4b)** layer of connective tissue, and an **IEL (membrane) (4c)**, which separates the tunica intima (4) from the next layer, the **tunica media (5)**.
- Tunica media (5) is composed predominantly of circular smooth muscle fibers. A loose network of fine elastic fibers is interspersed among the smooth muscle cells.
- **Tunica adventitia (6)** is the connective tissue layer that surrounds the vessel. This layer contains small nerves and blood vessels. In tunica adventitia (6), the blood vessels are collectively called **vasa vasorum (7)**, or "blood vessels of the blood vessel."

When arteries acquire about 25 or more layers of smooth muscle fibers in the tunica media, they are called muscular or distributing arteries. Elastic fibers become more numerous in the tunica media but are still present as thin fibers and networks.

A **venule (9)** and small vein (11) are also illustrated. Note the relatively thin wall and a large lumen. The thin wall, however, appears to have many cell layers when the vein is sectioned in an **oblique plane (9)**. In cross section, the wall of the vein exhibits the following layers:

- Tunica intima, which is composed of **endothelium (11a)** and an extremely thin layer of fine collagen and elastic fibers, which blend with the connective tissue of the **tunica media (11b)**.
- Tunica media (11b), which consists of a thin layer of circularly arranged smooth muscle loosely embedded in connective tissue. Tunica media (11b) is much thinner in veins than in arteries (5).
- **Tunica adventitia (11c)**, which contains a wide layer of connective tissue. In veins, the tunica adventitia (11c) layer is thicker than the tunica media (11b).

Two **arterioles (2, 8)**, cut in different planes, are also illustrated. The arterioles (2, 8) have a thin IEL and a layer of smooth muscle fibers in the tunica media. One **arteriole (8)** is shown cut in longitudinal plane with a branching **capillary (10)**. When an arteriole (8) is cut at an oblique angle, only the circular smooth muscle layer of the tunica media is seen. Also visible in the illustration are capillaries (10) sectioned in longitudinal and oblique planes, and small **nerves (1)** in transverse planes.

The **lymphatic vessels (12, 13)** are recognized by having the thinnest walls. When the lymphatic vessel is cut in a longitudinal plane, the flaps of a **valve (13)** are seen in its lumen. Many veins in the arms and legs have similar valves in their lumina.

Numerous **adipose cells (14)** are found in the surrounding connective tissue.

FIGURE 10.2 | Capillaries Sectioned in Transverse and Longitudinal Planes in the Mesentery of a Small Intestine

---

This high-magnification photomicrograph of the mesentery connective tissue shows the **capillaries (1, 3, 4, 5)** sectioned in both transverse (1, 5) and longitudinal planes (3, 4). Note that the lumen of the capillaries (1, 3, 4, 5) is about the size of a RBC. In the transverse plane (1, 5), the RBCs fill the lumina of the capillaries (1, 5), and in the longitudinal plane (3, 4), the RBCs are lined one behind the other in a row. Surrounding the capillaries (1, 3, 4, 5) are the **adipose cells (2)** of the intestinal mesentery, which appear empty due to the chemicals used for the preparation of this slide. Blue-staining collagen fibers of the **connective tissue (6)** surround the adipose cells (2) and the capillaries (1, 3, 4, 5).

1 Nerves (transverse sections)

2 Arteriole

3 Small artery

4 Tunica intima:
   a. Endothelium
   b. Subendothelial connective tissue
   c. IEL (membrane)

5 Tunica media

6 Tunica adventitia

7 Vasa vasorum

8 Arteriole (oblique and longitudinal sections)

9 Venule (oblique section)

10 Capillaries (longitudinal and transverse sections)

11 Small vein:
   a. Endothelium
   b. Tunica media
   c. Tunica adventitia

12 Lymphatic vessel (transverse and longitudinal sections)

13 Valve of lymphatic vessel

14 Adipose cells

FIGURE 10.1 ■ Blood and lymphatic vessels in the connective tissue. Stain: hematoxylin and eosin. Low magnification.

1 Capillaries (transverse plane)

2 Adipose cells

3 Capillary with RBCs (longitudinal plane)

4 Capillary with RBCs (longitudinal plane)

5 Capillary (transverse plane)

6 Connective tissue fibers

FIGURE 10.2 ■ Capillaries sectioned in transverse and longitudinal planes in a mesentery of the small intestine. Stain: Mallory-Azan. ×205.

FIGURE 10.3 | Ultrastructure of a Continuous Capillary Sectioned in Transverse Plane

This ultrastructure micrograph shows a capillary in the CNS, sectioned in a transverse plane. A layer of **continuous endothelium of the capillary** (6) surrounds the **capillary lumen**. Also visible on the left side of the capillary are the **nucleus of the endothelial cell** (3) and a section of a **pericyte process** (5) that is closely attached to the capillary wall. The capillary endothelium (6), the **nucleus of the endothelial cell** (3), and the section of the pericyte process (5) are surrounded by a **basal lamina** (2, 7). Adjacent to the capillary wall is a section of a **myelinated axon** (8). Also closely attached to the capillary wall in the CNS are a dense meshwork of fibers from axons, dendrites, and various processes of glial cells, such as the astrocytic endfeet, that fill the spaces in the CNS. This neural meshwork is called the **neuropil** (1, 4).

1 Neuropil

2 Basal lamina

3 Nucleus of
endothelial cell

4 Neuropil

Capillary lumen

5 Section of
pericyte process

6 Continuous
endothelium of
capillary

7 Basal lamina

8 Myelinated axon

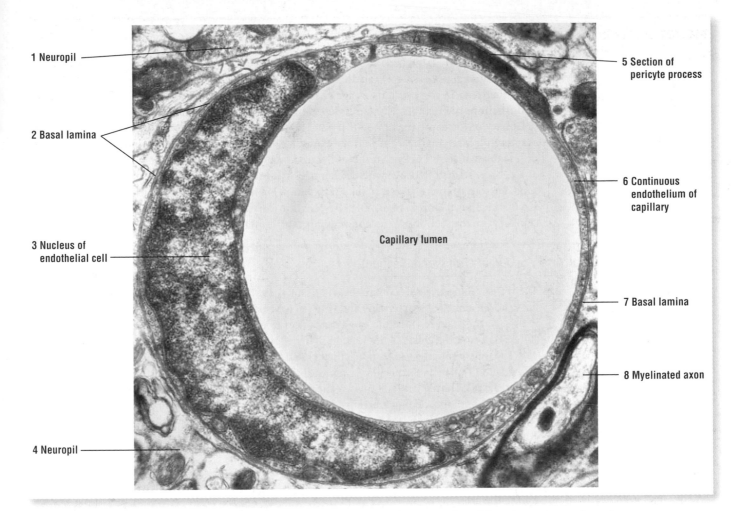

FIGURE 10.3 ■ Ultrastructure of a continuous capillary sectioned in a transverse plane in the CNS. Courtesy of Dr. Mark DeSantis, Professor Emeritus, WWAMI Medical Program, University of Idaho, Moscow, Idaho. ×25,000.

FIGURE 10.4 | Ultrastructure of a Fenestrated Capillary Sectioned in a Transverse Plane in the Choroid Plexus of a CNS Ventricle

The ultrastructure of a fenestrated capillary exhibits a distinctly different type of endothelium from that seen in the previous image of a continuous capillary (see Figure 10.3). The capillary **endothelium (3)** exhibits numerous opening or **fenestrations** (arrows) **(3)** around the entire periphery of the **capillary lumen (5)**. Note that the fenestrations (arrows) (3) are closed by thin diaphragms. Seen on the right side of the capillary is the **cytoplasm of an endothelia cell (7)** with different organelles. Located in the center and completely filling the capillary lumen is a section of a densely stained **RBC (2)** with its characteristic biconcave shape (see Figure 10.2 for comparison). Surrounding the fenestrated endothelium (3) and the cytoplasm of the endothelial cell (7) is a distinct **basal lamina (4, 6)**. In close proximity to the basal lamina (4, 6) and surrounding the capillary are the sections of the **ependymal cell cytoplasm (1, 8)** of the choroid plexus.

FIGURE 10.5 | Muscular Artery and Vein (Transverse Section)

The walls of blood vessels contain elastic tissue that allows them to expand and contract. In this illustration, a muscular **artery (1)** and **vein (4)** have been cut in the transverse plane and prepared with a plastic stain to illustrate the distribution of elastic fibers in their walls. The elastic fibers stain black, and the collagen fibers stain light yellow.

The wall of the artery (1) is much thicker and contains more smooth muscle fibers than the wall of the vein (4). The innermost layer tunica intima of the artery (1) is stained dark because of the thick **IEL (1a)**. The thick middle layer of the muscular artery, the **tunica media (1b)**, contains several layers of smooth muscle fibers, arranged in a circular pattern, and thin dark strands of **elastic fibers (1b)**. On the periphery of the tunica media (1b) is the less conspicuous **EEL (1c)**. Surrounding the artery is the connective tissue **tunica adventitia (1d)**, which contains both the light-staining **collagen fibers (2)** and the dark-staining **elastic fibers (3)**.

The wall of the vein (4) also contains the layers **tunica intima (4a)**, **tunica media (4b)**, and **tunica adventitia (4c)**. However, these three layers in the vein (4) are not as thick as those in the wall of the artery (1).

Surrounding both vessels are the **capillary (5)**, **arteriole (7)**, **venule (6)**, and cells of the **adipose tissue (8)**. Present in the lumina of both vessels (1, 4) are numerous erythrocytes and leukocytes.

1 Ependymal cell cytoplasm

2 RBC

3 Fenestrated endothelium

4 Basal lamina

5 Capillary lumen

6 Basal lamina

7 Cytoplasm of endothelial cell

8 Ependymal cell cytoplasm

Fenestrations

FIGURE 10.4 ■ Ultrastructure of a fenestrated capillary sectioned in a transverse plane in the choroid plexus of a CNS ventricle. ×25,000.

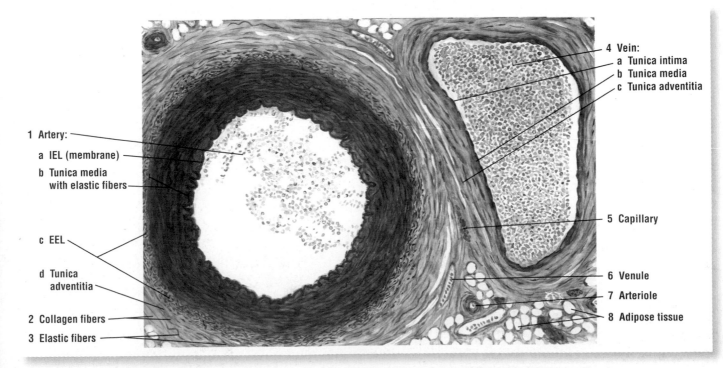

1 Artery:

a IEL (membrane)

b Tunica media with elastic fibers

c EEL

d Tunica adventitia

2 Collagen fibers

3 Elastic fibers

4 Vein:
a Tunica intima
b Tunica media
c Tunica adventitia

5 Capillary

6 Venule

7 Arteriole

8 Adipose tissue

FIGURE 10.5 ■ Muscular artery and vein (transverse section). Stain: elastic stain. Low magnification

---

FIGURE 10.6 | Artery and Vein in the Dense Irregular Connective Tissue of the Vas Deferens

This photomicrograph illustrates the structural differences between a **small artery (1)** and a small **vein (6)** in dense irregular **connective tissue (5)**. The small artery (1) has a relatively thick muscular wall and a small lumen. The arterial wall consists of the **tunica intima (2)**, composed of an inner layer of **endothelium (2a)**, a **subendothelial (2b)** layer of connective tissue, and an IEL **(membrane) (2c)**. This membrane (2c) separates the tunica intima (2) from the **tunica media (3)**, which consists predominantly of circular smooth muscle fibers. Surrounding the tunica media (3) is the connective tissue layer **tunica adventitia (4)**.

Adjacent to the small artery (1) is a small vein (6) with a much larger lumen that is filled with blood cells. The wall of the vein (6) is much thinner in comparison to that of the artery (1) but also consists of **tunica intima (7)** composed of **endothelium (7a)**, a thin layer of circular smooth muscle **tunica media (8)**, and the layer of connective tissue **tunica adventitia (9)**.

FIGURE 10.7 | Wall of an Elastic Artery: Aorta (Transverse Section)

The wall of the aorta is similar in morphology to that of the artery illustrated in Figure 10.6. Instead of smooth muscle fibers, the **elastic fibers (4)** constitute the bulk of the **tunica media (6)**, with **smooth muscle fibers (10)** less abundant than in the muscular arteries. The size and arrangement of the elastic fibers (4) in the tunica media (6) are demonstrated with the elastic stain. Other tissues in the wall of the aorta, such as fine elastic fibers and smooth muscle fibers (10), are either lightly stained or remain colorless.

The simple squamous **endothelium (1)** and the **subendothelial connective tissue (2)** in the **tunica intima (5)** are indicated but remain unstained. The first visible elastic membrane is the **IEL (membrane) (3)**.

The **tunica adventitia (7)**, somewhat less stained with elastic stain, is a narrow, peripheral zone of connective tissue. A **venule (9a)** and an **arteriole (9b)** of the **vasa vasorum (9)** supply the tunica adventitia (7). In such large blood vessels as the aorta and the pulmonary arteries, tunica media (6) occupies most of the vessel wall, whereas tunica adventitia (7) is reduced to a proportionately smaller area, as illustrated in this figure.

1 Small artery

2 Tunica intima:
   a. Endothelium
   b. Subendothelial
     connective tissue
   c. IEL (membrane)

3 Tunica media

4 Tunica adventitia

5 Connective tissue

6 Small vein

7 Tunica intima:
   a. Endothelium
8 Tunica media
9 Tunica adventitia

FIGURE 10.6 ■ Artery and vein in the dense irregular connective tissue of the vas deferens. Stain: iron hematoxylin and Alcian blue. ×64.

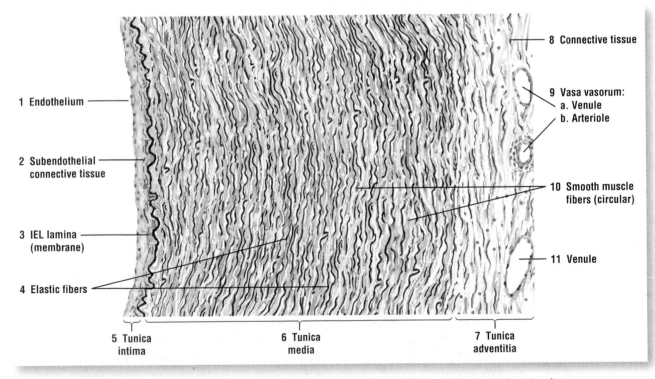

1 Endothelium

2 Subendothelial
   connective tissue

3 IEL lamina
   (membrane)

4 Elastic fibers

8 Connective tissue

9 Vasa vasorum:
   a. Venule
   b. Arteriole

10 Smooth muscle
    fibers (circular)

11 Venule

5 Tunica
  intima

6 Tunica
  media

7 Tunica
  adventitia

FIGURE 10.7 ■ Wall of a large elastic artery: aorta (transverse section). Stain: elastic stain. Low magnification.

FIGURE 10.8 | Wall of a Large Vein: Portal Vein (Transverse Section)

In contrast to the wall of a large artery (Figure 10.7), the wall of a large vein is characterized by thick, muscular **tunica adventitia (6)** in which the **smooth muscle fibers (7)** show a longitudinal orientation. In the transverse section of the portal vein, the smooth muscle fibers (7) are segregated into bundles and are seen mainly in cross section, surrounded by the connective tissue of the tunica adventitia (6). An **arteriole (8a)**, two **venules (8b)**, and a **capillary (8c)** in a longitudinal section of the **vasa vasorum (8)** are visible in the connective tissue of the tunica adventitia (6).

In contrast to the thick tunica adventitia (6), the **tunica media (5)** is thinner. The **smooth muscle fibers (3)** exhibit a circular orientation. In other large veins, the tunica media (5) may be extremely thin and compact.

The **tunica intima (4)** is part of the **endothelium (1)** and is supported by a small amount of **subendothelial connective tissue (2)**. In addition, large veins may exhibit an IEL that is not as well developed as in the arteries.

FIGURE 10.9 | Heart: Left Atrium, Atrioventricular Valve, and Left Ventricle (Longitudinal Section)

The wall of the heart consists of three layers: an inner **endocardium**, a middle **myocardium**, and an outer **epicardium**. The endocardium consists of a simple squamous endothelium and a thin subendothelial connective tissue. Deeper to the endocardium is the **subendocardial layer of connective tissue**. Here are found small blood vessels and Purkinje fibers. The subendocardial layer attaches to the endomysium of the cardiac muscle fibers. The myocardium is the thickest layer and consists of cardiac muscle fibers. The epicardium consists of a simple squamous mesothelium and an underlying **subepicardial layer** of connective tissue. The subepicardial layer contains **coronary blood vessels**, nerves, and **adipose tissue**.

A longitudinal section through the left side of the heart illustrates a portion of the **atrium (1)**, the **cusps of the atrioventricular (mitral) valve (5)**, and a section of the **ventricle (19)**. The endocardium (1, 9) lines the cavities of the atrium and the ventricle. Below the endocardium (1, 9) is the subendocardial connective tissue (2). The myocardium (3, 19) in both the atrium (3) and the ventricle (19) consists of cardiac muscle fibers.

The outer epicardium (13, 16) of the atrium (13) and the ventricle (16) is continuous and covers the heart externally with mesothelium. A subepicardial layer (17) contains connective tissue, adipose tissue (15), and numerous coronary blood vessels (15), which vary in amount in different regions of the heart. The epicardium (13, 16) also extends into the coronary (atrioventricular [AV]) sulcus and the interventricular sulcus of the heart.

Between the atrium (1) and the ventricle (19) is a layer of dense fibrous connective tissue called the **annulus fibrosus (4)**. A bicuspid (mitral) AV valve separates the atrium (1) from the ventricle (19). The cusps of the AV (mitral) valve (5) are formed by a double membrane of the **endocardium (6)** and a dense **connective tissue core (7)** that is continuous with the annulus fibrosus (4). On the ventral surface of each cusp (5) are the insertions of the connective tissue cords, the **chordae tendineae (8)**, which extend from the cusps of the valve (5) and attach to the **papillary muscles (11)** that project from the ventricle wall. The inner surface of the ventricle also contains prominent muscular (myocardial) ridges called **trabeculae carneae (10)** that give rise to the papillary muscles (11). The papillary muscles (11) via the chordae tendineae (8) hold and stabilize the cusps in the AV valves of the right and left ventricles during ventricular contractions.

The **Purkinje fibers (18)**, or impulse-conducting fibers, are located in the subendocardial connective tissue (2). They are distinguished from cardiac muscle fibers by their larger size and lighter-staining properties. The Purkinje fibers are illustrated in greater detail and higher magnification in Figures 10.11 and 10.12.

A large blood vessel of the heart, the **coronary artery (12)**, is found in the subepicardial connective tissue (17). Below the coronary artery is the **coronary sinus (14)**, a blood vessel that drains the heart. Entering the coronary sinus (14) is a **coronary vein (14)** with its valve. Smaller coronary blood vessels (15) are seen in the subepicardial connective tissue (17) and in the connective tissue septa that are found in the myocardium (19).

1 Endothelium

2 Subendothelial connective tissue

3 Smooth muscle fibers (circular)

7 Smooth muscle fibers (bundles, longitudinal section)

8 Vasa vasorum:
 a. Arteriole
 b. Venules
 c. Capillary

4 Tunica intima 5 Tunica media 6 Tunica adventitia

FIGURE 10.8 ■ Wall of a large vein: portal vein (transverse section). Stain: hematoxylin and eosin. Low magnification.

1 Endocardium of atrium

2 Subendocardial connective tissue

3 Myocardium of atrium

4 Annulus fibrosus

5 Cusps of atrioventricular (mitral) valve

6 Endocardium

7 Connective tissue core

8 Chorda tendinae

9 Endocardium of ventricle

10 Trabeculae carneae

11 Papillary muscle

12 Coronary artery

13 Epicardium of atrium

14 Coronary sinus and valve of coronary vein

15 Adipose tissue and coronary vein

16 Epicardium of ventricle

17 Subepicardial connective tissue

18 Purkinje fibers

19 Myocardium of ventricle

FIGURE 10.9 ■ Heart: a section of the left atrium, atrioventricular valve, and left ventricle (longitudinal section). Stain: hematoxylin and eosin. Low magnification.

FIGURE 10.10 | Heart: Right Ventricle, Pulmonary Trunk, and Pulmonary Valve (Longitudinal Section)

A section of the right ventricle and a lower portion of the **pulmonary trunk (5)** are illustrated. As in other blood vessels, the pulmonary trunk (5) is lined by the endothelium of the **tunica intima (5a)**. The **tunica media (5b)** constitutes the thickest portion of the wall of the pulmonary trunk (5); however, its thick, elastic laminae are not seen at this magnification. The thin connective tissue **tunica adventitia (5c)** merges with the surrounding **subepicardial connective tissue (2)**, which contains **adipose tissue** and **coronary arterioles and venules (3)**.

The pulmonary trunk (5) arises from the **annulus fibrosus (8)**. One cusp of its **semilunar (pulmonary) valve (6)** is illustrated. Similar to the AV valve (see Figure 10.9), the semilunar valve (6) of the pulmonary trunk (5) is covered with **endocardium (6)**. A **connective tissue core (7)** from the annulus fibrosus (8) extends into the base of the semilunar valve (6) and forms its central core.

The thick **myocardium (4)** of the right ventricle is lined internally by the **endocardium (9)**. The endocardium (9) extends over the pulmonary valve (6) and the annulus fibrosus (8) and blends in with the tunica intima (5a) of the pulmonary trunk (5).

The pulmonary trunk (5) is lined by the subepicardial connective tissue and adipose tissue (2), which, in turn, is covered by the **epicardium (1)**. Both of these layers cover the external surface of the right ventricle. Coronary arterioles and venules (3) are seen in the subepicardial connective tissue (2).

FIGURE 10.11 | Heart: Contracting Cardiac Muscle Fibers and Impulse-Conducting Purkinje Fibers

This figure illustrates a section of the heart stained with Mallory-Azan stain. With this preparation, the blue-stained collagen fibers accentuate the **subendocardial connective tissue (9)** that surrounds the **Purkinje fibers (6, 10)**. The characteristic features of Purkinje fibers (6, 10) are demonstrated in both longitudinal and transverse planes of section. In transverse plane (6), the Purkinje fibers exhibit fewer myofibrils that are distributed peripherally, leaving a perinuclear zone of comparatively clear sarcoplasm. A nucleus is seen in some transverse sections; in others, a central area of clear sarcoplasm is seen, with the plane of section bypassing the nucleus.

The Purkinje fibers (6, 10) are located under the **endocardium (7)**, which represents the endothelium of the heart cavities. The Purkinje fibers (6, 10) are different from typical **cardiac muscle fibers (1, 3)**. In contrast to cardiac muscle fibers (1, 3), the Purkinje fibers (6, 10) are larger and show less intense staining.

The cardiac muscle fibers (1, 3) are connected to each other via the prominent **intercalated disks (4)**. The intercalated disks (4) are not observed in the Purkinje fibers (6, 10). Instead, the Purkinje fibers (6, 10) are connected to each other via desmosomes and gap junctions and eventually merge with cardiac muscle fibers (1, 3).

The heart musculature has a rich blood supply. Seen in this illustration are a **capillary (8)**, **arteriole (5)**, and **venule (2)**.

1 Epicardium

5 Pulmonary trunk:
 a. Tunica intima
 b. Tunica media
 c. Tunica adventitia

2 Subepicardial connective tissue and adipose tissue

6 Endocardium of semilunar (pulmonary) valve

7 Connective tissue core

3 Coronary arteriole and venule

8 Annulus fibrosus

9 Endocardium of right ventricle

4 Myocardium

FIGURE 10.10 ■ Heart: a section of right ventricle, pulmonary trunk, and pulmonary valve (longitudinal section). Stain: hematoxylin and eosin. Low magnification.

1 Cardiac muscle fibers (transverse section)

6 Purkinje fibers (transverse section)

7 Endocardium

2 Venule

8 Capillary

3 Cardiac muscle fibers (longitudinal section)

4 Intercalated disks

9 Subendocardial connective tissue

5 Arteriole

10 Purkinje fibers (longitudinal section)

FIGURE 10.11 ■ Heart: contracting cardiac muscle fibers and impulse-conducting Purkinje fibers. Stain: Mallory-Azan. High magnification.

FIGURE 10.12 | Heart Wall: Purkinje Fibers

A photomicrograph of the ventricular heart wall illustrates the **endocardium (3)** of the heart chamber, **subendocardial connective tissue (4)**, and the underlying **Purkinje fibers (5)**. In comparison with the adjacent, red-stained **cardiac muscle fibers (1)**, the Purkinje fibers (5) are larger and exhibit less intense staining. Also, the Purkinje fibers (5) exhibit fewer myofibrils, which are peripherally distributed and which leave a perinuclear zone of clear sarcoplasm. Purkinje fibers (5) gradually merge with the cardiac muscle fibers (1). Surrounding both the Purkinje fibers (5) and the cardiac muscle fibers (1) are bundles of **connective tissue fibers (2)**.

1 Cardiac muscle fibers

2 Connective tissue fibers

3 Endocardium

4 Subendocardial connective tissue

5 Purkinje fibers

FIGURE 10.12 ■ A section of heart wall: Purkinje fibers. Stain: Mallory-Azan. ×64.

FUNCTIONAL CORRELATIONS 10.1	Circulatory System

BLOOD VESSELS

The **elastic arteries** transport the ejected blood from the heart and move it along the systemic vascular path. The presence of an increased number of **elastic fibers** in their walls allows the elastic arteries to greatly expand in diameter during **systole** (heart contraction), when a large volume of blood is forcefully ejected from the ventricles into their lumina. During **diastole** (heart relaxation), the expanded elastic walls recoil upon the volume of blood in their lumina and force the blood to move forward through the vascular channels. As a result, a less variable systemic blood pressure is maintained, and blood flows more evenly through the body during heartbeats.

In contrast, the **muscular arteries** control blood flow and blood pressure through **vasoconstriction** (narrowing) or **vasodilation** (expanding) of their lumina. Vasoconstriction and vasodilation, owing to a high proportion of **smooth muscle fibers** in the artery walls, are controlled by unmyelinated axons of the **sympathetic division** of the **autonomic nervous system (ANS)**. Similarly, by autonomic constriction or dilation of their lumina, the smooth muscle fibers in smaller muscular arteries or arterioles regulate blood flow into the capillary beds.

Terminal arterioles give rise to the smallest blood vessels, called **capillaries**. Because of their very thin walls, capillaries are major sites for the exchange of gases, metabolites, nutrients, and waste products between blood and interstitial tissues.

LYMPHATIC VESSELS

The main function of the **lymphatic vascular system** is to passively collect excess tissue fluid and proteins, called **lymph**, from the intercellular spaces of the connective tissue and return it into the venous portion of the blood vascular system. Lymph is a clear fluid and an **ultrafiltrate** of the blood plasma. Numerous lymph nodes are located along the route of the lymph vessels. In the maze of lymph node channels, the collected lymph is filtered of cells and particulate matter. Lymph that flows

(Continued)

FUNCTIONAL CORRELATIONS 10.1 | Circulatory System *(Continued)*

through the lymph nodes is also exposed to the numerous macrophages that reside here. These engulf any foreign microorganisms as well as other suspended matter. The lymph vessels also bring to the systemic bloodstream **lymphocytes**, **fatty acids** absorbed through the capillary lymph vessels called **lacteals** in the small intestine, and **immunoglobulins** (antibodies) produced in the lymph nodes. Thus, the lymphatic vessels serve as an important component of the immune system of the body.

ENDOTHELIUM

The endothelium lining the lumina of blood vessels performs important physiologic, metabolic, and secretory functions. The endothelial cells form a **semipermeable barrier** between blood and the interstitial tissue. The cells are anchored to the basal lamina and attached to each other by adhesion junctions. The presence of many **pinocytotic** vesicles in the endothelial cells indicates a bidirectional movement of molecules between blood and tissues. The smooth lining of the endothelium in the blood vessels and the secretion of **anticoagulants** by the endothelial cells perform an important role in preventing blood clotting. The endothelial cell surfaces are also lined by **glycocalyx** protein. In addition, endothelial cells secrete **prostacyclin**, which is an **antithrombotic** substance that prevents platelet adhesion in the blood vessels and blood clot formation.

Endothelial cells also produce vasoactive chemicals such as **nitrous oxide** and its related compounds, which induce **vasodilation** and increased blood flow. Conversely, the secretion of **endothelin proteins** by endothelial cells counteracts the nitrous oxide effects by causing vasoconstriction of blood vessels and decreased blood flow. The endothelium also induces the conversion of **angiotensin I** to **angiotensin II**, a powerful vasoconstrictor that increases blood pressure. Endothelium also converts such compounds as prostaglandins, bradykinin, serotonin, and other substances to biologically inactive compounds; degrades lipoproteins; and produces growth factors for fibroblasts, blood cell colonies, and platelets, as well as other functions. The cytoplasm of endothelial cells also contains small membrane-bound, electron-dense structures called **Weibel-Palade bodies**. These bodies store the glycoprotein **von Willebrand factor** that is synthesized by arterial endothelial cells. When the endothelium is damaged, von Willebrand factor is released into the blood to induce platelets adhesion and **blood clot formation**.

THE HEART WALL

Pacemaker of the Heart

Cardiac muscle is **involuntary** and contracts rhythmically and automatically. The **impulse-generating** and **impulse-conducting** portions of the heart are specialized or modified **cardiac muscle fibers** located in the **sinoatrial (SA) node** and the **AV node** in the wall of the **right atrium** of the heart. The modified cardiac muscle fibers in these nodes exhibit spontaneous rhythmic depolarization or impulse conduction, which sends a wave of stimulation throughout the myocardium of the heart. Because the fibers in the SA node depolarize and repolarize faster than those in the AV node, the SA node sets the pace for the heartbeat and is, therefore, called the **pacemaker**.

Intercalated disks bind all cardiac muscle fibers while stimulatory impulses from the SA node are conducted via **gap junctions** to the atrial musculature, causing rapid spread of stimuli throughout the entire heart muscle and cardiac muscle fiber contraction. Impulses from the SA node travel through the heart musculature via **internodal pathways** to stimulate the AV node that lies in the interatrial septum. From the AV node, the impulses spread along a bundle of specialized conducting cardiac fibers, called the **AV bundle (of His)**, located in the interventricular septum (between ventricles). The AV bundle divides into right and left bundle branches. Approximately halfway down the interventricular septum, the AV bundle branches become the **Purkinje fibers**, which branch further in order to transmit the stimulation throughout the ventricular musculature.

The pacemaker activities of the heart are influenced by the axons from the **ANS** and by certain **hormones**. Axons from both the parasympathetic division and the sympathetic division innervate the heart and form a wide plexus at its base. Although these axons innervate the heart myocardium, they do not affect the initiation of rhythmic activity of the nodes. Instead, they affect the heart rate. Stimulation by the sympathetic nerves accelerates the heart rate, whereas stimulation by the parasympathetic nerves produces the opposite effect and decreases the heart rate.

Purkinje Fibers

Purkinje fibers are thicker and larger than cardiac muscle fibers and contain a greater amount of **glycogen**. They also contain fewer contractile filaments. Purkinje fibers are part of the conduction system of the heart. These fibers are located beneath the **endocardium** on either side of the interventricular septum and are recognized as separate tracts. Because Purkinje fibers branch throughout the myocardium, they deliver continuous waves of stimulation from the atrial nodes (SA and AV) to the rest of the heart musculature via the **gap junctions**. This stimulation produces ventricular contractions (systole) and the ejection of blood from both ventricular chambers.

Atrial Natriuretic Hormone

Certain cardiac muscle fibers in the atria exhibit dense granules in their cytoplasm. These granules contain **atrial natriuretic hormone**, a chemical that is released in response to atrial distention or stretching. The main function of this hormone is to decrease blood pressure by regulating blood volume. The atrial natriuretic hormone inhibits the release of **renin** by the specialized cells in the kidney and **aldosterone** from the adrenal gland cortex. These inhibitions induce the kidney to lose more sodium ions and water (diuresis). As a result, the blood volume and blood pressure are reduced, and the distention of the atrial wall is relieved, which prevents further release of the atrial natriuretic hormone.

Circulatory System

Cardiovascular System

- Consists of heart, major arteries, arterioles, capillaries, veins, and venules
- Two major circuits are systemic circulation and pulmonary circulation
- Systemic circulation takes blood to all systems and back to the heart
- Pulmonary circulation takes blood to the lungs for gaseous exchange and back to the heart

Type of Arteries

Elastic Arteries

- Are the largest vessels and include aorta, pulmonary trunk, and their major branches
- Wall primarily composed of elastic connective tissue mixed with smooth muscle cells
- Exhibit resilience and flexibility; walls greatly expand during systole (heart contraction)
- During diastole (heart relaxation), walls recoil and force blood forward

Muscular Arteries, Arterioles, and Capillaries

- Most numerous vessels with their walls lined with smooth muscle fibers
- Control of blood flow through vasoconstriction or vasodilation of lumina
- Smooth muscles in arterial walls controlled by axons from the ANS
- Arterioles are the small blood vessels with one to five layers of smooth muscle
- Terminal arterioles deliver blood to the smallest blood vessels, the capillaries
- Capillaries are the sites of metabolic exchanges between blood and tissues
- Capillaries connect arterioles with venules

Structural Plan of Arteries

- Wall consists of three layers: inner tunica intima, middle tunica media, and outer tunica adventitia
- Tunica intima consists of endothelium and subendothelial connective tissue
- Tunica media is composed mainly of smooth muscle fibers with some elastic fibers
- In elastic and muscular arteries, smooth muscles produce elastic fibers and some collagen
- Tunica adventitia contains primarily collagen type I and elastic fibers

- IEL separates tunica intima from tunica media
- Fenestrations in IEL allow diffusion of nutrients to deeper cells
- EEL separates tunica media from tunica adventitia

Structural Plan of Veins

- Capillaries unite to form larger vessels called venules and postcapillary venules
- Thinner walls, larger diameters, and more structural variation than arteries
- Blood under low pressure and valves present to prevent backflow of blood in extremities
- Blood flow toward heart is due to muscular contractions around veins and valves
- Valves absent in veins of the viscera, the CNS, and the inferior and superior venae cavae
- Wall consists of three layers: tunica intima, tunica media, and tunica adventitia
- Tunica intima consists of endothelium and subendothelial connective tissue
- Tunica media is thin, and smooth muscle intermixes with connective tissue fibers
- Tunica adventitia is the thickest layer, with longitudinal smooth muscle fibers

Vasa Vasorum

- Found in the thicker walls of large arteries and veins that do not allow diffusion from lumina
- Small adjacent arterial blood vessels supply tunica media and tunica adventitia
- More extensive in the walls of veins than arteries due to poor oxygen content of veins

Types of Capillaries

- Average diameter is about the size of a RBC (about 8 μm)
- Consist of thin endothelium, basal lamina, and pericytes
- Continuous capillaries are most common; endothelium forms solid lining
- Continuous capillaries found in most organs
- Fenestrated capillaries contain pores or fenestrations in endothelium
- Fenestrated capillaries found in endocrine glands, small intestine, and kidney glomeruli
- Sinusoidal capillaries exhibit wide diameters with wide gaps between endothelial cells

- Basement membrane incomplete or absent in sinusoidal capillaries
- Sinusoidal capillaries found in liver, spleen, and bone marrow

Lymphatic Vascular System

- Associated with the circulatory system and drains extracellular fluid lymph from tissues
- Lymphatic capillaries start as blind dilations and form the lymph drainage system
- Lymph eventually returned to the circulatory system after filtering lymph in lymph nodes
- Vessels are very thin and show greater permeability than capillaries
- Lymph vessels contain valves, and lymph movement is due to muscular contractions
- Lymph flows through lymph nodes and is exposed to macrophages
- Lymph contains lymphocytes, fatty acids, and immunoglobulins (antibodies)
- Integral component of immune system of the body

Endothelium

- Forms a semipermeable barrier between blood and interstitial tissue
- Pinocytotic vesicles in endothelium allow bidirectional movement of molecules
- Provides smooth surface for blood flow without damage to the platelets
- Lined by glycocalyx and secretes prostacyclin, which prevents platelet adhesion and blood clotting
- Produces nitrous oxide, which induces vasodilation
- Produces endothelin proteins that counteract nitrous oxide and cause vasoconstriction
- Converts angiotensin I to angiotensin II, a vasoconstrictor that raises blood pressure
- Converts certain chemicals to inactive compounds, degrades lipoproteins, and produces growth factors
- Contains electron-dense Weibel-Palade bodies that store von Willebrand factor

- Releases von Willebrand factor during damage, which increases platelet adhesion and blood clotting

Heart Wall—Endocardium, Myocardium, and Epicardium

Pacemaker

- Impulse conduction by specialized cardiac cells located in SA and AV nodes
- SA and AV nodes located in the wall of the right atrium
- SA node sets the pace for the heart and is the pacemaker of the heart
- Impulse from SA node conducted via gap junctions to all heart musculature
- AV bundles located on right and left sides of the interventricular septum
- AV bundles become Purkinje fibers
- Pacemaker activities influenced by ANS and hormones
- Sympathetic axons stimulate heart rate; parasympathetic nerves decrease heart rate

Purkinje Fibers

- Larger than cardiac fibers with more glycogen and lighter staining
- Part of the conduction system of the heart
- Located beneath the endocardium on either side of the interventricular septum
- Branch throughout the myocardium and deliver stimuli via gap junctions to the rest of the heart

Atrial Natriuretic Hormone

- Certain atrial cells contain granules of atrial natriuretic hormone
- Released when atrial wall is stretched
- Decreases blood pressure by inhibiting renin and aldosterone release
- Kidney loses more sodium and water, which decreases blood volume and pressure

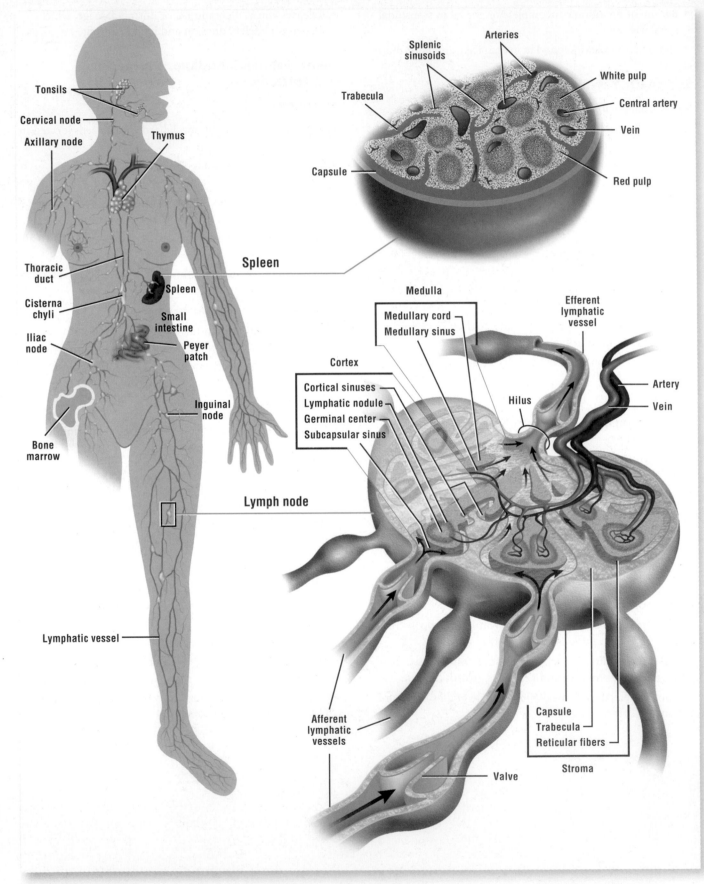

OVERVIEW FIGURE 11.1 ■ Location and distribution of the lymphoid organs and lymphatic channels in the body. Internal contents of the lymph node and the spleen are illustrated in greater detail.

CHAPTER 11

Immune System ▮

The main function of the **immune system** is to protect the organism against invading pathogens or antigens (bacteria, parasites, and viruses). The immune response occurs as soon as the organism detects the pathogens, which can enter the organism in numerous places in the body. For this reason, the cells, tissues, and organs of the immune system have wide distribution throughout the organism so that the immunologic response is quick to counteract the effects of invading foreign substances.

The lymphoid system includes all cells, tissues, and organs in the body that contain aggregates (accumulations) of immune cells called **lymphocytes**. Cells of the immune system, especially lymphocytes, are distributed throughout the body as single cells; as isolated accumulations of cells; as distinct nonencapsulated lymphatic nodules in the loose connective tissue of the **digestive**, **respiratory**, and **reproductive systems**; or as encapsulated individual lymphoid organs. The major organs of the immune system are the lymph nodes, tonsils, thymus, and spleen. Because bone marrow produces lymphocytes, it is also considered a lymphoid organ and part of the immune system.

Although it is important to study the histology of the different organs of the immune system, much of what takes place functionally within these organs and the body cannot be seen histologically and must be explained immunologically. It is known, however, that the cells, tissues, and organs of the immune system are constantly challenged by foreign substances.

Organs of the Immune System: Lymph Nodes, the Spleen, and the Thymus

The overview figure illustrates the distribution of the lymphoid system in the body and the general structures of two encapsulated lymphoid organs—the **lymph nodes** and **spleen**. The lymph nodes have a wide distribution and are primarily found along the paths of lymphatic vessels, which are most prominent in inguinal and axillary regions of the body. A connective tissue **capsule** surrounds the lymph node and sends its **trabeculae** into its interior. Each lymph node contains an outer **cortex** and an inner **medulla**. A network of reticular fibers and spherical, nonencapsulated aggregations of lymphocytes called **lymphoid nodules** characterize the cortex. Some lymphoid nodules exhibit lighter-staining central areas called **germinal centers**. The medulla consists of **medullary cords** and **medullary sinuses**. Medullary cords are networks of reticular fibers filled with plasma cells, macrophages, and lymphocytes separated by capillary-like channels called medullary sinuses.

The collected lymph enters the lymph node via **afferent lymphatic vessels** that penetrate the capsule on the convex surface. Lymph is then filtered as it slowly flows through the cortex and medullary sinuses to exit the lymph node on the opposite side via the **efferent lymphatic vessels** (see Overview Figure 11.1).

The spleen is a large lymphoid organ with a rich blood supply. A connective tissue capsule surrounds the spleen and divides its interior into incomplete compartments called the **splenic pulp**, which consists of white pulp and red pulp. They are so named because of their color when the spleen is cut open. **White pulp** consists of dark-staining lymphoid aggregations or **lymphatic nodules** that surround a blood vessel called the **central artery**. This is a misnomer because the central artery is located in an eccentric position in the white pulp. White pulp is located within the blood-rich red pulp. The arterial system ends in **red pulp**, which consists of **splenic cords** and **splenic (blood) sinusoids**. The splenic cords contain networks of reticular fibers in which are found numerous macrophages, lymphocytes, plasma cells, and different blood cells. In contrast, splenic sinuses are interconnected blood channels that drain splenic blood into larger sinuses that eventually leave the spleen via the splenic vein (see Overview Figure 11.1).

The **thymus gland** is a soft, lobulated lymphoepithelial organ located in the upper anterior mediastinum and lower part of the neck. The gland is most active during childhood, after which it undergoes slow involution, and, in adults, the lymphoid region is filled with adipose tissue. The thymus gland is surrounded by a connective tissue capsule, under which is the dark-staining **cortex** with an extensive network of interconnecting spaces. These spaces become colonized by **immature lymphocytes** that migrate here from hemopoietic tissues in the developing individual to undergo maturation and differentiation. The epithelial cells of the thymus gland provide structural support for the increased lymphocyte population. In the lighter-staining **medulla**, the epithelial cells form a coarser framework that contains fewer lymphocytes and whorls of epithelial cells that combine to form **thymic (Hassall) corpuscles**.

Cells of the Immune System

The cells that carry out immune response include lymphocytes and various supporting cells. Three major types of lymphocytes are recognized. These are **T lymphocytes (T cells)**, **B lymphocytes (B cells)**, and **natural killer (NK) cells**. Supporting cells are those that interact with lymphocytes and participate in the presentation of antigens to lymphocytes for immune response.

All components of the lymphoid system are an essential part of the **immune system**. Different types of lymphocytes are present in various organs of the body. Morphologically, all types of lymphocytes appear very similar, but, functionally, they are very different. The B cells and T cells are distinguished on the basis of where they differentiate and mature into immunocompetent cells and on the types of surface receptors present on their cell membranes. These two functionally distinct types of lymphocytes are found in blood, lymph, lymphoid tissues, and lymphoid organs. Like all blood cells, both types of lymphocytes originate from precursor **hemopoietic stem cells** in the **bone marrow** and then enter the bloodstream.

T cells arise from lymphocytes that are carried from the bone marrow to the **thymus gland**. Here, they mature, differentiate, and acquire surface receptors and **immunocompetence** before migrating to take up residence in peripheral lymphoid tissues and organs. The thymus gland produces mature T cells early in life. After their stay in the thymus gland, T cells are distributed throughout the body via the blood and populate lymph nodes, the spleen, and lymphoid aggregates or nodules in connective tissue. In these regions, the T cells carry out immune responses when stimulated. On encountering an antigen, T cells destroy the antigen either by cytotoxic action or by activating B cells. There are four main subtypes of differentiated T cells: **helper T cells**, **cytotoxic T cells**, **regulatory (suppressor) T cells**, and **memory T cells**.

When encountering an antigen, **helper T cells** assist other lymphocytes by secreting immune chemicals called **cytokines**, also called **interleukins**. Cytokines are protein hormones that stimulate the proliferation, secretion, differentiation, and maturation of B cells into **plasma cells**, which then produce immune proteins called **antibodies**, also called **immunoglobulins**. The helper T cells also activate macrophages to become phagocytic and activate cytotoxic T cells.

Cytotoxic T cells specifically recognize antigenically different cells, such as virus-infected cells, foreign cells, or malignant cells, and destroy them. These lymphocytes become activated when they combine with antigens that react with their receptors. The cytotoxic T cells then release lysosomes with lytic granules that contain pore-forming protein called **perforin**. Perforin creates channels in the membrane of the targeted cell, resulting in **apoptosis**, or cell death.

Regulatory (suppressor) T cells may decrease or inhibit the functions of helper T cells and cytotoxic T cells and, thus, functionally suppress immune response by influencing the activities of other cells in the immune system.

Memory T cells are the long-living progeny of T cells. They respond rapidly to the same antigens in the body and stimulate the immediate production of cytotoxic T cells. Memory T cells are the counterparts of memory B cells.

B cells mature and become immunocompetent in bone marrow. After maturation, blood carries B cells to the nonthymic lymphoid tissues, such as the lymph nodes, spleen, and connective tissue. B cells are able to recognize a particular type of antigen owing to the presence of **antigen**

receptors on the surface of their cell membrane. Immunocompetent B cells become activated when they encounter a specific antigen, and it binds to the surface antigen receptor of the B cell. The response of B cells to an antigen, however, is more intense when antigen-presenting cells (APCs), such as **helper T cells**, present the antigen to the B cells. Helper T cells secrete a cytokine (**interleukin 2**) that induces increased proliferation and differentiation of antigen-activated B cells. Numerous progeny of activated B cells enlarge, divide, proliferate, and differentiate into **plasma cells**. Plasma cells then secrete large amounts of **antibodies** specific to the antigen that triggered plasma cell formation. Antibodies react with the antigens and initiate a complex process that eventually destroys the foreign substance that activated the immune response. The dependence of B cells on helper T cells increases the antibody secretion and produces a strong immune response, such as activation of phagocytes and production of **memory B cells**. Other activated B cells do not become plasma cells. Instead, they persist in lymphoid organs as memory B cells. These memory cells produce a more rapid and longer-lasting immunologic response should the same antigen reappear.

NK cells develop from the same precursor cells as B and T cells and are the third type of lymphocytes that are especially genetically programmed to recognize and kill certain altered cells. NK cells attack virally infected cells and cancer cells and eliminate the target cells in a fashion similar to cytotoxic T cells.

In addition to T, B, and NK cells and macrophages, **APCs** perform important functions in immune responses, and they are found in most tissues. These cells phagocytose and process antigens and then present the antigen to T cells, inducing their activation. Most APCs belong to the mononuclear phagocytic system. Included in this group are the connective tissue **macrophages**, **perisinusoidal macrophages** in the liver (Kupffer cells), **Langerhans cells,** also called **dendritic** cells in the skin, and macrophages within the lymphoid organs.

Types of Immune Responses

An essential feature of the mammalian immune system is its ability to initiate different types of responses to foreign matter. The presence of foreign cells or antigens in the body stimulates a highly complex series of immune reactions. The immune responses to invading foreign organisms can be divided into two main types of responses, the innate immune response and the adaptive immune response.

The **innate immune response** is the first line of defense that limits the spread of infection. Its response to antigen invasion is composed of phagocytic functions, which are rapid and include the mobilization of neutrophils, mast cells, macrophages, and NK cells. Although the response of the innate immune system is fast, it is **nonspecific** and does not produce memory cells.

The **adaptive immune response** targets specific invading foreign organisms and provides **specific,** or adaptive, defenses. This response is slower than the innate immune response, but it produces and retains numerous memory cells, which can respond to the second encounter with the particular antigen in a manner that is rapid, stronger, and longer lasting. The two types of specific immune responses are the **humoral immune response** and the **cell-mediated immune response**. These responses result in the production of antibodies, which bind to the antigens, or the stimulation of cells that destroy foreign cells. Both the B cells and T cells respond to antigens by different means. These two types of closely related immune responses take place in the body, both of which are triggered by antigens and form an integral defense system of the body.

In the **humoral-mediated immune response**, exposure of **B cells** to an antigen induces the proliferation and transformation of some of the B cells into **plasma cells**. These, in turn, secrete specific **antibodies** into blood and lymph that bind to, inactivate, and destroy the specific foreign substance or antigens. The activation and proliferation of B cells against most antigens require the cooperation of helper T cells that respond to the same antigen and the production of certain cytokines. The presence of the B cells, plasma cells, and antibodies in the blood and lymph is the basis of the humoral immune response.

In the **cell-mediated immune response**, specific T cells are stimulated by the presence of antigens on the surface of **APCs**. The T cells proliferate and secrete **cytokines** that stimulate or activate other T cells, B cells, and cytotoxic T cells. On activation and directly binding to target cells, cytotoxic T cells destroy foreign cells by inducing **apoptosis,** or programmed cell death of the target cells. The activated T cells then destroy foreign microorganisms, parasites, tumor cells, or virus-infected cells by direct cell-to-cell contact. This is done by releasing lytic granules that contain perforin, which, in turn, creates pores in the plasma membrane and causes cell death. T cells may also attack indirectly by activating B cells and increasing their antibody production, or stimulating the **macrophages** of the immune system. T cells provide specific immune protection without secreting antibodies; instead, they have surface receptors for antigens.

 Supplemental micrographic images are available at **www.thePoint.com/Eroschenko12e** under Lymphoid System.

FIGURE 11.1 | Lymph Node (Panoramic View)

The lymph node consists of dense masses of lymphocyte aggregations intermixed with dilated lymphatic sinuses that contain lymph and are supported by a framework of fine reticular fibers. A lymph node has been sectioned in half to show the outer dark-staining **cortex (4)** and the inner light-staining **medulla (10)**. The lymph node is surrounded by a **pericapsular adipose tissue (1)** that contains numerous blood vessels, shown here as an **arteriole and venule (9)**. A dense connective tissue **capsule (2)** surrounds the lymph node. From the capsule (2), **connective tissue trabeculae (6)** extend into the node, initially between the lymphatic nodules, and then ramifying throughout the medulla (10) for a variable distance. The trabecular connective tissue (6) also contains the major **blood vessels (5, 8)** of the lymph node.

Afferent lymphatic vessels with **valves (7)** course in the connective tissue capsule (2) of the lymph node and, at intervals, penetrate the capsule to enter a narrow space called the **subcapsular sinus (3, 15)**. From here, the sinuses (cortical sinuses) extend along the trabeculae (6) to pass into the **medullary sinuses (11)**.

The cortex (4) of the lymph node contains numerous lymphocyte aggregations called **lymphatic nodules (16)**. When the lymphatic nodules (16) are sectioned through the center, lighter-stained areas become visible. These lighter areas are the **germinal centers (17)** of the lymphatic nodules (16) and represent the active sites of lymphocyte proliferation.

In the medulla (10) of the lymph node, the lymphocytes are arranged as irregular cords of lymphatic tissue called **medullary cords (14)**. Medullary cords (14) contain macrophages, plasma cells, and small lymphocytes. The dilated medullary sinuses (11) drain the lymph from the cortical region of the lymph node and course between the medullary cords (14) toward the **hilus** of the organ.

The concavity of the lymph node represents the hilus (12). Nerves, blood vessels, and veins that supply and drain the lymph node are located in the hilus (12). **Efferent lymphatic vessels (13)** drain the lymph from the medullary sinuses (11) and exit the lymph node in the hilus (12).

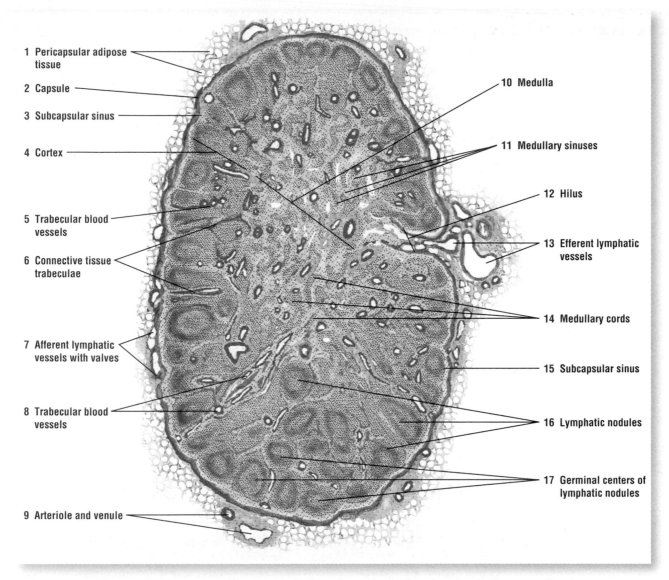

1 Pericapsular adipose tissue

2 Capsule

3 Subcapsular sinus

4 Cortex

5 Trabecular blood vessels

6 Connective tissue trabeculae

7 Afferent lymphatic vessels with valves

8 Trabecular blood vessels

9 Arteriole and venule

10 Medulla

11 Medullary sinuses

12 Hilus

13 Efferent lymphatic vessels

14 Medullary cords

15 Subcapsular sinus

16 Lymphatic nodules

17 Germinal centers of lymphatic nodules

FIGURE 11.1 ■ Lymph node (panoramic view). Stain: hematoxylin and eosin. Medium magnification.

FIGURE 11.2 | Lymph Node Capsule, Cortex, and Medulla (Sectional View)

A small section of a cortical region of the lymph node is illustrated at a higher magnification.

A layer of **connective tissue (1)** with a **venule** and an **arteriole (11)** surrounds the lymph node **capsule (3)**. Visible in the connective tissue (1) is an afferent **lymphatic vessel (2)** lined with endothelium and containing a **valve (2)**. Arising from the inner surface of the capsule (3), the connective tissue **trabeculae (5, 14)** extend through the cortex and medulla. Associated with the connective tissue trabeculae (5, 14) are numerous **trabecular blood vessels (16)**.

The cortex of the lymph node is separated from the connective tissue capsule (3) by the **subcapsular (marginal) sinus (4, 12)**. The cortex consists of **lymphatic nodules (13)** situated adjacent to each other but incompletely separated by internodular connective tissue trabeculae (5, 14) and **trabecular (cortical) sinuses (6)**. In this illustration, two complete lymphatic nodules (13) are illustrated. When sectioned through the middle, the lymphatic nodules exhibit a central, light-staining **germinal center (7, 15)** surrounded by a deeper-staining peripheral portion of the nodule (13). In the germinal centers (7, 15) of the lymphatic nodules (13), the cells are more loosely aggregated and the developing lymphocytes have larger and lighter-staining nuclei with more cytoplasm.

The deeper portion of the lymph node cortex is the **paracortex (8, 17)**. This area is the thymus-dependent zone and is primarily occupied by T cells. This is also a transition area from the lymphatic nodules (7, 13) to the **medullary cords (9, 19)** of the lymph node medulla. The medulla consists of anastomosing cords of lymphatic tissue, the medullary cords (9, 19), interspersed with **medullary sinuses (10, 18)** that drain the lymph from the node into the efferent lymphatic vessels that are located at the hilus (see Figure 11.1).

Fine reticular connective tissue provides the main structural support for the lymph node and forms the core of the lymphatic nodules (13) in the cortex, the medullary cords (9, 19), and all medullary sinuses (10, 18) in the medulla. Relatively few lymphocytes are seen in the medullary sinuses (10, 18); thus, it is possible to distinguish the reticular framework of the node in the lymphatic nodules (13) and the medullary cords (9, 19). The lymphocytes are so abundant that the fine reticulum is obscured, unless it is specifically stained, as shown in Figure 11.6. Most of the lymphocytes are small with large, deep-staining nuclei and condensed chromatin and exhibit either a small amount of cytoplasm or none at all.

FUNCTIONAL CORRELATIONS 11.1 | Lymph Nodes

Lymph nodes are important components of the defense mechanism. They have a strategic distribution throughout the body along the paths of **lymphatic vessels** and are most prominent in the **inguinal** and **axillary regions**. Their major functions are **lymph filtration** and the **phagocytosis** of bacteria or foreign substances from the filtered lymph, preventing them from reaching the general circulation. Trapped within the reticular fiber network of each lymph node are fixed or free macrophages that destroy any foreign substances. Thus, as lymph is filtered, the nodes participate in localizing and preventing the spread of infection into the general circulation and other organs.

Lymph nodes also produce, store, recirculate, and activate **B cells** and **T cells**. Here the lymphocytes can proliferate, and the B cells can transform into plasma cells. As a result, lymph that leaves the lymph nodes via the efferent vessels may contain increased amounts of antibodies that can then be distributed to the entire body. After entering the lymph node, the B cells congregate in the **lymphatic nodules** of lymph nodes that are located in the outer cortex. The T cells concentrate below the lymphatic nodules in the deep **cortical** or **paracortical (paracortex) regions**. Lymph nodes are also the sites of **antigenic recognition** and **antigenic activation** of B cells, which give rise to **plasma cells** and **memory B cells**. When B cells are activated by the APCs, as part of the immune response, these lymphocytes proliferate in the central region of the lymphatic nodule and are recognized as lighter-staining **germinal centers**.

FUNCTIONAL CORRELATIONS 11.1 | Lymph Nodes *(Continued)*

Continuous lymphocyte circulation between blood and lymph takes place in the lymph nodes, tonsils, Peyer patches, and spleen. Circulating B cells and T cells enter the lymph nodes through the incoming arteries. All lymph that is formed in the body eventually reaches the blood, and lymphocytes that leave the lymph nodes via the efferent lymph vessels also return to the bloodstream. The arteries that supply the lymph nodes and branch into capillaries in the cortex and paracortex regions also provide an entryway for lymphocytes into the lymph nodes. Most of the lymphocytes enter the lymph nodes through the thin-walled postcapillary venules located in the paracortex. Here, the postcapillary venules are lined by tall cuboidal or columnar endothelium containing specialized **lymphocyte-homing receptors**. Because these venules are lined by taller endothelium, they are called **high endothelial venules**. The circulating lymphocytes recognize the receptors on the endothelial cells and leave the bloodstream to enter the lymph node. Both B cells and T cells leave the bloodstream via the high endothelial venules. This pathway allows the movement of lymphocytes from blood to lymph nodes, from which they can again enter and travel in lymph to other lymph nodes, eventually entering the systemic circulation. Movement of B cells and T cells across the high endothelial venules into lymph nodes is considered **homing**. These specialized venules are also present in other lymphoid organs, such as Peyer patches in the small intestine, tonsils, appendix, and cortex of the thymus; high endothelial venules are absent from the spleen.

1 Connective tissue
2 Afferent lymphatic vessel with valve
3 Capsule
4 Subcapsular (marginal) sinus
5 Connective tissue trabecula
6 Trabecular (cortical) sinuses
7 Germinal center of lymphatic nodule
8 Paracortex (deep cortex)
9 Medullary cords
10 Medullary sinuses

11 Venule and arteriole
12 Subcapsular (marginal) sinus
13 Lymphatic nodule
14 Connective tissue trabecula
15 Germinal center of lymphatic nodule
16 Trabecular blood vessels
17 Paracortex (deep cortex)
18 Medullary sinuses
19 Medullary cords

FIGURE 11.2 ■ Lymph node: capsule, cortex, and medulla (sectional view). Stain: hematoxylin and eosin. Medium magnification.

FIGURE 11.3 | Cortex and Medulla of a Lymph Node

This low-power photomicrograph illustrates the cortex and medulla of the lymph node. A loose connective tissue **capsule (4)** with blood vessels and **adipose cells (7)** covers the lymph node. Inferior to the capsule (4) is the **subcapsular (marginal) sinus (5)**, which overlies the darker-staining and peripheral lymph node **cortex (3)**. In the cortex (3) are found numerous **lymphatic nodules (1, 6)**, some of which contain a lighter-staining **germinal center (2)**.

The central region of the lymph node is the lighter-staining **medulla (9)**. This region is characterized by the dark-staining **medullary cords (12)** and the light-staining lymphatic channels, the **medullary sinuses (11)**. The medullary sinuses (11) drain the lymph that enters the lymph node through the afferent lymphatic vessels in the capsule (see Figure 11.2) and converges toward the hilum of the lymph node (see Figure 11.1). In the hilum are found numerous **arteries (8)** and veins. The lymph leaves the lymph node via the **efferent lymphatic vessels** with **valves (10)** at the hilum.

FIGURE 11.4 | Lymph Node: Subcortical Sinus and Lymphatic Nodule

This figure illustrates, at a higher magnification and in greater detail, a portion of the lymph node with the connective tissue **capsule (3)**, **trabecula (4)**, and **subcapsular sinus (1)** that continue on both sides of the trabecula (4) as **trabecular sinuses (12)** into the interior of the lymph node.

The reticular connective tissue of the lymph node, the **reticular cells (8, 11)**, is seen in different regions of the node. Reticular cells (8, 11) are visible in the subcapsular sinus (1), trabecular sinuses (12), and the **germinal center (9)** of the **lymphatic nodule (14)**. Numerous free **macrophages (2, 6, 16)** are also seen in the subcapsular sinus (1), trabecular sinuses (12), and the germinal center (9) of the lymphatic nodule (14).

A lymphatic nodule with a small section of its **peripheral zone (14)** and a germinal center (9) with developing lymphocytes are also visible. **Endothelial cells (5, 13)** line the sinuses (1, 12) and form an incomplete cover over the surface of the lymphatic nodules (14).

The peripheral zone of the lymphatic nodule (14) stains dense because of the accumulation of **small lymphocytes (7)**. The small lymphocytes (7) are characterized by dark-staining nuclei, condensed chromatin, and little or no cytoplasm. Small lymphocytes (7) are also present in the subcapsular sinus (1) and trabecular sinuses (12).

The germinal center (9) of the lymphatic nodule (14) contains **medium-sized lymphocytes (10)**. These cells are characterized by larger, lighter nuclei and more cytoplasm than is seen in the small lymphocytes (7). The nuclei of medium-sized lymphocytes (10) exhibit variations in the size and density of the chromatin. The largest cells, with less condensed chromatin, are derived from **lymphoblasts (17)**. The lymphoblasts (17) are visible in small numbers in the germinal center (9) of the lymphatic nodules (14) as large, round cells with a broad band of cytoplasm and a large vesicular nucleus with one or more nucleoli. **Lymphoblasts (15)** produce other lymphoblasts and medium-sized lymphocytes (10). With successive mitotic divisions of lymphoblasts (15), the chromatin condenses and the cells decrease in size, resulting in the formation of small lymphocytes (7).

1 Lymphatic nodule
2 Germinal center
3 Cortex
4 Capsule
5 Subcapsular (marginal) sinus
6 Lymphatic nodule
7 Adipose cells

8 Arteries
9 Medulla
10 Efferent lymphatic vessel with valves
11 Medullary sinuses
12 Medullary cords

FIGURE 11.3 ■ Cortex and medulla of a lymph node. Stain: Mallory-Azan. ×25.

1 Subcapsular sinus
2 Macrophage
3 Capsule
4 Trabecula
5 Endothelial cell
6 Macrophage
7 Small lymphocytes
8 Reticular cells
9 Germinal center
10 Medium-sized lymphocytes

11 Reticular cells
12 Trabecular sinuses
13 Endothelial cell
14 Lymphatic nodule (peripheral zone)
15 Lymphoblasts undergoing mitosis
16 Macrophage
17 Lymphoblasts

FIGURE 11.4 ■ Lymph node: subcortical sinus, trabecular sinus, reticular cells, and lymphatic nodule. Stain: hematoxylin and eosin. High magnification.

FIGURE 11.5 | Lymph Node: High Endothelial Venule in Paracortex (Deep Cortex) of a Lymph Node

The paracortex region of lymph nodes contains postcapillary venules. These venules have an unusual morphology to facilitate the **migration of lymphocytes** from the blood into the lymph node. This image shows a **high endothelial venule (2)** that is lined by tall cuboidal endothelium, instead of the usual squamous endothelium. Several migrating lymphocytes (3) are seen moving through the venule wall between the high endothelium (2) into the **paracortex** of the lymph node. Surrounding the high endothelial venule (2) are **lymphocytes** in the paracortex (5), a **medullary sinus (1)**, and a **venule (4)** with blood cells.

FIGURE 11.6 | Lymph Node: Subcapsular Sinus, Trabecular Sinus, and Supporting Reticular Fibers

A section of a lymph node has been stained with the silver method to illustrate the intricate arrangement of the supporting **reticular fibers (6, 9)** of a lymph node. The thicker and denser collagen fibers in the connective tissue **capsule (3)** stain pink. Both the capsule and the rest of the lymph node are supported by delicate reticular fibers (6, 9) that stain black and form a fine meshwork throughout the organ.

The various zones that are illustrated in Figure 11.2 with hematoxylin and eosin stain are readily recognizable with the silver stain. A connective tissue **trabecula (4)** from the capsule (3) penetrates the interior of the lymph node between two **lymphatic nodules (8, 12)**. Inferior to the capsule (3) are **subcapsular (marginal) sinuses (1, 7)** that continue on each side of the trabecula (4) as **trabecular sinuses (2, 5)** into the medulla of the node and eventually exit through the efferent lymph vessels in the hilum. Also observed are **medullary cords (10)** and **medullary sinuses (11)**.

1 Medullary sinus

2 High endothelial venule

3 Migrating lymphocytes

4 Venule

5 Lymphocytes in paracortex

FIGURE 11.5 ■ Lymph node: high endothelial venule in the paracortex (deep cortex) of a lymph node. Stain: hematoxylin and eosin. High magnification.

1 Subcapsular (marginal) sinus

2 Trabecular sinus

3 Capsule

4 Trabecula

5 Trabecular sinus

6 Reticular fibers

7 Subcapsular (marginal) sinus

8 Lymphatic nodule

9 Reticular fibers

10 Medullary cords

11 Medullary sinuses

12 Lymphatic nodule

FIGURE 11.6 ■ Lymph node: subcapsular sinus, trabecular sinus, and supporting reticular fibers. Stain: Silver stain. Medium magnification.

FIGURE 11.7 | Thymus Gland (Panoramic View)

The thymus gland is a lobulated lymphoid organ enclosed by a connective tissue **capsule (1)** from which arise connective tissue **trabeculae (2, 10)**. The trabeculae (2, 10) extend into the interior of the organ and subdivide the thymus gland into numerous incomplete **lobules (8)**. Each lobule consists of a dark-staining outer **cortex (3, 13)** and a light-staining inner **medulla (4, 12)**. Because the lobules are incomplete, the medulla shows continuity between the neighboring lobules (4, 12). **Blood vessels (5, 14)** pass into the thymus gland via the connective tissue capsule (1) and the trabeculae (2, 10).

The cortex (3, 13) of each lobule contains densely packed lymphocytes that do not form lymphatic nodules. In contrast, the medulla (4, 12) contains fewer lymphocytes but more epithelial reticular cells (see Figure 11.7). The medulla also contains numerous **thymic (Hassall) corpuscles (6, 9)** that characterize the thymus gland.

The histology of the thymus gland varies with the age of the individual. The thymus gland attains its greatest development shortly after birth. By the time of puberty, thymus glands begin to involute or show signs of gradual regression and degeneration. As a consequence, lymphocyte production declines, and the thymic (Hassall) corpuscles (6, 9) become more prominent. In addition, the parenchyma or cellular portion of the gland is gradually replaced by loose **connective tissue (10)** and **adipose cells (7, 11)**. The thymus gland depicted in this illustration exhibits adipose tissue accumulation and the initial signs of involution associated with increasing age.

FIGURE 11.8 | Thymus Gland (Sectional View)

A small section of the **cortex** and medulla of a thymus gland lobule is illustrated at a higher magnification. The thymic lymphocytes in the cortex (1, 5) form dense aggregations. In contrast, the **medulla (3)** contains only a few lymphocytes but more **epithelial reticular cells (7, 10)**.

The **thymic (Hassall) corpuscles (8, 9)** are oval structures consisting of round or spherical aggregations (whorls) of flattened epithelial cells. The thymic corpuscles also exhibit calcification or **degeneration centers (9)** that stain pink or eosinophilic. The functional significance of these corpuscles remains unknown.

Blood vessels (6) and **adipose cells (4)** are present in both the thymic lobules and in a connective tissue **trabecula (2)**.

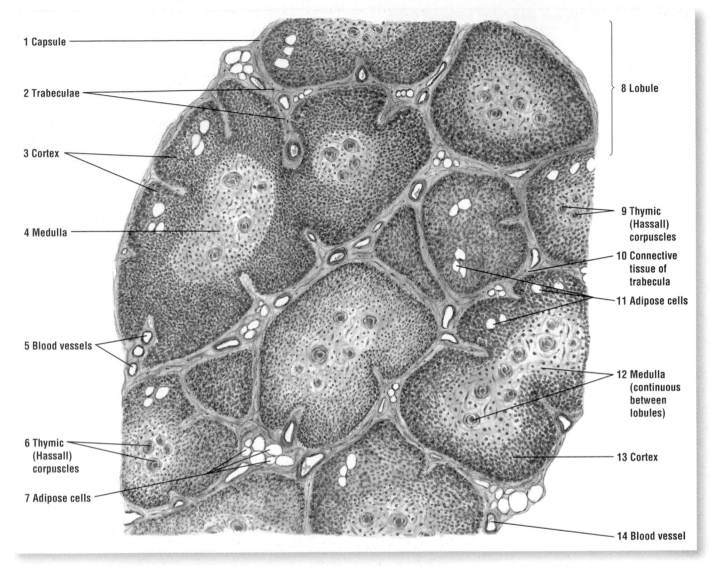

1 Capsule

2 Trabeculae

3 Cortex

4 Medulla

5 Blood vessels

6 Thymic (Hassall) corpuscles

7 Adipose cells

8 Lobule

9 Thymic (Hassall) corpuscles

10 Connective tissue of trabecula

11 Adipose cells

12 Medulla (continuous between lobules)

13 Cortex

14 Blood vessel

FIGURE 11.7 ■ Thymus gland (panoramic view). Stain: hematoxylin and eosin. Low magnification.

1 Cortex (with thymic lymphocytes)

2 Trabecula

3 Medulla

4 Adipose cells

5 Cortex (with thymic lymphocytes)

6 Blood vessels

7 Epithelial reticular cells

8 Thymic (Hassall) corpuscle

9 Degeneration centers of thymic (Hassall) corpuscles

10 Epithelial reticular cells

FIGURE 11.8 ■ Thymus gland (sectional view). Stain: hematoxylin and eosin. High magnification.

FIGURE 11.9 | Cortex and Medulla of a Thymus Gland

A low-magnification photomicrograph shows a portion of the lobule of the thymus gland. A **connective tissue trabecula (1)** subdivides the gland into incomplete lobules. Each lobule consists of the darker-staining **cortex (2)** and the lighter-staining **medulla (3)**. A characteristic **thymic (Hassall) corpuscle (4)** is present in the center of the medulla in one of the lobules.

FUNCTIONAL CORRELATIONS 11.2 | Thymus Gland

The **thymus gland** performs an important role early in childhood in **immune system development**. Its main function is to produce a diverse group of T cells that can respond to antigens. Undifferentiated **lymphocytes** are carried from the bone marrow via the bloodstream to the thymus gland. In much of the thymic cortex, the **epithelial reticular cells**, also called **thymic nurse cells**, surround the lymphocytes and promote their differentiation, proliferation, and maturation. Here, the lymphocytes mature into **immunocompetent T cells**, **helper T cells**, and **cytotoxic T cells**, whereby they acquire their surface receptors for the recognition of antigens. Furthermore, the developing lymphocytes are prevented from exposure to blood borne antigens by a physical **blood–thymus barrier**, formed by endothelial cells, epithelial reticular cells, and macrophages. Macrophages outside of the capillaries ensure that substances transported in the blood vessels do not interact with the developing T cells in the cortex and induce an autoimmune response against the body's own cells or tissues. After maturation, the T cells leave the thymus gland via the bloodstream and populate the **lymph nodes**, **spleen**, and other thymus-dependent **lymphatic tissues** in the organism.

The maturation and selection of T cells within the thymus gland is a very complicated process that includes the **positive** and **negative** selection of T cells. Only a small fraction of lymphocytes generated in the thymus gland reach maturity. As maturation progresses in the cortex, the T cells are presented by APCs with self and foreign antigens. Lymphocytes that are unable to recognize self-antigens or that recognize self-antigens die and are eliminated by macrophages (**negative selection**), which is about 95% of the total cells. Those lymphocytes that recognize the foreign antigens (**positive selection**) survive, reach maturity, enter the medulla from the cortex, and are then distributed in the bloodstream to other sites in the body.

In addition to forming the blood–thymus barrier, the epithelial reticular cells secrete hormones that are necessary for the proliferation, differentiation, and maturation of T cells and the expression of their surface markers. The hormones are **thymulin**, **thymopoietin**, **thymosin**, **thymic humoral factor**, **interleukins**, and **interferon**. The epithelial reticular cells also form distinctive whorls called **thymic (Hassall) corpuscles** in the medulla of the gland, which are characteristic features in identifying the thymus gland.

The thymus gland involutes after puberty, becomes filled with adipose tissue, and the production of T cells decreases. However, because T lymphocyte progeny has been established, immunity is maintained without the need for new T-cell production. If the thymus gland is removed from a newborn, the lymphoid organs will not receive the immunocompetent T cells and the individual will not acquire the immunologic competence to fight pathogens. Death may occur early in life as a result of complications of an infection and the lack of a functional immune system.

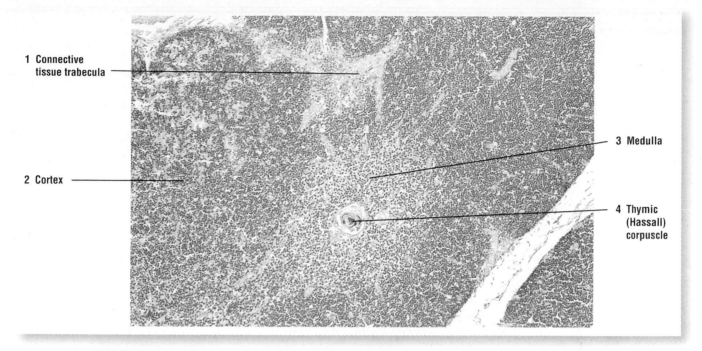

1 Connective
tissue trabecula

2 Cortex

3 Medulla

4 Thymic
(Hassall)
corpuscle

FIGURE 11.9 ■ Cortex and medulla of a thymus gland. Stain: hematoxylin and eosin. ×30.

FIGURE 11.10 | Spleen (Panoramic View)

The spleen is surrounded by a dense connective tissue **capsule (1)** from which arise connective tissue **trabeculae (3, 5, 11)** that extend deep into the spleen's interior. The main trabeculae enter the spleen at the hilus and extend throughout the organ. Located within the trabeculae (3, 5, 11) are **trabecular arteries (5b)** and **trabecular veins (5a)**. Trabeculae that are cut in transverse section (11) appear round or nodular and may contain blood vessels.

The spleen is characterized by numerous aggregations of **lymphatic nodules (4, 6)**. These nodules constitute the **white pulp (4, 6)** of the organ. The lymphatic nodules (4, 6) also contain **germinal centers (8, 9)** that decrease in number with age. Passing through each lymphatic nodule (4, 6) is a blood vessel called a **central artery (2, 7, 10)** that is located in the periphery of the lymphatic nodules (4, 6). Central arteries (2, 7, 10) are branches of trabecular arteries (5b) that become ensheathed with lymphatic tissue as they leave the connective tissue trabeculae (3, 5, 11). This periarterial lymphatic sheath also forms the lymphatic nodules (4, 6) that constitute the white pulp (4, 6) of the spleen.

Surrounding the lymphatic nodules (4, 6) and intermeshed with the connective tissue trabeculae (3, 5, 11) is a diffuse cellular meshwork that makes up the bulk of the organ. This meshwork collectively forms the **red** or **splenic pulp (12, 13)**. In fresh preparations, red pulp is red because of its extensive vascular tissue. The red pulp (12, 13) also contains **pulp arteries (14)**, **venous sinuses (13)**, and **splenic cords** (of Billroth) **(12)**. The splenic cords (12) appear as diffuse strands of lymphatic tissue between the venous sinuses (13) and form a spongy meshwork of reticular connective tissue, usually obscured by the density of other tissue.

The spleen does not exhibit a distinct cortex and a medulla, as seen in lymph nodes. However, lymphatic nodules (4, 6) are found throughout the spleen. In addition, the spleen contains venous sinuses (13), in contrast to lymphatic sinuses that are found in the lymph nodes. The spleen also does not exhibit subcapsular or trabecular sinuses. The capsule (1) and trabeculae (3, 5, 11) in the spleen are thicker than those around the lymph nodes and contain some smooth muscle cells.

FIGURE 11.11 | Spleen: Red and White Pulp

A higher magnification of a section of the spleen illustrates the red and white pulp and associated connective tissue trabeculae, blood vessels, venous sinuses, and splenic cords.

The large **lymphatic nodule (3)** represents the white pulp of the spleen. Each nodule normally exhibits a peripheral zone—the periarterial lymphatic sheath—with densely packed small lymphocytes. The **central artery (4)** in the lymphatic nodule (3) has a peripheral, or an eccentric, position. Because the artery occupies the center of the periarterial lymphatic sheath, it is called the central artery. The cells found in the periarterial lymphatic sheath are mainly T cells. A **germinal center (5)** may not always be present. In the more lightly stained germinal center (5) are found B cells, many medium-sized lymphocytes, some small lymphocytes, and lymphoblasts.

The red pulp contains the **splenic cords** (of Billroth) **(1, 8)** and **venous sinuses (2, 9)** that course between the cords. The splenic cords (1, 8) are thin aggregations of lymphatic tissue containing small lymphocytes, associated cells, and various blood cells. Venous sinuses (2, 9) are dilated vessels lined with the modified endothelium of elongated cells that appear cuboidal in transverse sections.

Also present in the red pulp are the **pulp arteries (10)**. These represent the branches of the central artery (4) after it leaves the lymphatic nodule (3). Capillaries and pulp veins (venules) are also present.

Connective tissue trabeculae with a **trabecular artery (6)** and **trabecular vein (7)** are evident. These vessels have endothelial tunica intima and muscular tunica media. The tunica adventitia is not apparent, because the connective tissue of the trabeculae surrounds the tunica media.

1 Capsule

2 Central artery

3 Trabeculae

4 Lymphatic nodule (white pulp)

9 Germinal center

10 Central artery

11 Trabeculae

5 Trabecular:
   a. Vein
   b. Artery

12 Splenic cords (in red pulp)

13 Venous sinuses (in red pulp)

6 Lymphatic nodule (white pulp)

7 Central artery

8 Germinal center

14 Pulp arteries

FIGURE 11.10 ■ Spleen (panoramic view). Stain: hematoxylin and eosin. Low magnification.

1 Splenic cord

2 Venous sinus

3 Lymphatic nodule

4 Central artery

5 Germinal center

6 Trabecular artery

7 Trabecular vein

8 Splenic cords

9 Venous sinuses

10 Pulp arteries

FIGURE 11.11 ■ Spleen: red and white pulp. Stain: hematoxylin and eosin. Medium magnification.

FIGURE 11.12 | Red and White Pulp of the Spleen

A low-magnification photomicrograph illustrates a section of the spleen. A dense irregular **connective tissue capsule (1)** covers the organ. From the capsule (1), **connective tissue trabeculae (3)** with blood vessels extend into the interior of the organ. The spleen is composed of white pulp and red pulp. **White pulp (2)** consists of lymphocytes and aggregations of **lymphatic nodules (2a)**. Within the lymphatic nodule (2a) are found the **germinal center (2b)** and a **central artery (2c)** that is located off-center. Surrounding the white pulp lymphatic nodules (2) is the **red pulp (4)**. It is primarily composed of **venous sinuses (4a)** and **splenic cords (4b)**.

FUNCTIONAL CORRELATIONS 11.3 | The Spleen

The **spleen** is the largest lymphoid organ with an extensive blood supply. It filters blood and is the site of immune responses to blood borne antigens. The spleen consists of red pulp and white pulp. **Red pulp** consists of a dense network of reticular fibers that contains numerous erythrocytes, lymphocytes, plasma cells, macrophages, and other granulocytes. The main function of the red pulp is to filter the blood. It removes antigens, microorganisms, platelets, and aged or abnormal erythrocytes from the blood. In contrast to other lymphoid organs, the spleen does not have a cortex and medulla.

The **white pulp** is the immune component of the spleen and consists mainly of accumulated lymphocytes in the lymphatic nodules that surround an artery, the central artery. Lymphocytes around the **central arteries** of the white pulp are primarily **T cells** that form the **periarteriolar lymphatic sheaths (PALS)**, whereas the lymphatic nodules contain mainly **B cells**. **APCs** and **macrophages** reside within the white pulp. These cells detect trapped bacteria and antigens and initiate immune responses against them. As a result, T cells and B cells interact, become activated, proliferate, and perform their immune response.

Macrophages in the spleen also break down the **hemoglobin** of worn-out **erythrocytes**. Iron from hemoglobin is recycled and returned to the **bone marrow**, where it is reused during the synthesis of new hemoglobin by developing erythrocytes. The **heme** from the hemoglobin is further degraded and excreted into **bile** by the liver cells.

During fetal life, the spleen is a **hemopoietic organ**, producing **granulocytes** and **erythrocytes**. This hemopoietic capability, however, ceases after birth. The spleen also serves as an important **reservoir** for blood. Because it has a sponge like microstructure, much blood can be stored in its interior. When needed, the stored blood is returned from the spleen to the general circulation. Although the spleen performs various important functions in the body, it is not an essential organ for life.

FIGURE 11.13 | Palatine Tonsil

The paired palatine tonsils consist of aggregates of lymphatic nodules located in the oral cavity. The palatine tonsils are not surrounded by a connective tissue capsule. As a result, the surface of the palatine tonsil is covered by a protective **stratified squamous nonkeratinized epithelium (1, 6)** that covers the rest of the oral cavity. Each tonsil is invaginated by deep grooves called **tonsillar crypts (3, 9)** that are also lined by stratified squamous nonkeratinized epithelium (1, 6).

Below the epithelium (1, 6) in the underlying connective tissue are numerous **lymphatic nodules (2)** that are distributed along the lengths of the tonsillar crypts (3, 9). The lymphatic nodules (2) frequently merge with each other and usually exhibit lighter-staining **germinal centers (7)**.

A dense connective tissue underlies the palatine tonsil and forms its **capsule (4, 10)**. The connective tissue **trabeculae**, some with **blood vessels (8)**, arise from the capsule (4, 10) and pass toward the surface of the tonsil between the lymphatic nodules (2).

Below the connective tissue capsule (10) are sections of **skeletal muscle (5)** fibers.

1 Connective tissue capsule

3 Connective tissue trabeculae

2 White pulp:
 a. Lymphatic nodule

 b. Germinal center

 c. Central artery

4 Red pulp:
 a. Venous sinuses

 b. Splenic cords

FIGURE 11.12 ■ Red and white pulp of the spleen. Stain: Mallory-Azan. ×21.

1 Stratified squamous nonkeratinized epithelium

6 Stratified squamous nonkeratinized epithelium

2 Lymphatic nodules

7 Germinal centers

8 Trabeculae with blood vessels

3 Tonsillar crypts

9 Tonsillar crypts

4 Capsule

5 Skeletal muscle

10 Capsule

FIGURE 11.13 ■ Palatine tonsil. Stain: hematoxylin and eosin. Low magnification.

Immune System

- Protects organism against invading pathogens and has wide distribution
- Contains aggregates of immune cells (lymphocytes) in nodules or lymphoid organs
- Major organs are the lymph nodes, tonsils, thymus, and spleen as well as bone marrow

Organs of Immune System: Lymph Nodes, Thymus, and Spleen

Lymph Nodes

- Distributed along the paths of lymphatic vessels
- Most prominent in inguinal and axillary regions
- Major function is lymph filtration and phagocytosis of foreign material from lymph
- Surrounded by connective tissue capsule that sends trabeculae into the interior of the organ
- Exhibit an outer dark-staining cortex and an inner light-staining medulla
- Lymphoid nodules, some with germinal centers, are aggregated in the cortex
- Afferent lymph vessels with valves penetrate the capsule and enter subcapsular sinus
- Major blood vessels present in connective tissue trabeculae
- Medullary cords in the medulla contain plasma cells, macrophages, and lymphocytes
- Medullary sinuses are capillary channels that drain lymph from cortical regions
- Efferent lymphatic vessels drain lymph from the medullary sinuses to exit at the hilus
- Produce, store, and recirculate B and T cells
- B cells accumulate in lymphatic nodules, and activated cells form germinal centers
- Deeper region of the cortex is the paracortex, occupied by T cells
- T cells concentrate in deep cortical or paracortex regions
- Activate B cells to give rise to plasma cells and memory B cells
- B and T cells enter lymph nodes through postcapillary venules
- Postcapillary venules contain lymphocyte-homing receptors and high endothelium
- Both B and T cells leave bloodstream through high endothelial venules
- High endothelial venules present in other lymphoid organs except the spleen

Cells of the Immune System

- Include lymphocytes and different supporting cells
- Three types of lymphocytes are T cells, B cells, and NK cells
- Originate from hemopoietic stem cells in the bone marrow

T Lymphocytes (T Cells)

- T cells arise from lymphocytes that were carried to and matured in the thymus gland
- After maturation, T cells are distributed to all lymph tissues and organs
- On encountering antigens, T cells destroy them by cytotoxic action or by activating B cells
- Four types of differentiated T cells: helper T cells, cytotoxic T cells, memory T cells, and suppressor T cells
- Helper T cells secrete cytokines or interleukins when they encounter antigens
- Cytokines stimulate B cells to differentiate into plasma cells and to secrete antibodies
- Cytotoxic T cells attack and destroy virus-infected, foreign, or malignant cells via perforating protein perforin
- Memory T cells are the long-living progeny of T cells and respond to the same antigens
- Suppressor T cells decrease or inhibit the functions of helper T cells and cytotoxic T cells
- Maturation of T cells is a very complicated process, involving positive and negative selection
- Most T cells recognize self-antigens and die (negative selection)
- T cells that recognize foreign antigens reach maturity and enter the bloodstream (positive selection)

B Lymphocytes (B Cells)

- B cells remain and mature in the bone marrow, then move to nonthymic lymphoid tissues and organs
- Recognize antigens as a result of antigen receptors on cell membranes and become activated
- Response is more intense when antigen-presenting helper T cells present antigens to B cells
- Cytokines secreted by helper T cells increase the proliferation of activated B cells
- B cells differentiate into plasma cells and secrete antibodies to destroy foreign substances
- Other activated B cells remain as memory B cells for future defense against the same antigens

Natural Killer Cells and Antigen-Presenting Cells

- Develop from the same precursors as B cells and T cells
- NK cells attack virally infected cells and cancer cells as do cytotoxic T cells
- APCs phagocytose and present antigens to T cells for response
- APCs belong to mononuclear phagocytic system
- APCs include connective tissue macrophages, perisinusoidal macrophages (Kupffer cells) in the liver, Langerhans cells (dendritic) in the skin, and macrophages in the lymphoid organs

Types of Immune Responses

Innate Immune Response

- First line of defense that limits the spread of infection
- Response composed of the rapid response of phagocytic cells and their functions
- Response is nonspecific and does not produce memory cells

Adaptive Immune Response

- Targets specific invading organisms and provides specific or adaptive response
- Response is slower than innate response but produces memory cells that can respond to secondary encounters
- Two types of specific responses are humoral and mediated immune responses
- In humoral-mediated response, antigens induce B cells to transform into plasma cells
- Plasma cells, in turn, secrete specific antibodies to destroy antigens
- In cell-mediated response, T cells are activated, then they bind to target cells, and destroy them

Spleen

- Largest lymphoid organ with extensive blood supply; filters blood and serves as a blood reservoir
- Surrounded by a connective tissue capsule that divides it into compartments called splenic pulp
- White pulp consists of lymphatic nodules with a germinal center around a central artery
- T cells form PALS around central arteries
- B cells are found in the lymphatic nodules
- Red pulp consists of splenic cords and splenic (blood) sinusoids
- Splenic cords contain macrophages, lymphocytes, plasma cells, and different blood cells
- Does not exhibit cortex and medulla but contains lymphatic nodules
- White pulp is the site of immune response to blood borne antigens
- T cells surround the central arteries, whereas B cells are mainly in the lymphatic nodules
- APCs and macrophages are found in white pulp
- Breaks down hemoglobin from worn-out erythrocytes and recycles iron to bone marrow
- Degrades heme from hemoglobin, which is then excreted in the bile
- During fetal life is an important hemopoietic organ

Thymus Gland

- Lobulated lymphoepithelial organ with dark-staining cortex and light-staining medulla
- Most active in childhood and has an important role early in life in immune system development
- Site where immature lymphocytes from the bone marrow mature into T cells, helper T cells, and cytotoxic T cells
- Thymic nurse cells promote lymphocyte differentiation, proliferation, and maturation
- Blood–thymus barrier prevents developing lymphocytes contacting blood borne antigens
- Sends mature T cells to populate the lymph nodes, the spleen, and the lymphatic tissues
- Epithelial reticular cells secrete numerous hormones needed for lymphocyte maturation
- Epithelial reticular cells form thymic (Hassall) corpuscles in the medulla
- Maturation of T cells involves positive and negative selection
- Involutes and becomes filled with adipose tissues as the individual ages
- Removal early in life results in loss of immunologic competence

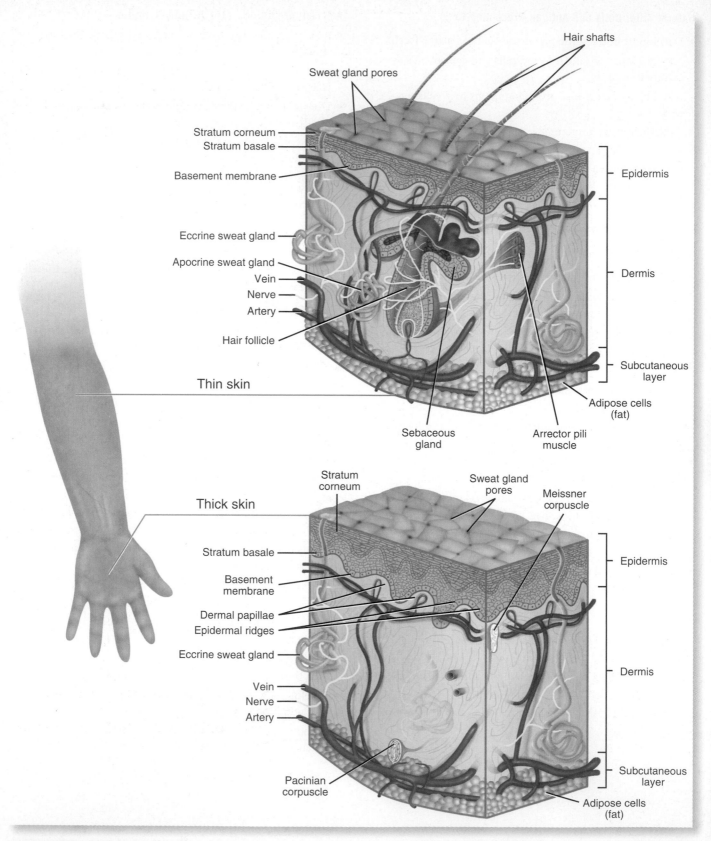

Hair shafts

Sweat gland pores

Stratum corneum

Stratum basale

Basement membrane

Epidermis

Eccrine sweat gland

Apocrine sweat gland

Vein

Nerve

Artery

Dermis

Hair follicle

Thin skin

Subcutaneous layer

Adipose cells (fat)

Sebaceous gland

Arrector pili muscle

Stratum corneum

Thick skin

Sweat gland pores

Meissner corpuscle

Stratum basale

Epidermis

Basement membrane

Dermal papillae

Epidermal ridges

Eccrine sweat gland

Vein

Nerve

Artery

Dermis

Pacinian corpuscle

Subcutaneous layer

Adipose cells (fat)

OVERVIEW FIGURE 12.1 ■ Comparison between thin skin in the arm and thick skin in the palm, including the contents of the connective tissue dermis.

CHAPTER 12

Integumentary System ■

General Overview

Skin is the largest organ in the body. Its derivatives and appendages form the **integumentary system**. In humans, skin derivatives include nails, hair, and several types of sweat and sebaceous glands. The surfaces of the body are covered either by thin skin or thick skin. Skin, or **integument**, consists of two distinct regions—the superficial epidermis and a deep dermis. The surface layer of the skin, or the **epidermis,** is nonvascular and is lined by **keratinized stratified squamous epithelium** with distinct cell types and different cell layers. Inferior to the epidermis is the vascular **dermis**, characterized by dense irregular connective tissue, blood vessels, nerves, and different glands. In some areas of the body, numerous hair follicles are visible in the dermis. Beneath the dermis is the **hypodermis,** or a **subcutaneous layer** of connective tissue and adipose tissue that forms the superficial fascia seen in gross anatomy.

Dermis: Papillary and Reticular Layers

Dermis is the inferior connective tissue layer that binds to the epidermis. A distinct **basement membrane** separates the epidermis from the dermis. In addition, the dermis contains epidermal derivatives, such as the sweat glands, sebaceous glands, and hair follicles.

The junction of the dermis with the epidermis is irregular. The superficial layer of the dermis forms numerous raised projections called **dermal papillae**, which interdigitate with evaginations of the epidermis, called **epidermal ridges**. This region of the skin is the **papillary layer** of the dermis. It contains loose irregular connective tissue fibers, capillaries, blood vessels, fibroblasts, macrophages, and other loose connective tissue cells.

The deeper layer of the dermis is called the **reticular layer**. This layer is thicker and is characterized by dense irregular connective tissue fibers (mainly type I collagen) and is less cellular than the papillary layer. Also, this layer of the dermis can withstand more mechanical stresses and can provide support for nerves, blood vessels, hair follicles, and all the sweat glands. There is no distinct boundary between the two dermal layers, and the papillary layer blends with the reticular layer. Also, the dermis blends inferiorly with the **hypodermis,** or the **subcutaneous layer**, which contains the superficial fascia and adipose tissue.

The connective tissue of the dermis is highly vascular and contains numerous blood vessels, lymph vessels, and nerves. Certain regions of the skin exhibit **arteriovenous anastomoses** used for temperature regulation. Here, blood passes directly from the arteries into the veins. In addition, the dermis contains numerous sensory receptors. **Meissner corpuscles** are located closer to the surface of the skin in dermal papillae, whereas **Pacinian corpuscles** are found deeper in the connective tissue of the dermis (Overview Fig. 12.1).

FUNCTIONAL CORRELATIONS 12.1 | Epidermal Cells and Cell Layers

There are four cell types in the epidermis of the skin, with the **keratinocytes** being the most dominant cells. Keratinocytes divide, grow, migrate up, undergo **keratinization,** or **cornification**, and form the protective epidermal and surface layer for the skin. The epidermis is composed of stratified keratinized squamous epithelium. There are other less abundant cell types in the epidermis. These are the melanocytes, Langerhans cells, and Merkel cells, which are interspersed among the keratinocytes in the epidermis. In thick skin, five distinct and recognizable cell layers can be identified.

Stratum Basale (Germinativum)—The Deepest Layer

The **stratum basale** is the deepest or basal layer in the epidermis. It consists of a single layer of columnar to cuboidal cells that rest on a **basement membrane** separating the dermis from the epidermis. The cells are attached to one another by cell junctions, called **desmosomes**, and to the underlying basement membrane by **hemidesmosomes**. Cells in the stratum basale serve as **stem cells** for the epidermis; thus, much increased mitotic activity is seen in this layer. The cells continually divide and mature as they migrate up toward the superficial layers. All cells in the stratum basale produce and contain **intermediate keratin filaments** that increase in number as the cells move superficially. These filaments eventually form the components of keratin in the superficial cell layer.

Stratum Spinosum—The Second Layer

As the keratinocytes divide by mitosis, they move upward in the epidermis and form the second cell layer of keratinocytes, or **stratum spinosum**. This layer consists of four to six rows of cells. Routine histologic preparations with different chemicals cause these cells to shrink. As a result, the developed intercellular spaces between cells appear to form numerous cytoplasmic extensions, or spines, that project from their surfaces. The spines represent the sites where **desmosomes** are anchored to bundles of intermediate keratin filaments, or tonofilaments, and to neighboring cells. The synthesis of keratin filaments continues in this layer, and they are assembled into bundles of **tonofilaments**. Tonofilaments maintain cohesion among cells and provide resistance to the abrasion of the epidermis; they terminate at various desmosomes.

Stratum Granulosum—The Third Layer

Maturing cells that move above the stratum spinosum accumulate dense basophilic **keratohyalin granules** and form the third layer, the **stratum granulosum**. Three to five layers of flattened cells form this layer. The secretory granules are not surrounded by a membrane and consist of the protein **filaggrin**, which associates and cross-links with bundles of keratin tonofilaments. The combination of keratin tonofilaments with the filaggrin protein of keratohyalin granules produces **keratin** through the process called **keratinization**. The keratin formed by this process is the soft keratin of the skin. In addition, the cytoplasm in the cells of stratum granulosum contains membrane-bound **lamellar granules** formed by lipid bilayers. These lamellar granules are then discharged into the intercellular spaces between the stratum granulosum and the next layer, the stratum corneum (or stratum lucidum if present), as a **lipid** that forms an impermeable water barrier and seals the skin.

Stratum Lucidum—The Fourth Layer

In thick skin only, the **stratum lucidum** is translucent and barely visible; it lies just superior to the stratum granulosum and inferior to the stratum corneum. The tightly packed cells lack nuclei or organelles and are dead. The flattened cells contain densely packed keratin filaments.

Stratum Corneum—The Fifth Layer

The **stratum corneum** is the fifth and most superficial layer of the skin. All nuclei and organelles have disappeared from the cells. Stratum corneum primarily consists of flattened, dead cells filled with soft **keratin filaments**. The keratinized, superficial cells from this layer are continually shed, or **desquamated,** and are replaced by new cells arising from the deep stratum basale. During the keratinization process, the hydrolytic enzymes disrupt the nucleus and all cytoplasmic organelles, which disappear as the cells fill with keratin.

Other Skin Cells

In addition to the **keratinocytes** that form and become the superficial layer of keratinized epithelium, the epidermis also contains three less abundant cell types. These are melanocytes, Langerhans cells, and Merkel cells. Unless the skin is prepared with special stains, these cells are normally not distinguishable in histologic slides prepared with only hematoxylin and eosin.

Melanocytes are derived from the neural crest cells. They have long, irregular cytoplasmic or dendritic extensions that branch into the epidermis. Melanocytes are located between the stratum basale and the stratum spinosum of the epidermis and synthesize the dark brown pigment **melanin**. Melanin is synthesized from the amino acid tyrosine by melanocytes. The formed melanin granules in the melanocytes then migrate to their cytoplasmic extensions, from which they are transferred to keratinocytes in the basal cell layers of the epidermis. Melanin imparts a dark color to the skin, and exposure of the skin to sunlight promotes increased synthesis of melanin. The main function of melanin is to protect the skin from the damaging effects of ultraviolet radiation.

Langerhans cells originate from bone marrow, migrate via the bloodstream, and reside in the skin, mainly in the stratum spinosum. These dendritic-type cells participate in the body's immune responses. Langerhans cells recognize, phagocytose, and process foreign **antigens** and then present them to T lymphocytes for an immune response. Thus, these cells function as **antigen-presenting** cells and are part of the immunologic defense of the skin.

Merkel cells are found in the stratum basale layer of the epidermis and are most abundant in the fingertips. Because these cells are closely associated with afferent (sensory) **unmyelinated axons**, they function as **mechanoreceptors** for cutaneous sensation.

Major Skin Functions

The skin comes in direct contact with the external environment. As a result, it performs numerous important functions, most of which are protective.

Protection

The **keratinized stratified epithelium** of the epidermis protects the body surfaces from mechanical abrasion and forms a physical barrier to pathogens or foreign microorganisms. Because a **glycolipid layer** is present between the cells of the stratum granulosum, the epidermis is also **impermeable** to water. This layer also prevents the loss of body fluids through dehydration. Increased synthesis of the pigment melanin by melanocytes further protects the skin against the damaging ultraviolet radiation.

Temperature Regulation

Physical exercise or a warm environment increases **sweating**. Sweating reduces the body temperature after **evaporation** of sweat from skin surfaces. In addition to sweating, temperature regulation also involves increased **dilation** of blood vessels that brings more blood to the superficial layers of the skin where cooling of the circulating blood increases heat loss. Conversely, in cold temperatures, body heat is conserved by **constriction** of superficial blood vessels, decreased blood flow to the skin, and maintaining more heat in the body core.

Sensory Perception

The skin is a large **sensory organ**, sensing the external environment. Numerous encapsulated and free **sensory nerve endings** within the skin respond to stimuli for temperature (heat and cold), touch, pain, and pressure.

Excretion

Through the production of sweat by the **sweat glands**, water, sodium salts, urea, and nitrogenous wastes are excreted through the surface of the skin.

Formation of Vitamin D

Vitamin D is formed from precursor molecules synthesized in the epidermis during exposure of the skin to **ultraviolet** rays from the sun. Vitamin D is essential for **calcium absorption** from the intestinal mucosa and for proper mineral metabolism.

SECTION 1   Thin Skin

Most surfaces of the body are not exposed to increased abrasion and wear and tear. As a result, these parts of the body are covered by **thin skin**. In these regions, the epidermis is thinner, and its cellular composition is simpler than that of thick skin. Present in thin skin are **hair follicles, sebaceous glands**, and different types of **sweat glands (apocrine** and **eccrine)**. Attached to the connective tissue sheath of hair follicles and the connective tissue of the dermis are smooth muscle fibers, called **arrector pili**. Also associated with the hair follicles are numerous sebaceous glands (see Overview Fig. 12.1). Thus, the terms "thick skin" and "thin skin" refer only to the thickness of the epidermis and do not include the layers below it, which can vary in thickness, depending on the location of the body.

 Supplemental micrographic images are available at **www.thePoint.com/Eroschenko12e** under Skin System.

FIGURE 12.1 | **Thin Skin: Epidermis and the Contents of the Dermis**

This illustration depicts a section of thin skin from the general body surface, where wear and tear is minimal. To differentiate between the cellular and connective tissue components of the skin, a special stain was used. With this stain, the collagen fibers of the connective tissue components stain blue, and the cellular components stain bright red.

The skin consists of two principal layers: the **epidermis (10)** and **dermis (14)**. The epidermis (10) is the superficial cellular layer with different cell types. The dermis (14), located directly below the epidermis (10), contains connective tissue fibers and cellular components of epidermal origin.

In thin skin, the epidermis (10) exhibits a stratified squamous epithelium and a thin layer of keratinized cells called the **stratum corneum (1)**. The most superficial cells in the stratum corneum (1) are constantly shed, or desquamate, from the surface. Also, the stratum corneum (1) of thin skin is much thinner in contrast to that of thick skin, in which the stratum corneum (1) is much thicker. In this illustration, a few rows of polygonal cells are visible in the epidermis (10). These cells form the layer **stratum spinosum (2)**.

The narrow zone of irregular, lighter-staining connective tissue directly below the epidermis (10) is the **papillary layer (11)** of the dermis (14). The papillary layer (11) indents the base of the epidermis to form the **dermal papillae (3)**. The deeper **reticular layer (12)** comprises the bulk of the dermis (14) and consists of dense irregular connective tissue. A small portion of the **hypodermis (13)**, the superficial region of the underlying subcutaneous **adipose tissue (9)**, is also illustrated.

Skin appendages, such as the **sweat gland (7)** and **hair follicles (8)**, develop from the epidermis (10) and are located in the dermis (14). The sweat gland (7) is illustrated in greater detail in Figure 12.3. The expanded terminal portion of the hair follicle (8) observed in the longitudinal section is the **hair bulb (8a)**. The base of the hair bulb (8a) is indented by the connective tissue to form a **dermal papilla (8b)**. Within each dermal papilla (8b) is a capillary network vital for sustaining the hair follicle (8). Attached to hair follicles (8) are thin strips of smooth muscle called the **arrector pili muscles (5)**. Also associated with hair follicles (8) are numerous **sebaceous glands (6)**.

In the reticular layer (12) of the dermis (14) are found examples of the cross sections of a coiled portion of the sweat gland (7). The elongated portions of the sweat gland (7) that continue to the surface of the skin are the excretory **ductal portions** of the **sweat glands (4, 7a)**. The more circular and deeper-lying parts of the sweat gland are the **secretory (7b)** portions of the sweat gland (7).

1 Stratum corneum
2 Stratum spinosum
3 Dermal papillae
4 Ducts of sweat glands
5 Arrector pili muscles
6 Sebaceous glands
7 Sweat gland:
   a. Ductal portion
   b. Secretory portion
8 Hair follicle:
   a. Bulb
   b. Dermal papilla
9 Adipose tissue

10 Epidermis
11 Papillary layer
12 Reticular layer
13 Hypodermis
14 Dermis

FIGURE 12.1 ■ Thin skin: epidermis and the contents of the dermis. Stain: Masson trichrome (blue stain). Low magnification.

FIGURE 12.2 | Skin: Epidermis, Dermis, and Hypodermis in the Scalp

This low-magnification section of the thin skin of the scalp is prepared with a routine histologic stain. It illustrates both the epidermis and dermis and some of the skin derivatives in the deeper connective tissue layers. The epidermis stains darker than the underlying connective tissue of the dermis. In the epidermis are visible the cell layers **stratum corneum (1)**, with desquamating superficial cells; the **stratum spinosum (2);** and the basal cell layer, the **stratum basale (3)**, with brown **melanin (pigment) granules (3)**.

The **connective tissue dermal papillae (4)** indent the underside of the epidermis. The thin connective tissue papillary layer of the dermis is located immediately under the epidermis. The thicker connective tissue **reticular layer (12)** of the dermis extends from just below the epidermis to the **subcutaneous layer (8)** with **adipose tissue (8)**. Located inferior to the subcutaneous layer (8) are **skeletal muscle fibers (9)**, sectioned in transverse and longitudinal planes.

Hair follicles (13) in the skin of the scalp are numerous, closely packed, and oriented at an angle to the surface. A complete hair follicle in longitudinal section is illustrated in the figure. Parts of other hair follicles (13), sectioned in different planes, are also visible. When the hair follicle (13) is cut in a transverse plane, the following structures are visible: the cuticle, **internal root sheath (13a), external root sheath (13b), connective tissue sheath (13c), hair bulb (13d)**, and the connective tissue dermal **papilla (13e)**. The hair passes upward through the follicle (13) to the skin surface. Numerous **sebaceous glands (11)** surround each hair follicle (13). The sebaceous glands (11) are aggregates of clear cells that are connected to a duct that opens into the hair follicle (13) (see Fig. 12.5).

The **arrector pili muscles (5, 10)** are smooth muscles aligned at an oblique angle to the hair follicles (13). The arrector pili muscles (5, 10) attach to the papillary layer of the dermis and to the connective tissue sheath (13c) of the hair follicle (13). The contraction of arrector pili muscles (5, 10) causes the hair shaft to move into a more vertical position.

Deep in the dermis or subcutaneous layer (8) are the basal portions of the highly coiled **sweat glands (6)**. Sections of the sweat gland (6) that exhibit lightly stained columnar epithelium are the **secretory portions (6b)** of the gland. These are distinct from the **excretory ducts (6a)** of the sweat glands (6), which are lined by the stratified cuboidal epithelium of smaller, darker-stained cells. Each sweat gland duct (6a) is coiled deep in the dermis but straightens out in the upper dermis and follows a spiral course through the epidermis to the surface of the skin (see Fig. 12.3).

The skin contains many **blood vessels (14)** and has rich sensory innervations. The sensory receptors for pressure and vibration are the **Pacinian corpuscles (7)**, located in the subcutaneous tissue (8). The Pacinian corpuscles (7) are illustrated in greater detail and higher magnification in Figure 12.10.

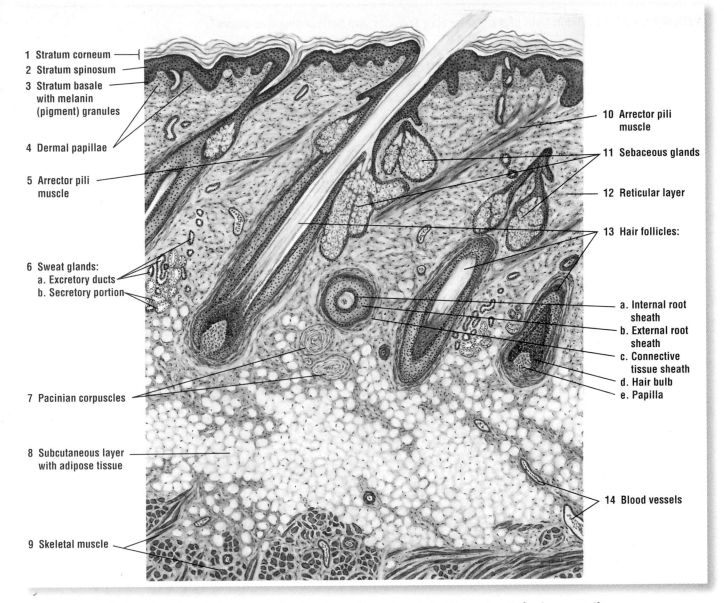

1 Stratum corneum
2 Stratum spinosum
3 Stratum basale with melanin (pigment) granules
4 Dermal papillae
5 Arrector pili muscle
6 Sweat glands:
   a. Excretory ducts
   b. Secretory portion
7 Pacinian corpuscles
8 Subcutaneous layer with adipose tissue
9 Skeletal muscle
10 Arrector pili muscle
11 Sebaceous glands
12 Reticular layer
13 Hair follicles:
   a. Internal root sheath
   b. External root sheath
   c. Connective tissue sheath
   d. Hair bulb
   e. Papilla
14 Blood vessels

FIGURE 12.2 ■ Skin: epidermis, dermis, and hypodermis in the scalp. Stain: hematoxylin and eosin. Low magnification.

FIGURE 12.3 | Hairy Thin Skin of the Scalp: Hair Follicles and Surrounding Structures

This low-power photomicrograph illustrates a section of the thin skin of the scalp. In the **epidermis (1)** of the thin skin, the **stratum corneum (1a), stratum granulosum (1b)**, and **stratum spinosum (1c)** layers are thinner than the same layers in the thick skin. In the dense irregular connective tissue of the **dermis (4)** are **hair follicles (3)** and associated **sebaceous glands (2, 5)**. An **arrector pili muscle (6)** extends from the deep connective tissue around the hair follicle (3) to the connective tissue of the papillary layer of the dermis (4).

1 Epidermis:
   a. Stratum corneum
   b. Stratum granulosum
   c. Stratum spinosum

2 Sebaceous gland

3 Hair follicles

4 Dermis

5 Sebaceous gland

6 Arrector pili muscle

FIGURE 12.3 ■ Hairy thin skin of the scalp: hair follicles and surrounding structures. Stain: hematoxylin and eosin. ×40.

FIGURE 12.4 | Section of a Hair Follicle with Surrounding Structures

This figure illustrates a longitudinal section of a hair follicle and surrounding glands and structures. The different layers of the hair follicle are identified on the right side. The hair follicle is surrounded by an outer **connective tissue sheath (15)** of the **dermis (7)**. Under the connective tissue sheath (15) is an **external root sheath (14)** composed of several cell layers. These cell layers are continuous with the epithelial layer of the epidermis. The **internal root sheath (13)** is composed of a thin, pale epithelial stratum (the Henle layer) and a thin, granular epithelial stratum (the Huxley layer). These two cell layers become indistinguishable as their cells merge with the cells in the expanded part of the hair follicle called the **hair bulb (21)**. Internal to the cell layers of the internal root sheath (13) are cells that produce the **cuticle (12)** of the hair and the keratinized **cortex (11)** of the hair follicle, which appears as a pale yellow layer. The **hair root (16)** and the **dermal papilla (18)** form the hair bulb (21). In the hair bulb (21), the external root sheath (14) and internal root sheath (13) merge into an undifferentiated group of cells called the **hair matrix (17)**, which is situated above the dermal papilla (18). Cell mitoses and **melanin pigment (19)** can be seen in the matrix cells (17). Numerous **capillaries (20)** supply the connective tissue of the dermal papilla (18).

In the connective tissue of the dermis (7) and adjacent to the hair follicle are visible transverse sections of the basal portion of a coiled **sweat gland (8, 9)**. The **secretory cells (9)** of the sweat gland are tall and stain light. Along the bases of the secretory cells (9) are flattened nuclei of the contractile **myoepithelial cells (10)**. The **excretory ducts (8)** of the sweat gland are smaller in diameter, are lined with a stratified cuboidal epithelium, and stain darker than the secretory cells (9).

A sebaceous **gland (4)** that is connected to the hair follicle is sectioned through the middle. The sebaceous gland (4) is lined with a stratified epithelium that has continuity with the external root sheath (14) of the hair follicle. The epithelium of the sebaceous gland is modified, and along its base is a row of columnar or cuboidal cells, the **basal cells (3)**, in which the nuclei may be flattened. These cells rest on a basement membrane, which is surrounded by the connective tissue of the dermis (7). The basal cells (3) of the sebaceous gland (4) divide and fill the acinus of the gland with larger, polyhedral **secretory cells (5)** that enlarge, accumulate secretory material, and become round. The secretory cells (5) in the interior of the acinus undergo **degeneration (2)**, a process in which the cells become the oily secretory product of the gland, called sebum. Sebum passes through the short **duct** of the **sebaceous gland (1)** into the lumen of the hair follicle.

Each hair follicle is surrounded by numerous sebaceous glands (4). The sebaceous glands lie in the connective tissue of the dermis (7) and in the angle between the hair follicle and the smooth muscle strip called the **arrector pili muscle (6)**. When the arrector pili muscle contracts, the hair stands up, forming a dimple or a goose bump on the skin and forcing the sebum out of the sebaceous gland (4) into the lumen of the hair follicle.

1 Duct of sebaceous gland

2 Degenerating secretory cells

3 Basal cells

4 Sebaceous gland

5 Nuclei of secretory cells

6 Arrector pili muscle

7 Connective tissue of dermis

8 Excretory ducts of sweat gland

9 Secretory cells of sweat gland

10 Myoepithelial cells

11 Cortex

12 Cuticle

13 Internal root sheath

14 External root sheath

15 Connective tissue sheath

16 Hair root

17 Hair matrix

18 Dermal papilla

19 Melanin pigment

20 Capillaries of dermal papilla

21 Hair bulb

FIGURE 12.4 ■ Hair follicle: bulb of the hair follicle, sweat gland, sebaceous gland, and arrector pili muscle. Stain: hematoxylin and eosin. Medium magnification.

SECTION 2 Thick Skin

The basic histology of skin is similar in different regions of the body, except in the thickness of the epidermis. **Palms** and **soles** are constantly exposed to increased wear, tear, and abrasion. As a protective measure, the epidermis in these regions is thick, especially the outermost stratified keratinized layer. Because of the increased thickness of the epidermis, the skin on the palms and soles is called **thick skin**. Thick skin also contains numerous **sweat glands**, but it lacks hair follicles, sebaceous glands, and smooth muscle fibers (see Overview Fig. 12.1).

 Supplemental micrographic images are available at **www.thePoint.com/Eroschenko12e** under Skin System.

FIGURE 12.5 | Thick Skin: Epidermis, Dermis, and Hypodermis of the Palm

A low-power photomicrograph illustrates the superficial and deep structures in the thick skin of the palm. The following cell layers are recognized in the **epidermis (6): stratum corneum (7), stratum granulosum (8)**, and **stratum basale (9)**. Inferior to the epidermis (6) is the dense irregular connective tissue **dermis (5). Dermal papillae (11)** from the dermis (5) indent the base of the epidermis (6). Deep in the dermis (5) and the **hypodermis (4),** are cross sections of the coiled simple tubular **sweat glands (3)** and the **excretory ducts of the sweat glands (10)**. A thick layer of **adipose tissue (1)** deep to the dermis (5) is the hypodermis (4), or the superficial fascia. The hypodermis (4) is not part of the integument. Two sensory receptors called the **Pacinian corpuscles (2)** are seen inferior to the adipose tissue (1) of the hypodermis (4).

FIGURE 12.6 | Thick Skin of the Palm, Superficial Cell Layers, and Melanin Pigment

Thick skin is best illustrated by examining a section from the palm. The epidermis of thick skin exhibits five distinct cell layers and is much thicker than that of the thin skin (see Figs. 12.1 to 12.3). The different cell layers of the epidermis are illustrated in greater detail and at higher magnification on the left.

The outermost layer of thick skin is the **stratum corneum (1, 9)**, a wide layer of flattened, dead, or keratinized cells that are constantly shed, or **desquamated (8),** from the skin surface. Inferior to the stratum corneum (1, 9) is a narrow, lightly stained **stratum lucidum (2)**. This thin layer is difficult to see in most slide preparations. At a higher magnification, the outlines of flattened cells and eleidin droplets in this layer are occasionally seen.

Located below the stratum lucidum (2) is the **stratum granulosum (3, 11)**, in which the cells are filled with dark-staining **keratohyalin granules (3)**. Directly under the stratum granulosum (3, 11) is the thick **stratum spinosum (4, 12)** composed of several layers of polyhedral cells. These cells are connected to each other by spinous processes or intercellular bridges that represent the attachment sites of desmosomes (macula adherens).

The deepest cell layer in the skin is the columnar **stratum basale (5, 13)** that rests on the connective tissue **basement membrane (6, 15)**. Mitotic activity and the brown melanin pigment (5, 13) are normally seen in the deeper layers of the stratum spinosum (4, 12) and stratum basale (5, 13).

The **excretory duct** of a **sweat gland (10)** located deep in the dermis penetrates the epidermis, loses its epithelial wall, and spirals through the epidermal cell layers (1 to 5) to the skin surface as small channels with a thin lining.

Dermal papillae (7) are prominent in thick skin. Some dermal papillae (7) may contain tactile or sensory **Meissner corpuscles (14)** and **capillary loops (16)**.

1 Adipose tissue

2 Pacinian corpuscles

3 Sweat glands

7 Stratum corneum

8 Stratum granulosum

9 Stratum basale

10 Excretory ducts of sweat glands

11 Dermal papillae

4 Hypodermis   5 Dermis   6 Epidermis

FIGURE 12.5 ■ Thick skin: epidermis, dermis, and hypodermis of the palm. Stain: hematoxylin and eosin. ×17.

1 Stratum corneum

2 Stratum lucidum

3 Stratum granulosum with keratohyalin granules

4 Stratum spinosum

5 Stratum basale with melanin pigment

6 Basement membrane

7 Dermal papillae

8 Desquamated cells

9 Stratum corneum

10 Excretory ducts of sweat glands

11 Stratum granulosum

12 Stratum spinosum

13 Stratum basale with melanin pigment

14 Meissner corpuscle

15 Basement membrane

16 Capillary loops

FIGURE 12.6 ■ Thick skin of the palm, superficial cell layers, and melanin pigment. Stain: hematoxylin and eosin. Medium magnification.

FIGURE 12.7 | Thick Skin: Epidermis and Superficial Cell Layers

A higher-magnification photomicrograph shows a clear distinction between the different cell layers in the **epidermis (1)** of the thick skin of the palm. The outermost and the thickest layer is the **stratum corneum (1a)**. Inferior to the stratum corneum (1a) are two to three layers of dark cells filled with granules. This is the **stratum granulosum (1b)**. Below the stratum granulosum (1b) is the **stratum spinosum (1c)**, a thicker layer of polyhedral cells. The deepest cell layer in the epidermis (1) is the **stratum basale (1d)**. The cells in this layer contain brown **melanin granules (6)**. The stratum basale (1d) is attached to a thin connective tissue **basement membrane (4)** that separates the epidermis (1) from the **dermis (2)**. The connective tissue of the dermis (2) indents the epidermis (1) to form **dermal papillae (5)**. Passing through the dermis (2) and the cell layers of the epidermis (1) is the **excretory duct (3)** of a sweat gland that is located deep in the dermis.

FIGURE 12.8 | Apocrine Sweat Glands: Secretory and Excretory Portions of the Sweat Gland

The apocrine glands are large, coiled sweat glands that deliver their secretions into the adjacent **hair follicle (7)**. This illustration shows numerous cross sections of an apocrine sweat gland and a few secretory units of an eccrine sweat gland for comparison. The **secretory portion** of the **apocrine sweat gland (3)** consists of wide and dilated lumina. The gland is embedded deep in the **connective tissue** of the **dermis (5)** or hypodermis with **adipose cells (4)** and numerous **blood vessels (8)**. In comparison, the **secretory portion** of an **eccrine sweat gland (6)** is smaller and exhibits much smaller lumina. The cuboidal secretory cells of the apocrine sweat gland (3) are surrounded by numerous **myoepithelial cells (2)** that are located at the base of the secretory cells. When cut at an oblique angle, the myoepithelial cells (2) loop over the secretory cells to surround them. The **excretory portion** of the **sweat gland (1)** is lined by a double layer of dark-staining cuboidal cells, which is similar to the excretory duct of the eccrine sweat gland.

1 Epidermis:

  a. Stratum corneum

  b. Stratum granulosum

  c. Stratum spinosum

  d. Stratum basale

2 Dermis

3 Excretory duct of sweat gland

4 Basement membrane

5 Dermal papillae

6 Melanin granules

FIGURE 12.7 ■ Thick skin: epidermis and superficial cell layers. Stain: hematoxylin and eosin. ×40.

1 Excretory portion of a sweat gland

2 Myoepithelial cells around secretory portion

3 Secretory portion of an apocrine sweat gland

4 Adipose cells of hypodermis

5 Connective tissue of dermis

6 Secretory portion of an eccrine sweat gland

7 Hair follicle

8 Blood vessels

FIGURE 12.8 ■ Apocrine sweat gland: secretory and excretory potions of the sweat gland. Stain: hematoxylin and eosin. Medium magnification.

FIGURE 12.9 | Cross Section and Three-Dimensional Appearance of an Eccrine Sweat Gland

The eccrine sweat gland is a simple, highly coiled tubular gland that extends deep into the dermis or the upper hypodermis. To illustrate this extension, the sweat gland is shown in both cross-sectional (*left side*) and three-dimensional views (*right side*) as it makes its way through the dermis and **epidermis (1, 6)**.

Part of the coiled portion of the sweat gland that lies deep in the dermis is the **secretory portion (9)**. Here, **secretory cells (4)** are large and columnar and stain lightly eosinophilic. Surrounding the bases of the secretory cells (4) are thin, spindle-shaped **myoepithelial cells (5)** that are located between the base of the secretory cells (4) and the basement membrane (not illustrated) that surrounds the cells. The area where the light-staining secretory cells (4, 9) give rise to the dark-staining **excretory duct (2, 7)** represents the **transition area (3, 8)** between the secretory and excretory regions of the sweat gland.

The cells of the excretory ducts (2, 7) are smaller than the secretory cells (4). Also, the excretory ducts (2, 7) have smaller diameters and are lined by denser-staining, stratified cuboidal cells. There are no myoepithelial cells around the excretory ducts (2, 7). As the excretory ducts (2, 7) ascend through the connective tissue of the dermis, they straighten out and penetrate the cell layers of the epidermis (1, 6), where they lose the epithelial wall and follow a spiral course through the cells to the surface of the skin.

FUNCTIONAL CORRELATIONS 12.2 | Skin Derivatives or Appendages

Nails, hairs, and **sweat glands** are derivatives of the skin that develop directly from the downgrowth of the surface epithelium of the epidermis. During development, these appendages grow into and reside deep within the connective tissue of the **dermis**. Sweat glands may also extend deeper into the **subcutaneous layer** or **hypodermis**.

Hairs are the hard, cornified, cylindrical structures that arise from **hair follicles** in the skin. One portion of the hair projects through the epithelium of the skin to the exterior surface; the other portion remains embedded in the dermis. Hair grows from the expanded portion at the base of the hair follicle called the **hair bulb,** which consists of a **matrix** of dividing cells that produce the growth of hair. Also present here are melanocytes that provide the pigment for the hair. The base of the hair bulb is indented by a **connective tissue papilla**, a highly vascularized region that brings essential nutrients to hair follicle cells. Here, the hair cells divide, grow, cornify, and form the hairs.

Associated with each hair follicle are one or more **sebaceous glands** that produce an oily secretion called **sebum**. Sebaceous glands also develop from epidermal cells. The secretory product, sebum, forms when cells die in sebaceous glands. Eventually, the secretory product sebum is expelled from the glands onto the shaft of the hair follicle. Also, extending from the connective tissue around the hair follicle to the **papillary layer** of the **dermis** are bundles of smooth muscle called **arrector pili**. The sebaceous glands are located between the arrector pili muscle and the hair follicle. Arrector pili muscles are controlled by the **autonomic nervous system** and contract during strong emotions, fear, and cold. Contraction of the arrector pili muscle erects the hair shaft, depresses the skin where it inserts, and produces a small bump on the surface of skin, often called a goose bump. In addition, this contraction forces the sebum from sebaceous glands onto the hair follicle and skin. Sebum oils keep the skin smooth, waterproof it, prevent it from drying, and give it some antibacterial protection.

Sweat glands are widely distributed in skin and are of two types: eccrine and apocrine. **Eccrine** sweat glands are simple, coiled tubular glands. Their **secretory portion** is found deep in the dermis, from which a coiled, stratified cuboidal **excretory duct** leads to the skin surface. The eccrine sweat glands contain two cell

(box continues on page 278)

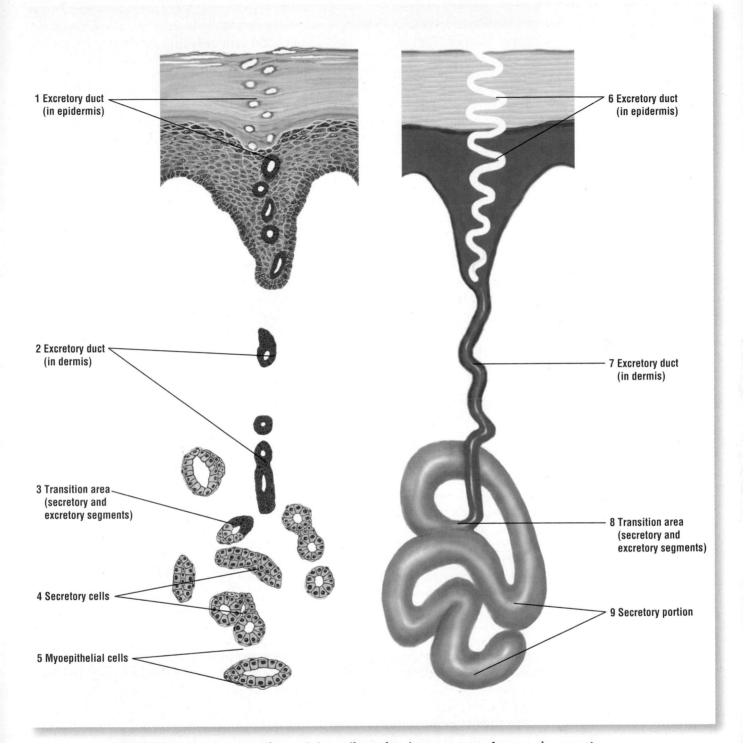

1 Excretory duct
(in epidermis)

2 Excretory duct
(in dermis)

3 Transition area
(secretory and
excretory segments)

4 Secretory cells

5 Myoepithelial cells

6 Excretory duct
(in epidermis)

7 Excretory duct
(in dermis)

8 Transition area
(secretory and
excretory segments)

9 Secretory portion

FIGURE 12.9 ■ Cross section and three-dimensional appearance of an eccrine sweat
gland. Stain: hematoxylin and eosin. Low magnification.

FUNCTIONAL CORRELATIONS 12.2 | Skin Derivatives or Appendages (Continued)

types: **clear cells** without secretory granules and **dark cells** with secretory granules. Secretion from the dark cells is primarily mucus, whereas secretion from clear cells contains water and electrolytes. Surrounding the basal region of the secretory portion of each sweat gland are **myoepithelial cells**, whose contraction expels the secretion (sweat) from sweat glands. Eccrine sweat glands are most numerous in the skin of the palms and soles. The eccrine sweat glands have an important role in assisting the organism in temperature regulation through evaporation of water from sweat on the body surfaces. Also, as excretory structures, sweat glands excrete water, sodium salts, ammonia, uric acid, and urea.

Apocrine sweat glands are also found in the dermis and are primarily limited to the axilla, anus, and areolar regions of the breast. These glands also develop from the downgrowth of the epidermis. These sweat glands are larger than eccrine sweat glands, and their ducts open into the **hair follicle** canal. The secretory portion of the gland is coiled and tubular. In contrast to eccrine sweat glands, the lumina of the secretory portion of the gland are wide and dilated, and the secretory cells are low cuboidal. The excretory ducts of the apocrine glands are also stratified cuboidal and are similar to eccrine sweat glands. Similarly, the secretory portions of the apocrine glands are surrounded by contractile **myoepithelial cells**. The apocrine sweat glands become functional at puberty, when the **sex hormones** are produced. The glands produce a **viscous secretion**, which acquires a distinct and unpleasant odor after bacterial decomposition.

FIGURE 12.10 | Glomus in the Dermis of Thick Skin

Arteriovenous anastomoses are numerous in the thick skin of the fingers and toes. In some arteriovenous anastomoses, there is a direct connection between the artery and vein. In others, the arterial portion of the anastomosis forms a specialized thick-walled structure called the **glomus** (2). The blood vessel in the glomus (2) is highly coiled, or convoluted, and, as a result, more than one lumen of the coiled vessel may be seen in a transverse section of the glomus (2).

The smooth muscle cells in the tunica media of the glomus artery (2) have enlarged and become **epithelioid cells (6)**. The tunica media of the glomus artery (2) becomes thin again before it empties into a venule at the **arteriovenous junction (5)**.

All arteriovenous anastomoses are richly innervated and supplied by blood vessels. A **connective tissue sheath (7)** encloses the glomus (2). The **dermis (4)** that surrounds the glomus (2) contains numerous **blood vessels (8)**, peripheral **nerves (1)**, and excretory **ducts** of **sweat glands (3)**.

FUNCTIONAL CORRELATIONS 12.3 | Arteriovenous Anastomoses and the Glomus

In numerous tissues, direct communications between arteries and veins called **arteriovenous anastomoses** bypass the capillaries. Their main functions are the regulation of blood pressure, blood flow, and temperature and conservation of body heat. A more complex structure that also forms shunts is called a **glomus**. A glomus consists of a highly coiled arteriovenous shunt that is surrounded by collagenous connective tissue. The function of the glomus is also to regulate blood flow and to conserve body heat. These structures are found in the fingertips, external ear, and other peripheral areas that are exposed to extremely cold temperatures and where arteriovenous shunts are needed.

1 Nerves with axons

2 Glomus

3 Duct of sweat gland

4 Dermis

5 Arteriovenous junction

6 Epithelioid cells of glomus

7 Connective tissue sheath around glomus

8 Venules

FIGURE 12.10 ■ Glomus in the dermis of thick skin. Stain: hematoxylin and eosin. High magnification.

FIGURE 12.11 | Pacinian Corpuscles in the Dermis of Thick Skin (Transverse and Longitudinal Sections)

Located deep in the **dermis (3)** of the thick skin and subcutaneous tissue are the **Pacinian corpuscles (2, 9).** One Pacinian corpuscle is illustrated in a longitudinal section (2) and the other in transverse section (9).

Each Pacinian corpuscle (2, 9) is an ovoid structure with an elongated central myelinated **axon (2b, 9b).** The axon (2b, 9b) in the corpuscle is surrounded by **concentric lamellae (2a, 9a)** of compact collagenous fibers that become denser in the periphery to form the **connective tissue capsule (2c, 9c).** Between the connective tissue lamellae (2c, 9c) is a small amount of lymphlike fluid. In a transverse section, the layers of connective tissue lamellae (9a) surrounding the central axon (9b) of the Pacinian corpuscle (9) resemble a sliced onion.

In the connective tissue of the dermis (3) and surrounding the Pacinian corpuscles (2, 9) are numerous **adipose cells (5),** blood vessels such as a **venule (10),** peripheral **nerves (4, 6),** and cross sections of an **excretory duct (1)** and the **secretory portion** of the **sweat gland (8).** The contractile **myoepithelial cells (7)** surround the secretory portion of the sweat gland (8).

The Pacinian corpuscles (2, 9) are important sensory receptors for pressure, vibration, and touch.

1 Excretory ducts of sweat glands

2 Pacinian corpuscle:
   a. Concentric lamellae
   b. Axon
   c. Connective tissue capsule

3 Dermis

4 Nerve

5 Adipose cells

6 Nerve

7 Myoepithelial cells

8 Secretory portion of sweat gland

9 Pacinian corpuscle:
   a. Concentric lamellae
   b. Axon
   c. Connective tissue capsule

10 Venule

FIGURE 12.11 ■ Pacinian corpuscles in the dermis of thick skin (transverse and longitudinal sections). Stain: hematoxylin and eosin. High magnification.

Integumentary System

General Overview

- Skin is the largest organ; skin and its derivatives form the integumentary system
- Consists of the superficial epidermis and deeper dermis
- Nonvascular epidermis is covered by keratinized stratified squamous epithelium
- Vascular dermis contains irregular connective tissue, blood vessels, nerves, and glands
- Beneath the dermis is the hypodermis, or subcutaneous, layer of connective tissue or fascia

Dermis: Papillary and Reticular Layers

Papillary Layer

- Basement membrane separates the dermis from the epidermis
- Is the superficial layer in the dermis and contains loose irregular connective tissue
- Dermal papillae and epidermal ridges form evaginations and interdigitations
- Connective tissue filled with fibers, cells, and blood vessels
- Sensory receptors (Meissner corpuscles) are present in the dermal papillae

Reticular Layer

- Is the deeper and thicker layer in dermis, filled with dense irregular connective tissue
- Few cells present and collagen is type I
- No distinct boundary between the papillary and reticular layers
- Blends inferiorly with the hypodermis or subcutaneous layer (hypodermis) of superficial fascia
- Contains arteriovenous anastomoses and sensory receptors in Pacinian corpuscles
- Concentric lamellae of collagen fibers surround myelinated axons in Pacinian corpuscles

Epidermal Cell Layers

Stratum Basale (Germinativum): The First Layer

- Deepest or basal single layer of cells that rests on the basement membrane
- Cells attached by desmosomes and by hemidesmosomes to the basement membrane
- Cells serve as stem cells for the epidermis and show increased mitotic activity
- Cells mature and migrate upward in the epidermis and produce intermediate keratin filaments

Stratum Spinosum: The Second Layer

- Is the layer above the stratum basale that consists of four to six rows of cells
- During histologic preparation, cells shrink and intercellular spaces appear as spines
- Cells synthesize keratin filaments that become assembled into tonofilaments
- Spines represent sites of desmosome attachments to keratin tonofilaments

Stratum Granulosum: The Third Layer

- Cells above the stratum spinosum and consists of three to five cell layers of flattened cells
- Cells filled with dense keratohyalin granules and membrane-bound lamellar granules
- Keratohyalin granules consist of the protein filaggrin that cross-links with keratin filaments
- Combination of keratin tonofilaments with keratohyalin granules produces soft keratin
- Lamellar granules discharge lipid material between cells and waterproof the skin

Stratum Lucidum: The Fourth Layer

- Lies superior to the stratum granulosum, found in thick skin only; translucent and barely visible
- Hydrolytic enzymes disrupt cell contents and pack them with keratin filaments

Stratum Corneum: The Fifth Layer

- Most superficial layer and consists of flat, dead cells filled with soft keratin
- Keratinized cells continually shed or desquamated from the surface and replaced by new cells
- During keratinization, hydrolytic enzymes eliminate the nucleus and organelles

Other Skin Cells

Melanocytes

- Arise from neural crest cells and are located between the stratum basale and stratum spinosum
- Long irregular cytoplasmic or dendritic extensions branch into the epidermis
- Synthesize from amino acid tyrosine a dark brown pigment: melanin
- Melanin transferred from cytoplasmic extensions to keratinocytes in basal cell layers
- Melanin darkens skin color and protects it from ultraviolet radiation

Langerhans Cells

- Dendritic-type cells originate from the bone marrow and migrate via the blood to the skin
- Reside primarily in the stratum spinosum and are part of the immune system of the skin
- Are antigen-presenting cells of the skin

Merkel Cells

- Present in the basal layer of the epidermis and function as mechanoreceptors for sensation

Epidermis: Thick Versus Thin Skin

- Palms and soles, because of wear and tear, are covered by thick skin
- Thick skin contains sweat glands but lacks hair, sebaceous glands, and smooth muscle
- Thin skin contains sebaceous glands, hair, sweat glands, and arrector pili smooth muscle
- Keratinocytes are the predominant cell type in the epidermis
- Less numerous epidermal cells are the melanocytes, Langerhans cells, and Merkel cells

Major Skin Functions

- Protection through the keratinized epidermis from abrasion and the entrance of pathogens
- Impermeable to water, owing to lipid layer in the epidermis
- Body temperature regulation as a result of sweating and changes in vessel diameters
- Sensory perception of touch, pain, pressure, and temperature changes because of nerve endings
- Excretions through sweat of water, sodium salts, urea, and nitrogenous waste
- Formation of vitamin D from precursor molecules produced in the epidermis when exposed to the sun

Skin Derivatives

Hairs

- Develop from the surface epithelium of the epidermis and reside deep in the dermis
- Are hard cylindrical structures that arise from hair follicles
- Surrounded by external and internal root sheaths
- Grow from the expanded hair bulb of the hair follicle

- Hair bulb indented by connective tissue (dermal) papilla that is highly vascularized
- Hair matrix situated above the papilla contains mitotic cells and melanocytes

Sebaceous Glands

- Numerous sebaceous glands associated with each hair follicle
- Cells in sebaceous glands grow, accumulate secretions, die, and become oily secretion sebum
- Smooth muscles arrector pili attach to the papillary layer of the dermis and to the sheath of the hair follicle
- Contraction of the arrector pili muscle stands hair up and forces sebum into the lumen of the hair follicle

Sweat Glands

- Widely distributed in the skin and are of two types: eccrine and apocrine
- Assist in temperature regulation and excretion of water, salts, and some nitrogenous waste

Eccrine Sweat Glands

- Are simple coiled glands located deep in the dermis in the skin of palms and soles
- Consist of clear and dark secretory cells and excretory duct
- Clear cells secrete watery product, whereas dark cells secrete mainly mucus
- Contractile myoepithelial cells surround only the secretory cells
- Excretory duct is thin, dark-staining, and lined by stratified cuboidal cells
- Excretory duct ascends, straightens, and penetrates the epidermis to reach the surface of the skin

Apocrine Sweat Glands

- Found coiled in the deep dermis of the axilla, anus, and areolar regions of the breast
- Ducts of glands open into hair follicles
- Lumina are wide and dilated, with low cuboidal epithelium
- Contractile myoepithelial cells surround the secretory portion of the glands
- Become functional at puberty when sex hormones are present
- Secretion has an unpleasant odor after bacterial decomposition

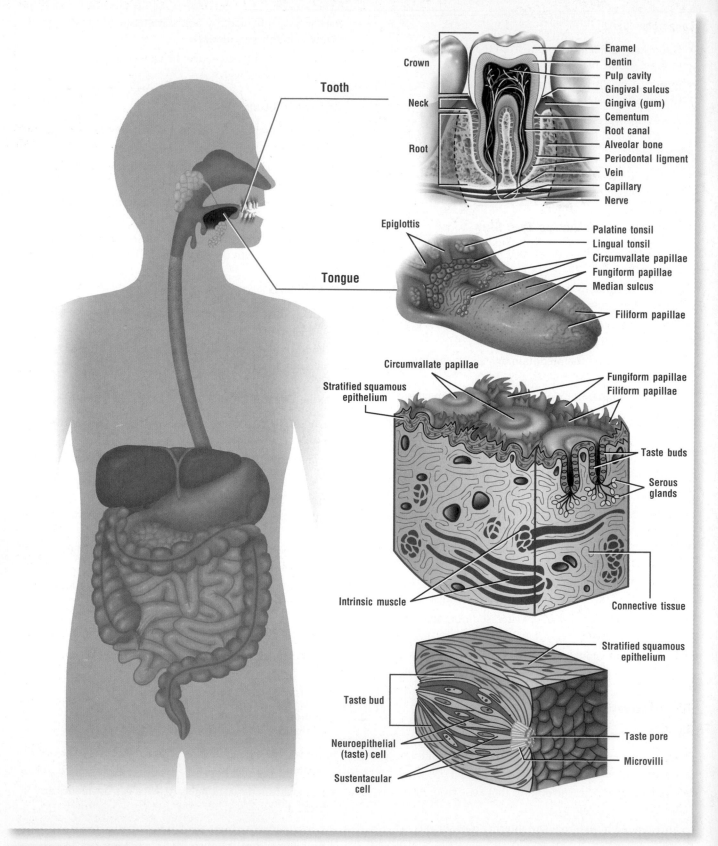

OVERVIEW FIGURE 13.1 ■ Oral cavity. The salivary glands and their connections to the oral cavity, morphology of the tongue in cross section, a tooth, and detail of a taste bud are illustrated.

CHAPTER 13

Digestive System Part I: Oral Cavity and Major Salivary Glands

The digestive system consists of a long **hollow tube,** or tract, that starts at the oral cavity and terminates at the anus. The system consists of the **oral cavity, esophagus, stomach, small intestine, large intestine, rectum**, and **anal canal**. Associated with the digestive tract are the accessory digestive organs, the **salivary glands, liver**, and **pancreas** that are located outside the digestive tract. Their secretory products are delivered to the digestive tract through excretory ducts that penetrate the digestive tract wall and deliver their secretory products into the digestive tube (Overview Fig. 13.1).

SECTION 1   Oral Cavity

In the oral cavity, food is ingested, masticated (chewed), and lubricated by saliva for swallowing. Because food is physically broken down in the oral cavity, this region is lined with a protective, nonkeratinized, **stratified squamous epithelium**, which also lines the inner or labial surface of the lips.

The Lips

The oral cavity is formed, in part, by the lips and cheeks. The lips are lined with a very thin skin covered by a stratified squamous keratinized epithelium. Blood vessels are close to the lip surface, imparting a red color to the lips. The outer surface of the lip contains hair follicles, sebaceous glands, and sweat glands. The lips also contain skeletal muscle called **orbicularis oris**. Inside the free margin of the lip, the outer lining changes to a thicker stratified squamous nonkeratinized oral epithelium. Beneath the oral epithelium are found mucus-secreting **labial glands**.

The Tongue

The **tongue** is a muscular organ located in the oral cavity. The core of the tongue consists of **connective tissue** and interlacing bundles of **skeletal muscle fibers**. The distribution and random orientation of individual skeletal muscle fibers in the tongue allows for its increased movement during chewing, swallowing, and speaking. The dorsal surface of the tongue is divided into an anterior two thirds and a posterior one third section by a V-shaped depression called the **sulcus terminalis**.

Papillae

The epithelium on the dorsal surface of the tongue is irregular or rough owing to numerous elevations or projections called **papillae**. These are indented by the underlying connective tissue called **lamina propria**. All papillae on the tongue are covered by **stratified squamous epithelium** that shows partial or incomplete **keratinization**. In contrast, the epithelium on the ventral surface of the tongue is smooth and nonkeratinized.

There are four types of projections or papillae on the dorsal surface of the tongue: filiform, fungiform, circumvallate, and foliate.

Filiform Papillae

The most numerous and smallest papillae on the surface of the tongue are the narrow, conical, or pointed, **filiform papillae**. They cover the entire anterior dorsal surface of the tongue and are keratinized. Filiform papillae of the tongue do not contain taste buds.

Fungiform Papillae

The less numerous but larger, broader, and taller than the filiform papillae are the **fungiform papillae**. These papillae exhibit a mushroom-like shape, project above the filiform papillae, and are more prevalent in the anterior region and tip of the tongue. Fungiform papillae are interspersed and scattered among the filiform papillae of the tongue surface.

Circumvallate Papillae

Circumvallate papillae are much larger than the fungiform or filiform papillae. About 8 to 12 circumvallate papillae are located in the posterior region of the tongue in humans. These papillae are characterized by deep moats or **furrows** that completely encircle them. Numerous excretory ducts from underlying **serous (von Ebner) glands** that are located in the connective tissue of the tongue empty their serous secretions into the base of these furrows. Numerous taste buds are located in the stratified epithelium on the lateral sides of each papilla.

Foliate Papillae

Foliate papillae are well developed in some animals but are rudimentary or poorly developed in humans.

Taste Buds

Located in the confines of the stratified epithelium of the foliate and fungiform papillae, and on the lateral sides of the circumvallate papillae, are barrel-shaped structures called the **taste buds**. In addition to the tongue, taste buds are found in the epithelium of the soft palate, pharynx, and epiglottis. The epithelial surface of each taste bud contains an opening called the **taste pore**. Each taste bud occupies the full thickness of the epithelium. Three main cell types are found in each taste bud.

Located within each taste bud are elongated **gustatory (neuroepithelial** or **taste) cells** that extend from the base of the taste bud to the taste pore. The apices of each taste cell exhibit numerous **microvilli** that protrude through the taste pore. The bases of the taste cells form **synapses** with the processes of small afferent axons. Also present within the confines of the taste buds are elongated, supporting **sustentacular cells**. These cells are less numerous and are not sensory. At the base of each taste bud are located the **basal cells**. These cells are undifferentiated and serve as **stem cells** for the other two cell types in taste buds (see Overview Fig. 13.1).

Lymphoid Aggregations: Tonsils (Palatine, Pharyngeal, and Lingual)

The tonsils are aggregates of diffuse lymphoid tissue and lymphoid nodules that are located in the oral pharynx. The **palatine tonsils** are located on the lateral walls of the oral part of the pharynx. These tonsils are lined with stratified squamous nonkeratinized epithelium and exhibit numerous **crypts**. A connective tissue capsule separates the tonsils from the adjacent tissue. The **pharyngeal tonsil** is a single structure situated in the superior and posterior portions of the pharynx. It is covered by pseudostratified ciliated epithelium. The **lingual tonsils** are located on the dorsal surface of the posterior third of the tongue. They are several in number and are seen as small bulges composed of masses of lymphoid aggregations. The lingual tonsils are lined with a stratified squamous nonkeratinized epithelium. Each lingual tonsil is invaginated by the covering epithelium to form numerous crypts, around which are found aggregations of lymphatic nodules with germinal centers.

 Supplemental micrographic images are available at **www.thePoint.com/Eroschenko12e** under Digestive System Part I: Oral Cavity.

FIGURE 13.1 | Lip (Longitudinal Section)

Thin skin, or thin, **epidermis (11),** lines the external surface of the lip. The epidermis (11) is composed of stratified squamous keratinized epithelium with **desquamating surface cells (10).** Beneath the epidermis (11) is the **dermis (14)** with **sebaceous glands (2, 12)** that are associated with **hair follicles (4, 15)** and the simple tubular **sweat glands (16)** located deeper in the dermis (14). The dermis (14) also contains the **arrector pili muscles (3, 13),** smooth muscles that attach to the hair follicles (4, 15). Also visible in the lip periphery are blood vessels, an **artery (6a)** and a **venule (6b).** The core of the lip contains a layer of striated muscles, the **orbicularis oris (5, 17).**

The **transition zone (1)** of the skin epidermis (11) to the oral epithelium illustrates a mucocutaneous junction. The internal or oral surface of the lip is lined with a moist, stratified, squamous nonkeratinized **oral epithelium (8)** that is thicker than the epithelium of the epidermis (11). The surface cells of the oral epithelium (8), without becoming cornified, are sloughed off (desquamated) into the fluids of the **mouth (10).** In the deeper connective tissue of the lip are found tubuloacinar, mucus-secreting **labial glands (9, 18).** The secretions from these glands moisten the oral mucosa. The small excretory ducts of the labial glands (9, 18) open into the oral cavity.

In the underlying connective tissue of the lip are also numerous **adipose cells (7),** blood vessels (6), and numerous capillaries. Because the blood vessels (6) are very close to the surface, the color of the blood shows through the overlying thin epithelium, giving the lips a characteristic red color.

1 Transition zone
2 Sebaceous glands
3 Arrector pili muscle
4 Hair follicle
5 Orbicularis oris
6 Blood vessels:
   a. Artery
   b. Vein
7 Adipose cells
8 Oral epithelium
9 Mucus-secreting labial glands
10 Desquamating surface cells
11 Epidermis
12 Sebaceous glands
13 Arrector pili muscle
14 Dermis
15 Hair follicle
16 Sweat gland
17 Orbicularis oris
18 Mucus-secreting labial glands

FIGURE 13.1 ■ Lip (longitudinal section). Stain: hematoxylin and eosin. Low magnification.

FIGURE 13.2 | Anterior Region of the Tongue: Apex (Longitudinal Section)

This illustration shows a longitudinal section of the anterior portion of the tongue. The oral cavity is lined with a protective **mucosa (5)** that consists of an outer epithelial layer (**epithelium) (5a)** and an underlying connective tissue layer called the **lamina propria (5b)**.

The dorsal surface of the tongue is rough and characterized by numerous mucosal projections called **papillae (1, 2, 6)**. In contrast, the mucosa (5) of the ventral surface of the tongue is smooth. The slender, cone-shaped **filiform papillae (2, 6)** are the most numerous papillae and cover the entire dorsal surface of the tongue. The tips of the filiform papillae (2, 6) show keratinization.

Less numerous are the **fungiform papillae (1)** with a broad, round surface of noncornified epithelium and a prominent core of **lamina propria (5b)**.

The core of the tongue consists of crisscrossing bundles of **skeletal muscle (3, 7)**. As a result, the skeletal muscles of the tongue are typically seen in longitudinal, transverse, or oblique planes of section. In the **connective tissue (9)** around the muscle bundles may be seen **blood vessels (4, 8)**, such as an **artery (4a, 8a)** and a **vein (4b, 8b)**, and **nerve fibers (11)**.

In the lower half of the tongue and surrounded by skeletal muscle fibers (3, 7) is a portion of the **anterior lingual gland (10)**. This gland is of a mixed type and contains both **mucous acini (10b)** and **serous acini (10c)**, as well as mixed acini. The **interlobular ducts (10a)** from the anterior lingual gland (10) pass into the larger **excretory duct** of the **lingual gland (12)** that opens into the oral cavity on the ventral surface of the tongue.

FIGURE 13.3 | Tongue: Circumvallate Papilla (Cross Section)

A cross section of a circumvallate papilla of the tongue is illustrated. The **lingual epithelium (2)** of the tongue that covers the circumvallate papilla is **stratified squamous epithelium (1)**. The underlying connective tissue, the **lamina propria (3)**, exhibits numerous **secondary papillae (7)** that project into the overlying stratified squamous epithelium (1, 2) of the papilla. A deep trench, or **furrow (5, 10),** surrounds the base of each circumvallate papilla.

The oval **taste buds (4, 9)** are located in the epithelium of the lateral surfaces of the circumvallate papilla and in the epithelium on the outer wall of the furrow (5, 10). (Fig. 13.5 illustrates the taste buds in greater detail with higher magnification.)

Located deep in the lamina propria (3) and core of the tongue are numerous, tubuloacinar **serous (von Ebner) glands (6, 11)**, whose **excretory ducts (6a, 11a)** open at the base of the circular furrows (5, 10) in the circumvallate papilla. The secretory product from the **serous secretory acini (6b, 11b)** acts as a solvent for taste-inducing substances.

Most of the core of the tongue consists of interlacing bundles of **skeletal muscles (12)**. Examples of skeletal muscle fibers sectioned in **longitudinal (12a)** and **transverse (12b) planes** are abundant. This interlacing arrangement of skeletal muscles (12) gives the tongue the necessary mobility for phonating and chewing and swallowing of food. The lamina propria (3) surrounding the serous glands (6, 11) and muscles (12) also contains an abundance of **blood vessels (8)**.

1 Fungiform papillae

2 Filiform papillae

3 Skeletal muscle

4 Blood vessels:
   a. Artery
   b. Vein

5 Mucosa:
   a. Epithelium
   b. Lamina propria

6 Filiform papillae

7 Skeletal muscle

8 Blood vessels:
   a. Artery
   b. Vein

9 Connective tissue

10 Anterior lingual gland:
   a. Interlobular ducts
   b. Mucous acinus
   c. Serous acinus

11 Nerve fibers

12 Excretory duct of the lingual gland

FIGURE 13.2 ■ Anterior region of the tongue: apex (longitudinal section). Stain: hematoxylin and eosin. Low magnification.

1 Stratified squamous epithelium

2 Lingual epithelium

3 Lamina propria

4 Taste buds

5 Furrow

6 Serous (von Ebner glands):
   a. Excretory ducts

   b. Serous secretory acini

7 Secondary papillae

8 Blood vessels

9 Taste buds

10 Furrow

11 Serous (von Ebner glands):
   a. Excretory ducts

   b. Serous secretory acini

12 Skeletal muscles:
   a. Longitudinal

   b. Transverse

FIGURE 13.3 ■ Tongue: circumvallate papilla (cross section). Stain: hematoxylin and eosin. Medium magnification.

FIGURE 13.4 | Tongue: Filiform and Fungiform Papillae

This low-power photomicrograph shows a section of the dorsal surface of the tongue. In the center is a large **fungiform papilla (2)**. The surface of the fungiform papilla (2) is covered by **stratified squamous epithelium (3)** that is not cornified, or keratinized. The fungiform papilla (2) also exhibits numerous **taste buds (4)** that are located in the epithelium on the apical surface of the papilla, in contrast to the circumvallate papillae, in which the taste buds are located in the peripheral epithelium (see Fig. 13.3).

The underlying connective tissue core, the **lamina propria (5)**, projects into the surface epithelium of the fungiform papilla (2) to form numerous indentations. Surrounding the fungiform papilla (2) are the slender **filiform papillae (1)**, whose conical tips are covered by stratified squamous epithelium that exhibits partial keratinization.

FIGURE 13.5 | Tongue: Taste Buds

The taste **buds (5, 12)** at the bottom of a **furrow (14)** of the circumvallate papilla are illustrated in greater detail. The taste buds (5, 12) are embedded within and extend the full thickness of the stratified **lingual epithelium (1)** of the circumvallate papilla. The taste buds (5, 12) are distinguished from the surrounding stratified epithelium (1) by their oval shapes and elongated cells (modified columnar) that are arranged perpendicular to the epithelium (1).

Several types of cells are found in the taste buds (5, 12). Three different types of cells can be identified in this illustration. The supporting, or **sustentacular cells (3, 8)**, are elongated and exhibit a darker cytoplasm and a slender, dark nucleus. The **taste**, or **gustatory cells (7, 11)**, exhibit a lighter cytoplasm and a more oval, lighter nucleus. The **basal cells (13)** are located at the periphery of the taste bud (5, 12) near the basement membrane. The basal cells (13) give rise to both the sustentacular cells (3, 8) and the gustatory cells (7, 11).

Each taste bud (5, 12) exhibits a small opening onto the epithelial surface called the **taste pore (9)**. The apical surfaces of both the sustentacular cells (3, 8) and the gustatory cells (7, 11) exhibit long **microvilli (taste hairs) (4)** that extend into and protrude through the taste pore (9) into the furrow (14) that surrounds the circumvallate papilla.

The underlying **lamina propria (2)** adjacent to the epithelium and the taste buds (5, 12) consists of a loose connective tissue with numerous **blood vessels (6, 10)** and nerve fibers.

FUNCTIONAL CORRELATIONS 13.1 | Tongue and Taste Buds

The main functions of the tongue during food processing are to perceive **taste** and to assist with mastication (chewing) and swallowing of the food mass, called a **bolus**. In the oral cavity, taste sensations are detected by receptor taste cells located in the **taste buds** of the **fungiform** and **circumvallate papillae** of the tongue. In addition to the tongue, where taste buds are most numerous, taste buds are found in the mucous membrane of the **soft palate, pharynx**, and **epiglottis**.

Substances to be tasted are first dissolved in the **saliva** that is present in the oral cavity during food intake. The dissolved substance then contacts the taste cells by entering through the taste pore. In addition to saliva, taste buds located in the epithelium of circumvallate papillae are continuously washed by watery secretions produced by the underlying **serous (von Ebner) glands**. This secretion enters the **furrow** at the base of the papillae and continues to dissolve different substances, which then enter the **taste pores** in taste buds. The receptor taste cells are then stimulated by coming in direct contact with the molecules of dissolved substances, which in turn conduct nerve impulses over the afferent nerve fibers that eventually reach the brain for taste interpretation and detection.

There are four basic taste sensations: **sour, salt, bitter**, and **sweet**. A fifth type of taste, called **unami** (savory), is sensed by certain amino acids such as glutamate. All remaining taste sensations are various combinations of the basic four tastes. It is now believed that the sensitivity to all tastes is equally distributed across the entire tongue. However, it is also believed that some areas of the tongue may be more sensitive to a certain specific type of taste than to others.

1 Filiform papillae

2 Fungiform papilla

3 Stratified squamous epithelium

4 Taste buds

5 Lamina propria

FIGURE 13.4 ■ Tongue: filiform and fungiform papillae. Stain: hematoxylin and eosin. ×25.

1 Lingual epithelium

2 Lamina propria

3 Sustentacular cell

4 Microvilli (taste hairs)

5 Taste bud

6 Blood vessel

7 Gustatory cell

8 Sustentacular cell

9 Taste pore

10 Blood vessel

11 Gustatory cell

12 Taste bud

13 Basal cells

14 Furrow

FIGURE 13.5 ■ Tongue: taste buds. Stain: hematoxylin and eosin. High magnification.

FIGURE 13.6 | Posterior Tongue: Behind Circumvallate Papilla and Near Lingual Tonsil (Longitudinal Section)

The anterior two thirds of the tongue is separated from the posterior third of the tongue by a depression or a sulcus terminalis. The posterior region of the tongue is located behind the circumvallate papillae and near the lingual tonsils. The dorsal surface of the posterior region typically exhibits large **mucosal ridges (1)** and elevations or **folds (7)** that resemble the large fungiform papillae of the anterior tongue. A **stratified squamous epithelium (6)** without keratinization covers the mucosal ridges (1) and the folds (7). The filiform and fungiform papillae that are normally seen in the anterior region of the tongue are absent from the posterior tongue. Lymphatic nodules of the lingual tonsils can be seen in these folds (7).

The lamina **propria (7)** of the mucosa is wider but similar to that in the anterior two thirds of the tongue. Under the stratified squamous epithelium (6) are seen aggregations of diffuse **lymphatic tissue (2)** and accumulations of **adipose tissue (4), nerve fibers (3)** (in longitudinal section), blood vessels, an **artery (8),** and a **vein (9).**

Deep in the connective tissue of the lamina propria (7) and between the interlacing **skeletal muscle fibers (5)** are found the mucous acini of the **posterior lingual glands (11).** The **excretory ducts (10)** of the posterior lingual glands (11) open onto the dorsal surface of the tongue, usually between bases of the mucosal ridges and folds (1, 7). The posterior lingual glands (11) come in contact with the serous (von Ebner) glands of the circumvallate papilla in the anterior region of the tongue. In the posterior region of the tongue, the posterior lingual glands (11) extend through the root of the tongue.

FIGURE 13.7 | Lingual Tonsils (Transverse Section)

Lingual tonsils are aggregations of small, individual tonsils, each with its own **tonsillar crypt (2, 8).** Lingual tonsils are situated on the dorsal surface of the posterior region or the root of the tongue. A nonkeratinized **stratified squamous epithelium (1)** lines the tonsils and their crypts (2, 8). The tonsillar crypts (2, 8) form deep invaginations on the surface of the tongue and may extend deep into the **lamina propria (5).**

Numerous lymphatic **nodules (3, 9),** some exhibiting **germinal centers (3, 9),** are located in the lamina propria (5) below the stratified squamous surface epithelium (1). Dense **lymphatic infiltration (4, 10)** surrounds the individual lymphatic nodules (3, 9) of the tonsils.

Located deep in the lamina propria (5) are fat cells of the **adipose tissue (7)** and the secretory **mucous acini** of the **posterior lingual glands (11).** Small excretory ducts from the lingual glands (11) unite to form larger **excretory ducts (6).** Most of the excretory ducts (6) open into the tonsillar crypts (2, 8), although some may open directly on the lingual surface. Interspersed among the connective tissue of the lamina propria (5), the adipose tissue (7), and the secretory mucous acini of the posterior lingual glands (11) are fibers of the **skeletal muscles (12)** of the tongue.

1 Mucosal ridges

2 Diffuse lymphatic tissue

3 Nerve fibers

4 Adipose tissue

5 Skeletal muscle fibers (transverse and longitudinal sections)

6 Stratified squamous epithelium

7 Lamina propria of mucosal fold

8 Artery

9 Vein

10 Excretory ducts of the posterior lingual glands

11 Mucous acini of the posterior lingual glands

FIGURE 13.6 ■ Posterior tongue: behind circumvallate papillae and near lingual tonsil (longitudinal section). Stain: hematoxylin and eosin. Low magnification.

1 Stratified squamous epithelium

2 Tonsillar crypts

3 Lymphatic nodules with germinal centers

4 Lymphatic infiltration

5 Lamina propria

6 Excretory ducts

7 Adipose tissue

8 Tonsillar crypts

9 Lymphatic nodules with germinal centers

10 Lymphatic infiltration

11 Mucous acini of the posterior lingual glands

12 Skeletal muscles

FIGURE 13.7 ■ Lingual tonsils (transverse section). Stain: hematoxylin and eosin. Low magnification.

FIGURE 13.8 | Dried Tooth (Longitudinal Section)

This illustration shows a longitudinal section of a dried, nondecalcified, and unstained tooth. The mineralized parts of a tooth are the enamel, dentin, and cementum. **Dentin (3)** is covered by **enamel (1)** in the region that projects above the gum. Enamel is not present at the root of the tooth, and here the dentin is covered by **cementum (6)**. Cementum (6) contains lacunae with the cementum-producing cells called cementocytes and their connecting canaliculi. Dentin (3) surrounds both the **pulp cavity (5)** and its extension into the root of the tooth as the **root canal (11)**. In living persons, the pulp cavity and root canal are filled with fine connective tissue, fibroblasts, histiocytes, and dentin-forming cells, the odontoblasts. Blood capillaries and nerves enter the pulp cavity (5) through an **apical foramen (13)** at the tip of each root.

Dentin (3) exhibits wavy, parallel dentinal tubules. The earlier, or primary, dentin is located at the periphery of the tooth. The later, or secondary, dentin lies along the pulp cavity, where it is formed throughout life by odontoblasts. In the crown of a dried tooth at the **dentinoenamel junction (2)** are numerous irregular, air-filled spaces that appear black in the section. These **interglobular spaces (4, 10)** are filled with incompletely calcified dentin (interglobular dentin) in living persons. Similar areas, but smaller and spaced closer together, are present in the root, close to the dentinal–cementum junction, where they form the **granular layer (of Tomes) (12)**.

The dentin in the crown of the tooth is covered with a thicker layer of enamel (1), composed of enamel rods or prisms held together by an interprismatic cementing substance. The **lines of Retzius (7)** represent the variations in the rate of enamel deposition. Light rays passing through a dried section of the tooth are refracted by twists that occur in the enamel rods as they course toward the surface of the tooth. These are the light **lines of Schreger (8)**. Poor calcification of enamel rods during enamel formation can produce **enamel tufts (9)** that extend from the dentinoenamel junction into the enamel (see Fig. 13.9).

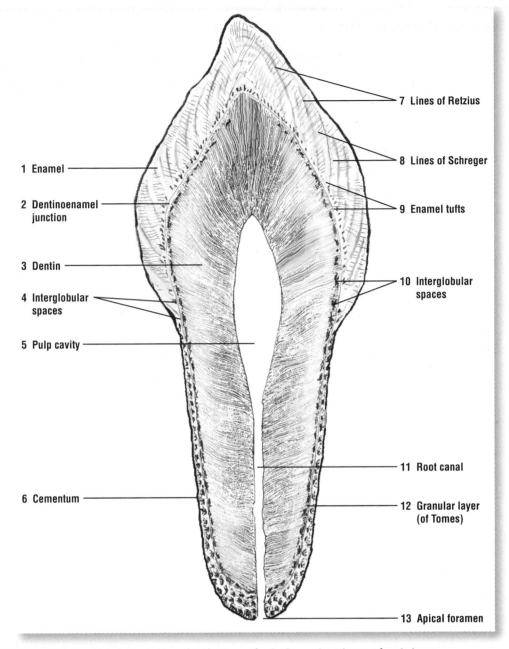

1 Enamel

2 Dentinoenamel junction

3 Dentin

4 Interglobular spaces

5 Pulp cavity

6 Cementum

7 Lines of Retzius

8 Lines of Schreger

9 Enamel tufts

10 Interglobular spaces

11 Root canal

12 Granular layer (of Tomes)

13 Apical foramen

FIGURE 13.8 ■ Dried tooth (longitudinal section). Ground and unstained. Low magnification.

FIGURE 13.9 | Dried Tooth: Dentinoenamel Junction

A section of the **dentin matrix (4)** and **enamel (5)** at the **dentinoenamel junction (1)** is illustrated at a higher magnification. The enamel is produced by cells called ameloblasts as successive segments that form elongated **enamel rods** or **prisms (7)**. The **enamel tufts (6)**, which are the poorly calcified, twisted enamel rods or prisms, extend from the dentinoenamel junction (1) into the enamel (5). The dentin matrix (4) is produced by cells called odontoblasts. The odontoblastic processes of the odontoblasts occupy tunnel-like spaces in the dentin, forming the clearly visible **dentin tubules (3)** and black, air-filled **interglobular spaces (2)**.

FIGURE 13.10 | Dried Tooth: Cementum and Dentin Junction

The junction between the **dentin matrix (5)** and **cementum (2)** is illustrated at a higher magnification at the root of a tooth. At the junction of the cementum (2) with the dentin matrix (5) is a layer of small interglobular spaces, the **granular layer of Tomes (7)**. Internal to this layer in the dentin matrix (5) are the large, irregular **interglobular spaces (4, 8)** that are commonly seen in the crown of the tooth, but may also be present in the root of the tooth.

Cementum (2) is a thin layer of bony material secreted by cells called cementoblasts (mature forms, cementocytes). The bonelike cementum exhibits **lacunae (1)** that house the cementocytes and numerous **canaliculi (3)** for the cytoplasmic processes of cementocytes.

1 Dentinoenamel junction

2 Interglobular spaces

3 Dentin tubules

4 Dentin matrix

5 Enamel

6 Enamel tufts

7 Enamel rods

FIGURE 13.9 ■ Dried tooth: dentinoenamel junction. Ground and unstained. Medium magnification.

1 Lacunae

2 Cementum

3 Canaliculi

4 Interglobular space

5 Dentin matrix

6 Dentin tubules

7 Granular layer (of Tomes)

8 Interglobular space

FIGURE 13.10 ■ Dried tooth: cementum and dentin junction. Ground and unstained. Medium magnification.

FIGURE 13.11 | Developing Tooth (Longitudinal Section)

A developing tooth is shown embedded in a socket, the **dental alveolus (23)** in the **bone (9)** of the jaw. The stratified squamous nonkeratinized **oral epithelium (1, 11)** covers the developing tooth. The underlying connective tissue in the digestive tube is called the **lamina propria (2, 12)**. A downgrowth from the oral epithelium (1, 11) invades the lamina propria (2, 12) and the primitive connective tissue as the **dental lamina (3)**. A layer of primitive **connective tissue (8, 17)** surrounds the developing tooth and forms a compact layer around the tooth, the **dental sac (8, 17)**.

The dental lamina (3) from the oral epithelium (1, 11) proliferates and gives rise to a cap-shaped enamel organ that consists of the **external enamel epithelium (4)**, the extracellular **stellate reticulum (5, 14)**, and the enamel-forming **ameloblasts** of the **inner enamel epithelium (6)**. The ameloblasts of the inner enamel epithelium (6) secrete the hard **enamel (7, 13)** around the **dentin (16)**. The enamel (7, 13) appears as a narrow band of dark, red-staining material.

At the concave or the opposite end of the enamel organ, the **dental papilla (21)** originates from the primitive connective tissue **mesenchyme (21)** and forms the dental pulp or core of the developing tooth. **Blood vessels (20)** and nerves extend into and innervate the dental papilla (21) from below. The mesenchymal cells in the dental papilla (21) differentiate into **odontoblasts (15, 19)** and form the outer margin of the dental papilla (21). The odontoblasts (15) secrete an uncalcified dentin called **predentin (18)**. As predentin (18) calcifies, it forms a layer of pink-staining dentin (16) that lies adjacent to the dark-staining enamel (7, 13).

At the base of the tooth, the external enamel epithelium (4) and the ameloblasts of the inner enamel epithelium (6) continue to grow downward and form the bilayered **epithelial root sheath (of Hertwig) (10, 22)**. The cells of the epithelial root sheath (10, 22) induce the adjacent mesenchyme (21) cells to differentiate into odontoblasts (15, 19) and to form dentin (16).

FIGURE 13.12 | Developing Tooth: Dentinoenamel Junction in Detail

A section of the dentinoenamel junction from a developing tooth is illustrated at high magnification. On the left side of the figure is a small area of **stellate reticulum (1)** of the enamel adjacent to the tall columnar **ameloblasts (2)** that secrete the **enamel (3)**. During enamel (3) formation, the apical extensions of ameloblasts become transformed into terminal processes (of Tomes). The mature enamel (3) consists of calcified, elongated **enamel rods (4)** or prisms that are barely visible in the dark-stained enamel (3). The enamel rods (4) extend through the thickness of the enamel (3).

The right side of the figure shows the nuclei of **mesenchymal cells** in the **dental papilla (5)**. The **odontoblasts (6)** are located adjacent to the dental papilla (5). The odontoblasts (6) secrete the uncalcified organic matrix of **predentin (8)**, which later calcifies into **dentin (9)**. The odontoblasts (6) exhibit slender apical extensions called **odontoblast processes (of Tomes) (7)**. These processes penetrate both the predentin (8) and the dentin (9).

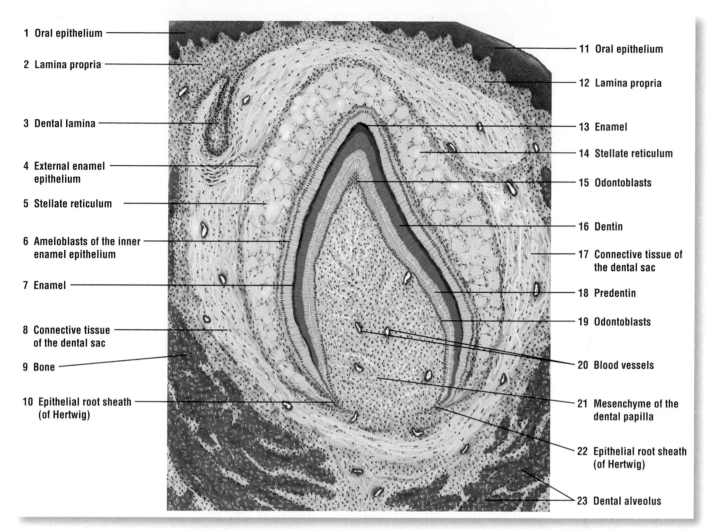

1 Oral epithelium
2 Lamina propria
3 Dental lamina
4 External enamel epithelium
5 Stellate reticulum
6 Ameloblasts of the inner enamel epithelium
7 Enamel
8 Connective tissue of the dental sac
9 Bone
10 Epithelial root sheath (of Hertwig)

11 Oral epithelium
12 Lamina propria
13 Enamel
14 Stellate reticulum
15 Odontoblasts
16 Dentin
17 Connective tissue of the dental sac
18 Predentin
19 Odontoblasts
20 Blood vessels
21 Mesenchyme of the dental papilla
22 Epithelial root sheath (of Hertwig)
23 Dental alveolus

FIGURE 13.11 ■ Developing tooth (longitudinal section). Stain: hematoxylin and eosin. Low magnification.

1 Stellate reticulum
2 Ameloblasts
3 Enamel
4 Enamel rods

5 Mesenchymal cells in dental papilla
6 Odontoblasts
7 Odontoblast processes (of Tomes)
8 Predentin
9 Dentin

FIGURE 13.12 ■ Developing tooth: dentinoenamel junction in detail. Stain: hematoxylin and eosin. High magnification.

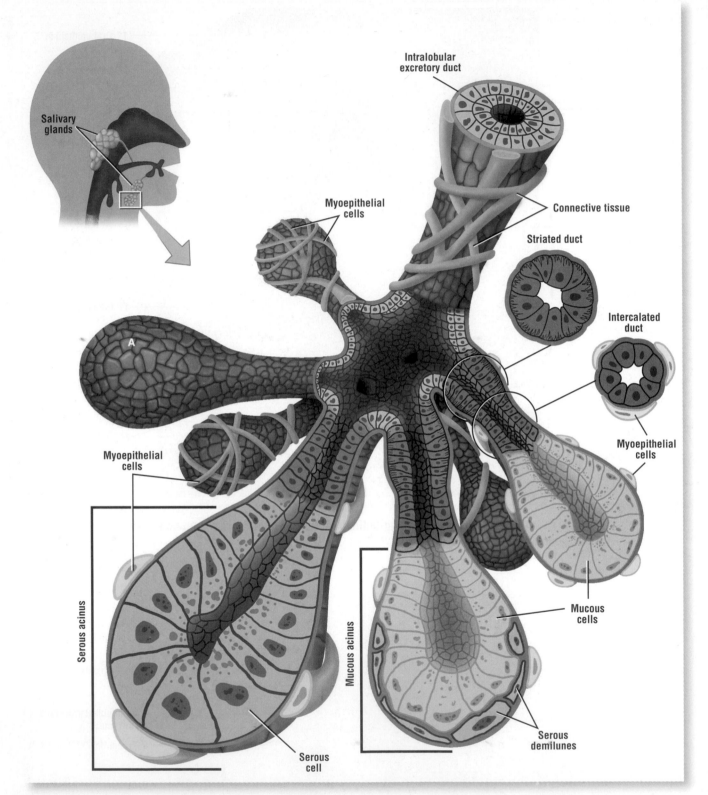

OVERVIEW FIGURE 13.2 ■ Salivary glands. The different types of acini (serous, mucous, and mixed, with serous demilunes), different duct types (intercalated, striated, and interlobular), and myoepithelial cells of a salivary gland are illustrated.

SECTION 2 Major Salivary Glands

There are three major **salivary glands** for the oral cavity: parotid, submandibular, and sublingual. Salivary glands are located outside the oral cavity and convey their secretions into the mouth via large and long **excretory ducts**. The paired **parotid glands** are the largest of the salivary glands, located anterior and inferior to the external ear. The smaller and also paired **submandibular (submaxillary) glands** are located inferior to the mandible in the floor of the mouth. The smallest salivary glands are the **sublingual glands**, which are aggregates of smaller glands located inferior to the tongue.

Salivary glands are surrounded by dense connective tissue capsules from which septa subdivide the secretory areas of the glands into lobes and lobules. Each salivary gland is composed of cellular **secretory units** called **acini** (singular, acinus) and numerous **excretory ducts** with variable histologic features, depending on their location in the gland. The secretory units are small, saclike dilations located at the beginning of the first segment of the excretory duct system called the **intercalated ducts**.

Cells of the Salivary Gland Acini

Cells that comprise the secretory acini of salivary glands are of two types: serous or mucous. The acini exhibit either serous cells that produce protein-rich watery secretions or mucous cells that secrete the viscous mucus or a mixture cells that produce both types of secretions (see Overview Fig. 13.2).

Serous cells in the acini are pyramidal in shape. Their spherical, or round, nuclei are displaced basally by secretory granules accumulated in the upper or apical regions of the cytoplasm.

Mucous cells are similar in shape to serous cells, except their cytoplasm is completely filled with a light-staining, secretory product called **mucus**. As a result, the accumulated secretory granules flatten the nucleus and displace it to the base of the cytoplasm.

In some salivary glands, both mucous and serous cells are present in the same secretory acinus. In these mixed acini, where mucous cells predominate, serous cells form a crescent, or moon-shaped, cap over the mucous cells. In routine histologic preparations, these serous crescent-like structures are called **serous demilunes**. With new rapid freezing techniques, however, it has been shown that these demilunes are apparently artifacts of fixation. This fact should be borne in mind when examining the histologic slides of mixed salivary glands that show the serous demilunes at the end of mucous acini that were prepared with routine histologic methods. The secretions from serous cells in the demilunes enter the lumen of the acinus through tiny intercellular canaliculi between mucous cells.

Myoepithelial cells are flattened cells that surround both the serous and mucous acini and the initial portion of the duct system. Myoepithelial cells are also highly branched and exhibit **contractile** functions. They are sometimes called "basket cells" because they surround the acini with their cytoplasmic branches like a basket. Myoepithelial cells are located between the cell membrane of the secretory cells in acini and the surrounding basement membrane.

Salivary Gland Ducts

Connective tissue fibers subdivide the salivary glands into numerous **lobules**, in which are found the secretory units and their excretory ducts.

Intercalated Ducts

Serous and mucous, as well as mixed secretory acini, initially empty their secretions into the **intercalated ducts**. These are the initial and smallest ducts in the salivary glands with tiny lumina lined with a low cuboidal epithelium. Contractile myoepithelial cells surround the acini and some portions of intercalated ducts.

Striated Ducts

Several intercalated ducts merge to form the larger **striated ducts**. These ducts are lined with a columnar epithelium and, with proper staining, exhibit tiny basal striations. The striations correspond to the basal infoldings of the cell membrane and the cellular interdigitations. Located in these basal infoldings of the cell membrane are numerous and elongated mitochondria.

Serous glands have well-developed intercalated ducts and striated ducts. In contrast, mucous glands exhibit poorly developed intercalated ducts and striated ducts.

Excretory Intralobular Ducts

Striated ducts, in turn, join to form larger **intralobular ducts** of gradually increasing size, surrounded by increasing layers of connective tissue fibers.

Interlobular and Interlobar Ducts

Intralobular ducts join to form the larger **interlobular ducts** and **interlobar ducts**. The terminal portion of these large ducts conveys saliva from salivary glands to the oral cavity and constitutes the main ducts of each salivary gland. As these interlobular and interlobar excretory ducts get larger and larger, the lining epithelium may be lined with either stratified low cuboidal or stratified columnar cells (see Overview Fig. 13.2).

 Supplemental micrographic images are available at **www.thePoint.com/Eroschenko12e** under Digestive System Part I: Oral Cavity.

FIGURE 13.13 | Parotid Salivary Gland

The parotid salivary gland is a large serous gland that is classified as a compound tubuloacinar gland. This illustration depicts a section of the parotid gland at a lower magnification, with details of specific structures represented at a higher magnification in separate boxes below.

The parotid gland is surrounded by a capsule from which arise numerous **interlobular connective tissue septa (6)** that subdivide the gland into lobes and lobules. Located in the connective tissue septa (6) between the lobules are **arteriole (9), venule (1),** and **interlobular excretory ducts (2, 13, IV)**.

Each salivary gland lobule contains secretory cells that form the **serous acini (5, 8, I)** and whose pyramid-shaped cells are arranged around a lumen. The spherical nuclei of the serous cells (I) are located at the base of the slightly basophilic cytoplasm. In certain sections, the lumen in serous acini (5, 8, I) is not always visible. At a higher magnification, small **secretory granules (I)** are visible in the cell apices of the serous acini (5, 8, I). The number of secretory granules in these cells varies with the functional activity of the gland. All serous acini (5, 8, I) are surrounded by thin, contractile **myoepithelial cells (7, I)** that are located between the basement membrane and the serous cells (5, 8, I). Because of their small size, in some sections only the nuclei are visible in the myoepithelial cells (7, I). Some parotid gland lobules may contain numerous **adipose cells (3)** that appear as clear oval structures surrounded by darker-staining serous acini (5, 8, I).

The secretory serous acini (5, 8, I) empty their product into narrow channels, the **intercalated ducts (10, 12, II)**. These ducts have small lumina, are lined with a simple squamous or a low cuboidal epithelium, and are often surrounded by myoepithelial cells (see Fig. 13.14). The secretory product from the intercalated ducts (10, 12, II) drains into larger **striated ducts (11, III)**. These ducts have larger lumina and are lined with simple columnar cells that exhibit basal striations (11, III). The striations that are seen in the striated ducts (11, III) are formed by deep infoldings of the basal cell membrane.

The striated ducts (11, III), in turn, empty their product into the **intralobular excretory ducts (4)** that are located within the lobules of the gland. These ducts join larger interlobular excretory ducts (2, 13, IV) in the connective tissue septa (6) that surround the salivary gland lobules. The lumina of interlobular excretory ducts (2, 13, IV) become progressively wider and the epithelium taller as the ducts increase in size. The epithelium of excretory ducts can increase from columnar to pseudostratified or even stratified columnar in large excretory (lobar) ducts that drain the lobes of the parotid gland.

1 Venule

2 Interlobular
 excretory duct

3 Adipose cells

4 Interlobular
 excretory duct

5 Serous acini

6 Interlobluar
 connective tissue
 septa

7 Myoepithelial
 cells

8 Serous acini

9 Arteriole

10 Intercalated duct

11 Striated ducts

12 Intercalated duct

13 Interlobular
 excretory ducts

I
Serous acinus

II
Intercalated duct

III
Striated duct

IV
Interlobular excretory duct

FIGURE 13.13 ■ Parotid salivary gland. Stain: hematoxylin and eosin. Upper: medium magnification. Lower: high magnification.

FIGURE 13.14 | Submandibular Salivary Gland

The submandibular salivary gland is also a compound tubuloacinar gland. However, the submandibular gland is a mixed gland, containing both serous and mucous acini, with serous acini predominating. The presence of both serous and mucous acini distinguishes the submandibular gland from the parotid gland, which is a purely serous gland.

This illustration depicts several lobules of the submandibular gland in which a few **mucous acini (5, 11, 13, II)** are intermixed with **serous acini (6, I)**. The detailed features of different acini and ducts of the gland are illustrated at a higher magnification in separate boxes below.

The serous acini (6, I) are similar to those in the parotid gland (Fig. 13.13). These acini are characterized by smaller, darker-stained pyramidal cells, spherical basal nuclei, and apical secretory granules. The mucous acini (5, 11, 13, II) are larger than the serous acini (6, I), have larger lumina, and exhibit more variation in size and shape. The mucous cells (5, 11, 13, II) are columnar with pale or almost colorless cytoplasm after staining. The nuclei of mucous cells (5, 11, 13, II) are flattened and pressed against the base of the cell membrane.

In mixed acini (serous and mucous), the mucous acini are normally surrounded or capped by one or more serous cells, forming a crescent-shaped **serous demilune (7, 10)**. The thin, contractile **myoepithelial cells (8)** surround the serous (I) and mucous (II) acini and the **intercalated ducts (III)**.

The duct system of the submandibular gland is similar to that of the parotid gland. The small intralobular **intercalated ducts (12, 14, 17, III)** have small lumina and are shorter, whereas the **striated ducts (4, 15, IV)** with distinct **basal striations (18)** in the cells are longer than in the parotid gland. This figure also illustrates a mucous acinus (13) that opens into an intercalated duct (14), which then joins a larger striated duct (15). Interlobular excretory ducts (16) are located in the **interlobular connective tissue septa (3)** that divide the gland into lobules and lobes. Also located in the connective tissue septa (3) are nerves, an **arteriole (1)**, a **venule (2)**, and **adipose cells (9)**.

1 Ateriole

2 Venule

3 Interlobular connective tissue septa

4 Striated ducts

5 Musouc acini

6 Serous acini

7 Serous demilune

8 Myoepithelial cells

9 Adipose cells

10 Serous demilune

11 Mucous acinus

12 Intercalated duct

13 Mucous acinus

14 Intercalated duct

15 Striated duct

16 Interlobular excretory ducts

17 Intercalated duct

18 Basal striations

I
Serous acinus

II
Mucous acinius

III
Intercalated duct

IV
Striated duct

FIGURE 13.14 ■ Submandibular salivary gland. Stain: hematoxylin and eosin. Upper: medium magnification. Lower: high magnification.

FIGURE 13.15 | Sublingual Salivary Gland

The sublingual salivary gland is also a compound, mixed tubuloacinar gland that resembles the submandibular gland because it contains both **serous (11)** and **mucous acini (9, I, II)**. Most of the acini, however, are mucous (9, I, II) that are capped with peripheral **serous demilunes (1, 13, II)**. The light-stained mucous acini (9, I) are conspicuous in this section. Purely serous acini (11) are less numerous in the sublingual gland; however, the composition of each gland varies. In this medium-magnification illustration, serous acini (11) appear frequently, whereas in other sections of the sublingual gland, serous acini (11) may be absent. At a higher magnification, the contractile **myoepithelial cells (7, I)** are seen around individual serous and mucous acini (I).

In comparison with other salivary glands, the duct system of the sublingual gland is somewhat different. The **intercalated ducts (2, III)** are short or absent, and not readily observed in a given section. In contrast, the nonstriated **intralobular excretory ducts (6, 8, IV)** are more prevalent in the sublingual glands. These excretory ducts (6, 8, IV) are equivalent to the striated ducts of the submandibular and parotid glands but lack the extensive membrane infolding and basal striations.

The **interlobular connective tissue septa (4)** are also more abundant in the sublingual glands than in the parotid and submandibular glands. An **arteriole (3)**, a **venule (5)**, nerve fibers, and **interlobular excretory ducts (12)** are seen in the septa. The epithelial lining of the interlobular excretory ducts (12) varies from low columnar in the smaller ducts to pseudostratified or stratified columnar in the larger ducts. In addition, the oval **adipose cells (10)** are seen scattered in the connective tissue of the gland.

1 Serous demilune

2 Intercalated duct

3 Arteriole

4 Interlobular connective tissue septal

5 Venule

6 Interlobular excretory duct

7 Myoepithelial cells

8 Intralobular excretory duct

9 Mucous acini

10 Adipose cells

11 Serous acini

12 Interlobular excretory duct

13 Serous demilune

I	II	III	IV
Mucous acinus	Mucous acinus with serous demilune	Intercalated duct	Interlobuar excretory duct

FIGURE 13.15 ■ Sublingual salivary gland. Stain: hematoxylin and eosin. Upper: medium magnification. Lower: high magnification.

FIGURE 13.16 | Serous Salivary Gland: Parotid Gland

This photomicrograph illustrates a section of the parotid salivary gland. In humans, the parotid gland is entirely composed of **serous acini (1)** and excretory ducts. In this illustration, the cytoplasm of serous cells in the serous acini (1) is filled with tiny secretory granules. A small **intercalated duct (2)** with its cuboidal epithelium is surrounded by the serous acini (1). Also visible on the right side of the illustration is a larger, lighter-stained excretory duct, the **striated duct (3)**.

FIGURE 13.17 | Mixed Salivary Gland: Sublingual Gland

The sublingual salivary gland exhibits both **mucous acini (2)** and **serous acini (3)**. The mucous acini (2) are larger and lighter staining than the serous acini (3), and their cytoplasm is filled with **mucus (1)**. The serous acini (3) are darker staining with tiny secretory granules located in the apical cytoplasm. The serous acini (3) that surround the mucous acini (2) form crescent-shaped structures called **serous demilunes (4)**. A tiny excretory **intercalated duct (5)**, lined with a cuboidal epithelium, and a larger **striated duct (6)** with columnar epithelium, are also visible in the gland.

FUNCTIONAL CORRELATIONS 13.2 | Salivary Glands, Saliva, and Salivary Ducts

Salivary glands produce about 1 L/day of a watery secretion called **saliva**, which enters the oral cavity via different large excretory ducts. **Myoepithelial cells** surround the secretory acini and the initial portions of intercalated ducts in the salivary glands. As a result of nervous stimulation, the myoepithelial cells contract and expel the secretory products from different acini into the oral cavity.

Saliva is a mixture of secretions produced by cells in different salivary glands. Although the major composition of saliva is **water**, it also contains ions, mucus, enzymes, and antibodies (immunoglobulins). The sight, smell, thought, taste, or actual presence of food in the mouth causes an **autonomic stimulation** of the salivary glands that increases production of saliva and stimulates its release into the oral cavity.

Saliva performs numerous important functions. It moistens the chewed food and provides solvents that allow it to be tasted. Saliva lubricates the bolus of chewed food for easier swallowing and assistance in its passage through the esophagus to the stomach. Saliva also contains numerous **electrolytes** (calcium, potassium, sodium, chloride, bicarbonate ions, and others). A digestive enzyme, **salivary amylase**, is also present in the saliva. It is mainly produced by the **serous acini** in the salivary glands. Salivary amylase initiates the breakdown of starch into smaller carbohydrates during the short time that food is present in the oral cavity. Once the bolus is delivered into the stomach, it is acidified by gastric juices, an action that decreases amylase activity and carbohydrate digestion.

Saliva also functions in controlling **bacterial flora** in the oral cavity and protecting it against oral pathogens. Another salivary enzyme, **lysozyme**, also secreted by serous cells of the salivary gland, hydrolyzes cell walls of bacteria and inhibits their growth in the oral cavity. In addition, saliva contains salivary **antibodies**. The antibodies, primarily immunoglobulin A, are produced by the **plasma cells** that are located in the connective tissue of salivary glands. The antibodies form complexes with antigens and assist in immunologic defense against oral bacteria. Salivary acinar cells secrete a protein component that binds to and transports the immunoglobulins from plasma cells in the connective tissue into saliva.

As saliva flows through the duct system of salivary glands, the different salivary ducts modify its ionic content by selective transport, resorption, or secretions of ions. The **intercalated ducts** secrete **bicarbonate ions** into the ducts and absorb **chloride** from its contents. The **striated ducts** actively reabsorb **sodium** from saliva, whereas **potassium** and bicarbonate ions are added to the salivary secretions.

The numerous infoldings of the basal cell membrane or striations seen in the striated ducts contain numerous elongated mitochondria. These structures are characteristic features of cells that transport fluids and electrolytes across cell membranes.

The striated ducts of each lobule drain into interlobular or excretory ducts that eventually form the main duct for each gland, which ultimately penetrates the wall and empties its contents into the oral cavity.

FIGURE 13.16 ■ Serous salivary gland: parotid gland. Stain: hematoxylin and eosin. ×165.

FIGURE 13.17 ■ Mixed salivary gland: sublingual gland. Stain: hematoxylin and eosin. ×165.

The Digestive System Part I: Oral Cavity and Salivary Glands

- Hollow tube consisting of oral cavity, esophagus, stomach, small intestine, large intestine, rectum, and anal canal
- Salivary glands, liver, and pancreas are accessory organs located outside the tube
- Secretory products from all accessory organs delivered to the tube via excretory ducts

SECTION 1 • Oral Cavity

- Lined with stratified squamous epithelium for protection
- Food masticated here, and saliva lubricates food for swallowing

Lips

- Lined with thin skin covered by stratified squamous keratinized epithelium
- Blood vessels close to the surface impart red color
- Contain hairs, sebaceous and sweat glands, and mucus-secreting labial glands
- Core contains skeletal muscle orbicularis oris

Tongue

- Consists of connective tissue and interlacing skeleton muscle fibers
- Dorsal surface divided into anterior two thirds and posterior third by sulcus terminalis
- Dorsal surface covered by elevations called filiform, fungiform, and circumvallate papillae
- Filiform papillae are most numerous, smallest, and keratinized; lack taste buds
- Fungiform papillae are less numerous, larger, mushroom-like, and contain taste buds
- Circumvallate papillae are largest, are in the back of tongue, and are encircled by furrows
- Numerous taste buds located on the lateral sides of each papilla
- Underlying serous glands empty serous secretions into the base of furrows
- Foliate papillae are rudimentary in humans
- Posterior lingual glands in the connective tissue open onto dorsal surface of tongue

Taste Buds

- Located in foliate, fungiform, and circumvallate papillae; pharynx; palate; and epiglottis
- Exhibit tastes pores and occupy thickness of epithelium; microvilli protrude through taste pore
- Neuroepithelial cells synapse with afferent axons and are the receptors for taste
- Also contain supportive sustentacular cells, whereas basal cells can serve as stem cells
- Substances that are tasted are first dissolved in saliva and then enter taste pore
- Serous glands wash peripheral taste buds in the furrows of circumvallate papillae
- Five basic taste sensations are sour, salt, bitter, sweet, and unami
- Sensitivity to all tastes distribute across entire tongue
- Some areas of tongue may be more sensitive to certain tastes

Lymphoid Aggregations: Tonsils

- Diffuse lymphoid tissue and nodules in the oral pharynx
- Palatine and lingual tonsils covered by stratified squamous epithelium and show crypts
- Pharyngeal tonsil is single and covered by pseudostratified ciliated epithelium
- Some lymphatic nodules contain germinal centers

Teeth

- Developing teeth found in dental alveolus in the jawbone
- Downward growth from oral epithelium forms dental lamina and gives rise to ameloblasts
- Mesenchyme gives rise to dental papilla and odontoblasts
- Odontoblasts secrete dentin, whereas ameloblasts produce enamel of tooth

Section 2 • Major Salivary Glands

- Parotid, submandibular, and sublingual are major salivary glands that produce saliva
- Composed of secretory acini and excretory ducts that bring saliva into oral cavity

- Cells are serous or mucous; serous cells form serous demi-lunes around mucous acini
- Myoepithelial cells surround serous and mucous acini and part of intercalated ducts
- Serous, mucous, and mixed secretory acini empty secretions into intercalated ducts
- Intercalated ducts merge into larger striated ducts with basal membrane infoldings
- Striated ducts form larger interlobular ducts that empty into interlobar excretory ducts
- Glands produce about 1 L of saliva per day, which is mostly water

- Saliva formed after autonomic stimulation
- Saliva contains electrolytes and carbohydrate-digesting enzyme salivary amylase
- Saliva contains antibodies produced by plasma cells and lysozyme to control oral bacteria
- Saliva is modified by transport of ions as it passes intercalated ducts and striated ducts
- Intercalated ducts secrete bicarbonate ions into ducts and remove chloride
- Striated ducts absorb sodium from saliva, whereas potassium and bicarbonate ions are added

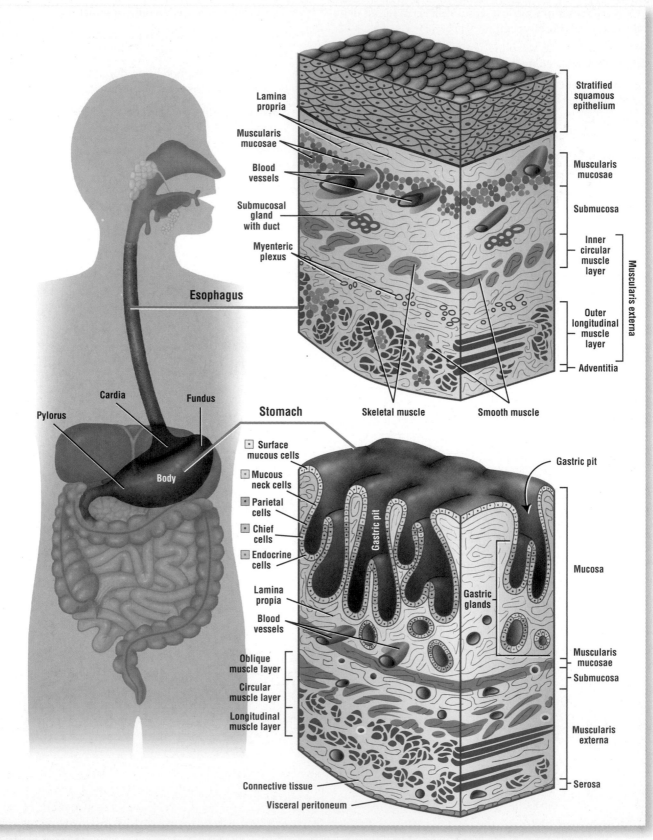

OVERVIEW FIGURE 14.1 ■ Detailed illustration comparing the structural differences of the four layers (mucosa, submucosa, muscularis externa, and adventitia or serosa) in the wall of the esophagus and stomach.

CHAPTER 14

Digestive System Part II: Esophagus and Stomach

General Plan of the Digestive System—An Overview

The digestive (gastrointestinal) tract is a long hollow tube that extends from the esophagus to the rectum. It includes the esophagus, stomach, small intestine (duodenum, jejunum, and ileum), large intestine (colon), and rectum. The wall of the digestive tube shows four distinct layers that represent the basic histologic organization of the entire tract. The four layers are the mucosa, submucosa, muscularis externa, and serosa (or adventitia). Because the digestive tract performs different functions during the digestive processes, the morphology of these layers exhibits variations relative to those functions. This difference is primarily evident in the epithelium that differs throughout the digestive tract and indicates the specific functions of each section of the tract.

Mucosa

The **mucosa** is the innermost layer of the digestive tube. It consists of a lining **epithelium** and glands that extend into the underlying layer of loose connective tissue called the **lamina propria**. An inner circular and an outer longitudinal layer of smooth muscle, called the **muscularis mucosae**, form the outer boundary of the mucosa.

Submucosa

The **submucosa** is located inferior to or underneath the mucosa. It consists of dense irregular connective tissue with numerous blood and lymph vessels, and a **submucosal (Meissner) nerve plexus**. This nerve plexus contains postganglionic parasympathetic neurons. The neurons and axons of the submucosal nerve plexus control the motility of the mucosa and secretory activities of associated mucosal glands. In the initial portion of the small intestine, the duodenum, the submucosa contains numerous branched mucous glands.

Muscularis Externa

The **muscularis externa** is a thick, smooth muscle layer located inferior to or below the submucosa. Except for the large intestine, this layer is composed of an inner layer of circular smooth muscle and an outer layer of longitudinal smooth muscle. Situated between the two smooth muscle layers of the muscularis externa are connective tissue and another nerve plexus called the **myenteric (Auerbach) nerve plexus**. This plexus also contains some postganglionic parasympathetic neurons and controls the motility of smooth muscles in the muscularis externa.

Serosa

The **serosa** is the outermost layer of the abdominal portion of the esophagus, stomach, and small intestine and is continuous with the mesentery and the lining of the abdominal cavity. The serosa is a serous membrane consisting of simple squamous epithelium called **mesothelium** and a thin layer of underlying loose connective tissue that surrounds the visceral organs. If mesothelium covers the visceral organs, the organs are within the abdominal or pelvic cavities (**intraperitoneal**) and the outermost layer is called serosa. Serosa also covers parts of the colon (ascending and descending colon) only on the anterior and lateral surfaces because their posterior surfaces are bound to the posterior abdominal body wall and are not covered by the mesothelium or suspended by a mesentery (Overview Fig. 14.1).

Adventitia

When the digestive tube is not covered by mesothelium, it lies outside the peritoneal cavity and is called **retroperitoneal**. In this case, the outermost layer adheres to the body wall and consists only of a connective tissue layer called **adventitia**.

The characteristic features of each layer of the digestive tube and their functions are discussed in detail with each illustration of the different parts of the digestive tract.

SECTION 1   Esophagus

Esophagus

The **esophagus** is a soft tube approximately 10 inches long that extends from the **pharynx** to the **stomach**. It is located posterior to the trachea and in the mediastinum of the **thoracic cavity**. After descending in the thoracic cavity, the esophagus penetrates the muscular **diaphragm**. A short section of the esophagus is present in the abdominal cavity before it terminates at the stomach. In the thoracic cavity, the esophagus is surrounded only by the connective tissue, which is called the **adventitia**. In the abdominal cavity, a simple squamous mesothelium covers the outermost wall of the short segment of the esophagus. This constitutes the **serosa**.

The esophageal lumen is lined with a moist, **nonkeratinized stratified squamous epithelium**. When the esophagus is empty, the lumen exhibits numerous but temporary **longitudinal folds** of mucosa that are due to the contractions of the esophageal muscles. The wall of the esophagus contains two types of glands that secrete **mucus** but are located in different parts of the organ. In the lamina propria of the proximal and distal parts of the esophagus near the stomach are the **esophageal cardiac glands**. They are so named because they resemble the mucous glands located in the cardia region of the stomach. In the submucosa are the **esophageal glands proper** that are scattered along the entire length of the esophagus. The released mucus from these glands lubricates the lumen of the esophagus, protects the mucosa, and facilitates smooth passage of food material (bolus) through the esophagus to the stomach.

The outer wall of the esophagus, the **muscularis externa**, is unusual because it contains both skeletal and smooth muscles fibers. In the upper third of the esophagus, both layers of the muscularis externa contain striated **skeletal muscle fibers**. In the middle third of the esophagus, the muscularis externa contains a mixture of both **skeletal** and **smooth muscle** fibers, whereas in the lower third of the esophagus, both layers are composed entirely of **smooth muscle fibers** (see Overview Fig. 14.1).

 Supplemental micrographic images are available at **www.thePoint.com/Eroschenko12e** under Digestive System Part II: Esophagus and Stomach.

FIGURE 14.1 | Wall of the Upper Esophagus (Transverse Section)

The esophagus is a long, hollow tube whose wall consists of the mucosa, submucosa, muscularis externa, and adventitia. In this illustration, the upper portion of the esophagus has been sectioned in a transverse plane.

The **mucosa (1)** of the esophagus consists of three parts: an inner lining of nonkeratinized **stratified squamous epithelium (1a)**; an underlying thin layer of fine connective tissue, the **lamina propria (1b)**; and a layer of longitudinal smooth muscle fibers, the **muscularis mucosae (1c)**, shown in this illustration in the transverse plane. The **connective tissue papillae (9)** of the lamina propria (1b) indent the epithelium (1a). Found in the lamina propria (1b) are small **blood vessels (8)**, diffuse lymphatic tissue, and a small **lymphatic nodule (7)**.

The **submucosa (3)** in the esophagus is a wide layer of moderately dense irregular connective tissue that often contains **adipose tissue (12)**. The **mucous acini** of **esophageal glands proper (2)** are present in the submucosa (3) at intervals throughout the length of the esophagus. The **excretory ducts (10)** of the esophageal glands (2) pass through the muscularis mucosae (1c) and the lamina propria (1b) to open into the esophageal lumen. The dark-staining ductal epithelium of the glands merges with the stratified squamous surface epithelium (1a) of the esophagus (see Fig. 14.2). Numerous blood vessels, such as the **vein** and **artery (11)**, are found in the connective tissue of the submucosa (3).

Located inferior to the submucosa (3) is the **muscularis externa (4)**, composed of two well-defined muscle layers, an **inner circular muscle layer (4a)** and the **outer longitudinal muscle layer (4b)**, whose muscle fibers are shown here sectioned in a transverse plane. A thin layer of **connective tissue (13)** lies between the inner circular muscle layer (4a) and the outer longitudinal muscle layer (4b).

The muscularis externa (4) of the esophagus is highly variable in different species. In humans, the muscularis externa (4) in the upper third of the esophagus consists primarily of striated skeletal muscles. In the middle third of the esophagus, the inner circular layer (4a) and the outer longitudinal layer (4b) exhibit a mixture of both smooth muscle and skeletal muscle fibers. In the lower third of the esophagus, only smooth muscle is present.

The **adventitia (5)** of the esophagus consists of a loose connective tissue layer that blends with the adventitia of the trachea and the surrounding structures. **Adipose tissue (14)**, large blood vessels, an **artery** and a **vein (15)**, and **nerve fibers (6)** are numerous in the connective tissue of the adventitia (5).

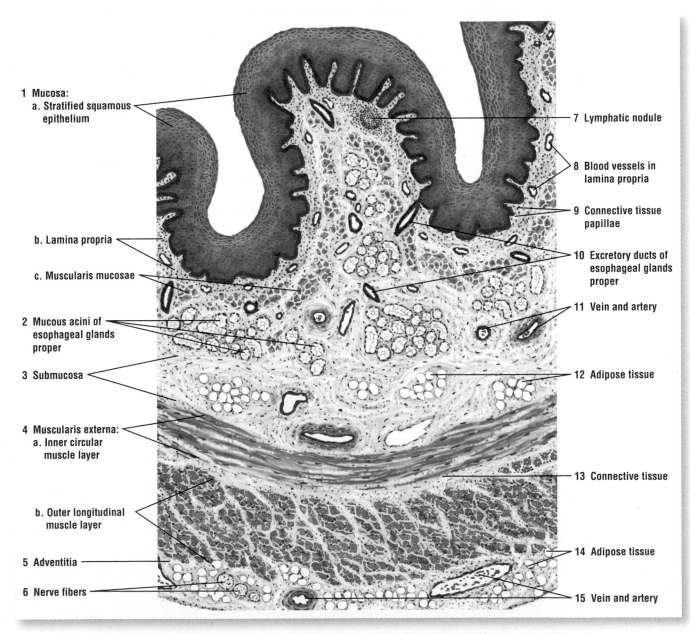

FIGURE 14.1 ■ Wall of the upper esophagus (transverse section). Stain: hematoxylin and eosin. Low magnification.

FIGURE 14.2 | Upper Esophagus (Transverse Section)

The next two histologic sections illustrate the difference between the upper and the lower esophageal wall.

The different layers of the esophagus are easily distinguishable. The mucosa of the upper esophagus (as in Fig. 14.1) consists of a stratified squamous nonkeratinized **epithelium (1)**, a connective tissue **lamina propria (2)**, and a layer of smooth muscle **muscularis mucosae (3)** (transverse plane). A small **lymphatic nodule (4)** is visible in the lamina propria (2). In the **submucosa (7)** are cells of adipose tissue and **mucous acini of esophageal glands proper (6)** with their **excretory ducts (5)**. The muscularis externa of the upper esophagus consists of an **inner circular layer (10)** and an **outer longitudinal layer (14)** of skeletal muscles, separated by a layer of **connective tissue (11)**. The outermost layer around the esophagus is the connective tissue **adventitia (8)** with adipose tissue, **nerves (13)**, a **vein (9)**, and an **artery (12)**.

FIGURE 14.3 | Lower Esophagus (Transverse Section)

This illustration shows the terminal portion of the esophagus after it has penetrated the diaphragm and entered the peritoneal cavity near the stomach.

The layers in the wall of the lower esophagus are similar to those in the upper region except for regional modifications (see Fig. 14.2). As in the upper esophagus, the **mucosa (1)** of the lower esophagus consists of stratified squamous nonkeratinized **epithelium (1a)**, the connective tissue **lamina propria (1b)**, and a smooth muscle layer **muscularis mucosae (1c)** (transverse section). Also visible are the **connective tissue papillae (2)** of the lamina propria (1b) that indent the lining epithelium (1a) and a **lymphatic nodule (3)**.

The connective tissue **submucosa (6)** also contains mucous acini of the **esophageal glands proper (5)**, their **excretory ducts (4)**, and **adipose tissue (7)**. In some regions of the esophagus, these glands may be absent.

The major differences between the upper and lower esophagus are seen in the next two layers. The **muscularis externa (10)** in the lower esophagus consists entirely of smooth muscle layers, an **inner circular muscle layer (10a)** and an **outer longitudinal muscle layer (10b)**. The outermost layer of the lower esophagus is the **serosa (8),** or visceral peritoneum. Serosa (8) consists of a connective tissue layer lined with a simple squamous layer mesothelium. In contrast, the adventitia that surrounds the esophagus in the thoracic region consists only of a connective tissue layer.

In the upper esophagus, less connective tissue is present in the lamina propria (1b), around the smooth muscle fibers of muscularis externa (10), and in the serosa (8).

1 Epithelium

2 Lamina propria

3 Muscularis mucosae

4 Lymphatic nodule

5 Excretory ducts of esophageal glands proper

6 Mucous acini of esophageal glands proper

7 Submucosa

8 Adventitia

9 Vein

10 Inner circular muscle layer (skeletal)

11 Connective tissue

12 Artery

13 Nerves

14 Outer longitudinal muscle layer (skeletal)

FIGURE 14.2 ■ Upper esophagus (transverse section). Stain: hematoxylin and eosin. Low magnification.

1 Mucosa:
   a. Epithelium
   b. Lamina propria
   c. Muscularis mucosae

2 Connective tissue papillae

3 Lymphatic nodule

4 Excretory ducts of esophageal glands proper

5 Esophageal glands proper

6 Submucosa

7 Adipose tissue

8 Serosa (mesothelium)

9 Vein and artery

10 Muscularis externa:
   a. Inner circular muscle layer (smooth)
   b. Outer longitudinal muscle layer (smooth)

FIGURE 14.3 ■ Lower esophagus (transverse section). Stain: hematoxylin and eosin. Low magnification.

FIGURE 14.4 | Upper Esophagus: Mucosa and Submucosa (Longitudinal Section)

This higher-magnification illustration of the upper esophagus has been sectioned longitudinally. The smooth muscle fibers of the muscularis mucosae (9) exhibit a longitudinal orientation, and the fibers of the inner circular muscle layer are cut in a transverse section.

The esophagus is lined with a stratified squamous **epithelium (7)**. Squamous cells form the outermost layers of the epithelium, the numerous polyhedral cells form the intermediate layers, and low columnar cells form the basal layer. Mitotic activity can be seen in the deeper layers of the epithelium. The connective tissue **lamina propria (8)** contains numerous blood vessels, aggregates of lymphocytes, and a small **lymphatic nodule (2)**. **Connective tissue papillae (1)** from the lamina propria (8) indent the surface epithelium (7). The **muscularis mucosae (9)** is illustrated as bundles of smooth muscle fibers sectioned in a longitudinal plane.

The underlying **submucosa (3, 10)** contains **mucous acini of esophageal glands proper (4)**. Small **excretory ducts (11)** from these glands (4), lined with a simple epithelium, join the larger excretory ducts that are lined with a stratified epithelium. One of the excretory ducts joins the stratified squamous epithelium (7) of the esophageal lumen. In the submucosa (3, 10) are also **blood vessels (12), nerves (5),** and **adipose cells (6)**.

In the upper esophagus, the **inner circular muscle layer (13)** is seen in the muscularis externa and it consists of skeletal muscle. A portion of this layer is illustrated in a transverse plane at the bottom of the figure.

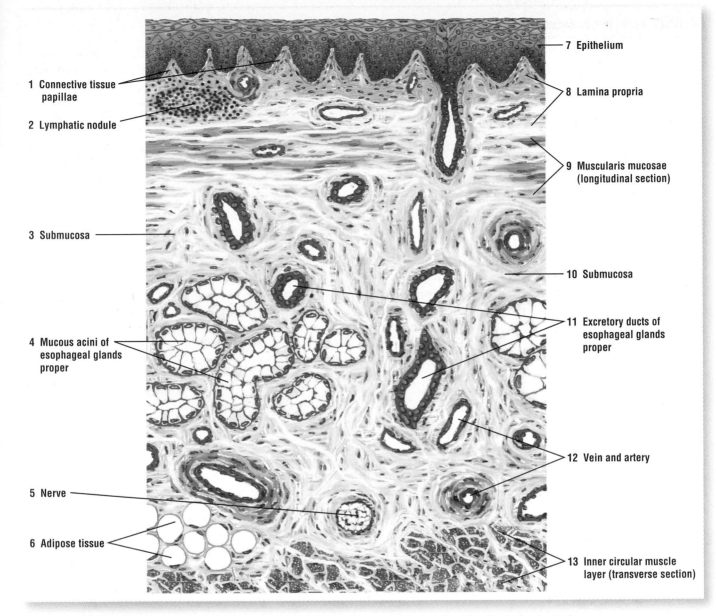

1 Connective tissue papillae

2 Lymphatic nodule

3 Submucosa

4 Mucous acini of esophageal glands proper

5 Nerve

6 Adipose tissue

7 Epithelium

8 Lamina propria

9 Muscularis mucosae (longitudinal section)

10 Submucosa

11 Excretory ducts of esophageal glands proper

12 Vein and artery

13 Inner circular muscle layer (transverse section)

FIGURE 14.4 ■ Upper esophagus: mucosa and submucosa (longitudinal view). Stain: hematoxylin and eosin. Medium magnification.

FIGURE 14.5 | Lower Esophagus Wall (Transverse Section)

This low-magnification photomicrograph illustrates the lower portion of the esophagus and all layers of the mucosa. The mucosa consists of a thick but nonkeratinized **stratified squamous epithelium (1)**, a connective tissue **lamina propria (2)**, and a thin strip of smooth muscle **muscularis mucosae (3)**. Below the muscularis mucosae are the esophageal glands in the submucosa, and closer to the stomach are the esophageal cardiac glands in the lamina propria.

FUNCTIONAL CORRELATIONS 14.1 | Esophagus

The major function of the esophagus is to convey liquids or a mass of chewed food (**bolus**) from the oral cavity to the stomach. For this function, the lumen of the esophagus is lined with a protective **nonkeratinized stratified squamous epithelium**. Aiding in this function are numerous esophageal glands located in the connective tissue of the wall. There are two types of glands in the wall of the esophagus. The **esophageal cardiac glands** are present in the **lamina propria** of the upper and lower regions of the esophagus. These glands have a morphology similar to those found in the cardia of the stomach, where the esophagus terminates. **Esophageal glands proper** are located in the connective tissue of the submucosa. Both types of glands produce the secretory product **mucus**, which is conducted in **excretory ducts** through the epithelium to lubricate the esophageal lumen and protect it during the passage of ingested solid material. The swallowed material is moved from one end of the esophagus to the other by strong muscular contractions called **peristalsis**. At the lower end of the esophagus, a muscular **gastroesophageal sphincter** constricts the lumen and prevents the regurgitation of swallowed material into the esophagus.

1 Stratified squamous epithelium

2 Lamina propria

3 Muscularis mucosae

FIGURE 14.5 ■ Lower esophageal wall (transverse section). Stain: Mallory-Azan. ×30.

FIGURE 14.6 | Esophageal–Stomach Junction

At its terminal end, the esophagus joins the stomach and forms the esophageal–stomach junction. The nonkeratinized **stratified squamous epithelium (1)** of the **esophagus** abruptly changes to simple columnar, mucus-secreting **gastric epithelium (10)** of the cardia region of the **stomach**.

At the esophageal–stomach junction, the **esophageal glands proper (7)** may be seen in the **submucosa (8)**. **Excretory ducts (4, 6)** from these glands course through the **muscularis mucosae (5)** and the **lamina propria (2)** of the esophagus into its lumen. In the lamina propria (2) of the esophagus near the stomach region are the **esophageal cardiac glands (3)**. Both the esophageal glands proper (7) and the cardiac glands (3) secrete mucus.

The lamina propria of the esophagus (2) continues into the **lamina propria** of the **stomach (12)**, where it becomes filled with **glands (16, 17)** and diffuse lymphatic tissue. The lamina propria of the stomach (12) is penetrated by shallow **gastric pits (11)** into which empty the gastric glands (16, 17).

The upper region of the stomach contains two types of glands. The simple tubular **cardiac glands (17)** are limited to the transition region, the cardia of the stomach. These glands are lined with pale-staining, mucus-secreting columnar cells. Below the cardiac region of the stomach are the simple tubular **gastric glands (16)**, some of which exhibit basal branching.

In contrast to the cardiac glands (17), the gastric glands (16) contain four different cell types: the pale-staining **mucous neck cells (13)**; large, eosinophilic **parietal cells (14)**; basophilic **chief** or **zymogenic cells (15)**; and several different types of endocrine cells (not illustrated), collectively called the enteroendocrine cells.

The **muscularis mucosae** of the **stomach (18)** also continue with the muscularis mucosae of the esophagus (5). In the esophagus, the muscularis mucosae (5) are usually a single layer of longitudinal smooth muscle fibers, whereas in the stomach, a second layer of smooth muscle is added, called the inner circular layer.

The **submucosa (8, 19)** and the **muscularis externa (9, 21)** of the esophagus are continuous with those of the stomach. **Blood vessels (20)** are found in the submucosa (8, 19) from which smaller blood vessels are distributed to other regions of the stomach.

FIGURE 14.7 | Esophageal–Stomach Junction (Transverse Section)

This low-magnification photomicrograph illustrates the esophagus–stomach junction. The esophagus is characterized by a thick, protective, nonkeratinized **stratified squamous epithelium (1)**. Inferior to the epithelium (1) is the **lamina propria (2)**, below which is the smooth muscle **muscularis mucosae (3)**. The lamina propria (2) indents the undersurface of the esophageal epithelium to form the connective tissue papillae. The esophageal–stomach junction is characterized by an abrupt transition from the stratified epithelium (1) of the esophagus to the **simple columnar epithelium (4)** of the stomach. The surface of the stomach also exhibits numerous **gastric pits (5)** into which open the **gastric glands (6)**. The **lamina propria (7)** of the stomach, in contrast to that of the esophagus, is seen as thin strips of connective tissue between the tightly packed gastric glands (6).

Esophagus | Stomach

1 Stratified squamous epithelium

2 Lamina propria (esophagus)

3 Esophageal cardiac glands

4 Excretory duct

5 Muscularis muscosae (esophagus)

6 Excretory duct

7 Esophageal glands proper

8 Submucosa

9 Muscularis externa (esophagus)

10 Gastric epithelium

11 Gastric pits

12 Lamina propria (stomach)

13 Mucous neck cells

14 Parietal cells

15 Zymogen (chief) cells

16 Gastric glands

17 Cardiac glands (stomach)

18 Muscularis mucoasae (stomach)

19 Submucosa

20 Blood vessels (venule and arteriole)

21 Muscularis externa

FIGURE 14.6 ■ Esophageal–stomach junction. Stain: hematoxylin and eosin. Low magnification.

Stomach
4 Simple columnar epithelium

5 Gastric pits

Esophagus

1 Stratified squamous epithelium

2 Lamina propria

3 Muscularis mucosae

6 Gastric glands

7 Lamina propria

FIGURE 14.7 ■ Esophageal–stomach junction (transverse section). Stain: Mallory-Azan. ×30.

SECTION 2 Stomach

Stomach

The stomach is an expanded hollow organ situated between the esophagus and the small intestine. At the esophageal–stomach junction, there is an abrupt transition from the stratified squamous nonkeratinized epithelium of the esophagus to the **simple columnar epithelium** of the stomach, cells that produce a large quantity of mucus. The released mucus adheres to the surface epithelium and provides a very effective protective layer for the stomach lining against the corrosive gastric juices from the gastric glands.

Anatomically, the stomach is divided into the narrow strip called **cardia,** where the esophagus terminates. The upper dome-shaped portion of the stomach is the **fundus**, below which is located the **body** or **corpus** of the stomach. The funnel-shaped, lower terminal region of the stomach is called the **pylorus** (see Overview Fig. 14.1). The fundus and the body comprise about two thirds of the stomach, have identical histology, and form the major portions of the stomach. As a result, the stomach has only three distinct histologic regions: cardia, fundus/body, and pylorus. Also, all stomach regions exhibit **rugae**, the longitudinal folds of the mucosa and submucosa. These folds are temporary and disappear when the stomach is distended with fluid or solid material.

The luminal surface of the stomach is pitted with numerous tiny openings called **gastric pits**. These pits are formed by the luminal epithelium that invaginates the underlying connective tissue **lamina propria** of the **mucosa**. The stomach mucosa also consists of different cell types and deep **gastric glands** that produce most of the **gastric secretions** or juices for digestion. The tubular **gastric glands** are located below the luminal epithelium and open directly into the gastric pits to deliver their secretions into the stomach lumen. The gastric glands descend through the lamina propria to the **muscularis mucosae**.

Below the mucosa of the stomach is the dense connective tissue **submucosa** containing large blood vessels and nerves. The thick muscular wall of the stomach, the **muscularis externa**, exhibits three muscle layers instead of the two that are normally seen in the esophagus and the small intestine. The outer layer of the stomach is covered by the **serosa,** or visceral peritoneum (see Overview Fig. 14.1).

 Supplemental micrographic images are available at **www.thePoint.com/Eroschenko12e** under Digestive System Part II: Esophagus and Stomach.

FIGURE 14.8 | Stomach: Fundus and Body Regions (Transverse Section)

The three histologic regions of the stomach are the cardia, the fundus and body, and the pylorus. The fundus and body constitute the most extensive region in the stomach. The stomach wall exhibits four general regions: **mucosa (1, 2, 3), submucosa (4), muscularis externa (5, 6, 7),** and **serosa (8)**.

The **mucosa** consists of the **surface epithelium (1), lamina propria (2),** and **muscularis mucosae (3)**. The surface of the stomach is lined with a **simple columnar epithelium (1, 11)** that extends into and lines the **gastric pits (10)**, which are tubular infoldings of the surface epithelium (11). In the fundus, the gastric pits (10) are not deep and extend into the mucosa about one fourth of its thickness. Beneath the epithelium is the loose connective tissue **lamina propria (2, 12)** that fills the spaces between the gastric glands. A thin, smooth muscle **muscularis mucosae (3, 15),** consisting of an inner circular and an outer longitudinal layer, forms the outer boundary of the mucosa. Thin strands of smooth muscle from the muscularis mucosae (3, 15) extend into lamina propria (2, 12) between the **gastric glands (13, 14)** toward the surface epithelium (1, 11), which are illustrated at a higher magnification in Figure 14.9, label 8.

The gastric glands (13, 14) are packed in the lamina propria (2, 12) and occupy the entire mucosa (1, 2, 3). The gastric glands open into the bottom of the gastric pits (10). The surface epithelium of the gastric mucosa, from the cardiac to the pyloric region, consists of the same cell type. However, the cells that constitute the gastric glands distinguish the regional differences of the stomach. Two distinct cell types can be identified in the gastric glands. The acidophilic **parietal cells (13)** are located in the upper portions of the glands, whereas the basophilic **chief (zymogenic) (14)** cells occupy the lower regions. The subglandular regions of the lamina propria (2, 12) may contain either lymphatic tissue or small **lymphatic nodules (16)**.

The mucosa of the empty stomach exhibits temporary folds called **rugae (9)**. Rugae (9) are formed during the contractions of the smooth muscle layer, the muscularis mucosae (3, 15). As the stomach fills, the rugae disappear and form a smooth mucosa.

The **submucosa (4)** lies below the muscularis mucosae (3, 15). In the empty stomach, submucosa (4) can extend into the rugae (9). The submucosa (4) contains dense irregular connective tissue and more **collagen fibers (17)** than do the lamina propria (2, 12). In addition, the submucosa (4) contains lymph vessels, **capillaries (21)**, large **arterioles (18)**, and **venules (19)**. Isolated clusters of parasympathetic ganglia of the **submucosal (Meissner) nerve plexus (20)** can be seen deeper in the submucosa.

The **muscularis externa (5, 6, 7)** consists of three layers of smooth muscle, each oriented in a different plane: an inner **oblique (5)**, a middle **circular (6)**, and an outer **longitudinal (7)** layer. The oblique layer is not complete and is not always seen in sections of the stomach wall. In this illustration, the circular layer has been sectioned longitudinally and the longitudinal layer transversely. Located between the circular and longitudinal smooth muscle layers is a **myenteric (Auerbach) nerve plexus (22)** of parasympathetic ganglia and nerve fibers.

The **serosa (8)** consists of a thin outer layer of connective tissue that overlies the muscularis externa (5, 6, 7) and is covered by a simple squamous mesothelium of the **visceral peritoneum (8)**. The serosa can contain **adipose cells (23)**.

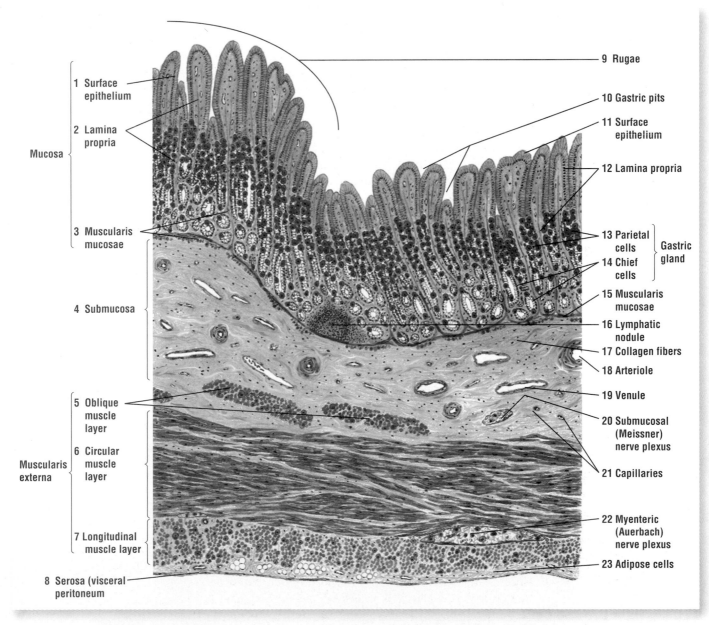

FIGURE 14.8 ■ Stomach: fundus and body regions (transverse section). Stain: hematoxylin and eosin. Low magnification.

FIGURE 14.9 | Stomach: Mucosa of the Fundus and Body (Transverse Section)

The mucosa and submucosa of the fundic region of the stomach are illustrated at a higher magnification. The simple columnar **surface epithelium (1, 13)** extends into the **gastric pits (11)** into which open the tubular **gastric glands (5)**. The **lamina propria (6)** fills the spaces between the packed gastric glands (5) and extends from the surface epithelium (1) to the **muscularis mucosae (9)**.

The lamina propria (6), which consists of fine reticular and collagen fibers, is better seen in the **mucosal ridges (2)**. Scattered throughout the lamina propria (6) are the fibroblast nuclei, accumulations of lymphoid tissue in the form of a **lymphatic nodule (17)**, lymphocytes, and other loose connective tissue cells.

The gastric glands (5) extend the length of the mucosa. In the deeper regions of the mucosa, the gastric glands may branch. As a result, the gastric glands appear as transverse and oblique sections. Each gastric gland consists of three regions. At the junction of the gastric pit with the gastric gland is the **isthmus (14)**, lined with surface epithelial cells (1, 13) and **parietal cells (4)**. Lower in the gland is the **neck (15)**, containing mainly **mucous neck cells (3)** and some parietal cells (4). The base or **fundus (16)** is the deep portion of the gland, composed predominantly of **chief (zymogenic) cells (7)** and a few parietal cells (4). The fundic glands also contain undifferentiated cells and enteroendocrine cells (not illustrated) that secrete different hormones to regulate the digestive system.

Three types of cells can be identified in the fundic gastric glands. The mucous neck cells (3) are located just below the gastric pits (11) and are interspersed between the parietal cells (4) in the neck region of the glands. The parietal cells (4) stain uniformly acidophilic (pink), which distinguishes them from other cells in the fundic glands. In contrast, the chief cells (zymogenic) (7) are basophilic and are distinguishable from the acidophilic parietal cells (4).

The muscularis mucosae (9) in the stomach is composed of two thin strips of smooth muscle: the **inner circular layer (9a)** and **outer longitudinal layer (9b)**. In this illustration, the inner circular layer (9a) is sectioned longitudinally, and the outer layer (9b) is sectioned transversely. Extending upward from the muscularis mucosae (9) to the surface epithelium (1, 13) are strands of **smooth muscle (8, 12)**.

Below the muscularis mucosa (9) is the **submucosa (10)** with denser connective tissue. **Collagen fibers (18)** and the nuclei of **fibroblasts (19)** are seen in the submucosa (10). The submucosa (10) also contains **arterioles (20), venules (21)**, lymphatics, and capillaries in addition to adipose cells.

1 Surface epithelium

2 Mucosal ridges

3 Mucous neck cells

4 Parietal cells

5 Gastric glands

6 Lamina propria

7 Chief (zymogenic) cells

8 Smooth muscle strands

9 Muscularis mucosae:
   a. Inner circular layer

   b. Outer longitudinal
      layer

10 Submocosa

11 Gastric pits

12 Smooth muscle
   strands

13 Surface epithelium

14 Isthmus

15 Neck

Gastric
glands

16 Base (fundus)

17 Lymphatic nodule

18 Collagen fibers

19 Fibroblasts

20 Arteriole

21 Venule

FIGURE 14.9 ■ Stomach: mucosa of the fundus and body (transverse section). Stain: hematoxylin and eosin. Medium magnification.

FIGURE 14.10 | Stomach: Fundus and Body Regions (Plastic Section)

This low-magnification photomicrograph illustrates the mucosa of the stomach wall. The fundus and body regions of the stomach have identical histology. The stomach surface is lined with a mucus-secreting, **simple columnar epithelium (1)** that extends down into the **gastric pits (2)**. In the fundus and body, the gastric pits (2) are shallow. Draining into the gastric pits (2) are the **gastric glands (5)** with different cell types. The cells of the gastric glands (5) are packed, and their lumina are not clearly visible. The large, pale-staining cells in the gastric glands (5) are the acid-secreting **parietal cells (3)**, which are more numerous in the upper regions of the gastric glands (5). The darker-staining cells are the **chief (zymogenic) cells (6)**, and they are mostly located in the basal regions of the gastric glands (5). Between the gastric glands (5) are strips of the connective tissue **lamina propria (7)**. A thin strip of the smooth muscle, the **muscularis mucosae (8)**, separates the mucosa from the **submucosa (4)** of the stomach.

FUNCTIONAL CORRELATIONS 14.2	Gastric Pits and Cells of Gastric Glands in the Stomach

The **cardia** and **pylorus** are located at opposite ends of the stomach. The cardia surrounds the entrance of the esophagus into the stomach. At the esophageal–stomach junction are the **cardiac glands**. The pylorus is the most inferior, funnel-shaped region of the stomach. It terminates at the border of the initial portion of the small intestine called the duodenum. In the cardia, the **gastric pits** are shallow, whereas in the pylorus, the gastric pits are deep. However, the gastric glands in both regions have similar histology, and their cells are predominantly **mucus secreting**.

In contrast, the gastric glands in the fundus and body of the stomach exhibit different histology from the other regions and contain three major cell types. Located in the upper region of gastric glands near the gastric pits are the **mucous neck cells**. The large polygonal cells with a distinctive eosinophilic cytoplasm are the **parietal cells**. These cells are primarily located in the upper half of the gastric glands and are squeezed between other gastric gland cells. Located predominantly in the lower region of the gastric glands are basophilic staining cuboidal **chief (zymogenic) cells**.

In addition to cells that are present in gastric glands, the mucosa of the digestive tract also contains a wide distribution of **enteroendocrine,** or gastrointestinal endocrine cells. These cells are widely distributed in different digestive organs and are located among and between existing exocrine cells. Unless sections of digestive organs are prepared with special stains, these cells are poorly seen in normal histologic sections.

1 Simple columnar epithelium

2 Gastric pits

5 Gastric glands

3 Parietal cells

6 Chief (zymogenic) cells

7 Lamina propria

8 Muscularis mucosae

4 Submucosa

FIGURE 14.10 ■ Stomach: fundus and body regions (plastic section). Stain: hematoxylin and eosin. ×50.

FIGURE 14.11 | Stomach: Superficial Region of Gastric (Fundic) Mucosa

Higher magnification of the superficial region of the stomach shows the cells that constitute the mucosa of the fundus and body.

The columnar **surface epithelium (1)** exhibits basal oval nuclei and a lightly stained cytoplasm owing to the presence of mucigen droplets. The surface epithelium (1) is separated from the **lamina propria (3, 7, 8)** by a thin **basement membrane (2)**. The lamina propria (3, 7, 8) is vascular and contains **blood vessels (9)**. The surface epithelium (1) also extends downward into the **gastric pits (4)**.

The **gastric glands (5)** lie in the lamina propria (3, 7, 8) below the gastric pits (4). The neck region of the gastric glands (5) is lined with **mucous neck cells (10)** that have round, basal nuclei. The constricted necks of the gastric glands (5) open by a short transition region into the bottom of the gastric pits (4).

The **parietal cells (6, 11)** are large cells with a pyramidal shape, round nuclei, and highly acidophilic cytoplasm that are interspersed among the mucous neck cells (10). Some pyramidal cells (6, 11) may be binucleate (two nuclei). The free surfaces of parietal cells (6, 11) open into the lumen of the gastric glands (5). The parietal cells (6, 11) are the most conspicuous cells in the gastric mucosa and are found predominantly in the upper third to upper half of the gastric glands (5).

Deeper in the lower half of the gastric glands (5) are found the basophilic **chief (zymogenic) cells (12)**, which also border on the lumen of the gland. Parietal cells (6, 11) are also seen here.

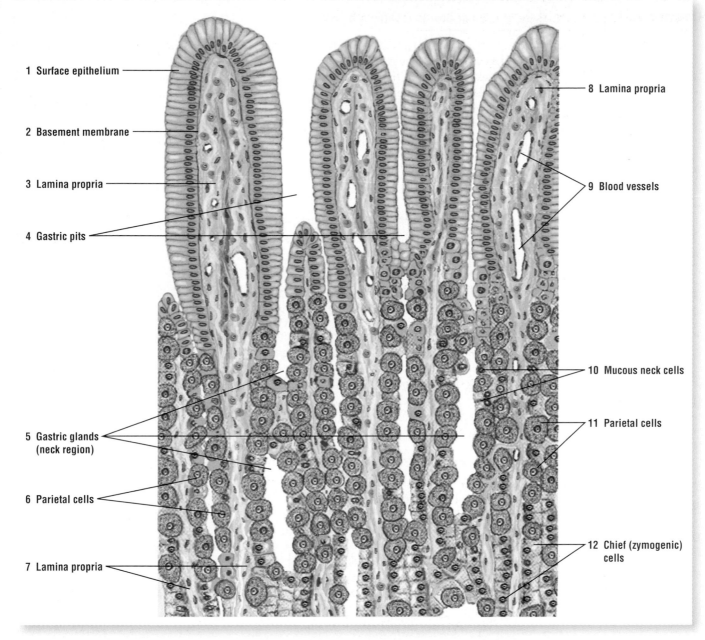

1 Surface epithelium

2 Basement membrane

3 Lamina propria

4 Gastric pits

5 Gastric glands
(neck region)

6 Parietal cells

7 Lamina propria

8 Lamina propria

9 Blood vessels

10 Mucous neck cells

11 Parietal cells

12 Chief (zymogenic)
cells

FIGURE 14.11 ■ Stomach: superficial region of gastric (fundic) mucosa. Stain: hematoxylin and eosin. High magnification.

FIGURE 14.12 | Stomach: Basal Region of Gastric (Fundic) Mucosa

The **gastric glands (1, 9)** in the body and fundus of the stomach show **basal branching (9)**. In the upper regions of the gastric glands, the **chief** or **zymogenic cells (6, 10)** border the lumen of gastric glands (1, 9). In the basal region of the gastric mucosa, the **parietal cells (2)** are wedged against the basement membrane and are not always in direct contact with the lumen.

The connective tissue **lamina propria (3, 7)** surrounds the gastric glands (1). A small **lymphatic nodule (4)** is located in the lamina propria (3) adjacent to the gastric glands (1, 9). The two layers of the **muscularis mucosae (5)**, the inner circular layer and the outer longitudinal layer, are seen below the gastric glands (1, 9). **Strands of smooth muscle (8)** extend upward from the muscularis mucosae (5) into the lamina propria (3, 7) between the gastric glands (1, 9).

Adjacent to the muscularis mucosae (5) is the connective tissue **submucosa (11)**.

FUNCTIONAL CORRELATIONS 14.3 | Stomach

The stomach has numerous important functions. The stomach **receives, stores, mixes, digests,** and **absorbs** some of the ingested products. In addition, the stomach cells secrete different hormones that regulate digestive functions. Some functions are **mechanically** and **chemically** designed specifically to reduce the mass of ingested food material, or **bolus**, to a semiliquid mass called **chyme**. The mechanical reduction of the bolus is performed by strong, muscular peristaltic contractions of the stomach wall when food enters the stomach. With the pylorus closed, the muscular contractions churn and mix the stomach contents with **gastric juices** produced by the **gastric glands**. **Neurons** and **axons** located in the **submucosal nerve plexus** and **myenteric nerve plexus** of the stomach wall regulate the peristaltic activity. The stomach also performs some absorptive functions; however, these are primarily limited to absorption of water, alcohol, salts, and certain drugs.

GASTRIC GLAND CELLS IN THE CARDIA, BODY, AND FUNDUS OF THE STOMACH

Cardiac glands are limited to the narrow cardia region of the stomach that surrounds the esophageal opening. They are composed primarily of mucous cells. The mucus produced by these glands and the cardiac glands of the esophagus neutralize the gastric reflux and protect the esophageal lining.

Chemical reduction or digestion of food in the stomach is the main function of gastric secretions produced by different cells in the gastric glands, especially cells located in the fundus and body regions of the stomach. The main components of the gastric secretions are **pepsin, hydrochloric acid, mucus, intrinsic factor, water, lysozyme,** and different **electrolytes**.

The **surface**, or **luminal epithelial cells** that line the stomach lumen and the mucous neck cells of the gastric pits secrete thick layers of **mucus**, whose main function is to cover, lubricate, and protect the stomach surface from the corrosive actions of acidic gastric juices secreted by different cells in the gastric glands and the ingested material that enters the stomach.

The major component of gastric juice is the **hydrochloric acid**, produced by **parietal cells** that are located in the upper regions of the gastric glands. In humans, parietal cells also produce **gastric intrinsic factor**, a glycoprotein that is necessary for the absorption of **vitamin B12** from the small intestine. Vitamin B12 is necessary for **erythrocyte** (red blood cell) production (**erythropoiesis**) in the red bone marrow. Deficiency of this vitamin leads to the development of **pernicious anemia**, a disorder of erythrocyte formation.

FUNCTIONAL CORRELATIONS 14.3 | Stomach *(Continued)*

Chief, or **zymogenic**, **cells** are filled with secretory granules that contain the pro-enzyme **pepsinogen**, an inactive precursor of **pepsin**. Release of pepsinogen during gastric secretion into the acidic environment of the stomach converts the inactive pepsinogen into the highly active, proteolytic enzyme pepsin. This enzyme digests large protein molecules into smaller peptides, converting almost all of the proteins into smaller molecules. Pepsin is primarily responsible for converting the solid food material into fluid chyme. The secretory activities of the chief and parietal cells are controlled by the autonomic nervous system and the hormone **gastrin**, secreted by the enteroendocrine cells of the pyloric region of the stomach.

Enteroendocrine cells secrete a variety of **polypeptides** and **proteins** with hormonal activity that influences different functions of the digestive tract. They are called enteroendocrine cells because they produce gastric hormones and are located in the digestive organs. The enteroendocrine cells are also called **APUD (amine precursor uptake and decarboxylation) cells** because they can take up the precursors of amines and decarboxylate them. These cells are not confined to the gastrointestinal tract; they are also found in the respiratory organs and other organs of the body where they are also known by different names. Additional details, description, and illustration of known enteroendocrine (APUD) cells are found in Chapter 15, "Digestive System Part III: Small and Large Intestines."

1 Gastric glands

2 Parietal cells

3 Lamina propria

4 Lymphatic nodule

5 Muscularis mucosae

6 Chief (zymogenic) cells

7 Lamina propria

8 Smooth muscle strand

9 Gastric glands (basal branching)

10 Chief (zymogenic) cells

11 Submucosa

FIGURE 14.12 ■ Stomach: basal region of gastric (fundic) mucosa. Stain: hematoxylin and eosin. High magnification.

FIGURE 14.13 | Pyloric Region of the Stomach

In the mucosa of the pyloric region of the stomach, the **gastric pits (3, 8)** are deeper than those in the body or fundus regions. The gastric pits (3, 8) extend into the mucosa to about one half or more of its thickness. The surface of the stomach is lined with a simple **columnar mucous epithelium (1)** that also extends into and lines all the gastric pits (3, 8).

The **pyloric glands (5, 9)** open into the bottom of the gastric pits (3, 8). The pyloric glands (5, 9) are either branched or coiled tubular glands containing mucous secretions, illustrated in both transverse (5) and longitudinal (9) sections. Similar to the cardia region of the stomach, only one type of cell is found in the epithelium of these glands. The tall columnar cell stains lightly because of its mucigen content. As seen in other mucous cells, the flattened or oval nuclei are located at the base. Enteroendocrine cells are also present in this region and can be demonstrated with a special stain.

The remaining structures in the pyloric region of the stomach are similar to those of other regions. The **lamina propria (4)** contains diffuse lymphatic tissue and an occasional **lymphatic nodule (11)**. Located below the lymphatic nodule (11) is the smooth muscle **muscularis mucosae (6)**. Individual **smooth muscle fibers (2, 10)** from the circular layer of the **muscularis mucosae (6)** pass upward between the pyloric glands (5, 9) into the lamina propria (4) and the upper region of the mucosa. Located below the muscularis mucosae (6) is the dense irregular connective tissue **submucosa (7)**, in which are found blood vessels—**arteriole (13)** and **venule (12)**—of different sizes.

FUNCTIONAL CORRELATIONS 14.4 | Cells in Pyloric Gastric Glands

Pyloric glands contain the same cell types as those present in cardiac glands in the cardia region of the stomach. Mucus-secreting cells predominate in these glands, and the secreted mucus covers and protects the pyloric mucosa. In addition to mucus, these cells also produce the enzyme **lysozyme** that destroys bacteria in the stomach.

1 Surface columnar mucous epithelium

2 Muscle fibers from muscularis mucosae

3 Gastric pits

4 Lamina propria

5 Pyloric glands (transverse section)

6 Muscularis mucosae

7 Submucosa

8 Gastric pits

9 Pyloric glands (longitudinal section)

10 Muscle fibers from muscularis mucosae

11 Lymphatic nodule

12 Venule

13 Arteriole

FIGURE 14.13 ■ Pyloric region of the stomach. Stain: hematoxylin and eosin. Medium magnification.

FIGURE 14.14 | Pyloric–Duodenal Junction (Longitudinal Section)

The **pylorus (1)** of the stomach is separated from the **duodenum (11)** of the small intestine by a thick smooth muscle layer called the **pyloric sphincter (8)** that is formed by the thickened circular layer of the muscularis externa of the **stomach (9)**.

At the junction with the duodenum (11), the **mucosal ridges (4)** of the stomach around **gastric pits (3)** become broader and more irregular and their shape more variable. Coiled tubular **pyloric (mucous) glands (6)**, located in the **lamina propria (5)**, open at the bottom of the gastric pits (3). **Lymphatic nodules (16)** are seen between the stomach (1) and the duodenum (11).

The mucus-secreting **stomach epithelium (2)** changes to the **intestinal epithelium (12)** in the duodenum. The intestinal epithelium (12) consists of goblet cells and columnar cells with striated borders (microvilli) that are present throughout the length of the small intestine. The duodenum (11) contains **villi (13)**, a specialized surface modification. Each villus (singular) (13) is a leaf-shaped surface projection. Between individual villi are **intervillous spaces (14)** of the intestinal lumen.

Short, simple tubular **intestinal glands (crypts of Lieberkühn) (15)** are present in the lamina propria of the duodenum. These glands consist primarily of goblet cells and cells with striated borders (microvilli) of the surface epithelium.

Duodenal glands (Brunner glands) (18) occupy most of the **submucosa (19)** in the upper duodenum (11) and are the characteristic features of the duodenum. The ducts of the duodenal glands (18) penetrate the **muscularis mucosae (17)** of the duodenum and enter the base of the intestinal glands (15), disrupting the muscularis mucosae (17) in this region. Except for the esophageal (submucosal) glands proper, the duodenal glands (18) are the only submucosal glands in the digestive tract. In the **muscularis externa of the stomach (9)** and in the **muscularis externa of the duodenum (20)** are neurons and axons of the **myenteric nerve plexuses (10, 21)**.

1 Pylorus

11 Duodenum

2 Stomach epithelium

3 Gastric pits

4 Mucosal ridges

5 Lamina propria (stomach)

6 Pyloric (mucous) glands

7 Muscularis mucosae

8 Pyloric sphincter

9 Muscularis externa (stomach)

10 Myenteric nerve plexus (stomach)

12 Intestinal epithelium

13 Villi

14 Intervillous spaces

15 Intestinal glands (crypts of Lieberkühn)

16 Lymphatic nodule

17 Muscularis mucosae

18 Duodenal glands (Brunner glands)

19 Submucosa

20 Muscularis externa (duodenum)

21 Myenteric nerve plexus (duodenum)

FIGURE 14.14 ■ Pyloric–duodenal junction (longitudinal section). Stain: hematoxylin and eosin. Low magnification.

Digestive System Part II: Esophagus and Stomach

General Plan of the Digestive System: An Overview

- Hollow tube extending from oral cavity to rectum
- Wall exhibits basic organization of the entire tube
- Morphology of the wall and epithelium varies due to different functions

Mucosa

- Is the innermost layer of digestive tract and consists of epithelium and glands
- Loose connective tissue around glands is the lamina propria
- Smooth muscle layer muscularis mucosae forms outer layer of mucosa
- Muscularis mucosa has an inner circular and an outer longitudinal smooth muscle layer

Submucosa

- Located inferior to mucosa
- Consists of dense irregular connective tissue with blood vessels, nerves, and lymphatics
- Contains submucosal nerve plexus that controls muscularis mucosae

Muscularis Externa

- Thick, smooth muscle layer inferior to or below submucosa
- Normally contains an inner circular and an outer longitudinal smooth muscle layer
- Myenteric nerve plexus located between inner and outer smooth muscle layers
- Myenteric nerve plexus controls motility of smooth muscles in muscularis externa

Serosa

- Most superficial layer of abdominal portions of the digestive tract
- Thin layer of connective tissue and mesothelium that cover the visceral organs
- Covers abdominal esophagus, stomach, small intestine, and anterior wall of colon

Adventitia

- Consists only of connective tissue layer without mesothelium lining
- Covers thoracic part of esophagus and posterior wall of ascending and descending colon

Esophagus

- Soft tube that extends from pharynx to stomach, posterior to the trachea
- Penetrates diaphragm, and a short portion is in abdominal cavity before entering stomach
- In thoracic cavity, outside layer is connective tissue or adventitia
- Lumen lined with moist, nonkeratinized stratified squamous epithelium
- Mucous esophageal glands are in both the lamina propria and the submucosa for lubrication
- In the upper third, muscularis externa contains skeletal muscle
- In the middle, both smooth and skeletal muscles found in muscularis externa
- In the lower third, muscularis externa contains smooth muscle only
- Muscularis mucosae and submucosa continue with those of stomach layers

Stomach

- Transition from esophagus to stomach is abrupt; stratified squamous to simple columnar
- Consists of cardia, fundus, body, and pyloric regions
- When contracted or empty, temporary rugae are seen in the wall
- Fundus and body form the major regions and are histologically identical
- Receives, stores, mixes, digests, and absorbs some food products to form liquid chyme
- Converts bolus of ingested food into semiliquid mass called chyme
- Surface is pitted by gastric pits, which are connected to gastric glands in the lamina propria
- Surface is lined with mucus-secreting, simple columnar epithelium for protection
- Gastric glands produce gastric juices rich in hydrochloric acid and protein-digesting enzymes
- Muscularis externa shows internal oblique, middle circular, and outer longitudinal muscle layers
- Submucosal and myenteric nerve plexuses regulate peristaltic activity
- Serosa or visceral peritoneum covers the outer layer of the stomach

Gastric Pits and Cells of Gastric Glands

- In cardia, gastric pits are shallow; in pylorus, gastric pits are deep; both produce mucus
- In body and fundus, parietal cells are large, acidophilic, and are in the upper gland region
- Deeper regions of the gastric glands contain chief or zymogen cells
- In cardia and pylorus, epithelium and simple tubular gastric glands produce mucus
- Glands in the pylorus also produce mucus and the bacteria-destroying enzyme lysozyme

- Parietal cells in fundus and body produce hydrochloric acid and gastric intrinsic factor
- Gastric intrinsic factor is essential for absorption of vitamin B12 and erythropoiesis
- Chief, or zymogen, cells produce pepsinogen that is converted to pepsin in acid environment
- Enteroendocrine cells secrete a variety of polypeptides and proteins for digestive functions
- Mucus-secreting stomach cells change to intestinal epithelium in the duodenum

OVERVIEW FIGURE 15.1 ■ Structural differences between the wall of the small intestine and the large intestine, with emphasis on different layers of the wall.

CHAPTER 15

Digestive System Part III:
Small Intestine and Large Intestine

SECTION 1 Small Intestine

Small Intestine

The **small intestine** is a convoluted tube about 5 to 7 meters long; it is the longest section of the digestive tract. The small intestine extends from the junction with the stomach to join with the **large intestine**, or **colon**. For descriptive purposes, the small intestine is divided into three parts: the **duodenum, jejunum**, and **ileum**. Although the microscopic differences among these three segments are minor, these differences nevertheless allow for identification of the segments.

The main function of the small intestine is the digestion of gastric contents and absorption of nutrients into blood capillaries and lymphatic lacteals.

Surface Modifications of the Small Intestine for Absorption

The mucosa of the small intestine exhibits specialized structural modifications that increase the cellular surface areas for the absorption of nutrients and fluids. These modifications include three structures: plicae circulares, villi, and microvilli.

In contrast to the rugae of the stomach, the **plicae circulares** are permanent spiral folds or elevations of the mucosa (with a submucosal core) that extend into the intestinal lumen. The plicae circulares are most prominent in the proximal portion of the small intestine, the jejunum, where most absorption takes place; they decrease in prominence toward the ileum.

Villi are permanent fingerlike projections of lamina propria of the mucosa that extend into the intestinal lumen. They are covered by **simple columnar epithelium** and are also more prominent in the proximal portion of the small intestine. The height of the villi also decreases toward the ileum of the small intestine. The connective tissue core of each villus contains a lymphatic capillary called a **lacteal**, blood capillaries, and individual strands of smooth muscles (Overview Fig. 15.1).

Each villus has a core of **lamina propria** that contains blood vessels, lymphatic capillaries, nerves, smooth muscle, and loose irregular connective tissue. In addition, the lamina propria is a storehouse for **immune cells**, such as lymphocytes, plasma cells, tissue eosinophils, macrophages, and mast cells.

Smooth muscle fibers from the muscularis mucosae extend into the core of individual villi and can induce movements in the villi. This action increases the contacts of the villi with the digested food products in the intestinal lumen.

Microvilli are cytoplasmic extensions that cover the apices of the intestinal absorptive cells. They are visible under a light microscope as a **striated (brush) border**. With transmission electron microscopy, they appear as regular and dense fingerlike extensions of the absorptive cells cytoplasm. The microvilli are coated by a glycoprotein coat (glycocalyx), which contains **brush border enzymes**.

Glands, Cells, and Lymphatic Cells and Nodules in the Small Intestine

Intestinal Glands

Located throughout the small intestine are the **intestinal glands (crypts of Lieberkühn)**. These glands open into the intestinal lumen at the base of the villi. The simple columnar epithelium that lines the villi is continuous with that of the intestinal glands. In these intestinal glands are found stem cells, absorptive cells, goblet cells, Paneth cells, and some enteroendocrine cells.

Intestinal Cells

- **Absorptive cells** are the most common cell types in the intestinal epithelium. These cells are tall and columnar with a prominent striated (brush) border of **microvilli**. A thick **glycocalyx** coat covers and protects the microvilli from the corrosive digestive chemicals.

- **Goblet cells** are interspersed among the columnar absorptive cells of the intestinal epithelium. They increase in number toward the distal region of the small intestine (ileum).

- **Enteroendocrine** or **APUD (amine precursor uptake and decarboxylation) cells** are scattered throughout the epithelium of the villi and intestinal glands.

- **Duodenal (Brunner) glands** are primarily found in the **submucosa** of the initial portion of the duodenum and are highly characteristic of this region of the small intestine. These are branched, tubuloacinar glands with light-staining **mucous cells**. The ducts of duodenal glands penetrate the muscularis mucosae and discharge their secretory products at the base of intestinal glands that are located between the villi.

- **Undifferentiated cells** are located at the base of intestinal glands, and they exhibit increased mitotic activity. They function as **stem cells** and replace all worn-out columnar absorptive cells, goblet cells, and intestinal gland cells in the small intestine.

- **Paneth cells** are located at the base of intestinal glands. They are characterized by the presence of deep-staining and unique eosinophilic granules in their cytoplasm.

Lymphatic Nodules and Lymphocytic Cells

Peyer patches are numerous aggregations of closely packed, permanent **lymphatic nodules**. They are found primarily in the wall of the terminal portion of the small intestine, the ileum. These nodules occupy a large portion of the lamina propria and submucosa of the ileum. The dispersed lymphocytes and the Peyer patches constitute the **gut-associated lymphoid tissue (GALT)**. This tissue serves as an important immunologic barrier throughout the entire gastrointestinal tract.

M cells are highly specialized epithelial cells that cover the Peyer patches and other large lymphatic nodules; they are not found anywhere else in the intestine. Instead of microvilli, these cells exhibit numerous microfolds. M cells phagocytose luminal antigens and transport them to the lymphocytes and macrophages that are located in the lamina propria, which are then stimulated to produce specific antibodies against the antigens.

Regional Differences in the Small Intestine

The **duodenum** is the shortest segment of the small intestine. The villi in this region are broad, tall, and numerous, with fewer goblet cells in the epithelium. Branched **duodenal (Brunner) glands** with mucus-secreting cells in the submucosa characterize this region. The glands, however, diminish in number toward the end of the duodenum.

The **jejunum** is much longer than the duodenum and contains the largest surface area for the absorption of the digested material. The villi in the jejunum are tall and lined with simple columnar epithelium composed mainly of absorptive cells and some mucus-secreting goblet cells. There are also more goblet cells in the epithelium of the jejunum than in the duodenum. The jejunum does not contain any duodenal (Brunner) glands or lymphatic nodule aggregations (Peyer patches).

The **ileum** contains scant villi that are narrow and short. In addition, the epithelium contains significantly more goblet cells than in the duodenum or the jejunum. Besides increased numbers of lymphocytes in the lamina propria, the aggregated lymphatic nodules (Peyer patches), are particularly large and most numerous in the distal ileum. Lymphatic nodules aggregate in the lamina propria and submucosa to form the prominent Peyer patches.

Supplemental micrographic images are available at **www.thePoint.com/Eroschenko12e** under Digestive System Part III: Small Intestine and Large Intestine.

FIGURE 15.1 | Small Intestine: Duodenum (Longitudinal Section)

The wall of the duodenum consists of four layers: the mucosa with the **lining epithelium (7a)**, the **lamina propria (7b)**, and the **muscularis mucosae (9, 12)**; the underlying connective tissue **submucosa** with the mucous **duodenal (Brunner) glands (3, 13)**; the two smooth muscle layers of the **muscularis externa (14)**; and the visceral peritoneum **serosa (15)**. These layers are continuous with those of the stomach, small intestine, and large intestine (colon).

The small intestine is characterized by fingerlike extensions called **villi (7)** (singular, villus); a lining epithelium **(7a)** of columnar cells lined with the microvilli that form the striated borders; light-staining **goblet cells (2)**; and short, tubular **intestinal glands (crypts of Lieberkühn) (4, 8)** in the lamina propria **(7b)**. Duodenal glands **(3, 13)** in the submucosa **(13)** characterize the duodenum. These glands are absent in the rest of the small intestine (jejunum and ileum) and the large intestine.

The villi **(7)** are mucosal surface modifications. Between the villi **(7)** are the **intervillous spaces (1)**. The lining epithelium **(7a)** covers each villus and the intestinal glands **(4, 8)**. Each villus **(7)** contains a core of lamina propria **(7b)**, strands of **smooth muscle fibers (10)** that extend upward into the villi from the muscularis mucosae **(9, 12)**, and a central lymphatic vessel called **lacteals (11)** (see Fig. 15.7 for details).

The intestinal glands **(4, 8)** are located in the lamina propria **(7b)** and open into the intervillous spaces **(1)**. In certain sections of the duodenum, the submucosal duodenal glands **(13)** extend into the lamina propria **(3)**. The lamina propria **(7b)** also contains fine connective tissue fibers with reticular cells, diffuse lymphatic tissue, and **lymphatic nodules (5)**.

The submucosa **(13)** in the duodenum is almost completely filled with branched, tubular duodenal glands **(13)**. The duodenal glands **(13)** disrupt the muscularis mucosae **(9, 12)** when they penetrate into the lamina propria **(3)**. The secretions from the duodenal glands **(3)** enter at the bottom of the intestinal glands **(3, 4, 8)**.

In a cross section of the duodenum, the muscularis externa **(14)** consists of an **inner circular layer (14a)** and an **outer longitudinal layer (14b)** of smooth muscle. However, in this figure, the duodenum has been cut in a longitudinal plane, and the direction of fibers in these two smooth muscle layers is reversed. Parasympathetic ganglion cells of the **myenteric (Auerbach) nerve plexus (6)**, found in the small and large intestines, are visible in the connective tissue between the two muscle layers of the muscularis externa **(14)**. Similar but smaller plexuses of ganglion cells are also found in the submucosa (not illustrated) in the small and large intestines.

The serosa (visceral peritoneum) **(15)** contains the connective tissue cells, blood vessels, and adipose cells. The serosa forms the outermost layer of the first part of the duodenum.

1 Intervillous spaces

2 Goblet cells

3 Duodenal glands in lamina propria

4 Intestinal glands

5 Lymphatic nodule

6 Myenteric nerve plexus

7 Villus
　a. Lining epithelium
　b. Lamina propria

8 Intestinal glands

9 Muscularis mucosae

10 Smooth muscle fibers

11 Lacteals

12 Muscularis mucosae

13 Duodenal glands in submucosa

14 Muscularis externa:
　a. Inner circular
　b. Outer longitudinal

15 Serosa

FIGURE 15.1 ■ Small intestine: duodenum (longitudinal section). Stain: hematoxylin and eosin. Low magnification.

FIGURE 15.2 | Small Intestine: Duodenum (Transverse Section)

This low-magnification photomicrograph illustrates a transverse section of the duodenum. The luminal surface of the duodenum exhibits **villi (2)** that are covered by **simple columnar epithelium (1)** with a brush border. The core of each villus (2) contains the **lamina propria (4, 6)** in which are found connective tissue cells, lymphatic cells, plasma cells, macrophages, smooth muscle cells, and others. In addition, the lamina propria (4, 6) contains blood vessels and the dilated, blind-ending lymphatic channels called **lacteals (3)**. Between the villi (2) are the **intestinal glands (7)** that extend to the **muscularis mucosae (8)**. Inferior to the muscularis mucosae (8) is the dense irregular connective tissue of **submucosa (9)**. In the duodenum, the submucosa (9) is filled with light-staining, mucus-secreting **duodenal glands (5)**, whose ducts pierce the muscularis mucosae (8) to deliver their secretory product at the base of the intestinal glands (7). Surrounding the submucosa (9) and the duodenal glands (5) is the **muscularis externa (10)**.

FUNCTIONAL CORRELATIONS 15.1 | Duodenum

A characteristic feature of the duodenum are the branched tubuloacinar **duodenal (Brunner) glands** in the submucosa. Their excretory ducts penetrate the muscularis mucosae to deliver their secretions at the base of intestinal glands. Duodenal glands secrete or release their product into the intestinal lumen in response to the entrance of **acidic chyme** from the stomach and parasympathetic stimulation by the vagus nerve.

The main function of the duodenal glands is to protect the duodenal mucosa from the highly corrosive action of the acidic gastric contents. Thus, alkaline **mucus** and **bicarbonate secretions** from the duodenal glands that enter the duodenum lumen buffer or neutralize the acidic chyme. This action also provides a more favorable environment for the activity of the digestive enzymes that are released into the duodenum from the pancreas.

Duodenal (Brunner) glands are also believed to produce a polypeptide hormone called **urogastrone**. This hormone inhibits hydrochloric acid secretion by the parietal cells in the stomach and increases epithelial proliferation in the small intestine.

1 Simple columnar epithelium
2 Villi
3 Lacteals
4 Lamina propria
5 Duodenal glands
6 Lamina propria
7 Intestinal glands
8 Muscularis mucosae
9 Submucosa
10 Muscularis externa

FIGURE 15.2 ■ Small intestine: duodenum (transverse section). Stain: hematoxylin and eosin. ×25.

FIGURE 15.3 | Small Intestine: Jejunum (Transverse Section)

The histology of the lower duodenum, jejunum, and ileum is similar to that of the upper duo-denum (see Fig. 15.1). The only exception is the duodenal (Brunner) glands; these are usually limited to the submucosa in the upper part of the duodenum and are not found in the jejunum and the ileum.

This figure illustrates the prominent and permanent fold of the **plica circularis (10)** that extends into the jejunal lumen. The core of the plica circularis (10) is formed by the dense irregular connective tissue **submucosa (3, 15)** that contains numerous **arteries** and **veins (13).** Numerous fingerlike extensions, the **villi (12),** cover the plica (10). Between the villi (12) are the **intervillous spaces (11),** and at the bottom of the villi (12) are the **intestinal glands (14)** located in the **lamina propria (5).** The intestinal glands (crypts of Lieberkühn) (4) open into the intervil-lous spaces (11).

In the lumen, each villus (12) exhibits a columnar **lining epithelium (1)** with striated border and goblet cells. Below the lining epithelium (1) in the lamina propria (5) is a **lymphatic nod-ule (6)** with a germinal center. Individual strands of smooth muscle fibers from the **muscularis mucosae (2)** extend in the lamina propria of the villi (12). Each villus also contains a central **lacteal (4)** and capillaries (see Fig. 15.7).

The small intestine is surrounded by the **muscularis externa** that contains an **inner circular smooth muscle (7)** layer and an **outer longitudinal smooth muscle (8)** layer. Parasympathetic ganglion cells of the **myenteric plexus (16)** are present in the connective tissue between the mus-cle layers of the muscularis externa (7, 8). A similar submucosal plexus is present in the submu-cosa of the small intestine, but it is not illustrated in this figure.

A visceral peritoneum, or **serosa (17),** surrounds the small intestine. Under the serosal lining are connective tissue fibers, blood vessels, and **adipose cells (9).**

FIGURE 15.4 | Intestinal Glands with Paneth Cells and Enteroendocrine Cells

Extending from the intervillous spaces of the intestinal lumen through the **lamina propria (6)** to the smooth muscle **muscularis mucosae (5)** are the **intestinal glands (1, 8).** This high-magnification illustration shows the bases of the intestinal glands (1, 8) sectioned in longitu-dinal (1) and cross sections (8). Located in the bases of the intestinal glands (1, 8) are different cell types. The most obvious are the pyramid-shaped cells with large, acidophilic granules that fill most of the cytoplasm and displace the nucleus toward the base of the cell. These are the **Paneth cells (4, 10)** and are found in the intestinal glands throughout the length of the small intestine. As in the villi of the intestinal lumen, there are also numerous **goblet cells (2)** in the intestinal glands (1, 8).

In addition to the goblet cells (2), there are numerous **mitotic cells (7)** that serve as stem cells for cells that are lost from the intestinal glands (1, 8). Also present are the **enteroendocrine cells (3, 9)** that are interspersed among the intestinal gland cells, goblet cells (2), and Paneth cells (4, 10). Enteroendocrine cells (3, 9) contain fine secretory granules that are located in the basal cytoplasm and are close to the connective tissue of the lamina propria (6) and the numer-ous blood vessels. Most enteroendocrine cells take up and decarboxylate precursors of biogenic monoamines and are, therefore, designated as amine precursor uptake and decarboxylation (APUD) cells. The APUD cells are found in the epithelia of different systems, such as the gastro-intestinal tract (the stomach and the small and large intestines), the respiratory tract, pancreas, and thyroid glands.

10 Plica circularis

1 Lining epithelium (with goblet cells)

2 Muscularis mucosae

3 Submucosa

4 Lacteal

5 Laminal propria

6 Lymphatic nodule with germinal center

Muscularis externa

7 Inner circular smooth muscle

8 Outer longitudinal smooth muscle

9 Adipose cells

11 Intervillous spaces

12 Villi

13 Artery and vein in submucosa

14 Intestinal glands

15 Submucosa

16 Myenteric nerve plexus

17 Serosa

FIGURE 15.3 ■ Small intestine: jejunum (transverse section). Stain: hematoxylin and eosin. Low magnification.

1 Intestinal gland

2 Goblet cells

3 Enteroendocrine cells

4 Paneth cells

5 Muscularis mucosae

6 Lamina propria

7 Mitotic cell

8 Intestinal gland

9 Enteroendocrine cell

10 Paneth cells

FIGURE 15.4 ■ Intestinal glands with Paneth cells and enteroendocrine cells. Stain: hematoxylin and eosin. High magnification.

FIGURE 15.5 | Small Intestine: Jejunum with Paneth Cells

This low-magnification photomicrograph illustrates the mucosa of the jejunum. The **villi (1)** are lined with a **simple columnar epithelium (2)** with a brush border. Between the columnar cells are the mucus-filled **goblet cells (3)**. Located in the **lamina propria (6)** of each villus are lymphatic cells, macrophages, smooth muscle cells, **blood vessels (7)**, and lymphatic lacteals (not visible). Between the villi are the **intestinal glands (8)**, whose bases contain red-staining or eosinophilic secretory granules of **Paneth cells (9)**. The intestinal glands (8) end near the **muscularis mucosae (4)**, inferior to which is the **submucosa (5)**.

FUNCTIONAL CORRELATIONS 15.2	Paneth Cells and Enteroendocrine Cells in the Small Intestine

Paneth cells, located in the bases of intestinal glands, are exocrine cells that produce **lysozyme**, an antibacterial enzyme that digests the bacterial cell walls and membranes of microorganisms and destroys them. Paneth cells may also have some **phagocytic** functions. Thus, these cells have an important function in controlling the microbial flora in the small intestine and regulating the microenvironment of the intestinal crypts.

Enteroendocrine cells in the small intestine secrete numerous **regulatory hormones** for the digestive system, including gastric inhibitory peptide, secretin, and cholecystokinin (pancreozymin). To release these hormones into the proximity of the capillaries, the secretory granules in these cells are located in the base of the cells, which are adjacent to the lamina propria and the capillaries.

Gastric inhibitory peptide affects the parietal cells in the stomach and inhibits or reduces their production of hydrochloric acid. Entrance of acidic chyme into the duodenum also produces a release of the hormone **secretin**, which then influences the exocrine cells of the pancreas to secrete a bicarbonate-rich fluid into the intestine. The bicarbonate fluid neutralizes the luminal acidity and establishes a more favorable environment for the action of digestive enzymes in the small intestine. **Cholecystokinin** increases the secretion of pancreatic enzymes into the small intestine and induces gall bladder contractions to release the stored bile.

FIGURE 15.6 | Small Intestine: Ileum with Lymphatic Nodules (Peyer Patches) (Transverse Section)

A characteristic feature of the ileum is the aggregations of **lymphatic nodules (5, 12)** called **Peyer patches (5, 12)**. Each Peyer patch is an aggregation of numerous lymphatic nodules that are located in the wall of the ileum opposite the mesenteric attachment. Most of the lymphatic nodules (5, 12) exhibit **germinal centers (5)**. The lymphatic nodules (5, 12) usually coalesce, and the boundaries between them become indistinct.

The lymphatic nodules (5, 12) originate in the diffuse lymphatic tissue of the **lamina propria (10)**. Villi are absent in the area of the intestinal lumen where the nodules reach the surface of the mucosa. Typically, the lymphatic nodules (5, 12) extend into the **submucosa (6)**, disrupt the **muscularis mucosae (13)**, and spread out in the loose connective tissue of the submucosa (6).

Also illustrated are the surface epithelium (1) that covers the villi (2, 8), intestinal glands (4, 11), lacteals in the villi (3, 9), the inner circular layer (14a) and the outer longitudinal layer (14b) of the muscularis externa (14), and the serosa (7).

1 Villi

2 Simple columnar
  epithelium

3 Goblet cells

4 Muscularis
  mucosae

5 Submucosa

6 Lamina propria

7 Blood vessels

8 Intestinal
  glands

9 Paneth cells

FIGURE 15.5 ■ Small intestine: jejunum with Paneth cells. Stain: Mallory-Azan. ×40.

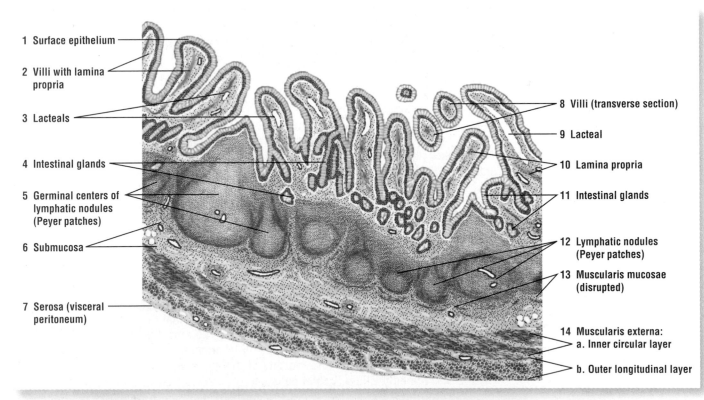

1 Surface epithelium

2 Villi with lamina
  propria

3 Lacteals

4 Intestinal glands

5 Germinal centers of
  lymphatic nodules
  (Peyer patches)

6 Submucosa

7 Serosa (visceral
  peritoneum)

8 Villi (transverse section)

9 Lacteal

10 Lamina propria

11 Intestinal glands

12 Lymphatic nodules
   (Peyer patches)

13 Muscularis mucosae
   (disrupted)

14 Muscularis externa:
   a. Inner circular layer

   b. Outer longitudinal layer

FIGURE 15.6 ■ Small intestine: ileum with lymphatic nodules (Peyer patches) (transverse
section). Stain: hematoxylin and eosin. Low magnification.

FIGURE 15.7 | Small Intestine: Villi (Longitudinal and Transverse Sections)

Several **villi (1)** are sectioned longitudinally and transversely and illustrated at a higher magnification. The simple columnar **surface epithelium (2)** that covers the villi (1) contains mucus-secreting **goblet cells (7)** and absorptive cells with **striated borders (microvilli) (3)**. To show mucus, the section was stained for carbohydrates. As a result, the goblet cells (7) are stained magenta.

A thin **basement membrane (8)** is visible between the surface epithelium (2) and the **lamina propria (4)**. In the core of the lamina propria (4) are found connective tissue cells and collagen fibers, blood cells, and **smooth muscle fibers (5)**. Also present in each villus (but not always seen in sections) is a **central lacteal (6)**, a lymphatic vessel lined with endothelium. Arterioles, one or more venules, and **capillaries (9)** are also visible in the villi.

FIGURE 15.8 | Ultrastructure of Microvilli in an Absorptive Cell in the Small Intestine

Microvilli are tiny surface projections that appear as a pink-staining brush border on absorptive cells in the intestine, especially when the slides are stained for carbohydrates and examined with a light microscope. With a transmission electron microscope, the brush border is seen as numerous, dense fingerlike **microvilli (1, 5)** that project from the apical plasma membrane of absorptive cells. Microvilli (1, 5) are seen in different cell types but are most prevalent lining the **intestinal lumen** of the small intestine.

The core of the microvilli (1, 5) consists of vertical actin microfilaments that are attached to the cytoplasm by a network of actin microfilaments called the **terminal web (2, 6)**. Also seen in the absorptive cell are numerous **cytoplasmic vesicles (4)** and **secretory granules (3)**. In addition, the cytoplasm contains numerous mitochondria (7), sectioned in different planes.

FUNCTIONAL CORRELATIONS 15.3 | Peyer Patches in the Ileum

The lamina propria and submucosa in the ileum contain numerous and large aggregates of large lymphatic nodules called **Peyer patches**. Overlying these lymphatic patches are specialized epithelial cells called the **M cells**. The cell membranes of M cells show deep invaginations or microfolds that contain both macrophages and lymphocytes. The lymphatic nodules of Peyer patches contain numerous **B lymphocytes**, some **T lymphocytes, macrophages**, and **plasma cells**. M cells continually sample the **antigens** of the intestinal lumen, ingest the antigens, and present them to the underlying lymphocytes and macrophages in the lamina propria. The antigens that reach the underlying lymphocytes and macrophages then initiate the proper immunologic responses to these foreign molecules.

SMALL INTESTINE: FUNCTIONAL OVERVIEW

The small intestine performs numerous digestive functions, including (1) continuation and completion of **digestion** (initiated in the oral cavity and the stomach) of food products (chyme) by chemicals and enzymes produced in the liver and pancreas and by cells in its own mucosa, (2) selective **absorption** of nutrients into the blood and lymph capillaries, (3) **transportation** of chyme and digestive waste material to the large intestine, and (4) release of different **hormones** into the bloodstream to regulate the secretory functions and motility of digestive organs.

On the surface epithelium, **goblet cells** secrete **mucus** that lubricates, coats, and protects the intestinal surface from the corrosive actions of digestive chemicals and enzymes. The outer **glycocalyx** coat on absorptive cells not only protects the intestinal surface from digestion but also contains numerous **brush border enzymes** required for the final breakdown of ingested food products before absorption into the system. These enzymes, such as disaccharidases, peptidases, sucrase, lipase, lactase, and others, are produced by absorptive epithelial cells and are an integral part of the membrane proteins of the glycocalyx.

(box continues on page 354)

1 Villi

2 Surface epithelium

3 Striated border (microvilli)

4 Lamina propria

5 Smooth muscle fibers

6 Central lacteal

7 Goblet cells

8 Basement membrane

9 Capillaries

FIGURE 15.7 ■ Small intestine: villi (longitudinal and transverse sections). Stain: periodic acid–Schiff. Medium magnification.

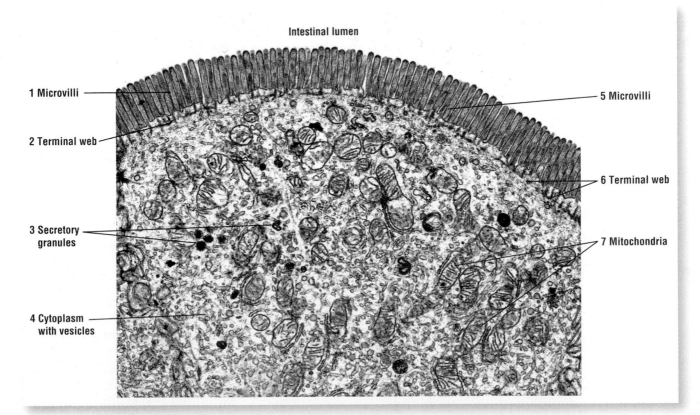

Intestinal lumen

1 Microvilli

2 Terminal web

3 Secretory granules

4 Cytoplasm with vesicles

5 Microvilli

6 Terminal web

7 Mitochondria

FIGURE 15.8 ■ Ultrastructure of microvilli in an absorptive cell in the small intestine. Courtesy of Dr. Rex A. Hess, Professor Emeritus, Comparative Biosciences, College of Veterinary Medicine, University of Illinois, Urbana, Illinois. ×6,150.

| FUNCTIONAL CORRELATIONS 15.3 | Peyer Patches in the Ileum *(Continued)* |

Absorption of nutrients into the cell interior in the small intestine occurs via diffusion, facilitated diffusion, osmosis, and active transport. Intestinal cells absorb **amino acids, glucose**, and **fatty acids**—the end products of protein, carbohydrate, and fat digestion, respectively. Amino acids, water, various ions, and glucose are transported through intestinal cells into the **blood capillaries** present in the lamina propria of each villus, from which they pass to the liver via the portal vein. Most of the long-chain fatty acids and monoglycerides, however, do not enter the capillaries, but instead enter the tiny, blind-ending lymphatic vessels, called **lacteals**, that are also located in the lamina propria of each villus. The presence of smooth muscle fibers in the villi causes movement and contractions of the villi. This action moves or forces the contents of the lacteals from the villi into larger lymph vessels in the submucosa and into the mesenteries.

SECTION 2   Large Intestine (Colon)

The large intestine is situated between the anus and the terminal end of the ileum. It is shorter and less convoluted than the small intestine. The large intestine consists of the following parts: the cecum; ascending, transverse, descending, and sigmoid colon; as well as the rectum and anus.

Chyme enters the large intestine from the ileum through the ileocecal valve. Unabsorbed and undigested food residues from the small intestine are forced into the large intestine by strong peristaltic actions of smooth muscles in the muscularis externa. The residues that enter the large intestine are in a semifluid state; however, by the time they reach the terminal portion of the large intestine, these residues become semisolid **feces**.

 Supplemental micrographic images are available at **www.thePoint.com/Eroschenko12e** under Digestive System Part III: Small Intestine and Large Intestine.

FIGURE 15.9 | Large Intestine: Colon and Mesentery (Panoramic View, Transverse Section)

The wall of the colon has the same basic layers as the small intestine. The **mucosa (4–7)** consists of simple columnar **epithelium (4)**, **intestinal glands (5)**, **lamina propria (6)**, and **muscularis mucosae (7)**. The underlying **submucosa (8)** contains connective tissue cells and fibers, various blood vessels, and nerves. Two smooth muscle layers make up the **muscularis externa (13)**. The **serosa (visceral peritoneum** and **mesentery) (3, 17)** covers the transverse colon and the sigmoid colon. There are several modifications in the colon wall that distinguish it from other regions of the digestive tract (tube).

The colon does not have villi or plicae circulares, and the luminal surface of the mucosa is smooth. In the undistended colon, the mucosa (4–7) and the submucosa (8) exhibit **temporary folds (12)**. In the lamina propria (6) and the submucosa (8) of the colon are **lymphatic nodules (9, 11)**.

The smooth muscle layers in the muscularis externa (13) of the colon are modified. The **inner circular muscle layer (16)** is continuous in the colon wall, whereas the outer muscle layer is condensed into three broad, longitudinal bands called **taeniae coli (1, 10)**. A very thin **outer longitudinal muscle layer (15)**, which is often discontinuous, is found between the taeniae coli (1, 10). The parasympathetic ganglion cells of the **myenteric (Auerbach) nerve plexus (2, 14)** are found between the two smooth muscle layers of the muscularis externa (13).

The transverse and sigmoid colon are attached to the body wall by a **mesentery (18)**. As a result, the serosa (3, 17) is the outermost layer.

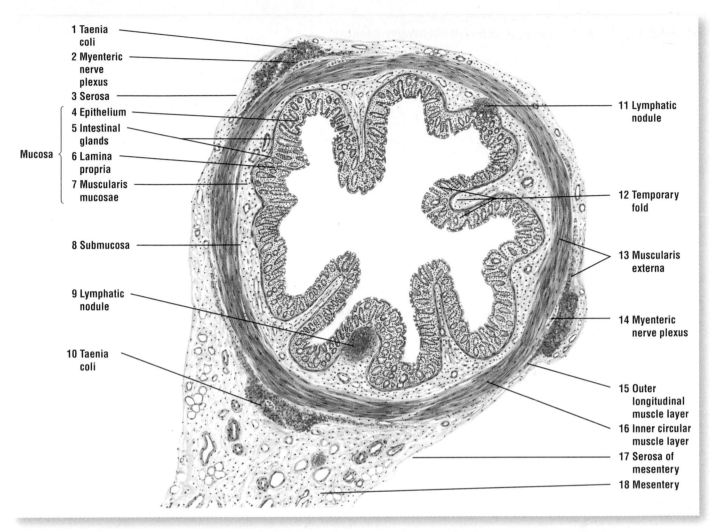

1 Taenia coli
2 Myenteric nerve plexus
3 Serosa
4 Epithelium
5 Intestinal glands
6 Lamina propria
7 Muscularis mucosae
Mucosa
8 Submucosa
9 Lymphatic nodule
10 Taenia coli

11 Lymphatic nodule
12 Temporary fold
13 Muscularis externa
14 Myenteric nerve plexus
15 Outer longitudinal muscle layer
16 Inner circular muscle layer
17 Serosa of mesentery
18 Mesentery

FIGURE 15.9 ■ Large intestine: colon and mesentery (panoramic view, transverse section). Stain: hematoxylin and eosin. Low magnification.

FIGURE 15.10 | Large Intestine: Colon Wall (Transverse Section)

This low-magnification photomicrograph illustrates a portion of the colon wall. The simple columnar epithelium contains the **absorptive columnar cells (1)** and the mucus-filled **goblet cells (2, 6)**, which increase in number toward the terminal end of the colon. The **intestinal glands (4)** in the colon are deep and straight and extend through the **lamina propria (3)** to the **muscularis mucosae (8)**. The lamina propria (3) and the **submucosa (9)** are filled with aggregations of lymphatic cells and **lymphatic nodules (5, 7)**.

1 Absorptive columnar cells

2 Goblet cells

3 Lamina propria

4 Intestinal glands

5 Lymphatic nodule

6 Goblet cells

7 Lymphatic nodule

8 Muscularis mucosae

9 Submucosa

FIGURE 15.10 ■ Large intestine: colon wall (transverse section). Stain: hematoxylin and eosin. ×30.

FIGURE 15.11 | Large Intestine: Colon Wall (Transverse Section)

The wall of an undistended colon normally exhibits **temporary folds (8)** that consist of both the **mucosa (10–12)** and **submucosa (13)** layers. The four layers of the colon wall that are continuous with those of the small intestine are the mucosa (10–12), submucosa (13), **muscularis externa (14)**, and **serosa (5)**.

Villi are not present in the colon. The connective tissue **lamina propria (11)** contains long **intestinal glands (1, 9)** (crypts of Lieberkühn) that continue through the lamina propria (11) to the smooth muscle layer **muscularis mucosae (2, 12)**.

The lining **epithelium (10)** in the colon is characterized by numerous **goblet cells (10)**. The lining epithelium (10) is simple columnar that continues to also line the intestinal glands (1, 9). Visible in the illustration are intestinal glands (1, 9) that are sectioned both longitudinally and in cross sections (9).

As in the small intestine, the lamina propria (11) contains abundant and diffuse lymphatic tissues. A distinct **lymphatic nodule (3)** is visible deep in the connective tissue of the lamina propria (11). Some of the larger lymphatic nodules may extend through the muscularis mucosae (2, 12) into the connective tissue of the submucosa (13).

In contrast to the small intestine, the muscularis externa (14) of the colon is atypical. The longitudinal layer of the muscularis externa (14) is arranged into strips or bands of smooth muscle called the **taeniae coli (16)**. As in the circular layer, the taeniae coli are supplied by **blood vessels (6)**. The parasympathetic ganglia of the **myenteric nerve plexus (4, 15)** are located between the muscle layers of the muscularis externa (14).

The outermost layer, serosa (5), covers the connective tissue and **adipose (fat) cells** (7). However, the serosa (5) covers only the transverse and sigmoid colon. The ascending and descending colon are retroperitoneal, and their posterior surface is lined with the connective tissue adventitia.

FUNCTIONAL CORRELATIONS 15.4 | Large Intestine

The principal functions of the large intestine are to absorb **water** and **minerals (electrolytes)** from the remaining indigestible material that was transported from the ileum of the small intestine and to compact it into feces for elimination from the body. Consistent with these functions, the epithelium of the large intestine contains **columnar absorptive cells** (similar to those in the epithelium of the small intestine) and numerous mucus-secreting **goblet cells**, which produce mucus for lubricating the lumen of the large intestine to facilitate passage of the feces. No digestive enzymes are produced by the cells of the large intestine.

HISTOLOGIC DIFFERENCES BETWEEN THE SMALL AND LARGE INTESTINES (COLON)

The large intestine lacks both plicae circulares and villi that characterize the small intestine. Intestinal glands are present in the large intestine and are similar to those of the small intestine. However, they are deeper (longer) and lack the Paneth cells in their bases. The epithelium of the large intestine also contains different enteroendocrine cells.

Also present in the small intestine are the **goblet cells** that are more numerous in the large intestine epithelium than in the small intestine. Moreover, the number of goblet cells increases from the cecum toward the terminal portion of the sigmoid colon. The lamina propria of the large intestine contains many solitary lymphatic nodules, lymphocyte accumulations, plasma cells, and macrophages.

In contrast to the small intestine, the muscularis externa of the large intestine and the cecum shows a unique arrangement. The inner circular smooth muscle layer is present. However, the outer longitudinal muscle layer is arranged into three longitudinal muscle strips called **taeniae coli**. The contraction, or tonus, in the taeniae coli forms sacculations or compartments in the large intestine, called **haustra** (see Overview Fig. 15.1).

8 Temporary fold (mucosa and submucosa)

1 Intestinal glands

2 Muscularis mucosae

3 Lymphatic nodule

4 Myenteric nerve plexus

5 Serosa

6 Blood vessels

7 Adiopose cells

9 Intestinal glands (longitudinal and cross section)

10 Lining epithelium with goblet cells

11 Lamina propria

12 Muscularis mucosae

13 Submucosa

Mucosa

14 Muscularis externa

15 Myenteric nerve plexus

16 Taenia coli

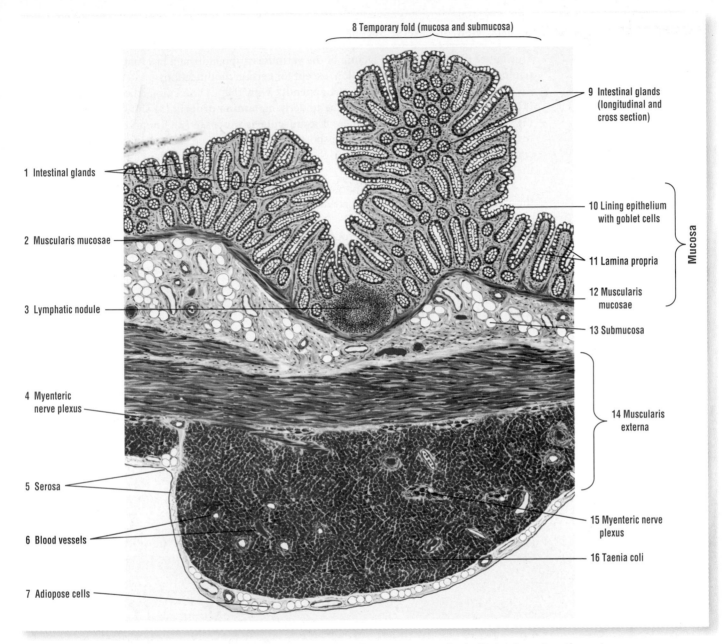

FIGURE 15.11 ■ Large intestine: colon wall (transverse section). Stain: hematoxylin and eosin. Medium magnification.

FIGURE 15.12 | Appendix (Panoramic View, Transverse Section)

This figure illustrates a cross section of the vermiform appendix at a low magnification. Its morphology is similar to that of the colon, except for certain modifications.

In comparing the mucosa of the appendix with that of the colon, the **lining epithelium (1)** contains numerous goblet cells, the underlying **lamina propria (3)** shows **intestinal glands (5)** (crypts of Lieberkühn), and there is a **muscularis mucosae (2)**. The intestinal glands (5) in the appendix are less well developed, shorter, and often spaced farther apart than those in the colon. **Diffuse lymphatic tissue (6)** in the lamina propria (3) is abundant and is present often in the **submucosa (8)**.

Lymphatic nodules **(4, 9)** with germinal centers are numerous and highly characteristic of the appendix. These nodules originate in the lamina propria (3) and may extend from the surface epithelium (1) to the submucosa (8).

The submucosa (8) has numerous blood vessels (11). The muscularis externa (7) consists of the inner circular layer (7a) and the outer longitudinal layer (7b). The parasympathetic ganglia (12) of the myenteric plexus (12) are located between the inner (7a) and outer (7b) smooth muscle layers of the muscularis externa.

The outermost layer of the appendix is the **serosa (10)** under which are seen **adipose cells (13)**.

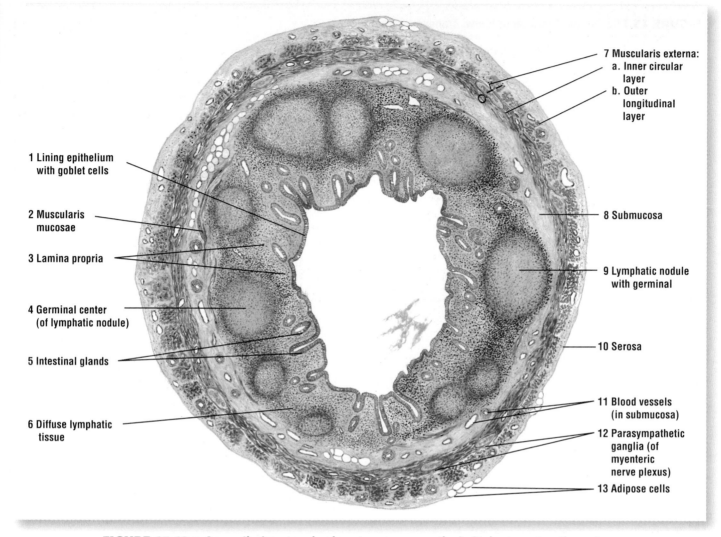

1 Lining epithelium with goblet cells

2 Muscularis mucosae

3 Lamina propria

4 Germinal center (of lymphatic nodule)

5 Intestinal glands

6 Diffuse lymphatic tissue

7 Muscularis externa:
   a. Inner circular layer
   b. Outer longitudinal layer

8 Submucosa

9 Lymphatic nodule with germinal

10 Serosa

11 Blood vessels (in submucosa)

12 Parasympathetic ganglia (of myenteric nerve plexus)

13 Adipose cells

FIGURE 15.12 ■ Appendix (panoramic view, transverse section). Stain: hematoxylin and eosin. Low magnification.

FIGURE 15.13 | Rectum (Panoramic View, Transverse Section)

The histology of the upper rectum is similar to that of the colon.

The surface **epithelium (1)** of the **lumen (5)** is lined with simple columnar cells with striated borders and goblet cells. The **intestinal glands (4), adipose cells (12),** and **lymphatic nodules (10)** in the **lamina propria (2)** are similar to those in the colon. The intestinal glands are longer, closer together, and filled with goblet cells. Beneath the lamina propria (2) is the **muscularis mucosae (11)**.

The longitudinal **folds (3)** in the upper rectum and colon are temporary. These folds (3) contain a core of **submucosa (8)** covered by the mucosa. Permanent longitudinal folds (rectal columns) are found in the lower rectum and the anal canal.

Taeniae coli of the colon continue into the rectum, where the **muscularis externa (13)** acquires the typical **inner circular (13a)** and **outer longitudinal (13b)** smooth muscle layers. Between these two smooth muscle layers are the **parasympathetic ganglia** of the **myenteric (Auerbach) plexus (14)**.

Adventitia (9) covers a portion of the rectum, and serosa covers the remainder. Numerous **blood vessels (6, 7, 15)** are found in both the submucosa (8) and the adventitia (9).

FIGURE 15.14 | Anorectal Junction (Longitudinal Section)

The portion of the anal canal above the **anorectal junction (7)** represents the lowermost part of the rectum. The part of the anal canal below the anorectal junction (7) shows the transition from the **simple columnar epithelium (1)** to the **stratified squamous epithelium (8)** of the skin. The change from the rectal mucosa to the anal mucosa occurs at the anorectal junction (7).

The rectal mucosa is similar to the mucosa of the colon. The **intestinal glands (3)** are somewhat shorter and spaced farther apart. As a result, the **lamina propria (2)** is more prominent, diffuse lymphatic tissue is more abundant, and solitary **lymphatic nodules (11)** are more numerous.

The **muscularis mucosae (4)** and the intestinal glands (3) of the digestive tract terminate in the vicinity of the anorectal junction (7). The lamina propria (2) of the rectum is replaced by the dense irregular connective tissue of the **lamina propria of the anal canal (9)**. The **submucosa (5)** of the rectum merges with the connective tissue in the lamina propria of the anal canal, a region that is highly vascular. The **internal hemorrhoidal plexus (10)** of veins lies in the mucosa of the anal canal. Blood vessels from this region continue into the submucosa (5) of the rectum.

The circular smooth muscle layer of the **muscularis externa (6)** increases in thickness in the upper region of the anal canal and forms the **internal anal sphincter (6)**. Lower in the anal canal, the internal anal sphincter (6) is replaced by skeletal muscles of the **external anal sphincter (12)**. External to the external anal sphincter (12) is the skeletal **levator ani muscle (13)**.

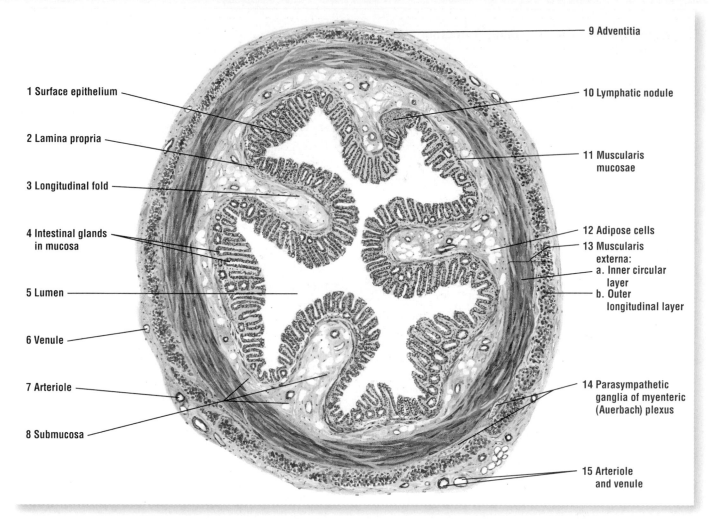

1 Surface epithelium

2 Lamina propria

3 Longitudinal fold

4 Intestinal glands in mucosa

5 Lumen

6 Venule

7 Arteriole

8 Submucosa

9 Adventitia

10 Lymphatic nodule

11 Muscularis mucosae

12 Adipose cells

13 Muscularis externa:
   a. Inner circular layer
   b. Outer longitudinal layer

14 Parasympathetic ganglia of myenteric (Auerbach) plexus

15 Arteriole and venule

FIGURE 15.13 ■ Rectum (panoramic view, transverse section). Stain: hematoxylin and eosin. Low magnification.

1 Simple columnar epithelium

2 Lamina propria

3 Intestinal glands

4 Muscularis mucosae

5 Submucosa

6 Muscularis externa (internal anal sphincter)

7 Anorectal junction

8 Stratified squamous epithelium

9 Lamina propria of anal canal

10 Internal hemorrhoidal plexus

11 Lymphatic nodules

12 External anal sphincter (skeletal muscle)

13 Levator ani muscle (skeletal)

FIGURE 15.14 ■ Anorectal junction (longitudinal section). Stain: hematoxylin and eosin. Low magnification.

Digestive System Part III: Small Intestine and Large Intestine

SECTION 1 • Small Intestine

- Long, convoluted tube divided into duodenum, jejunum, and ileum
- Duodenum is the shortest segment with broad, tall, and numerous villi
- Digests gastric contents and absorbs nutrients into blood capillaries and lymphatic lacteals
- Transports chyme and waste products to large intestine
- Releases numerous hormones to regulate secretory functions and motility of digestive organs
- Amino acids, water, ions, glucose, and other substances are absorbed and transported in blood capillaries
- Long-chain fatty acids and monoglycerides are transported by lymphatic lacteals
- Contains numerous permanent surface modifications that increase cellular contact for absorption
- Plicae circulares are spiral folds with submucosa core that extend into intestinal lumen
- Villi are fingerlike projections of lamina propria that extend into the intestinal lumen
- Microvilli are cytoplasmic extensions of absorptive cells that extend into the intestinal lumen
- Microvilli are coated with brush border enzymes that digest food products before absorption
- Villi contain a core of connective tissue with capillaries, lacteal, and smooth muscle strands
- Lamina propria is filled with lymphocytes, plasma cells, macrophages, eosinophils, and mast cells
- Smooth muscle strands in lamina propria of villi induce their movement and contractions

Cells of the Small Intestine

- Absorptive cells with microvilli covered by glycocalyx are most common in intestinal epithelium
- Goblet cells, interspersed between absorptive cells, increase in number toward distal region
- Enteroendocrine cells are scattered throughout the epithelium and intestinal glands
- Secretory granules of enteroendocrine cells located at the base of cells and close to capillaries
- Enteroendocrine cells secrete numerous regulatory hormones for the digestive system
- Undifferentiated cells in the base of intestinal glands replace worn-out luminal cells

- Paneth cells with pink eosinophilic granules in cytoplasm are located in the intestinal glands
- Paneth cells produce the antibacterial enzyme lysozyme to control microbial flora in the intestine
- M cells are specialized cells that cover the lymphatic Peyer patches

Glands of the Small Intestine

- Intestinal glands located between villi throughout the small intestine
- Intestinal glands open into the intestinal lumen at the base of the villi
- Duodenal glands in the submucosa of duodenum are characteristic of this region
- Duodenal glands penetrate muscularis mucosae to discharge mucus and bicarbonate secretions
- Bicarbonate secretions enter base of intestinal glands and protect duodenum from acidic chyme
- Polypeptide urogastrone from duodenal glands inhibits hydrochloric acid secretions

Lymphatic Accumulations in the Small Intestine

- Peyer patches are numerous aggregations of permanent lymphatic nodules
- Peyer patches found primarily in the lamina propria and submucosa of the terminal part of the intestine
- Overlying Peyer patches are specialized M cells, which are not anywhere else in the intestine
- M cells show deep invaginations that contain macrophages and lymphocytes
- M cells sample intestinal antigens and present them to underlying lymphocytes for response

SECTION 2 • Large Intestine

- Situated between anus and the terminal end of ileum
- Shorter and less convoluted than small intestine
- Consists of cecum and ascending, transverse, descending, and sigmoid sections
- Semifluid chyme enters through ileocecal valve
- At terminal end, semifluid residues become hardened or semisolid feces
- Main function is the absorption of water and electrolytes
- Epithelium consists of simple columnar epithelium with increased number of goblet cells

- Goblet cells produce mucus for lubricating the canal to facilitate passage of feces
- No enzymes or chemicals produced, but enteroendocrine cells are present in the epithelium
- No plicae circulares, villi, or Paneth cells are present; intestinal glands are deeper

- Increased numbers of solitary lymphatic nodules with cells are present in lamina propria
- Muscularis externa contains inner circular layer with outer layer arranged in three strips, the taeniae coli
- Contractions of taeniae coli form sacculations or haustra

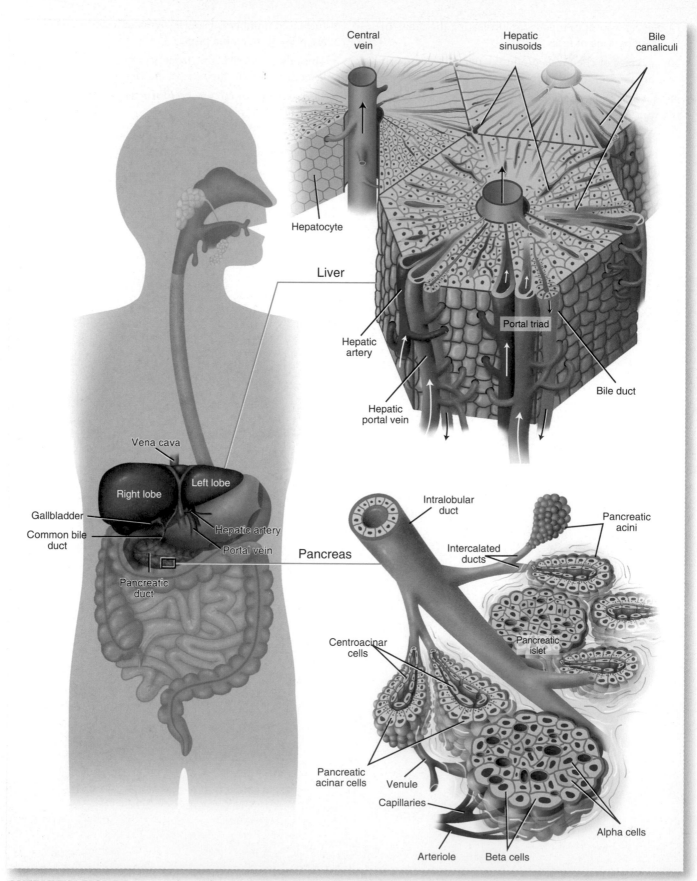

OVERVIEW FIGURE 16.1 ■ A section from the liver and the pancreas is illustrated, with emphasis on the details of the liver lobule and the duct system of the exocrine pancreas.

CHAPTER 16

Digestive System Part IV: Accessory Digestive Organs (Liver, Pancreas, and Gallbladder)

The accessory organs of the digestive system are located outside of the digestive tube. Excretory glands from the salivary glands open into the oral cavity. The **liver, gallbladder**, and **pancreas** that are located in the abdominal cavity deliver their secretory products to the duodenum also via excretory ducts. The **common bile duct** from the liver and the **main pancreatic duct** from the pancreas join in the duodenal loop to form a single duct common to both organs. This duct then penetrates the entire duodenal wall and enters the lumen of the duodenum. The gallbladder joins the common bile duct via the cystic duct. Thus, **bile** from the gallbladder and **digestive secretions** and **enzymes** from the pancreas enter the duodenum via a common duct.

SECTION 1 Liver

Liver

The liver is one of the largest digestive organs and is located in a very strategic position. All nutrients and liquids that are absorbed from the intestines enter the liver through the **hepatic portal vein**, except the complex lipid products, which enter and are transported by the **lymph vessels**. The absorbed products first percolate through the liver capillaries called **sinusoids**. Nutrient-rich blood in the hepatic portal vein is first brought to the liver before it enters the general circulation. Because venous blood from the digestive organs in the hepatic portal vein is poor in oxygen, a **hepatic artery** from the aorta supplies liver cells with oxygenated blood, forming a **dual blood supply** to the liver.

In hisotologic sections, liver exhibits repeating hexagonal units called **liver (hepatic) lobules**. In the center of each hepatic lobule is the **central vein**, from which radiate plates of liver cells, called **hepatocytes**, and the blood vessels sinusoids toward the periphery. In the periphery, the surrounding connective tissue contains **portal canals**, also called **portal areas** or **portal triads**, where branches of the **hepatic artery, hepatic portal vein, bile duct**, and **lymph vessels** can be seen. In human liver, three to six portal areas can be seen per hepatic lobule. Venous and arterial blood from the vessels in the peripheral portal area first mix in the liver sinusoids as it flows toward the central vein. From here, blood enters the general circulation through the hepatic veins that leave the liver and enter the inferior vena cava.

The hepatic sinusoids are tortuous, dilated blood channels lined with a discontinuous layer of **fenestrated endothelial cells** that also exhibit discontinuous basal lamina. The hepatic sinusoids are separated from the underlying hepatocytes by a subendothelial **perisinusoidal space of Disse**. Located in this space are the microvilli of individual hepatocytes and delicate strands of connective tissue fibers. The microvilli increase the surface area for exchange of metabolites that are present in the flowing blood and the hepatocytes. As a result, ingested material carried in the sinusoidal blood has direct access to hepatocytes through the discontinuous endothelial wall. The structure and the tortuous path of sinusoids through the liver allows for an efficient exchange of materials between hepatocytes and blood. In addition to the endothelial cells, the hepatic sinusoids also contain macrophages called **Kupffer cells** that form part of the lining endothelium.

These cells are large, and their processes may extend across or span the entire lumen of the sinusoid. Other cells that are found in the subendothelial perisinusoidal spaces are the **hepatic stellate cells**, also called the **Ito cells**. These cells are primary storage sites for fat and much of the body's vitamin A.

Hepatocytes also secrete bile into tiny channels called **bile canaliculi** located between individual hepatocytes. The canaliculi converge at the periphery of liver lobules in the portal areas to form **bile ducts**. From the portal areas, the bile ducts then drain into gradually larger hepatic ducts that carry bile out of the liver. Within the liver lobules, bile flows in bile canaliculi toward the bile duct in the peripheral portal area, whereas blood in the sinusoids flows in the opposite direction toward the central vein.

 Supplemental micrographic images are available at **www.thePoint.com/Eroschenko12e** under Digestive System Part IV: Liver, Gallbladder, and Pancreas.

FIGURE 16.1 | Pig Liver (Panoramic View, Transverse Section)

In the pig liver, connective tissue from the hilus extends between the liver lobes as **interlobular septa (5, 9)** and defines the **hepatic (liver) lobules (7)**. To illustrate the connective tissue boundaries that form each hepatic lobule (7), a section of pig's liver was stained with Mallory-Azan stain, which stains the connective tissue septa (5, 9) dark blue.

A complete hepatic lobule (on the left) and parts of adjacent hepatic lobules (7) are illustrated. The blue-staining interlobular septa (5, 9) contain interlobular branches of the **portal vein (4, 11)**, **bile duct (2, 12)**, and **hepatic artery (3, 13)**, which are collectively considered **portal areas**, portal canals, or portal triads. At the periphery of each lobule can be seen several portal areas within the interlobular septa (5, 9). Within the interlobular septa (5, 9) are also found small lymphatic vessels and nerves, which are small and only occasionally seen.

In the center of each hepatic lobule (7) is the **central vein (1, 8)**. Radiating from each central vein (1, 8) toward the lobule periphery are **plates of hepatic cells (6)**. Located between the hepatic plates (6) are blood channels called **hepatic sinusoids (10)**. Arterial and venous blood mixes in the hepatic sinusoids (10) and then flows toward the central vein (1, 8) of each lobule (7).

Bile is produced by the liver cells. Bile flows through the very small bile canaliculi between the hepatocytes into the interlobular **bile ducts (2, 12)** (see Fig. 16.5).

The interlobular vessels and bile ducts (2 to 4, 11 to 13) are highly branched in the liver. In a cross section of the liver lobule, more than one section of these structures can be seen within a portal area.

FIGURE 16.1 ■ Pig liver (panoramic view, transverse section). Stain: Mallory-Azan. Low magnification.

FIGURE 16.2 | Primate Liver (Panoramic View, Transverse Section)

In the primate or human liver, the connective tissue septa between individual **hepatic lobules (8)** are not as conspicuous as in the pig, and the liver sinusoids are continuous between lobules. Despite these differences, **portal areas** containing interlobular branches of the **portal veins (2, 11), hepatic arteries (3, 13), and bile ducts (1, 12)** are visible around the lobule (8) peripheries in the **interlobular septa (4, 10)**.

This figure illustrates numerous hepatic lobules (8). In the center of each hepatic lobule (8) is the **central vein (6, 9)**. The **hepatic sinusoids (5)** appear between the **plates of hepatic cells (7)** that radiate from the central veins (6, 9) toward the periphery of the hepatic lobule (8). As illustrated in Figure 16.1, branches of the interlobular vessels and bile ducts are seen within the portal areas of a hepatic lobule (8).

FUNCTIONAL CORRELATIONS 16.1 | Liver

The liver performs hundreds of functions. In fact, the liver hepatocytes perform more functions than any other cell in the body. In addition, the liver cells exhibit both endocrine and exocrine roles by secreting substances into a duct and into the blood sinusoids, respectively. In addition, the liver performs vital functions early in life during embryogenesis. In the fetus, the liver is the site of **hemopoiesis,** or blood cell production.

EXOCRINE FUNCTIONS

One major **exocrine function** of hepatocytes is to synthesize and release about 500 to 1,200 ml of **bile** per day. The secreted bile enters the very tiny channels called **bile canaliculi**. From these canaliculi, bile flows through the liver via a system of small ductules and larger ducts that eventually carry the bile from the liver and deliver it to the **gallbladder**. The gallbladder stores and concentrates bile by removal of water. Release of bile from the liver and gallbladder is primarily regulated by regulatory hormones of the digestive tract. Bile flow from the bile duct is increased when a hormone such as **cholecystokinin** is released by the mucosal enteroendocrine cells that are stimulated by dietary fats or fatty meal in the duodenum. Cholecystokinin hormone causes intermittent contraction of smooth muscles in the gallbladder wall and relaxation of the sphincter, expelling the bile and allowing it to enter the duodenum.

Bile salts in the bile do not digest, but instead **emulsify fats** that may have been partially digested in the small intestine (duodenum). This emulsification breaks down the fat into smaller molecules that allows for more efficient digestion of fats by the fat-digesting **pancreatic lipases** that are produced by the pancreas. The digested fats are subsequently absorbed by cells in the small intestine, and the long fatty acid chains eventually enter the blind-ending lymphatic **lacteal** channels located in the lamina propria of individual villi. From the lacteals, fats are carried into larger lymphatic ducts that eventually drain into the major veins and systemic circulation.

Hepatocytes also excrete **bilirubin**, a toxic chemical formed in the body after degradation of worn-out erythrocytes by liver macrophages called **Kupffer cells**. Bilirubin is taken up by hepatocytes from the blood and excreted into bile.

Hepatocytes also have an important role in the immune system. **Antibodies** produced by plasma cells in the intestinal lamina propria are taken up from blood by hepatocytes and transported into bile canaliculi and bile. From here, antibodies enter the intestinal lumen, where they control the intestinal bacterial flora.

ENDOCRINE FUNCTIONS

Hepatocytes are also **endocrine cells**, releasing substances directly into the bloodstream. The arrangement of hepatocytes in a liver lobule allows them to take up, metabolize, accumulate, and store numerous products from the blood. Hepatocytes then release many of the metabolized or secreted products back into the bloodstream, as the blood flows through the sinusoids and comes in direct contact with individual hepatocytes.

FUNCTIONAL CORRELATIONS 16.1 | **Liver** *(Continued)*

The endocrine functions of the liver hepatocytes involve synthesis of most **plasma proteins**, including albumins, lipoproteins, glycoproteins, and the blood-clotting factors prothrombin and fibrinogen. The liver cells also store fats, various vitamins, and carbohydrates as **glycogen**. When the cells of the body need **glucose**, glycogen that is stored in the liver is converted back into glucose and released into the bloodstream.

PHAGOCYTIC FUNCTIONS

Hepatocytes also **detoxify** the blood of drugs and harmful substances as it percolates through the sinusoids. **Kupffer cells** in the sinusoids are specialized liver phagocytes that have originated from blood monocytes. These large, branching cells are filled with lysosomes. They span the sinusoids and filter and phagocytose the particulate material, bacteria, cellular debris, and worn-out or damaged erythrocytes that flow through the sinusoids.

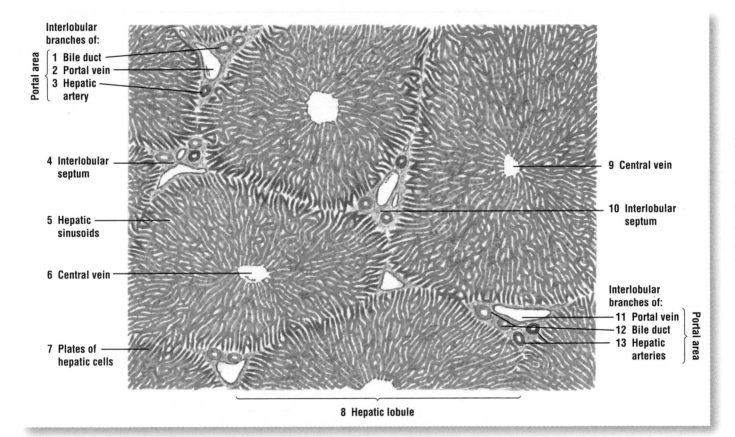

Portal area
- 1 Bile duct
- 2 Portal vein
- 3 Hepatic artery

Interlobular branches of:

4 Interlobular septum

5 Hepatic sinusoids

6 Central vein

7 Plates of hepatic cells

8 Hepatic lobule

9 Central vein

10 Interlobular septum

Interlobular branches of:
- 11 Portal vein
- 12 Bile duct
- 13 Hepatic arteries

Portal area

FIGURE 16.2 ■ Primate liver (panoramic view, transverse section). Stain: hematoxylin and eosin. Low magnification.

FIGURE 16.3 | Bovine Liver: Liver Lobule (Transverse Section)

This lower-magnification photomicrograph of a bovine liver illustrates several hepatic (liver) lobules. The portal area of the hepatic lobule contains the branches of the **portal vein (5)**; the **hepatic artery (6)**; and, normally, a bile duct, which is not seen in this micrograph. From the **central vein (1)** radiate the **plates of hepatic cells (2)** toward the lobule periphery. Located between the plates of hepatic cells (2) are the blood channels called **sinusoids (3)**. The sinusoids (3) convey blood from the portal vein (5) and hepatic artery (6) to the central vein (1). Both the central vein (1) and the sinusoids (3) are lined with a discontinuous and fenestrated type of **endothelium (4)**.

FIGURE 16.4 | Hepatic (Liver) Lobule (Sectional View, Transverse Section)

A section of the hepatic lobule between the **central vein (9)** and the peripheral connective tissue **interlobular septum (1, 6)** of the portal area is illustrated in greater detail. In the interlobular septum (1, 6) are transverse sections of a **portal vein (4), hepatic arteries (3), bile ducts (5)**, and a **lymphatic vessel (2)**. Multiple cross sections of hepatic arteries (3) and bile ducts (5) are attributable either to their branching in the septum or their passage into and out of the septum.

Branches of the portal vein (4) and hepatic artery (3) penetrate the interlobular septum (1, 6) and form the **sinusoids (8, 10)**. The sinusoids (8, 10) are situated between **plates of hepatic cells (7)** and follow their branchings and anastomoses. Discontinuous **endothelial cells (10)** line the sinusoids (8, 10) and the central vein (9). **Blood cells** (erythrocytes and leukocytes) in **sinusoids (8)** drain toward the central vein (9) of each lobule. Also present in the sinusoids (10) are fixed macrophages called Kupffer cells (see Fig. 16.6).

1 Central vein

2 Plates of
hepatic cells

3 Sinusoids

4 Endothelium

5 Portal vein

6 Hepatic artery

FIGURE 16.3 ■ Bovine liver: liver lobule (transverse section). Stain: hematoxylin and eosin. ×30.

7 Plates of hepatic cells

1 Interlobular septum

8 Blood cells in sinusoids

2 Lymphatic vessel

3 Hepatic arteries

9 Central vein

4 Portal vein

5 Bile ducts

6 Interlobular septum

10 Endothelial cells in
sinusoids

FIGURE 16.4 ■ Hepatic (Liver) lobule (sectional view, transverse section). Stain: hematoxylin and eosin. High magnification.

FIGURE 16.5 | Bile Canaliculi in Liver Lobule (Osmic Acid Preparation)

Preparation of a liver section with osmic acid and staining with hematoxylin and eosin reveals the **bile canaliculi (3, 5)**. Bile canaliculi (3, 5) are tiny channels between individual liver (hepatic) cells in the **hepatic plates (4)**. The canaliculi (3, 5) follow an irregular course between the hepatic plates (4) and branch freely within the hepatic plates (4).

The **sinusoids (6)** are lined with discontinuous **endothelial cells (1)**. All sinusoids (6) drain toward and open into the **central vein (2)**.

FIGURE 16.6 | Kupffer Cells in Liver Lobule (India Ink Preparation)

The majority of cells that line the liver **sinusoids (5)** are **endothelial cells (2)**. These small cells have an attenuated cytoplasm and a small nucleus. To demonstrate the phagocytic cells in the liver sinusoids (5), an animal was intravenously injected with India ink. The phagocytic **Kupffer cells (3, 7)** ingest the carbon particles from the ink, which fill their cytoplasm with dark deposits. As a result, Kupffer cells (3, 7) become prominent in the sinusoids (5) between the **hepatic plates (6)**. Kupffer cells (3, 7) are large cells with several processes and an irregular or stellate outline that protrudes into the sinusoids (5). The nuclei of Kupffer cells (3, 7) are obscured by the ingested carbon particles.

On the periphery of the lobule is visible a section of the connective tissue **interlobular septum (1)** and a part of the **bile duct (4)** that is lined with cuboidal cells.

FIGURE 16.7 | Glycogen Granules in Liver Cells (Hepatocytes)

The cytoplasm of liver cells varies in appearance depending on nutritional status. After a meal, liver **hepatocytes (1)** store increased amounts of glycogen in their cytoplasm. With the periodic acid–Schiff stain, the **glycogen granules (2, 4)** in the hepatocyte (1) cytoplasm stain bright red and exhibit an irregular distribution within the cytoplasm.

Also visible in this illustration are hepatic **sinusoids (3)** and flattened **endothelial cells (5)** that line their lumina.

1 Endothelial cells

2 Central vein

3 Bile canaliculi

4 Hepatic plates

5 Bile canaliculi

6 Sinusoids

FIGURE 16.5 ■ Bile canaliculi in liver lobule (osmic acid preparation). Stain: hematoxylin and eosin. High magnification.

1 Interlobular septum

2 Endothelial cells

3 Kupffer cells

4 Bile duct

5 Sinusoids

6 Hepatic plates

7 Kupffer cells

FIGURE 16.6 ■ Kupffer cells in liver lobule (India ink preparation). Stain: hematoxylin and eosin. High magnification.

1 Hepatocytes

2 Glycogen granules

3 Sinusoids

4 Glycogen granules

5 Endothelial cells

FIGURE 16.7 ■ Glycogen granules in liver cells (hepatocytes). Stain: periodic acid–Schiff with blue counterstain for nuclei. Oil immersion.

FIGURE 16.8 | Reticular Fibers in Liver Lobule

Fine reticular **fibers (6, 8)** provide most of the supporting connective tissue of the liver. In this illustration, the reticular fibers stain black, and the liver cells stain pale pink or violet. The reticular fibers **(6, 8)** line the **sinusoids (8)**, support the endothelial cells, and form a denser network of reticular fibers in the wall of the **central vein (7)**. The reticular fibers (6, 8) also merge with the **collagen fibers** in the **interlobular septum (1)**, where they surround the **portal vein (2)** and the **bile duct (3)**.

Also visible in the reticular network are the pink-staining **nuclei of hepatocytes (4)** and the **hepatic plates (5)** that radiate from the central vein (7) toward the interlobular septum (1).

FIGURE 16.9 | Liver Sinusoids, Space of Disse, Hepatocytes, and Endothelial Cells in a Liver Lobule

This high-magnification micrograph shows greater details of the cells and structures that are found in a liver lobule. The **sinusoids (1, 7)** are lined with discontinuous **endothelial cells (6, 8)**. As a result of some shrinkage during the slide preparation, the narrow separations between the endothelial cells (6, 8) and **hepatocytes (9)** show the **space of Disse (3, 5)**. Also visible in the sinusoids (1, 7) are the larger phagocytic **Kupffer cells (4, 10)** that can span the sinusoid (1, 7). Located between the hepatocytes (9) are very tiny channels in the cross section that appear as dots. These are the **bile canaliculi (2)**.

SECTION 2 Pancreas

Exocrine Pancreas

The pancreas is a soft, elongated organ located posterior to the stomach. The **head** of the pancreas lies in the duodenal loop, and the **tail** extends across the abdominal cavity to the spleen. Most of the pancreas is an **exocrine gland**. The exocrine secretory units or acini contain pyramid-shaped **acinar cells**, whose apices are filled with secretory granules. These granules contain the precursors of several pancreatic **digestive enzymes** that are secreted into the intestinal lumen via the excretory duct in an **inactive form**.

The secretory acini of the pancreas are subdivided into **lobules** and bound together by loose connective tissue. The **excretory ducts** in the exocrine pancreas start from within the center of individual acini as pale-staining **centroacinar cells**, which continue with the lining cells of the short **intercalated ducts** that are located outside of the acini. Intercalated ducts from different acini merge to form **intralobular ducts** in the connective tissue, which, in turn, join to form larger **interlobular ducts** that empty into the **main pancreatic duct**. Excretory ducts of the pancreas do not exhibit striations in their cells, and there are no striated ducts.

Endocrine Pancreas

The endocrine units of the pancreas are scattered among the exocrine acini as isolated, pale-staining, and highly vascularized units called **pancreatic islets (of Langerhans)**. Each islet is surrounded by fine fibers of the reticular connective tissue. With special immunocytochemical staining processes, four cell types can be identified in each pancreatic islet: **alpha, beta, delta**, and **pancreatic polypeptide (PP) cells**. The principal cells are the alpha, beta, and delta. Other cells in the pancreatic islets, including the PP cells, are considered minor cells.

Alpha cells constitute about 20% of the islets and are located primarily around the islet periphery. The beta cells are most numerous, constituting about 70% of the islet cells, and are primarily concentrated in the center of the islet. The remaining cell types are few in number and are located in various places throughout the islets.

Supplemental micrographic images are available at **www.thePoint.com/Eroschenko12e** under Digestive System Part IV: Liver, Gallbladder, and Pancreas.

1 Collagen fibers in interlobular septum

2 Portal vein

3 Bile duct

4 Nuclei of hepatocytes

5 Hepatic plates

6 Reticular fibers in wall of central vein

7 Central vein

8 Reticular fibers in wall of sinusoids

FIGURE 16.8 ■ Reticular fibers in liver lobule. Stain: reticulin method. Medium magnification.

1 Sinusoid

2 Bile canaliculi

3 Space of Disse

4 Kupffer cell

5 Space of Disse

6 Endothelial cell

7 Sinusoid

8 Endothelial cell

9 Hepatocytes

10 Kupffer cell

FIGURE 16.9 ■ Liver sinusoids, space of Disse, hepatocytes, and endothelial cells in a liver lobule. Stain: hematoxylin and eosin. ×205.

FIGURE 16.10 | Exocrine and Endocrine Pancreas (Sectional View)

The pancreas is a mixed organ; it contains both endocrine and exocrine components. The exocrine component forms the majority of the pancreas and consists of closely packed secretory **serous acini** and **zymogenic cells (5)** arranged in small lobules. The lobules are surrounded by thin intralobular and **interlobular connective tissue septa (1)** that contain numerous **blood vessels (2, 10); interlobular ducts (6);** nerves; and, occasionally, a sensory receptor called a **Pacinian corpuscle (8)**. Within the mass of serous acini **(5)** are the isolated **cells of pancreatic islets** (of Langerhans) **(3, 11)**. The pancreatic islets **(3, 11)** represent the endocrine portion of the organs and are the characteristic features of the pancreas.

Each pancreatic acinus **(5)** consists of pyramid-shaped, protein-secreting **zymogenic** cells **(5)** that surround a small central lumen. The initial parts of the excretory ducts of the individual acinus **(5)** are visible as pale-staining **centroacinar cells (7, 9)** in the middle of the acinus. The secretory products leave the acini via **intercalated (intralobular) ducts (4)** that have small lumina lined with a low cuboidal epithelium. The centroacinar cells **(7, 9)** are continuous with the epithelium that lines the intercalated ducts **(4)**.

The intercalated ducts **(4)** drain into interlobular ducts **(6)** located in the interlobular connective tissue septa **(4)**. The interlobular ducts **(6)** are lined with a simple cuboidal epithelium that becomes taller and stratified as the ducts increase in size.

Pancreatic islets **(3, 11)** are demarcated from the surrounding exocrine acini **(5)** tissue by a thin layer of reticular fibers. The islets **(3, 11)** are larger than the acini and are compact clusters of epithelial cells permeated by numerous fenestrated **capillaries (11)**. The cells of a pancreatic islet **(3, 7)** are illustrated at a higher magnification in Figures 16.11 and 16.12.

FUNCTIONAL CORRELATIONS 16.2 | Exocrine Pancreas

The exocrine and endocrine functions of the pancreas are performed by separate exocrine and endocrine cells, respectively. The pancreas produces numerous digestive enzymes that exit the gland through a major excretory duct, whereas the different hormones produced by the pancreatic islets are transported from the pancreas via numerous blood vessels.

Both hormones and vagal stimulation regulate pancreatic exocrine secretions. Two intestinal hormones, **secretin** and **cholecystokinin (CCK)**, secreted by the **enteroendocrine (APUD) cells** in the duodenal mucosa into the bloodstream, are the principal hormones that regulate exocrine pancreatic secretions.

In response to the presence of acidic chyme in the small intestine (duodenum), the release of the hormone **secretin** stimulates exocrine pancreatic cells to produce large amounts of a watery fluid rich in **sodium bicarbonate ions**. This fluid, which has little or no enzymatic activity, is primarily produced by **centroacinar cells** in the pancreatic acini and by cells that line the smaller **intercalated ducts**. The main function of this bicarbonate fluid is to neutralize the acidic chyme, stop the action of the proteolytic enzyme pepsin secreted by gastric glands in the stomach, and create a neutral pH in the duodenum for the action of the digestive pancreatic enzymes.

In response to the presence of fats and proteins in the small intestine, CCK is released into the bloodstream. CCK stimulates the acinar cells in the pancreas to secrete large amounts of digestive enzymes: **pancreatic amylase** for carbohydrate digestion, **pancreatic lipase** for lipid digestion, **deoxyribonuclease** and **ribonuclease** for digestion of nucleic acids, and the **proteolytic enzymes trypsinogen, chymotrypsinogen**, and **procarboxypeptidase**.

Pancreatic enzymes are first produced in the acinar cells in an **inactive form**, released after hormonal stimulation, and are activated only in the lumen of the duodenum through the action of the hormone **enterokinase** secreted by the intestinal mucosa. Enterokinase converts trypsinogen to trypsin, and trypsin then converts all other inactive pancreatic enzymes into active digestive enzymes for digestion of food products in the chyme.

1 Interlobular connective tissue

2 Blood vessel

3 Cells of pancreatic islet

4 Intercalated duct

5 Serous acini and zymogenic cells

6 Interlobular duct

7 Centroacinar cell

8 Pacinian corpuscle

9 Centroacinar cell

10 Blood vessel

11 Capillaries in pancreatic islet

FIGURE 16.10 ■ Exocrine and endocrine pancreas (sectional view). Stain: hematoxylin and eosin. Low magnification.

FIGURE 16.11 | Pancreatic Islet

A pale-staining, **pancreatic islet** (of Langerhans) **(2)** is illustrated at a higher magnification. The endocrine cells of the islet (2) are arranged in cords and clumps, between which are found fine connective tissue fibers and an extensive **capillary (3)** network. A thin **connective tissue capsule (5)** separates the endocrine pancreas from the surrounding exocrine **serous acini (4, 6)**. Some of the serous acini (4, 6) exhibit a centrally located cell, the **centroacinar cells (4, 6)**, which form the initial part of the duct system that leads to the excretory intercalated duct. In contrast to secretory acini in other glands, there are no myoepithelial cells that surround the secretory acini in the pancreas.

In routine histologic preparations, the cells that secrete different hormones from the pancreatic islet (2) cannot be identified. However, using different staining techniques, the hormone-secreting cells can be identified. These cells are illustrated in Figures 16.12 and 16.14.

FIGURE 16.12 | Pancreatic Islet (Special Preparation)

This pancreas has been prepared with a special stain to distinguish the glucagon-secreting **alpha** (A) **cells (1)** from the insulin-secreting **beta** (B) **cells (3)**. The cytoplasm of alpha cells (1) stains pink, whereas the cytoplasm of beta cells (3) stains blue. The alpha cells (1) are situated more peripherally in the islet, and the beta cells (3) more in the center. Also, beta cells (3) predominate, constituting about 70% of the islet. Delta (D) cells (not illustrated) are also present in the islets. These cells are least abundant, have a variable cell shape, and may occur anywhere in the pancreatic islet.

Capillaries (2) around the endocrine cells demonstrate the rich vascularity of the pancreatic islets. The thin **connective tissue capsule (4)** separates the islet cells from the **serous acini (6)**. **Centroacinar cells (5)** are visible in some of the acini.

FUNCTIONAL CORRELATIONS 16.3 | Endocrine Pancreas

The endocrine components of the pancreas are scattered throughout the organ as islands of endocrine cells called **pancreatic islets (of Langerhans)**. Pancreatic islets secrete two major hormones that regulate blood glucose levels and glucose metabolism.

Alpha cells in the pancreatic islets produce the hormone **glucagon**, which is released in response to low levels of glucose in the blood. Glucagon elevates blood glucose levels by accelerating the conversion of glycogen, amino acids, and fatty acids in the liver cells into glucose, which is then released into the bloodstream.

Beta cells in pancreatic islets produce the hormone **insulin**, whose release is stimulated by elevated blood glucose levels after a meal. Insulin lowers blood glucose levels by accelerating membrane transport of glucose into liver cells, muscle cells, and adipose cells. Insulin also accelerates the conversion of glucose into glycogen in liver cells. The effects of insulin on blood glucose levels are exactly opposite to that of glucagon

Delta cells secrete the hormone **somatostatin**. This hormone decreases and inhibits secretory activities of both alpha (glucagon-secreting) and beta (insulin-secreting) cells through local action within the pancreatic islets.

Pancreatic polypeptide cells produce the hormone **pancreatic polypeptide**, which inhibits the production of pancreatic enzymes and alkaline secretions from the acinar cells.

1 Intercalated duct

2 Endocrine cells of pancreatic islet

3 Capillaries

4 Centroacinar cell in serous acinus

5 Connective tissue capsule

6 Centroacinar cell in serous acinus

FIGURE 16.11 ■ Pancreatic islet. Stain: hematoxylin and eosin. High magnification.

1 Alpha cells

2 Capillary

3 Beta cells

4 Connective tissue capsule

5 Centroacinar cells

6 Serous acini

FIGURE 16.12 ■ Pancreatic islet (special preparation). Stain: Gomori chrome alum hematoxylin and phloxine. High magnification.

FIGURE 16.13 | Pancreas: Endocrine (Pancreatic Islet) and Exocrine Regions

This high-magnification photomicrograph of the pancreas illustrates both exocrine and endocrine components. In the center is the light-staining endocrine **pancreatic islet (3)**. A thin **connective tissue capsule (2)** separates the pancreatic islet (3) from the exocrine **secretory acini (5)**. The pancreatic islet (3) is vascularized by blood vessels and **capillaries (6)**. The exocrine secretory acini (5) consist of pyramid-shaped cells arranged around small lumina in whose centers are seen one or more light-staining **centroacinar cells (4)**.

The smallest excretory duct in the pancreas is the **intercalated duct (1)** lined with a simple cuboidal epithelium.

FIGURE 16.14 | Immunohistochemical Preparation of Mammalian Pancreatic Islet

With immunohistochemical preparation, it is possible to differentiate the major cell types in a pancreatic islet. This high-magnification image shows a more precise distribution of the two major cell types in the pancreatic islet. The **glucagon-producing cells**, the **A cells**, are stained bright **red**; they line the periphery of the islet. The **insulin-producing cells**, the **B cells**, are stained bright **green**. They are located on the inside of the islet and are surrounded by the peripheral A cells.

1 Intercalated duct

2 Connective tissue capsule

3 Pancreatic islet

4 Centroacinar cells

5 Secretory acini

6 Capillaries

FIGURE 16.13 ■ Pancreas: endocrine (pancreatic islet) and exocrine regions. Stain: periodic acid–Schiff and hematoxylin. ×80.

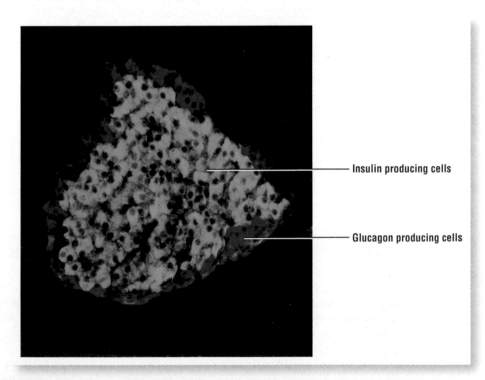

Insulin producing cells

Glucagon producing cells

FIGURE 16.14 ■ Immunohistochemical preparation of mammalian pancreatic islet. Courtesy of Dr. Ernest Adeghate, Professor and Chairman, Department of Anatomy, Faculty of Medicine and Health Sciences, UAE University, Al Ain, United Arab Emirates. ×200.

SECTION 3   Gallbladder

Gallbladder

The gallbladder is a small, hollow organ attached to the inferior surface of the liver. Bile is produced by liver hepatocytes that leaves the liver and flows to, is stored, and concentrated in the gallbladder. Upon hormonal stimulation, bile leaves the gallbladder via the cystic duct and enters the duodenum via the **common bile duct** through the **major duodenal papilla**, a fingerlike protrusion of the duodenal wall into the lumen.

The gallbladder is not a gland, because its main function is to store and concentrate bile by absorbing its water. Bile is released into the digestive tract as a result of hormonal stimulation after a meal that contains fatty foods. When the gallbladder is empty, the mucosa exhibits deep **folds**.

 Supplemental micrographic images are available at **www.thePoint.com/Eroschenko12e** under Digestive System Part IV: Liver, Gallbladder, and Pancreas.

FIGURE 16.15 | Wall of the Gallbladder

The gallbladder is a muscular sac. Its wall consists of the mucosa, the muscularis externa, and the adventitia or serosa. The wall of the gallbladder does not contain a muscularis mucosae or submucosa.

The mucosa consists of a **simple columnar epithelium (1)** and the underlying connective tissue **lamina propria (2)** that contains loose connective tissue, some diffuse lymphatic tissue, and blood vessels—**venule and arteriole (9)**. In the nondistended state, the gallbladder wall shows temporary **mucosal folds (7)** that disappear when the gallbladder becomes distended with bile. The mucosal folds (7) resemble the villi in the small intestine; however, they vary in size and shape and display an irregular arrangement. Between the mucosal folds (7) are found **diverticula, or crypts (3, 8)** that often form deep indentations in the mucosa. In cross section, the diverticula, or crypts (3, 8) in the lamina propria (2) resemble tubular glands. However, there are no glands in the gallbladder proper, except in the neck region of the organ.

External to the lamina propria (2) is the muscularis of the gallbladder with bundles of randomly oriented **smooth muscle fibers (10)** that do not show distinct layers and interlacing **elastic fibers (4)**.

Surrounding the bundles of smooth muscle fibers (10) is a thick layer of dense **connective tissue (6)** that contains large blood vessels—**artery and vein (11)**—lymphatics, and **nerves (5)**.

Serosa (12) covers the entire unattached gallbladder surface. Where the gallbladder is attached to the liver surface, this connective tissue layer is the adventitia.

FUNCTIONAL CORRELATIONS 16.4 | Gallbladder

The primary functions of the gallbladder are to collect, store, concentrate, and expel **bile** when it is needed for emulsification of fat. Bile is continually produced by liver hepatocytes and transported via the excretory ducts to the gallbladder for storage. Here, sodium is actively transported through the simple columnar epithelium of the gallbladder into the extracellular connective tissue, creating a strong osmotic pressure. Water and chloride ions passively follow, producing a highly concentrated bile.

Release of bile into the duodenum is under hormonal control. In response to the entrance of dietary fats into the proximal duodenum, the hormone **cholecystokinin (CCK)** is released into the bloodstream by **enteroendocrine cells** located in the intestinal mucosa. CCK is carried in the bloodstream to the gallbladder, where it causes strong, rhythmic contractions of the smooth muscle in the gallbladder wall. At the same time, the smooth **sphincter muscles** around the neck of gallbladder relax. The combination of these two actions forces the bile to flow into the duodenum via the common bile duct.

1 Simple columnar epithelium

2 Lamina propria

3 Diverticula, or crypts

4 Elastic fibers

5 Nerves

6 Connective tissue

7 Mucosal folds

8 Diverticula, or crypts

9 Venule and arteriole

10 Smooth muscle fibers

11 Artery and vein

12 Serosa

FIGURE 16.15 ■ Wall of the gallbladder. Stain: hematoxylin and eosin. Low magnification.

Digestive System Part IV: The Accessory Organs

Liver

- Located outside the digestive tube in strategic position
- All absorbed nutrients pass through liver via portal vein and hepatic sinusoids
- Has dual blood supply: portal vein and hepatic artery
- Is organized into repeating liver lobules, with central vein in the center of lobule
- Plates of liver cells (hepatocytes) radiate to lobule periphery from central vein
- Portal vein, hepatic artery, and bile duct in lobule periphery are portal areas
- Venous and arterial blood mix in sinusoids and flow toward central vein
- Hepatic sinusoids lined with discontinuous and fenestrated endothelium
- Substances in blood contact hepatocytes via subendothelial perisinusoidal space of Disse
- Phagocytic Kupffer cells and fat-storing hepatic stellate (Ito) cells are associated with sinusoids
- Performs more functions than any other organ
- In fetus is the site for hemopoiesis or blood cell formation
- Individual liver cells perform both exocrine and endocrine functions

Exocrine Functions

- Hepatocytes secrete bile into tiny channels, the bile canaliculi
- Bile flows in bile canaliculi toward bile ducts in portal areas in opposite direction to blood
- Bile is stored in gallbladder, where water is removed and bile is concentrated
- Hormone cholecystokinin regulates the release of bile from liver and gallbladder
- Enteroendocrine cells in intestinal mucosa release cholecystokinin as fats in chyme enter duodenum
- Cholecystokinin causes gallbladder contraction and expulsion of bile
- Bile emulsifies fats for more efficient digestion by pancreatic lipases
- Fats are absorbed into lymphatic lacteals in the villi of small intestine
- Hepatocytes excrete bilirubin into bile and move antibodies from blood into bile

Endocrine Functions

- Take up, metabolize, accumulate, and store products from blood

- Synthesize and release most plasma proteins, including blood-clotting factors
- Store glycogen and release as glucose when needed

Phagocytic Functions

- Detoxify drugs and harmful substances that flow through sinusoids
- Specialized liver macrophages, Kupffer cells, line the sinusoids
- Kupffer cells filter and phagocytose debris and worn-out red blood cells

Pancreas

Exocrine

- Head of organ lies in the duodenal loop and tail extends to the spleen
- Exocrine component forms majority of the organ and is composed of serous acini
- Acinar cells filled with granules that contain digestive enzymes
- Acini contain pale-staining centroacinar cells in their lumina from which excretory ducts start
- Centroacinar cells continuous with cells of short intercalated ducts
- Excretory ducts do not have striations in their cells and no striated ducts
- Neural and hormones secretin and cholecystokinin regulate exocrine secretions
- Intestinal enteroendocrine cells release hormones when acidic chyme is present
- Secretin stimulates sodium bicarbonate production by centroacinar cells and intercalated duct cells
- Alkaline sodium bicarbonate fluid neutralizes acidic chyme for pancreatic enzymes
- Cholecystokinin released when fats and proteins are present in chyme
- Cholecystokinin stimulates production and release of numerous pancreatic digestive enzymes
- Enzymes produced and released in inactive form and activated first in duodenum
- Trypsinogen from pancreas converted to trypsin by intestinal mucosa hormone enterokinase
- Trypsin converts all pancreatic enzymes into active digestive enzymes

Endocrine

- Endocrine portion in the form of isolated pancreatic islets among exocrine acini

- Each pancreatic islet is surrounded and separated by fine reticular fibers
- Four cell types present in pancreatic islets: alpha, beta, delta, and pancreatic polypeptide cells
- Alpha cells produce glucagon in response to low sugar levels
- Glucagon elevates blood glucose by accelerating conversion of glycogen in liver
- Beta cells produce insulin during elevated glucose levels
- Insulin lowers blood glucose by inducing glucose transport into liver, muscle, and adipose cells
- Delta cells produce somatostatin, which inhibits the activity of both alpha and beta cells

- Pancreatic polypeptide cells inhibit enzymatic and alkaline pancreatic secretions

Gallbladder

- Hollow organ inferior to the liver designed to store and concentrate bile
- Bile produced by liver hepatocytes is delivered by major excretory ducts
- Sodium is actively transported out, water and chloride follow, and bile is concentrated
- Bile is released in response to fats in the duodenum due to action of cholecystokinin
- Sphincter muscles relax and gallbladder contraction forces bile into the duodenum

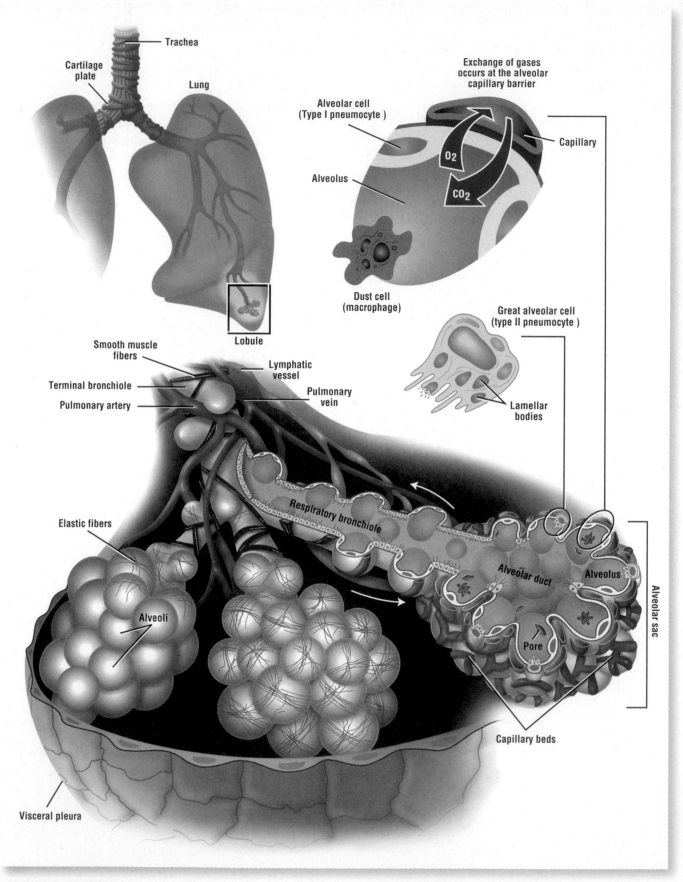

OVERVIEW FIGURE 17.1 ■ A section of the lung is illustrated in three dimensions and in transverse section, with emphasis on the internal structure of the respiratory bronchiole and alveolar cells.

Respiratory System

CHAPTER 17

Components of the Respiratory System

The respiratory system consists of **lungs** and numerous **air passages**, or tubes, of various sizes that lead to and from each lung. In addition, the system consists of a conducting portion and a respiratory portion. Also, located in the air passages of the nose are neuroepithelial sensory cells that detect odor, or smell, as the air passes to the lungs.

The **conducting portion** of the respiratory system consists of passageways outside (extrapulmonary) and inside (intrapulmonary) of the lungs that conduct air for gaseous exchange to and from the lungs. In contrast, the **respiratory portion** consists of passageways within the lungs that not only conduct the air but also allow for **respiration** or gaseous exchange.

The extrapulmonary passages, which include the trachea and different sizes of bronchi, are lined with a distinct **pseudostratified ciliated epithelium** containing numerous **goblet cells**. As the passageways enter the lungs, the bronchi undergo extensive branching, and their diameters become progressively smaller. There is also a gradual decrease in the height of the lining epithelium, the amount of cilia, and the number of goblet cells in these tubules. The **bronchioles** represent the terminal portion of the conducting passageways. These give rise to the **respiratory bronchioles**, which represent the **transition zone** between air conduction and respiratory portions.

The **respiratory portion** consists of respiratory bronchioles, alveolar ducts, alveolar sacs, and alveoli. Gaseous exchange in the lungs takes place in the **alveoli**, the very thin terminal air spaces of the respiratory system. In the alveoli, goblet cells are absent and the lining epithelium is thin **simple squamous.** The alveoli are in very close proximity to the capillaries.

Olfactory Epithelium

As the air enters the lungs, it first passes either through the mouth or through the nasal cavity. Located in the superior and lateral regions in the roof of the nose are the bony nasal shelves called **conchae**. Lining this region is a highly specialized pseudostratified epithelium called the **olfactory epithelium**, which detects and transmits odors to the brain. This epithelium consists of three cell types: supportive (sustentacular), basal, and olfactory (sensory). Located below the epithelium in the connective tissue are the **serous olfactory (Bowman) glands**. In contrast to the respiratory epithelium that can be located adjacent to the olfactory epithelium, the pseudostratified olfactory epithelium is distinguished by its lack of goblet cells or the presence of motile cilia on the surface of its cells.

Olfactory cells are the **sensory bipolar neurons** that are distributed between the more **apical supportive cells** and the **basal cells** of the olfactory epithelium. The olfactory cells span the thickness of the olfactory epithelium and end at the surface of the olfactory epithelium as small, round bulbs called the **olfactory vesicles**. Radiating from each olfactory vesicle are long, **nonmotile olfactory cilia** that lie parallel to the epithelial surface. These cilia are nonmotile and function as odor receptors. The base of the olfactory cells convert to axons that leave the epithelium by continuing through the basement membrane, converge in the connective tissue below the epithelium to form bundle of nerve fibers that pass through the ethmoid bone of the skull, and synapse in the olfactory bulb of the brain (olfactory, or cranial nerve I).

In the connective tissue directly below the olfactory epithelium are visible **olfactory nerves, olfactory (Bowman) glands**, blood vessels, lymphatic vessels, and other cellular components of the connective tissue. Olfactory (Bowman) glands produce a serous fluid that continually bathes the olfactory cilia and serves as a solvent to dissolve the odor molecules for stimulation of the olfactory cells and odor detection.

Respiratory System—The Conducting Portion

The conducting portion of the respiratory system consists of the nasal cavities, the pharynx, the larynx, the trachea, the extrapulmonary bronchi, and a series of solid intrapulmonary bronchi and bronchioles with decreasing diameters that eventually end as **terminal bronchioles**. **Hyaline cartilage** provides structural support and ensures that the larger air passageways are always patent (open). Starting with the trachea, incomplete C-shaped **hyaline cartilage rings** encircle the tube. Elastic and smooth muscle fibers, called the trachealis muscle, bridge the space between the ends of the hyaline cartilage. The ends of the C-shaped cartilage rings of the trachea face posteriorly and are located adjacent to the esophagus.

As the trachea divides into **bronchi** and the bronchi enter the lungs, the C-shaped hyaline cartilage rings are replaced by irregular **hyaline cartilage plates** that encircle the lumen of the intrapulmonary bronchi. As the bronchi continue to divide and decrease in size, the cartilage plates also decrease in size and number. When the diameters of bronchioles decrease to about 1 mm, cartilage plates completely disappear from conducting passageways. Terminal bronchioles represent the final and solid conducting passageways and have diameters ranging from 0.5 to 1.0 mm. There are between 20 and 25 generations of branching of intrapulmonary bronchi before the passageways reach the size of terminal bronchioles.

The larger bronchioles are lined with a tall, **ciliated pseudostratified epithelium** that is similar to that of the trachea and bronchi. As the tubular size decreases, the epithelial height is gradually reduced, and the epithelium becomes a **simple ciliated epithelium**. The epithelium of larger bronchioles also contains numerous **goblet cells**. The number of these cells, however, gradually decreases with the decreasing tubule size; the goblet cells are absent in the epithelium of terminal bronchioles.

Smaller terminal bronchioles are lined only with a **simple cuboidal epithelium**. In place of the goblet cells, another type of cells, called **Clara cells**, is found with the ciliated cells in the terminal and respiratory bronchioles. Clara cells are nonciliated, secretory cuboidal cells with dome-shaped apices that protrude into the lumen. Clara cells increase in number as ciliated cells decrease in the small bronchioles.

Respiratory System—The Respiratory Portion

The respiratory portion of the respiratory system is the distal continuation of the conducting portion and starts with the air passageways where respiration or gaseous exchange can occur. Terminal bronchioles branch to give rise to **respiratory bronchioles**, which are characterized by thin-walled outpockets called **alveoli**. This is the first region of the respiratory tube where respiration can take place. The respiratory bronchioles represent the **transitional zone** where air conduction and gaseous exchange or respiration can take place.

Respiration can occur only in **alveoli** because the barrier between inspired air in the alveoli and venous blood in capillaries is extremely thin. Alveoli are the final air spaces of the respiratory system and each alveolus is surrounded by capillary plexuses that bring blood close to the inspired air inside the alveoli for gaseous exchange. Other intrapulmonary structures in which respiration occurs are the **alveolar ducts** and **alveolar sacs**.

In addition to the cells in the passageways, there are other cell types in the lung. The alveoli contain two cell types. The most abundant cells are the squamous **type I alveolar cells, or type I pneumocytes**. These are extremely squamous cells that line all alveolar surfaces. Interspersed among the squamous alveolar cells either singly or in small groups are the **type II alveolar cells, or type II pneumocytes**. Lung **macrophages**, derived from circulating blood monocytes, are also found both in the connective tissue of alveolar walls, or interalveolar septa (**alveolar macrophages**), and in the alveoli (**dust cells**). Also present in the interalveolar septa are extensive capillary networks, pulmonary arteries, pulmonary veins, lymphatic ducts, and nerves (Overview Fig. 17.1).

 Supplemental micrographic images are available at **www.thePoint.com/Eroschenko12e** under Respiratory System.

FIGURE 17.1 | Olfactory Mucosa and Superior Concha (Panoramic View)

The olfactory mucosa is located in the roof of the nasal cavity, on each side of the dividing septum, and on the surface of the **superior concha (1)**, one of the bony shelves in the nasal cavity.

The olfactory **epithelium (2, 6)** (see Figs. 17.2 and 17.3) is specialized for the reception of smell. As a result, it appears different from the respiratory epithelium. The olfactory epithelium (2, 6) is a pseudostratified tall columnar epithelium without goblet cells and without motile cilia, in contrast to the respiratory epithelium.

The underlying lamina propria contains the branched tubuloacinar **olfactory (Bowman) glands (4, 5)**. These glands produce a serous secretion, in contrast to the mixed mucous and serous secretions produced by glands in the rest of the nasal cavity. Small nerves that are located in the lamina propria are the **olfactory nerves (3, 7)**. The olfactory nerves (3, 7) represent the aggregated afferent axons that leave the olfactory cells and continue into the cranial cavity, where they synapse in the olfactory (cranial) nerves.

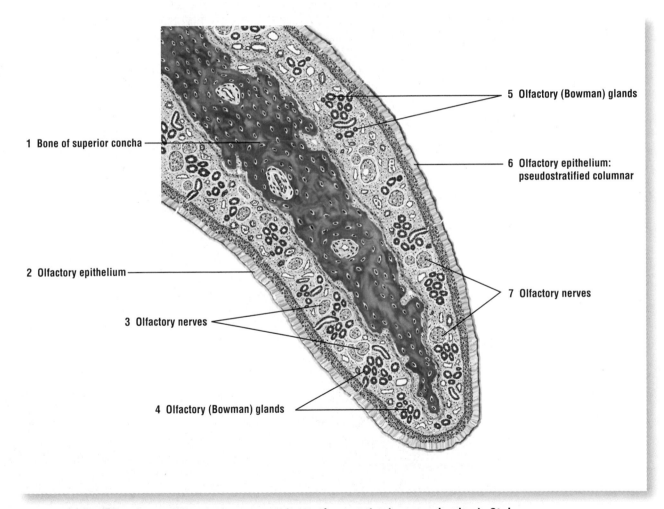

1 Bone of superior concha

2 Olfactory epithelium

3 Olfactory nerves

4 Olfactory (Bowman) glands

5 Olfactory (Bowman) glands

6 Olfactory epithelium: pseudostratified columnar

7 Olfactory nerves

FIGURE 17.1 ■ Olfactory mucosa and superior concha (panoramic view). Stain: hematoxylin and eosin. Low magnification.

FIGURE 17.2 | Olfactory Mucosa: Details of a Transitional Area

This illustration depicts a transition between the **olfactory epithelium (1)** and the **respiratory epithelium (9)**. In the transition region, the histologic differences between these epithelia are obvious. The olfactory epithelium (1) is a tall, pseudostratified columnar epithelium composed of three different cell types: supportive, basal, and neuroepithelial olfactory cells. The individual cell outlines are difficult to distinguish in a routine histologic preparation; however, the location and shape of nuclei allow identification of the cell types.

The supportive, or **sustentacular cells (3),** are elongated, with oval nuclei situated more apically (or superficially) in the epithelium. The **olfactory cells (4)** have oval or round nuclei that are located between the nuclei of the supportive cells (3) and the **basal cells (5)**. The apices and bases of the olfactory cells (4) are slender. The apical surfaces of the olfactory cells (4) contain slender, nonmotile microvilli that extend into the **mucus (2)** that covers the epithelial surface. The basal cells (5) are short cells located at the base of the epithelium between the supportive (3) and olfactory cells (4).

Extending from the bases of the olfactory cells (4) are axons that pass into the **lamina propria (6)** as bundles of unmyelinated **olfactory nerves,** or **fila olfactoria (14)**. The olfactory nerves (14) leave the nasal cavity and pass into the olfactory bulbs at the base of the brain.

The transition from the olfactory epithelium (1) to the respiratory epithelium (9) is abrupt. The respiratory epithelium (9) is a pseudostratified columnar epithelium with distinct **cilia (10)** and many **goblet cells (11)**. Also, in the illustrated transition area, the height of the respiratory epithelium (9) is similar to that of the olfactory epithelium (1). In other regions of the tract, the respiratory epithelium (9) is reduced in comparison to the olfactory epithelium (1).

The underlying lamina propria (6) contains capillaries, lymphatic vessels, **arterioles (8), venules (13)**, and branched, tubuloacinar serous **olfactory (Bowman) glands (7)**. The olfactory glands (7) deliver their secretions through narrow excretory **ducts (12)** that penetrate the olfactory epithelium (1). The secretions from the olfactory glands (7) moisten the epithelial surface, dissolve the molecules of odoriferous substances, and stimulate the olfactory cells (4).

1 Olfactory epithelium

2 Surface mucus

3 Nuclei of supportive cells

4 Nuclei of olfactory cells

5 Nuclei of basal cells

6 Lamina propria

7 Olfactory (Bowman) glands

8 Arteriole

9 Respiratory epithelium

10 Cilia

11 Goblet cells

12 Ducts of olfactory (Bowman) glands

13 Venule

14 Olfactory nerves (fila olfactoria)

FIGURE 17.2 ■ Olfactory mucosa: details of a transitional area. Stain: hematoxylin and eosin. High magnification.

FIGURE 17.3 | Olfactory Mucosa in the Nose: Transition Area

In the superior region of the nasal cavity, the **respiratory epithelium** changes abruptly into the **olfactory epithelium**, as shown in this higher-power photomicrograph.

The respiratory epithelium is lined with motile **cilia (1)** and contains **goblet cells (2)**. The olfactory epithelium lacks cilia (1) and goblet cells (2). Instead, it exhibits nuclei of **supportive cells (5)**, located near the epithelial surface; nuclei of odor receptive **olfactory cells (6)**, located more in the center of the epithelium; and **basal cells (7)**, located close to the **basement membrane (3)**.

Below the olfactory epithelium in the connective tissue lamina propria (4) are blood vessels (9), olfactory nerves (10), and olfactory (Bowman) glands (8).

FUNCTIONAL CORRELATIONS 17.1 | Olfactory Epithelium

To detect odors, odoriferous substances must first be dissolved. The dissolved odor molecules then bind to odor receptor molecules on the **olfactory cilia** and stimulate the odor-binding **receptors** on the nonmotile cilia of the olfactory epithelium to conduct impulses. The unmyelinated afferent axons of olfactory cells leave the olfactory epithelium at the base to form numerous small **olfactory nerve bundles** in the connective tissue of the lamina propria. Impulses from olfactory cells are conducted in these nerve bundles through the ethmoid bone in the skull and synapse in the **olfactory bulbs** of the brain, which are located in the skull above the nasal cavity. From here, neurons relay the information to higher centers in the cortex of the brain for odor interpretation.

Olfactory epithelium is kept moist by a watery secretion produced by serous tubuloacinar **olfactory (Bowman) glands** located directly below the epithelium in the lamina propria. This secretion, delivered via ducts through the olfactory epithelium, continually washes the surface of olfactory epithelium. In this manner, odor molecules are trapped, dissolved in the secreted fluid, and are then washed away by the new fluid, allowing the receptor cells to detect and respond to new odors.

The supportive cells form junctional complexes with the adjacent olfactory cells and provide structural support for the olfactory cells, whereas the basal cells function as stem cells. Basal cells serve as stem cells and can give rise to new olfactory cells and supportive cells of the olfactory epithelium.

Respiratory epithelium   Olfactory epithelium

1 Cilia

2 Goblet cells

3 Basement
  membrane

5 Supportive cells

6 Olfactory cells

7 Basal cells

8 Olfactory
  (Bowman) glands

9 Blood vessel

10 Olfactory
   nerves

4 Lamina
  propria

FIGURE 17.3 ▪ Olfactory mucosa in the nose: transition area. Stain: Mallory-Azan. ×80.

FIGURE 17.4 | Epiglottis (Longitudinal Section)

The epiglottis is the superior portion of the larynx that projects upward from the larynx's anterior wall. It has both a lingual and a laryngeal surface.

A central **elastic cartilage of the epiglottis (3)** forms the framework of the epiglottis. Its **lingual mucosa (2)** (anterior side) is lined with a **stratified squamous nonkeratinized epithelium (1)**. The underlying lamina propria merges with the connective tissue **perichondrium (4)** of the elastic cartilage of the epiglottis (3).

The lingual mucosa (2) with its stratified squamous epithelium (1) covers the apex of the epiglottis and about half of the **laryngeal mucosa (7)** (posterior side). Toward the base of the epiglottis on the laryngeal surface (7), the lining stratified squamous epithelium (1) changes to **pseudostratified ciliated columnar epithelium (8)**. Located below the epithelium in the **lamina propria (6)** on the laryngeal side (7) of the epiglottis are tubuloacinar **seromucous glands (6)**.

In addition to the tongue, **taste buds (5)** and solitary lymphatic nodules may be observed in the lingual epithelium (2) or laryngeal epithelium (7).

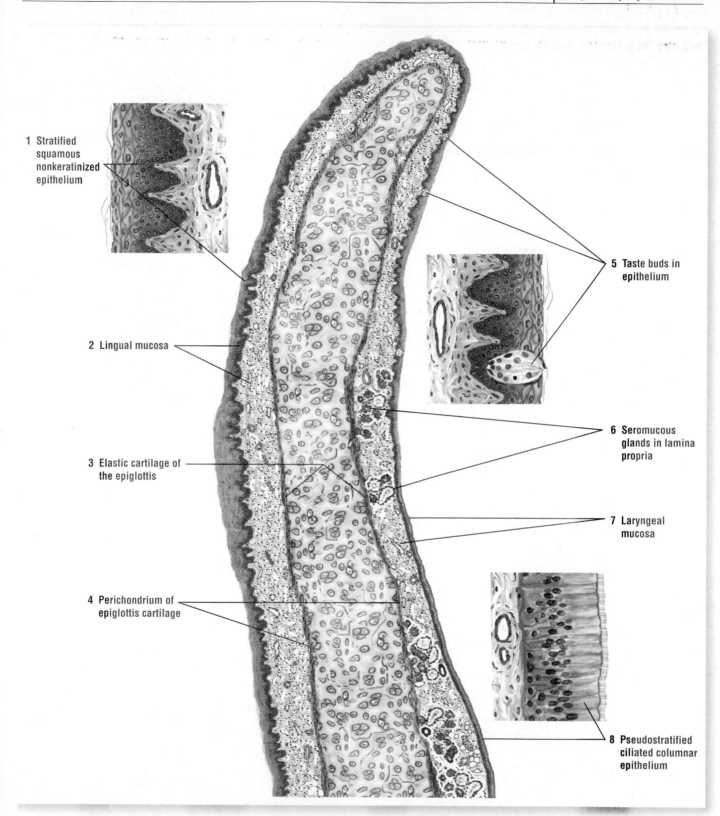

1 Stratified squamous nonkeratinized epithelium

2 Lingual mucosa

3 Elastic cartilage of the epiglottis

4 Perichondrium of epiglottis cartilage

5 Taste buds in epithelium

6 Seromucous glands in lamina propria

7 Laryngeal mucosa

8 Pseudostratified ciliated columnar epithelium

FIGURE 17.4 ■ Epiglottis (longitudinal section). Stain: hematoxylin and eosin. Low magnification. Insets: high magnification.

FIGURE 17.5 | Larynx (Frontal Section)

This image illustrates a vertical section through one half of the larynx.

The false **(superior) vocal fold (9)**, also called the vocal cord, is covered by the mucosa that is continuous with the posterior surface of the epiglottis. As in the epiglottis, the false vocal fold (9) is lined with a **pseudostratified ciliated columnar epithelium (7)** with goblet cells. In the **lamina propria (3)** are numerous and mixed **seromucous glands (8)**. Excretory ducts from these mixed glands (8) open onto the epithelial surface (7). Numerous **lymphatic nodules (2), blood vessels (1)**, and **adipose cells (1)** are also located in the lamina propria (3) of the false vocal fold (9).

The **ventricle (10)** is a deep indentation and recess that separates the false (superior) vocal fold (9) from the **true (inferior) vocal fold (11 to 13)**. The mucosa in the wall of the ventricle (10) is similar to that of the false vocal fold (9). Lymphatic nodules (2) are more numerous in this area and are sometimes called the laryngeal tonsils. The lamina propria (3) blends with the **perichondrium (5)** of the hyaline **thyroid cartilage (4)**. There is no distinct submucosa. The lower wall of the ventricle (10) makes the transition to the true vocal fold (11 to 13).

The mucosa of the true vocal fold (11 to 13) is lined with a nonkeratinized **stratified squamous epithelium (11)** and a thin, dense lamina propria devoid of glands, lymphatic tissue, or blood vessels. At the apex of the true vocal fold is the **vocalis ligament (12)** with dense elastic fibers that extend into the adjacent lamina propria and the skeletal **vocalis muscle (13)**. The skeletal thyroarytenoid muscle and the thyroid cartilage (4) constitute the remaining wall.

The epithelium in the lower larynx changes to **pseudostratified ciliated columnar epithelium (15)**, and the lamina propria contains mixed **seromucous glands (14)**. The hyaline **cricoid cartilage (6)** is the lowermost cartilage of the larynx.

1 Arteriole, venule, and adpiose cells

7 Pseudostratified ciliated epithelium

8 Seromucous glands

2 Lymphatic nodules

9 False vocal cord

3 Lamina propria

10 Ventricle

4 Thyroid cartilage

11 Stratified squamous epithelium

12 Vocalis ligament

True vocal fold

13 Vocalis muscle

5 Perichondrium

14 Seromucous glands

15 Pseudostratified ciliated epithelium

6 Cricoid cartilage

FIGURE 17.5 ■ Larynx (frontal section). Stain: hematoxylin and eosin. Low magnification.

FIGURE 17.6 | Trachea (Panoramic View, Transverse Section)

The wall of the trachea consists of mucosa, submucosa, hyaline cartilage, and adventitia. The trachea is kept patent (open) by C-shaped **hyaline cartilage (3)** rings. Hyaline cartilage (3) is surrounded by the dense connective tissue **perichondrium (9)**, which merges with the **submucosa (4)** on one side and the **adventitia (1)** on the other. Numerous **nerves (6), blood vessels (8)**, and **adipose tissue (2)** are located in the adventitia.

The gap between the posterior ends of the hyaline cartilage (3) is filled by the smooth **trachealis muscle (7)**. The trachealis muscle (7) lies in the connective tissue deep to the **elastic membrane (14)** of the mucosa. Most of the trachealis muscle (7) fibers insert into the perichondrium (9) that covers the hyaline cartilage (3).

The lumen of the trachea is lined with a **pseudostratified ciliated columnar epithelium (12)** with goblet cells. The underlying **lamina propria (13)** contains fine connective tissue fibers, diffuse lymphatic tissue, and occasional solitary lymphatic nodules. Located deeper in the lamina propria (13) is the longitudinal elastic membrane (14) formed by elastic fibers. The elastic membrane (14) divides the lamina propria (13) from the submucosa (4), which contains loose connective tissue that is similar to that of lamina propria (13). In the submucosa (4) are found the tubuloacinar **seromucous tracheal glands (10)** whose **excretory ducts (11)** pass through the lamina propria (13) to the tracheal lumen.

The mucosa exhibits **mucosal folds (5)** along the posterior wall of the trachea where the hyaline cartilage (3) is absent. The seromucous tracheal glands (10) that are present in the submucosa can extend and be seen in the adventitia (1).

FIGURE 17.7 | Tracheal Wall (Sectional View)

A section of tracheal wall between the **hyaline cartilage (1)** and the lining **pseudostratified ciliated columnar epithelium (8)** with **goblet cells (10)** is illustrated at a higher magnification. A thin **basement membrane (9)** separates the lining epithelium (8) from the **lamina propria (11)**.

Below the lamina propria (11) is the connective tissue **submucosa (6)**, in which are found the **seromucous tracheal glands (3)**. A **serous demilune (7)** surrounds a mucous acinus of the seromucous tracheal glands (3). The **excretory duct (5)** of the tracheal glands (3) is lined with a simple cuboidal epithelium and extends through the lamina propria (11) to the epithelial surface (8).

The adjacent hyaline cartilage (1) is surrounded by the connective tissue **perichondrium (2)**. The larger **chondrocytes in lacunae (4)** that are located in the interior of the hyaline cartilage (1) become progressively flatter toward the perichondrium (2), which gradually blends with the surrounding connective tissue of the submucosa (6). An **arteriole** and a **venule (12)** supply the connective tissue of the submucosa (6) and the lamina propria (11).

1 Adventitia

2 Adipose tissue

3 Hyaline cartilage

4 Submucosa

5 Mucosal folds

6 Nerves

7 Trachealis muscle (smooth)

8 Blood vessels

9 Perichondrium

10 Seromucous tracheal glands

11 Excretory ducts of seromucous tracheal glands

12 Pseudostratified ciliated columnar epithelium

13 Lamina propria

14 Elastic membrane

FIGURE 17.6 ■ Trachea (panoramic view, transverse section). Stain: hematoxylin and eosin. Low magnification.

1 Hyaline cartilage

2 Perichondrium

3 Seromucous tracheal glands

4 Chondrocytes in lacunae

5 Excretory duct of seromucous tracheal glands

6 Submucosa

7 Serous demilune

8 Pseudostratified ciliated columnar epithelium

9 Basement membrane

10 Goblet cells

11 Lamina propria

12 Arteriole and venule

FIGURE 17.7 ■ Tracheal wall (sectional view). Stain: hematoxylin and eosin. Medium magnification.

FIGURE 17.8 | Lung (Panoramic View)

This illustration shows the major structures in the lung for air conduction and gaseous exchange (respiration).

The histology of the intrapulmonary bronchi is similar to that of the trachea and extrapulmonary bronchi, except that in the intrapulmonary bronchi, the C-shaped cartilage rings of the trachea are replaced by cartilage plates. All cartilage in the trachea and lung is hyaline cartilage.

The wall of an **intrapulmonary bronchus (5)** is identified by the surrounding **hyaline cartilage plates (7)**. The bronchus (5) is also lined with a pseudostratified columnar ciliated epithelium with goblet cells. The wall in the intrapulmonary bronchus (5) consists of a thin **lamina propria (4)**, a narrow layer of **smooth muscle (3)**, a **submucosa (2)** with **bronchial glands (6)**, hyaline cartilage plates (7), and an **adventitia (1)**.

As the intrapulmonary bronchus (5) branches into smaller bronchi and bronchioles, the epithelial height and the cartilage around the bronchi decrease until only an occasional piece of cartilage is seen. Cartilage disappears from the bronchi walls when their diameters decrease to about 1 mm.

In the **bronchiole (17)**, pseudostratified columnar ciliated epithelium with occasional goblet cells lines the lumen. The lumen shows **mucosal folds (18)** caused by the contractions of the surrounding **smooth muscle (19)** layer. Bronchial glands and cartilage plates are no longer present, and the bronchiole (17) is surrounded by the **adventitia (16)**. In this illustration, a **lymphatic nodule (15)** and a **vein (15)** adjacent to the adventitia (16) accompany the bronchiole (17).

The terminal **bronchioles (8, 10)** exhibit **mucosal folds (10)** and are lined with a columnar ciliated epithelium that lacks goblet cells. A thin layer of lamina propria and **smooth muscle (11)** and an adventitia surround the terminal bronchioles (8, 10).

The respiratory **bronchioles (12, 22)** with alveoli outpocketings are directly connected to the **alveolar ducts (13, 20)** and the **alveoli (23)**. In the respiratory bronchioles (12, 22), the epithelium is low columnar, or cuboidal, and may be ciliated in the proximal portion of the tubules. A thin connective tissue layer supports the smooth muscle, the elastic fibers of the lamina propria, and the accompanying **blood vessels (21)**. The **alveoli (12)** in the walls of the respiratory bronchioles (12, 22) appear as small evaginations, or outpockets.

Each respiratory bronchiole (12, 22) divides into several alveolar ducts (13, 20). The walls of the alveolar ducts (13, 20) are lined with alveoli (23) that directly open into the alveolar duct. Clusters of alveoli (23) that surround and open into alveolar ducts (13, 20) are called **alveolar sacs (24)**. In this illustration, a plane of section passes from a terminal bronchiole (8) to the respiratory bronchiole and into alveolar ducts (20).

The **pulmonary vein (9)** and **pulmonary artery (9)** also branch as they accompany the bronchi and bronchioles into the lung. Small blood vessels are also seen in the connective tissue **trabeculae (25)** that separates the lungs into different segments.

The **serosa (14)** or visceral pleura surrounds the lungs. Serosa (14) consists of a thin layer of pleural **connective tissue (14a)** and a simple squamous layer of pleural **mesothelium (14b)**.

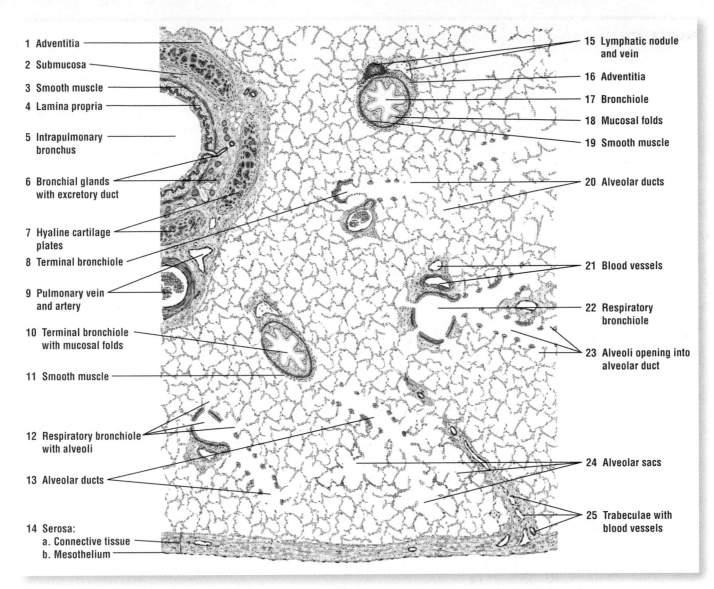

1 Adventitia

2 Submucosa

3 Smooth muscle

4 Lamina propria

5 Intrapulmonary bronchus

6 Bronchial glands with excretory duct

7 Hyaline cartilage plates

8 Terminal bronchiole

9 Pulmonary vein and artery

10 Terminal bronchiole with mucosal folds

11 Smooth muscle

12 Respiratory bronchiole with alveoli

13 Alveolar ducts

14 Serosa:
   a. Connective tissue
   b. Mesothelium

15 Lymphatic nodule and vein

16 Adventitia

17 Bronchiole

18 Mucosal folds

19 Smooth muscle

20 Alveolar ducts

21 Blood vessels

22 Respiratory bronchiole

23 Alveoli opening into alveolar duct

24 Alveolar sacs

25 Trabeculae with blood vessels

FIGURE 17.8 ■ Lung (panoramic view). Stain: hematoxylin and eosin. Low magnification.

FIGURE 17.9 | Intrapulmonary Bronchus (Transverse Section)

The trachea divides outside the lungs and gives rise to primary, or extrapulmonary, bronchi. On entering the lungs, the primary bronchi divide and give rise to a series of smaller or intrapulmonary bronchi.

The intrapulmonary bronchi are lined with a pseudostratified columnar ciliated **bronchial epithelium (6)** supported by a thin layer of **lamina propria (7)** of fine connective tissue with elastic fibers (not illustrated) and a few lymphocytes. A thin layer of **smooth muscle (10, 16)** surrounds the lamina propria (7) and separates it from the **submucosa (8)**. The submucosa (8) contains numerous **seromucous bronchial glands (5, 18)**. An **excretory duct (18)** from the bronchial gland (5, 18) passes through the lamina propria (7) to open into the bronchial lumen. In mixed seromucous bronchial glands (5, 18), serous demilunes may be seen.

In the lung, the hyaline cartilage rings of the trachea are replaced by the **hyaline cartilage plates (11, 14)** that surround the bronchus. A connective tissue **perichondrium (12, 15)** covers each cartilage plate (11, 14). The hyaline cartilage plates (11, 14) become smaller and farther apart as the bronchi continue to divide and decrease in size. Between the cartilage plates (11, 14), the submucosa (8) blends with the **adventitia (3)**. Bronchial glands (5, 18) and **adipose cells (2)** are present in the submucosa (8) of larger bronchi.

Bronchial blood vessels (19) and a **bronchial arteriole (4)** are visible in the connective tissue around the bronchus. Accompanying the bronchus are also a larger **vein (9)** and an **artery (17)**.

Surrounding the intrapulmonary bronchus, its connective tissue, and the hyaline cartilage plates (11, 14) are the lung **alveoli (1, 13)**.

FIGURE 17.10 | Intrapulmonary Bronchus, Cartilage Plates, and Surrounding Alveoli of the Lung

This medium-power micrograph of a small, intrapulmonary bronchus cut in cross section shows the characteristic **cartilage plates (5, 9)** that surround the **lumen of bronchus (2)**. The characteristic **respiratory epithelium (1)** consisting of ciliated cells and goblet cells lines the lumen of bronchus (2). Even at this low magnification, the epithelium appears to be pseudostratified columnar ciliated. Surrounding each cartilage plate (5, 9) is the connective tissue **perichondrium (3)**. Located below the respiratory epithelium (1) is a layer of **smooth muscle (7)** that encircles the bronchus and controls its diameter during respiration. In the connective tissue below the respiratory epithelium are found **seromucous tracheal glands (8)**, some of which directly open into the lumen of the bronchus (1). Also present in the connective tissue of the bronchus is a **lymphatic nodule (11)** that is filled with lymphocytes. Also visible is the connective tissue **adventitia (10)** that surrounds the bronchus and its associated tissue. Outside and surrounding the adventitia of the intrapulmonary bronchus are numerous, thin-walled **alveoli (4, 6)**.

1 Alveoli
2 Adipose cells
3 Adventitia
4 Bronchial arteriole
5 Seromucous bronchial glands
6 Bronchial epithelium
7 Lamina propria
8 Submucosa
9 Vein
10 Smooth muscle
11 Hyaline cartilage plate
12 Perichondrium

13 Alveoli
14 Hyaline cartilage plate
15 Perichondrium
16 Smooth muscle
17 Artery
18 Seromucous bronchial glands with excretory duct
19 Bronchial blood vessels

FIGURE 17.9 ■ Intrapulmonary bronchus (transverse section). Stain: hematoxylin and eosin. Low magnification.

1 Respiratory epithelium
2 Lumen of bronchus
3 Perichondrium
4 Alveoli
5 Cartilge plate

6 Alveoli
7 Smooth muscle
8 Seromucous tracheal glands
9 Cartilage plate
10 Adventitia
11 Lymphatic nodule

FIGURE 17.10 ■ Intrapulmonary bronchus, cartilage plates, and surrounding alveoli of the lung. Stain: hematoxylin and eosin. From: Gartner LP, Hiatt JM. BRS Cell Biology & Histology, 6th Edition. Baltimore: Lippincott Williams & Wilkins, 2011. ×75.

FIGURE 17.11 | Terminal Bronchiole (Transverse Section)

The bronchioles subdivide into smaller terminal bronchioles, whose diameters are approximately 1 mm or less. The terminal bronchioles are lined with a **simple columnar epithelium (3)**. In the smallest bronchioles, the epithelium may be simple cuboidal. The cartilage plates, bronchial glands, and goblet cells are absent from the terminal bronchioles. The terminal bronchioles represent the smallest passageways for conducting air.

Owing to smooth muscle contractions, **mucosal folds (7)** are prominent in the bronchioles. A well-developed **smooth muscle (5)** layer surrounds the thin **lamina propria (6)**, which, in turn, is surrounded by the **adventitia (8)**.

Adjacent to the bronchiole is a small branch of the **pulmonary artery (2)**. The terminal bronchiole is surrounded by the lung **alveoli (1)**. Surrounding the alveoli are the thin **interalveolar septa with capillaries (4)**.

FIGURE 17.12 | Respiratory Bronchiole, Alveolar Duct, and Lung Alveoli

The terminal bronchioles give rise to the respiratory bronchioles. The **respiratory bronchiole (2)** represents a transition zone between the conducting and respiratory portions of the respiratory system.

The wall of the respiratory bronchiole (2) is lined with a **simple cuboidal epithelium (3)**. Single **alveolar outpocketings (1, 6)** are found in the wall of each respiratory bronchiole (2). Cilia may be present in the epithelium of the proximal portion of the respiratory bronchiole (2) but disappear in the distal portion. A thin layer of **smooth muscle (7)** surrounds the epithelium. A small branch of the **pulmonary artery (4)** accompanies the respiratory bronchiole (2) into the lung.

Each respiratory bronchiole (2) gives rise to an **alveolar duct (9)** into which open numerous **alveoli (8)**. In the lamina propria that surrounds the rim of alveoli (8) in the alveolar duct (10) are **smooth muscle bundles (5)**. These smooth muscle bundles (5) appear as knobs between adjacent alveoli.

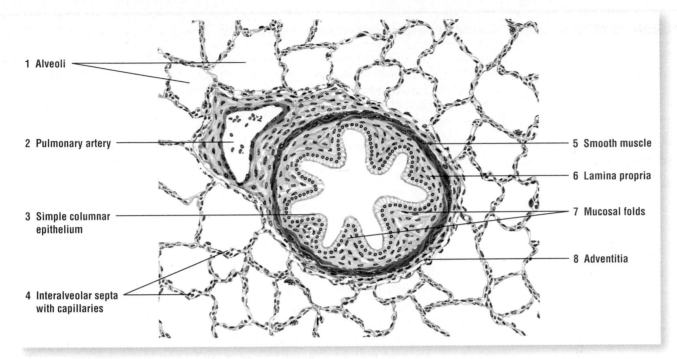

1 Alveoli

2 Pulmonary artery

3 Simple columnar epithelium

4 Interalveolar septa with capillaries

5 Smooth muscle

6 Lamina propria

7 Mucosal folds

8 Adventitia

FIGURE 17.11 ■ Terminal bronchiole (transverse section). Stain: hematoxylin and eosin. Low magnification.

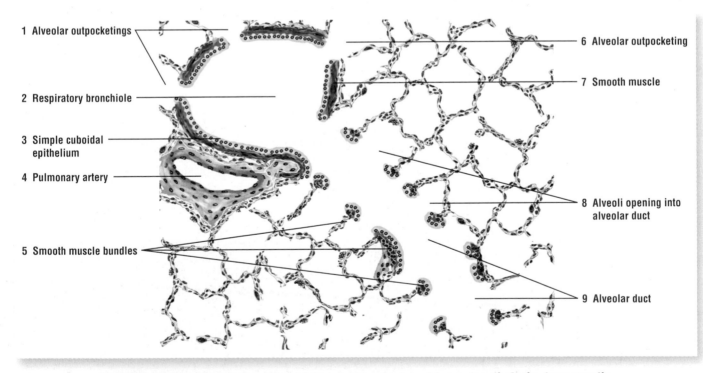

1 Alveolar outpocketings

2 Respiratory bronchiole

3 Simple cuboidal epithelium

4 Pulmonary artery

5 Smooth muscle bundles

6 Alveolar outpocketing

7 Smooth muscle

8 Alveoli opening into alveolar duct

9 Alveolar duct

FIGURE 17.12 ■ Respiratory bronchiole, alveolar duct, and lung alveoli. Stain: hematoxylin and eosin. Low magnification.

FIGURE 17.13 | Lung: Terminal Bronchiole, Respiratory Bronchiole, Alveolar Ducts, Alveoli, and Blood Vessel

This photomicrograph of the lung shows the smallest air-conducting passage, the **terminal bronchiole (7)**. The terminal bronchiole (7) gives rise to thinner **respiratory bronchioles (3)**, whose walls are characterized by numerous **alveoli (2)**. Each respiratory bronchiole (3) gives rise to an **alveolar duct (1, 4, 8)** that continues into the **alveolar sacs (5)**. The terminal bronchiole (7) and the adjacent **blood vessel (6)** are surrounded by the alveoli (2).

FIGURE 17.14 | Alveolar Walls and Alveolar Cells

The **alveoli (3)** are evaginations or outpocketings of the respiratory bronchioles, alveolar ducts, and alveolar sacs, the terminal ends of the alveolar ducts. The alveoli (3) are lined with a layer of thin, simple squamous **alveolar cells (type I pneumocytes) (7)**. The adjacent alveoli (3) share a common **interalveolar septum (4)**, or alveolar wall.

The interalveolar septa (4) consist of simple squamous alveolar cells (7), fine connective tissue fibers and fibroblasts, and numerous **capillaries (1)** located in the thin interalveolar septa (4). The thin interalveolar septa (4) bring the capillaries (1) close to the squamous alveolar cells (7) of the adjacent alveoli (3).

In addition, the alveoli (3) contain **alveolar macrophages (6)**, or dust cells. Normally, the alveolar macrophages (6) contain several carbon or dust particles in their cytoplasm. Also found in the alveoli (3) are the **great alveolar cells (2, 5)**, or type II pneumocytes. The greater alveolar cells (2, 5) are interspersed among the simple squamous alveolar cells (6) in the alveoli (3).

At the free ends of the interalveolar septa (4) and around the open ends of the alveoli (3) are narrow bands of **smooth muscle fibers (8)**. These muscle fibers are continuous with the muscle layer that lines the respiratory bronchioles.

1 Alveolar duct
2 Alveoli
3 Respiratory bronchiole
4 Alveolar duct
5 Alveolar sacs
6 Blood vessel
7 Terminal bronchiole
8 Alveolar duct

FIGURE 17.13 ■ Lung: terminal bronchiole, respiratory bronchiole, alveolar ducts, alveoli, and blood vessel. Stain: hematoxylin and eosin. ×40.

1 Capillaries
2 Great alveolar cell (type II pneumocyte)
3 Alveoli
4 Interalveolar septa
5 Great alveolar cell (type II pneumocyte)
6 Alveolar macrophages (dust cells)
7 Alveolar cells (type I pneumocytes)
8 Smooth muscle fibers

FIGURE 17.14 ■ Alveolar walls and alveolar cells. Stain: hematoxylin and eosin. High magnification. ×205.

FIGURE 17.15 | A Section of Lung Alveoli Adjacent to a Bronchiole Wall

This high-magnification micrograph shows the different cells and structures of the lung at a higher magnification. One **alveolus (2)** is clear with air, whereas adjacent alveoli contain **alveolar macrophages (dust cells) (1)** in their spaces. Also visible are the very thin-walled **capillaries with blood cells (3, 5)** that are located adjacent to the alveoli. Lining the inner surface of the alveoli are the simple squamous **alveolar cells (type I pneumocytes) (4)**. Also found lining the alveoli lumina are the more prominent and cuboidal **alveolar cells (type II pneumocytes) (6)**. An elongated **alveolar duct (8)** exhibits some **smooth muscle (7)** in its wall. Situated adjacent to the numerous thin-walled alveoli is a section of a wall from a terminal/respiratory **bronchiole** with its clear **lumen (9)** that is lined with a simple cuboidal **epithelium (10)**.

1 Alveolar macrophages (dust cells)

2 Alveolus

3 Capillaries with blood cells

4 Alveolar cells (type I pneumocytes)

5 Capillary with blood cells

6 Alveolar cells (type II pneumocytes)

7 Smooth muscle

8 Alveolar duct

9 Lumen of bronchiole

10 Lining epithlium of terminal bronchiole

FIGURE 17.15 ■ A section of lung alveoli adjacent to bronchiole wall. Stain: hematoxylin and eosin. ×205.

FIGURE 17.16 | A Low-Power Ultrastructure of the Lung Showing a Portion of a Bronchiole Wall and Adjacent Alveoli

This low-power ultrastructure of the lung shows a small section of the bronchiole wall and the surrounding alveoli. The **lumen of the bronchiole (14)** is lined with the secretory, dome-shaped **Clara cells (1, 8)** and **ciliated cells (2, 9)** with long cilia. Seen in the cytoplasm of the Clara cells (1, 8) are numerous and dense-staining secretory granules. This lung was perfused with fixatives, and, as a result, the capillaries are empty and do not contain any blood cells. However, the very thin, clear **capillaries (5, 11)** with their empty lumina are visible adjacent to the very thin and attenuated **cytoplasm of alveolar cells (6, 13)** (type I pneumocytes) that line the lumina of different **alveoli (7, 12)**. Surrounding the wall of the bronchiole is a thin layer of **connective tissue (10)**, containing some **smooth muscle cells (3)** and a **blood vessel with a white blood cell (4)** in its lumen.

FUNCTIONAL CORRELATIONS 17.2 | Cells in the Lung

RESPIRATORY SYSTEM—THE CONDUCTING PORTION

The conducting portions of the respiratory system condition the inhaled air. **Mucus** that is continuously produced by **goblet cells** in the pseudostratified ciliated respiratory epithelium and **mucous glands** in the lamina propria contain antimicrobial substances. The serous secretions contain immunoglobulins, lysozymes, and enzymes that destroy bacteria. These secretions form a mucous layer that covers the luminal surfaces in most conducting tubes. As a result, the **moist mucosa** in the conducting portion of the respiratory system **humidifies** the air. The mucus and ciliated epithelium also filter and clean the air of particulate matter, infectious microorganisms, and other airborne matter. These secretions are moved toward the pharynx by the motility of cilia where they are either swallowed or expelled. In addition, a rich and extensive **capillary network** beneath the epithelium in the connective tissue **warms** the inspired air as it passes the conducting portion and before it reaches the respiratory portion in the lungs. In the nasal cavities, the warming and humidifying of air is aided by projecting bones, the conchae, which are located on the lateral walls of the nasal cavity.

CLARA CELLS

Clara cells are most numerous in the terminal bronchioles. These cells also become the predominant cell type in the most distal part of the respiratory bronchioles. Clara cells have several important functions. They secrete one of the **surfactant-like** lipoproteins that coat the bronchial epithelium and break down (via proteolytic enzymes) the luminal stickiness of mucus produced in the larger bronchioles for more efficient respiration. These lipoproteins also serve as tension-reducing agents that are also found in the alveoli and that help to reduce the collapse of the airway walls. Clara cells may also function as **stem cells** that replace lost or injured bronchial ciliated and nonciliated epithelial cells. These cells also secrete proteins and lysozymes into the bronchial tree to protect the lung from inhaled toxic substances, oxidative pollutants, or inflammation and transfer immunoglobulins into bronchiolar lumina.

CELLS OF LUNG ALVEOLI

The lung alveoli contain numerous cell types. **Type I alveolar cells**, also called **type I pneumocytes**, are extremely thin simple squamous cells that line the alveoli in the lung and are the main sites for gaseous exchange. A thin **interalveolar septum** is located between adjacent alveoli. Located within the interalveolar septum between the delicate reticular and elastic fibers is a network of capillaries. Type I alveolar cells are in very close contact with the endothelial lining of capillaries, forming a very thin **blood–air barrier**, across which gaseous exchange takes place. The blood–air barrier consists of a thin layer of the secreted material surfactant, cytoplasm of type I pneumocyte, the fused basal lamina of the pneumocyte and the endothelial cell, and the thin cytoplasm of the capillary endothelium.

FUNCTIONAL CORRELATIONS 17.2 | Cells in the Lung (*Continued*)

Type II alveolar cells, also called **type II pneumocytes,** or **septal cells**, are fewer in number and cuboidal in shape. They are found singly or in groups adjacent to the squamous type I alveolar cells within the alveoli. Their rounded apices project into the alveoli above the type I alveolar cells. These type II alveolar cells are secretory and contain dense-staining **lamellar bodies** in their apical cytoplasm. These cells synthesize and secrete a phospholipid-rich product called **pulmonary surfactant**. When it is released into the alveolus, surfactant spreads as a thin layer over the surfaces of type I alveolar cells, lowering the alveolar **surface tension**. The reduced surface tension in the alveoli decreases the force that is needed to inflate alveoli during inspiration. Therefore, surfactant stabilizes the alveolar diameters, facilitates their expansion, and prevents their collapse during respiration by minimizing the collapsing forces. During fetal development, the great alveolar cells secrete a sufficient amount of surfactant for respiration during the last 28 to 32 weeks of gestation. In addition to producing surfactant, the type II cells can divide and function as **stem cells** for type I squamous alveolar cells in the alveoli. Surfactant also has some **bactericidal** effects and induces immune responses in the alveoli to counteract potentially dangerous inhaled pathogens, fungi, viruses, and bacteria.

Alveolar macrophages, or **dust cells,** are blood monocytes that have entered the pulmonary connective tissue septa and alveoli, and they function as phagocytes in both of these areas. The primary function of these macrophages is to clean the alveoli of invading microorganisms and inhaled particulate matter by **phagocytosis**. These cells are seen either in the individual alveoli or in the thin alveolar septa. They can be recognized in the alveoli or in the connective tissue septa by the contents of their cytoplasm, which normally contains numerous phagocytosed particulate or carbon particles.

1 Clara cell
2 Ciliated cell
3 Smooth muscle cells
4 Blood vessel with blood cell
5 Capillary
6 Cytoplasm of alveolar cell
7 Alveolus

14 Lumen of a bronchiole
15 Lumen of an alveolus

8 Clara cell
9 Ciliated cell
10 Connective tissue
11 Capillary
12 Alveolus
13 Cytoplasm of alveolar cells

FIGURE 17.16 ■ A low-power ultrastructure of the lung, showing a portion of a bronchiole wall and adjacent alveoli. From: Gartner LP, Hiatt JM. BRS Cell Biology & Histology, 6th Edition. Baltimore: Lippincott Williams & Wilkins, 2011. ×1,500.

Respiratory System

Components of Respiratory System—An Overview

- Conducting portion consists of solid passageways that move air in and out of lungs
- Extrapulmonary passages include the trachea and bronchi
- Pseudostratified ciliated epithelium with numerous goblet cells line the larger passageways
- As passageways branch and enter lung, there is a decrease in epithelium height and tubule size
- Terminal bronchioles represent the terminal portion of conducting portion
- Respiratory bronchioles represent the transition zone between conducting and respiratory zones

Olfactory Epithelium

- Located in the roof of the nasal cavity and laterally on each side of the superior conchae
- Specialized pseudostratified epithelium consisting of three cell types without goblet cells
- Contains supportive, basal, and olfactory cells, the sensory bipolar neurons
- Olfactory cells are the sensory bipolar neurons that respond to smell
- Olfactory cells span the thickness of epithelium and end as olfactory vesicles
- Surface of vesicles shows radiating nonmotile olfactory cilia that are receptors for odor
- Olfactory cilia contain odor-binding receptors that are stimulated by odor molecules
- Unmyelinated axons leave bases of olfactory cells to form nerve bundles
- Nerve bundles continue through skull bone to synapse in the olfactory bulbs of the brain
- Below epithelium, serous olfactory glands bathe olfactory cilia and provide odor solvents
- Supportive cells provide structural support, whereas basal cells serve as stem cells for the olfactory epithelium
- Transition from olfactory to respiratory epithelium is abrupt

Respiratory System—The Conducting Portion

- Extrapulmonary structures are the nose, pharynx, larynx, trachea, and extrapulmonary bronchi
- Intrapulmonary structures include bronchi, bronchioles, and terminal bronchioles
- Conditions air by humidifying, warming, and filtering it due to cilia and mucus
- Secretions from glands contain immunoglobulins, lysozyme, and enzymes to kill bacteria

- Incomplete hyaline cartilage C rings encircle and keep trachea patent (open)
- In the lungs, hyaline cartilage plates replace C rings and encircle the larger bronchi
- Bronchioles of about 1 mm diameter no longer have cartilage plates
- As tubular size decreases, epithelium becomes simple ciliated and goblet cells disappear

Clara Cells

- Replace goblet cells and become predominant cells in terminal and respiratory bronchioles
- Are secretory, nonciliated cells that increase in number as ciliated cells decrease
- Secrete surfactant-like lipoproteins components of that breakdown mucus stickiness and reduces surface tension
- May also function as stem cells to replace lost or injured bronchial epithelial cells
- Secrete proteins and lysozymes into bronchial tree to protect lung from inflammation or toxic pollutants

Respiratory System—The Respiratory Portion

- Starts with a passageway where initial respiration can take place
- Terminal bronchioles give rise to respiratory bronchioles, a transition zone for respiration
- Respiratory bronchioles exhibit thin-walled alveoli, where respiration can take place
- Gaseous exchange can take place only when alveoli are present
- Alveoli are final airspaces and are surrounded by capillary plexus for gaseous exchange
- Consists of respiratory bronchioles, alveolar ducts, alveolar sacs, and alveoli
- Goblet cells are absent from alveoli and the lining is very thin where respiration occurs

Cells of Lung Alveoli

- Type I alveolar cells (type I pneumocytes) are very thin that line the lung alveoli
- Capillary endothelium and type I alveolar cells form the thin blood–air barrier
- Type II alveolar cells (type II pneumocytes) are adjacent to type I alveolar cells
- Type II alveolar cells are secretory cells, whose apices project above type I alveolar cells
- Contain numerous secretory lamellar bodies
- Synthesize phospholipid surfactant for alveoli to reduce surface tension

- Surfactant reduces alveolar surface tension, allowing expansion and preventing collapse
- During fetal development, sufficient amount of surfactant produced for respiration
- Surfactant has bactericidal effects to counteract inhaled pathogens

Alveolar Macrophages

- Are blood monocytes that enter pulmonary connective tissue and alveoli
- Clean alveoli of invading organisms and phagocytose particular matter

Epiglottis

- Superior part of larynx that projects upward from larynx wall
- A central elastic cartilage forms core of the epiglottis
- Stratified squamous epithelium lines lingual (anterior) and part of laryngeal (posterior) surface
- Base of epiglottis lined with pseudostratified ciliated columnar epithelium
- Taste buds may be present in lingual or laryngeal epithelium

Larynx

- Pseudostratified ciliated columnar epithelium lines false vocal fold, as posterior epiglottis
- Mixed seromucous glands, blood vessels, lymphatic nodules, and adipose cells in lamina propria
- Ventricle, a deep indentation, separates false vocal fold from true vocal fold
- True vocal fold lined with stratified squamous nonkeratinized epithelium
- Vocalis ligament is at the apex of true vocal fold and skeletal vocalis muscle is adjacent
- Hyaline thyroid cartilage and cricoid cartilage provide support for the larynx
- Epithelium in lower larynx changes back to pseudostratified ciliated columnar epithelium

Trachea

- Wall consists of mucosa, submucosa, hyaline cartilage, and adventitia
- Cartilage C rings keep trachea open with gaps between rings filled with trachealis muscle
- Lining is pseudostratified ciliated columnar epithelium with goblet cells
- Submucosa contains seromucous tracheal glands with ducts opening into trachea lumen

OVERVIEW FIGURE 18.1 ■ A sagittal section of the kidney shows the cortex and medulla, with blood vessels and the excretory ducts, including the pelvis and the ureter and a histologic comparison of blood vessels, the different tubules of the nephron, and the collecting ducts.

CHAPTER 18

Urinary System

The Kidney

The urinary system consists of two **kidneys**, two **ureters** that lead to a single urinary **bladder**, and a single **urethra** that continues from the bladder to the exterior of the body. The kidneys are large, bean-shaped organs located retroperitoneally adjacent to the posterior body wall. Superior to each kidney is the **adrenal gland** embedded in renal fat and connective tissue. The concave, medial border of the kidney is the **hilum**, which contains three large structures, the **renal artery, renal vein**, and the funnel-shaped **renal pelvis** that becomes the ureter. Surrounding these structures is loose connective tissue and a fat-filled space called the **renal sinus**.

Each kidney is covered by a dense irregular connective tissue capsule. A sagittal section through the kidney shows a darker outer **cortex** and a lighter inner **medulla**, which consists of numerous cone-shaped **renal pyramids**. The base of each pyramid faces the cortex and forms the corticomedullary boundary. The round apex of each pyramid extends downward to the renal pelvis to form the domelike **renal papilla**. A portion of the cortex also extends on each side of the renal pyramids to form the **renal columns**.

Each renal papilla is surrounded by a funnel-shaped **minor calyx**, which collects urine from the papilla. The minor calyces join in the renal sinus to form a **major calyx**. Major calyces, in turn, join to form a single and a larger funnel-shaped renal pelvis. The renal pelvis leaves each kidney through the hilum, narrows to become a muscular **ureter**, and descends toward the bladder on each side of the posterior body wall.

Uriniferous Tubules

The functional unit of each kidney is the microscopic **uriniferous tubule**. It consists of a **nephron** and a **collecting duct** into which empty the filtered contents of the nephron. Millions of nephrons are present in each kidney cortex. The nephron, in turn, is subdivided into two components: a renal corpuscle and renal tubules.

Nephrons of the Kidney

There are two types of nephrons, based on their location in the kidney. **Cortical nephrons** are located in the cortex of the kidney, whereas the **juxtamedullary nephrons** are situated near the junction of the cortex and medulla of the kidney. Although all nephrons participate in urine formation, juxtamedullary nephrons produce a hypertonic environment in the interstitium of the kidney medulla that results in the production of concentrated (hypertonic) urine.

Renal Corpuscle

The renal corpuscle consists of a tuft of capillaries, called the **glomerulus**, surrounded by a double layer of epithelial cells called the **glomerular (Bowman) capsule**. The inner or **visceral layer** of the capsule consists of unique and highly specialized branching epithelial cells called **podocytes**. The podocytes are adjacent to the capillaries, and their long cytoplasmic processes completely invest the fenestrated glomerular capillaries. From these processes arise numerous smaller foot processes or **pedicles** that interdigitate with pedicles from adjacent podocytes and form tight-fitting **filtration slits**. A thin, semipermeable **filtration slit diaphragm** spans each filtration slit. The **outer**, or **parietal, layer** of the glomerular capsule consists of simple squamous epithelium.

The renal corpuscle is the initial segment of each nephron. The entry point of the glomerular capillaries into the renal corpuscle is called the **vascular pole**. Here, the afferent arteriole enters and the efferent arteriole exits the renal corpuscle. On the opposite end of the vascular pole of the renal corpuscle is the **urinary pole**, where the filtrate produced by the glomerulus leaves the renal corpuscle.

Blood Filtration

Blood flowing through the kidneys is filtered in renal corpuscles through the glomerular capillaries. The produced filtrate then enters the **capsular (urinary) space** that is located between the parietal and visceral cell layers of the glomerular capsule of the renal corpuscle. The filtrate leaves each renal corpuscle at the urinary pole, a site where the proximal convoluted tubule originates. The filtration barrier for blood in the renal corpuscles consists of three different components: the glomerular **capillary endothelium**; the underlying thicker glomerular **basement membrane**; and the visceral layer (of Bowman) of the capsule, **podocytes,** and **pedicles**.

Filtration Barrier in the Glomerulus

Blood filtration is facilitated by the glomerular endothelium of the capillaries, which is thin, **porous** (fenestrated), and highly permeable to many substances in the blood, except to the formed blood elements or large plasma proteins. Located between the capillary endothelium and the visceral podocytes is the denser **glomerular basement membrane** formed by the fusion of the endothelium and the podocytes. The glomerular basement membrane is a selective physical barrier that acts as a blood filter and restricts the movement of macromolecules about the size of albumin from the blood. The semipermeable slit diaphragms between the individual pedicles of the podocytes are highly specialized junctional complexes containing a transmembrane protein called **nephrin**. This protein connects firmly with the actin filaments in the adjacent pedicles of the podocytes. The filtration slit acts like a fine sieve in the renal corpuscle and prevents the passage of smaller molecules through the diaphragm. Thus, although each component of the filtration barrier in the glomerulus contributes to blood filtration, the podocyte slit diaphragms appear to be the main structures responsible for glomerular permeability and filtration because they are believed to be **size-selective molecular filters**. Thus, the filtrate that enters the capsular (urinary) space in the renal corpuscle is not urine. Instead, it is an ultrafiltrate that is similar to plasma, except for the absence of proteins.

Renal Tubules

The glomerular filtrate that leaves the renal corpuscle first enters the **renal tubule**, which extends from the glomerular capsule to the collecting tubule. This renal tubule has several distinct histologic and functional regions.

The portion of the renal tubule that starts at the renal corpuscle is highly twisted, or tortuous, and is therefore called the **proximal convoluted tubule**. Initially, this tubule is located in the cortex but then descends into the medulla to become continuous with another tubule, the loop of Henle. The **loop of Henle** consists of several parts: a thick descending portion of the proximal convoluted tubule, a thin descending and ascending segment, and a thick ascending portion called the **distal convoluted tubule**. The distal convoluted tubule is shorter and less convoluted than the proximal convoluted tubule, and it ascends back into the kidney cortex. Because the proximal convoluted tubule is longer than the distal convoluted tubule, it is more frequently observed near the renal corpuscles and in the renal cortex. From the distal convoluted tubule, the glomerular filtrate then flows to the **collecting tubule**. In juxtamedullary nephrons, the loop of Henle is very long. It descends from the kidney cortex deep into the medulla and then loops back to ascend into the cortex (Overview Fig. 18.1).

The collecting tubule and the collecting duct are not part of the nephron. A number of short collecting tubules join to form several larger **collecting ducts**. As the collecting ducts become larger and descend further toward the papillae of the medulla, they are called **papillary ducts**. Smaller collecting ducts are lined with a light-staining cuboidal epithelium. Deeper in the medulla, the epithelium in these ducts changes to columnar. At the tip of each papilla, the papillary ducts empty their contents into the minor calyx. The area on the papilla that exhibits openings of the numerous papillary ducts is called the **area cribrosa** (see Overview Fig. 18.1).

The kidney cortex also exhibits numerous, lighter-staining **medullary rays** that extend vertically from the bases of the pyramids into the cortex. Medullary rays consist primarily of collecting ducts, blood vessels, and straight portions of a number of nephrons that penetrate the cortex from the base of the pyramids.

Renal Blood Supply

To understand the functional correlation of the kidney, it is important to understand the blood supply of the organ. Each kidney is supplied by a large **renal artery** that divides in the hilum into several segmental branches, which branch into several **interlobar arteries**. The interlobar arteries continue in the kidney between the pyramids toward the cortex. At the corticomedullary junction, the interlobar arteries branch into **arcuate arteries**, which arch over the base of the pyramids and give rise to **interlobular arteries**. These arteries branch further into the **afferent arterioles**, which give rise to the **capillaries** in the **glomeruli** of renal corpuscles. **Efferent arterioles** leave the renal corpuscles and form a complex **peritubular capillary network** around the tubules in the cortex and long, straight capillary vessels, or **vasa recta**, in the medulla that loops back to the corticomedullary region. The vasa recta form loops that are parallel to the long loops of Henle that contain the urinary filtrate. The interstitium around these tubules and blood vessels is drained by interlobular veins that continue toward the arcuate veins.

 Supplemental micrographic images are available at **www.thePoint.com/Eroschenko12e** under Urinary System.

FIGURE 18.1 | Kidney: Cortex, Medulla, Pyramid, Renal Papilla, and Minor Calyx (Panoramic View)

In this sagittal section, the kidney is subdivided into an outer darker-staining **cortex** and an inner lighter-staining **medulla**. Externally, the cortex is covered with a dense irregular connective tissue **renal capsule (1)**.

The cortex contains both distal and **proximal convoluted tubules (4, 11), glomeruli (2)**, and **medullary rays (3)**. Present also in the cortex are the **interlobular arteries (12)** and **interlobular veins (13)**. The medullary rays (3) are formed by the straight portions of nephrons, blood vessels, and collecting tubules that join in the medulla to form the larger **collecting ducts (6)**. The medullary rays do not extend to the kidney capsule (1) because of the **subcapsular convoluted tubules (10)**.

The medulla comprises the renal pyramids. The **base** of each **pyramid (5)** is adjacent to the cortex and its apex forms the pointed **renal papilla (7)** that projects into the surrounding funnel-like structure, the **minor calyx (16)**, which represents the dilated portion of the ureter. The **area cribrosa (9)** is pierced by small holes, which are the openings of the collecting ducts (6) into the minor calyx (16).

The tip of the renal papilla (7) is usually covered with a simple **columnar epithelium (8)**. As the columnar epithelium of the renal papilla (7) reflects onto the outer wall of the minor calyx (16), it becomes a **transitional epithelium (16)**. A thin layer of connective tissue and smooth muscle (not illustrated) under this epithelium then merges with the connective tissue of the **renal sinus (15)**.

Present in the renal sinus (15) are branches of the renal artery and vein called the **interlobar artery (17)** and the **interlobar vein (18)**. The interlobar vessels (17, 18) enter the kidney and arch over the base of the pyramid (5) at the corticomedullary junction as the **arcuate artery and vein (14)**. The arcuate vessels (14) give rise to smaller interlobular arteries (12) and interlobular veins (13) that pass radially into the kidney cortex and give rise to the afferent glomerular arteries that give rise to the capillaries of the glomeruli (3).

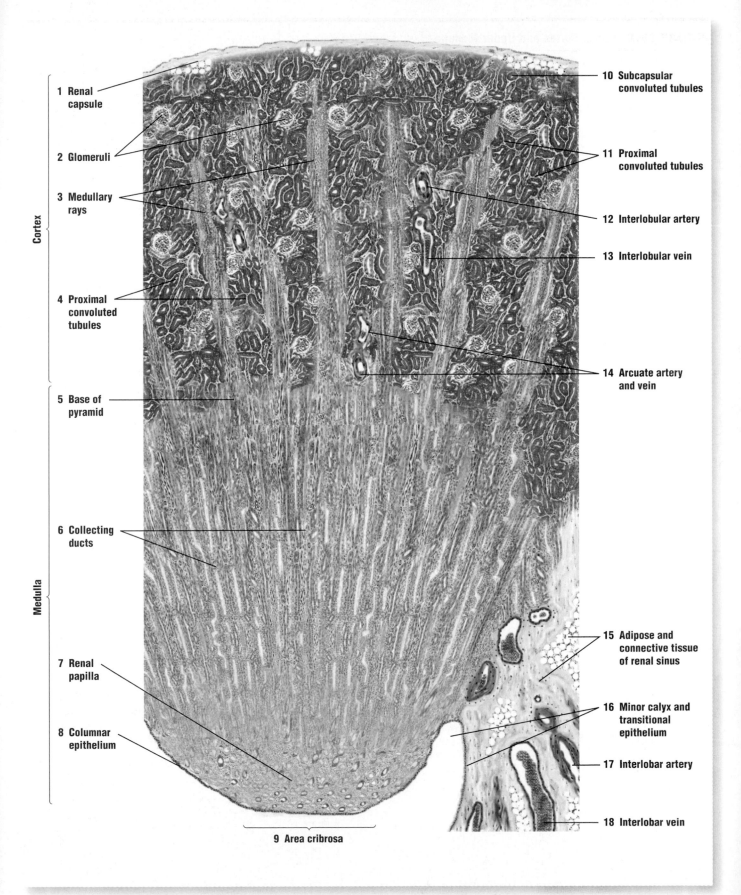

1 Renal capsule

2 Glomeruli

3 Medullary rays

4 Proximal convoluted tubules

5 Base of pyramid

6 Collecting ducts

7 Renal papilla

8 Columnar epithelium

9 Area cribrosa

10 Subcapsular convoluted tubules

11 Proximal convoluted tubules

12 Interlobular artery

13 Interlobular vein

14 Arcuate artery and vein

15 Adipose and connective tissue of renal sinus

16 Minor calyx and transitional epithelium

17 Interlobar artery

18 Interlobar vein

Cortex

Medulla

FIGURE 18.1 ■ Kidney: cortex, medulla, pyramid, renal papilla, and minor calyx (panoramic view). Stain: hematoxylin and eosin. Low magnification.

FIGURE 18.2 | Kidney Cortex and Upper Medulla

A higher magnification of the kidney shows greater detail of the cortex. The **renal corpuscles (5, 9)** consist of a **glomerulus (5a)** and the **glomerular (Bowman) capsule (5b)**. The glomerulus (5a) is a tuft of capillaries that is formed from the afferent **glomerular arteriole (11)**, is supported by fine connective tissue, and is surrounded by the glomerular capsule (5b).

The internal, or **visceral layer (9a)** of the glomerular capsule (5b) surrounds the glomerular capillaries with modified epithelial cells called **podocytes (9a)**. At the **vascular pole (8)** of the renal corpuscle (9), the epithelium of the visceral layer (9a) turns back to form the simple squamous **parietal layer (9b)** of the glomerular capsule (5b). The space between the visceral layer (9a) and the parietal layer (9b) of the renal corpuscle (9) is the **capsular space (10)**.

Two types of convoluted tubules, sectioned in various planes, surround the renal corpuscles (5, 9). These are the **proximal convoluted tubules (1)** and **distal convoluted tubules (2, 4)**. The convoluted tubules are the initial and terminal segments of the nephron. The proximal convoluted tubules (1) are longer than the distal convoluted tubules (2, 4) and are, therefore, more numerous in the cortex. The proximal convoluted tubules (1) exhibit a small, uneven lumen and a single layer of cuboidal cells with eosinophilic granular cytoplasm. A brush border (microvilli) lines the cells but is not always well preserved in the sections. Also, the cell boundaries in the proximal convoluted tubules (1) are not distinct because of the extensive basal and lateral cell membrane interdigitations with the neighboring cells.

The urinary capsular space (10) in the renal corpuscle (5, 9) is continuous with the lumen of the proximal convoluted tubule at the urinary pole (see Fig. 18.3). At the urinary pole, the squamous epithelium of the parietal layer (9b) of the glomerular capsule (5b) changes to the cuboidal epithelium of the proximal convoluted tubule (1).

The distal convoluted tubules (2, 4) are shorter and are fewer in number in the cortex. The distal convoluted tubules (2, 4) also exhibit larger lumina with smaller cuboidal cells. The cytoplasm stains less intensely than that in the proximal convoluted tubules (1), and the brush border is not present on the cells. Similar to the proximal convoluted tubules (1), the distal convoluted tubules (2, 4) show deep basal and lateral cell membrane infoldings and interdigitations.

Also found in the cortex are the medullary rays. The medullary rays include the following three types of tubules: **straight (descending) segments of the proximal tubules (14)**, **straight (ascending) segments of the distal tubules (6)**, and **collecting tubules (12)**. The straight (descending) segments of the proximal tubules (14) are very similar to the proximal convoluted tubules (1), and the straight (ascending) segments of the distal tubules (6) are very similar to distal convoluted tubules (2, 4). The collecting tubules (12) in the cortex are distinct because of their lightly stained cuboidal cells and cell membranes.

The medulla contains only straight portions of the tubules and the segments of the loop of Henle (thick and thin descending segments, and thin and thick ascending segments). The **thin segments of the loops of Henle (15)** are lined with a simple squamous epithelium and resemble the **capillaries (13)**. The distinguishing features of the thin loops of Henle (15) are the thicker epithelial lining and the absence of blood cells in their lumina. In contrast, most capillaries (13) have blood cells in the lumina.

Also visible in the cortex are the **interlobular blood vessels (3)** and the larger **interlobar vein and artery (7)**. The interlobular blood vessels (3) give rise to the afferent glomerular arteriole (11) that enters the glomerular capsule (5b) at the vascular pole (8) and forms the capillary tuft of the glomerulus (5a).

1 Proximal convoluted tubules

2 Distal convoluted tubules

3 Interlobular blood vessels

4 Distal convoluted tubules

5 Renal corpuscle:
 a. Glomerulus
 b. Glomerular (Bowman) capsule

6 Straight (ascending) segment of the distal tubule

7 Interlobar vein and artery

8 Vascular pole

9 Renal corpuscle:
 a. Visceral layer
 b. Parietal layer

10 Capsular space

11 Glomerular arteriole

12 Collecting tubules

13 Capillaries

14 Straight (descending) segment of the proximal tubule

15 Thin segments of the loop of Henle

FIGURE 18.2 ■ Kidney cortex and upper medulla. Stain: hematoxylin and eosin. Low magnification.

FUNCTIONAL CORRELATIONS 18.1 | Kidney Cells and Kidney Tubules

MESANGIAL CELLS

In addition to podocytes that surround the capillaries, there are other specialized cells in the glomerulus called **mesangial cells**. These cells are also attached to the capillaries and perform several important functions. Mesangial cells synthesize the extracellular matrix and provide structural support for the glomerular capillaries. As the blood is filtered through the glomerular capillaries, numerous proteinaceous macromolecules are trapped in the glomerular basement membrane and filtration slit diaphragms. Mesangial cells function as **macrophages** in the intraglomerular regions and phagocytose antigen–antibody complexes and the material that accumulate on the glomerular filter, thus preventing its clogging with filtered matter and keeping the glomerular filter free of debris. These cells also appear to be contractile and can regulate glomerular blood flow as a result of the presence of receptors for vasoactive substances. Some of the mesangial cells are also located outside the renal corpuscle in the vascular pole region, between the afferent and efferent arterioles. Here, they are called the **extraglomerular mesangial cells**, also called lacis cells, and form part of the juxtaglomerular apparatus.

THE KIDNEY CELLS

The kidneys are vital organs for maintaining the body's stable internal environment, or **homeostasis**. This function is performed by regulating the body's blood pressure; blood composition; and pH, fluid volume, and acid–base balance. The kidneys also produce urine, which is formed as a result of three main functions: (1) **filtration** of blood in the glomeruli; (2) **reabsorption** of nutrients and other valuable substances from the ultrafiltrate that enters the proximal and distal convoluted tubules; and (3) **secretion,** or **excretion,** of metabolic waste products, or unwanted chemicals or substances into the filtrate that eventually become urine. Approximately 99% of the glomerular ultrafiltrate produced by the kidneys that enters the tubules is reabsorbed into the system in the nephrons; the remaining 1% of the filtrate is conveyed to the bladder and is voided as urine.

In addition, kidney cells produce two important substances, the enzyme renin and the glycoprotein erythropoietin. **Renin** regulates blood pressure to maintain proper filtration pressure in the kidney glomeruli. **Erythropoietin** is synthesized and released by the endothelial cells of the peritubular capillary network in the renal cortex. Erythropoietin is a growth factor that stimulates erythrocyte production in red bone marrow.

KIDNEY TUBULES

Proximal Convoluted Tubules

All nephrons participate in the formation of urine. As the ultrafiltrate passes through the uriniferous and collecting tubules of the kidneys, it undergoes significant changes in its content and volume. The remaining fluid becomes concentrated urine, containing increased amounts of metabolic waste products. The cells of the proximal convoluted tubules show numerous deep **infoldings** of the basal cell membrane, between which are located numerous elongated mitochondria, and lateral **interdigitations** with its neighboring cells. These features are highly characteristic of cells that are involved in active transport of molecules and electrolytes from the filtrate across the cell membrane into the interstitium. The mitochondria supply the necessary ATP (energy) for active transport of sodium by **Na^+/K^+ ATPase** (sodium pump) that is located in the basolateral regions of the cell membrane.

Reabsorption of most of the substances from the glomerular filtrate takes place in the proximal convoluted tubules, which receives the glomerular ultrafiltrate from the capsular (urinary) space of the Bowman capsule. As the glomerular filtrate enters the proximal convoluted tubules, all **glucose, proteins**, and **amino acids**; almost all carbohydrates; and about 75% to 85% of water and sodium chloride ions are absorbed from the glomerular filtrate into the surrounding interstitium and **peritubular capillaries**. The presence of long and closely spaced **microvilli** (brush border) on proximal convoluted tubule cells greatly increases the surface area and facilitates absorption of the filtered material. In addition, the proximal convoluted tubules secrete certain metabolites, hydrogen, ammonia, dyes, and drugs such as penicillin from the body into the glomerular filtrate. The metabolic waste products urea and uric acid remain in the filtrate of the proximal convoluted tubules and are eliminated from the body in the urine.

The proximal convoluted tubule is longer than the distal convoluted tubule. As a result, the sections of this tubule are more frequently seen in the cortex near the renal corpuscles than those of distal convoluted tubules.

Loops of Henle

The descending and ascending **loops of Henle** of the juxtaglomerular nephrons are long, extend deep into the medulla, have different permeabilities, and have different functions. As a result, **hypertonic urine** is produced in the tubules by an osmotic gradient in the interstitium from the cortex of the kidney to the tips of the renal papillae. Sodium chloride and urea are transported and concentrated in the interstitial tissue of the kidney medulla by means of a complex **countercurrent multiplier system**, which creates a high interstitial osmolarity deep in the medulla. The descending loop of Henle is highly permeable to water but much less to sodium chloride, whereas the thin ascending limb is permeable to sodium chloride but not to water. The hypertonicity (high osmotic pressure) of the extracellular fluid created in the medulla interstitium removes water from the glomerular filtrate as it flows through these tubules. The water that enters the interstitium is then quickly removed by the capillary loops of the **vasa recta**, thus helping to maintain the osmotic concentration gradient in the medulla, conserving water, and concentrating the urine. These capillary loops are permeable to water and take up the water from the medullary interstitium to return it to the systemic circulation.

Distal Convoluted Tubules

The **distal convoluted tubules** are shorter and less convoluted than the proximal tubules. Therefore, these tubules are less frequently observed in the cortex and near the renal corpuscles. In comparison with the proximal convoluted tubules, the distal convoluted tubules do not exhibit brush borders, the cells are smaller, and more nuclei are seen per tubule. The basolateral membranes of distal convoluted tubule cells also show increased interdigitations and the presence of elongated mitochondria within these infoldings. The main function of the distal convoluted tubules is to actively **reabsorb sodium** ions from the tubular filtrate. This activity is directly linked with **excretion** of hydrogen, potassium, and ammonium ions into the tubular fluid. The excretion of hydrogen ions into the tubular fluid is connected with the absorption of bicarbonate ions, causing further acidification of urine.

Sodium reabsorption in the distal convoluted tubules is controlled by the hormone **aldosterone** that is secreted by the adrenal cortex. In the presence of aldosterone hormone, cells of the distal convoluted tubules begin to actively absorb sodium and chloride ions from the filtrate and transport them across the cell membrane into the interstitium. Here, these ions are quickly absorbed by the **peritubular capillaries** and returned back to the systemic circulation, thereby decreasing sodium loss in urine. These functions of the distal convoluted tubules are vital for maintaining the proper acid–base balance of body fluids and blood.

FIGURE 18.3 | Kidney Cortex: Juxtaglomerular Apparatus

A higher magnification of the kidney cortex illustrates in more detail the renal corpuscle, the surrounding convoluted tubules, and the juxtaglomerular apparatus.

In the middle of the illustration is the renal corpuscle with **glomerular capillaries (5), parietal (8a)** and **visceral (8b) layers** (epithelium) of the **glomerular (Bowman) capsule (8)**, and the **capsular space (10)** around the glomerulus. Surrounding the renal corpuscle are numerous tubules with brush borders and acidophilic cells. These are the **proximal convoluted tubules (7)**. These tubules are distinguished from the **distal convoluted tubules (1, 6)** that exhibit smaller and less intensely stained cells that lack the brush borders. In contrast to the convoluted tubules, the cuboidal cells of the **collecting tubule (11)** exhibit pale cytoplasm and distinct cell outlines. **Basement membrane (12)** surrounds the collecting tubules (11).

Each renal corpuscle exhibits a vascular pole where the afferent **glomerular arteriole (4)** enters and the efferent glomerular arteriole exits the renal corpuscle. Inside the renal corpuscle, the glomerular arteriole forms an extensive network of glomerular capillaries (5). On the opposite side of the vascular pole in the renal corpuscle is the **urinary pole (9)**. Here, the capsular space (10) becomes continuous with the lumen of the proximal convoluted tubule (7). The plane of section through both the vascular and urinary poles is only occasionally seen in the kidney cortex. This illustration shows the glomerular arteriole (4) on one end and the urinary pole (9) at the opposite end of the renal corpuscle.

At the vascular pole, modified epithelioid cells with cytoplasmic granules replace the smooth muscle cells in the tunica media of the afferent glomerular arteriole (4). These cells are the **juxtaglomerular cells (3)**. In the adjacent distal convoluted tubule, the cells that border the juxtaglomerular cells (3) are narrow and more columnar. This area of darker, more compact cell arrangement in the distal convoluted tubule is called the **macula densa (2)**. The juxtaglomerular cells (3) in the afferent glomerular arteriole (4) and the macula densa (2) cells in the distal convoluted tubule form the juxtaglomerular apparatus.

1 Distal convoluted tubule

2 Macula densa

3 Juxtaglomerular cells

4 Glomerula arteriole

5 Glomerula capillaries

6 Distal convoluted tubule

7 Proximal convoluted tubules

8 Glomerular capsule:
a. Parietal layer
b. Visceral layer

9 Urinary pole

10 Capsular space

11 Collecting tubule

12 Basement membrane

FIGURE 18.3 ■ Kidney cortex: juxtaglomerular apparatus. Stain: hematoxylin and eosin. Medium magnification.

FIGURE 18.4 | Kidney: Renal Corpuscle, Juxtaglomerular Apparatus, and Convoluted Tubules

This high-magnification photomicrograph shows a renal corpuscle with surrounding tubules. The renal corpuscle consists of the **glomerulus (1)** and the **glomerular capsule (2)** with a **parietal layer (2a)** and a **visceral layer (2b)**. Between these layers is the **capsular space (5)**, with **podocytes (4, 7)** located on the surface of the visceral layer (2b). At the vascular pole of the renal corpuscle, blood vessels enter and leave the renal corpuscle. Adjacent to the vascular pole is the **juxtaglomerular apparatus (3)**. The juxtaglomerular apparatus (3) consists of modified smooth muscle cells of the afferent arteriole in the vascular pole, the **juxtaglomerular cells (3a)**, and the **macula densa (3b)** of the **distal convoluted tubule (6, 9)**. Surrounding the renal corpuscle are the darker-staining **proximal convoluted tubules (8)** and the distal convoluted tubules (6, 9).

FUNCTIONAL CORRELATIONS 18.2 | Juxtaglomerular Apparatus

Adjacent to the renal corpuscles and distal convoluted tubules lies a special group of cells called **juxtaglomerular apparatus**. This apparatus consists of three components: the juxtaglomerular cells, the macula densa, and the extraglomerular mesangial cells (or lacis cells).

Juxtaglomerular cells are a group of modified **smooth muscle cells** located in the wall of the **afferent arteriole** of the vascular pole of the renal corpuscle before it penetrates the glomerular capsule to form the glomerulus. The cytoplasm of these cells contains membrane-bound **secretory granules** of the enzyme **renin**, which is synthesized, stored, and released into the blood stream when needed. Opposite the afferent arteriole is the **macula densa**, a group of modified distal convoluted tubule cells that form a dense cluster. The macula densa cells and juxtaglomerular cells are in close proximity to each other and are separated only by a thin basement membrane. This proximity of juxtaglomerular cells to the macula densa allows for integration of their functions.

The main function of the juxtaglomerular apparatus is to maintain the necessary blood pressure in the kidney for glomerular filtration. The cells of this apparatus act as both baroreceptors and chemoreceptors. The juxtaglomerular cells monitor changes in the **systemic blood pressure** by responding to stretching in the walls of the afferent arterioles. The cells in the macula densa are sensitive to changes in and monitor **sodium chloride concentrations** in the tubular fluid. A decrease in the blood pressure results in a decreased amount of glomerular filtrate and, consequently, a decreased sodium ion concentration in the filtrate as it flows past the macula densa in the distal convoluted tubule.

A decrease in systemic blood pressure or a decreased sodium concentration in the filtrate induces the juxtaglomerular cells to release the enzyme renin into the bloodstream. Renin, in turn, converts the blood plasma protein **angiotensinogen** to **angiotensin I**, which, in turn, is converted to **angiotensin II** by another enzyme present in the **endothelial cells** of lung capillaries. Angiotensin II is an active hormone and a powerful **vasoconstrictor** that initially produces arterial constriction, thereby increasing the systemic blood pressure. In addition, angiotensin II stimulates the release of the hormone **aldosterone** from the adrenal gland cortex.

Aldosterone acts primarily on the cells of distal convoluted tubules to increase their reabsorption of sodium and chloride ions from the glomerular filtrate. Water follows sodium chloride by osmosis and increases fluid volume in the circulatory system. The combination of these effects raises the systemic blood pressure, increases the glomerular filtration rate in the kidney, and decreases the secretion of renin by juxtaglomerular cells. Aldosterone also facilitates the elimination of potassium and hydrogen ions and is an essential hormone for maintaining electrolyte balance in the body.

1 Glomerulus

2 Glomerular capsule
  a. Parietal layer
  b. Visceral layer

3 Juxtaglomerular
  apparatus
  a. Juxtaglomerular
     cells
  b. Macula densa

4 Podocyte

5 Capsular space

6 Distal convoluted
  tubules

7 Podocyte

8 Proximal convoluted
  tubules

9 Distal convoluted
  tubule

FIGURE 18.4 ■ Kidney cortex: renal corpuscle, juxtaglomerular apparatus, and convoluted tubules. Stain: hematoxylin and eosin. ×130.

FIGURE 18.5 | Ultrastructure of Cells in the Proximal Convoluted Tubule of the Kidney

This medium-power ultrastructure image shows cells that form the proximal convoluted tubules in the kidney. The very long and closely packed **microvilli (1)** that line the apices are recognized as the brush border in the light microscopic images. The apices also exhibit an increased number of clear **pinocytotic vesicles (6)** and dense-staining **lysosomes (2, 5)**. Note that the cytoplasm of these cells is packed with numerous **mitochondria (4, 7)** that are needed for the energy to transport the nutrients from the ultrafiltrate. In the center of these cells is a **nucleus (3)**.

1 Microvilli

2 Lysosomes

3 Nucleus

4 Mitochondria

5 Lysosomes

6 Vesicles

7 Mitochondria

FIGURE 18.5 ■ Ultrastructure of cells in the proximal convoluted tubule of the kidney. Courtesy of Dr. Rex A. Hess, Professor Emeritus, Comparative Biosciences, College of Veterinary Medicine, University of Illinois, Urbana, Illinois. ×55,000.

FIGURE 18.6 | Ultrastructure of Apical Cell Surface in the Proximal Convoluted Tubule of the Kidney

This high-power ultrastructure image shows in greater detail the apical cell surface of the proximal convoluted tubules of the kidney. Note the long and closely packed **microvilli (1, 6)** of the brush border that extends into the lumen. In the cytoplasm are also numerous and clear **pinocytotic vesicles (2, 7)**. A tight **junctional complex (3)** is visible as a dark strip near the base of the microvilli, or the apical region of the cell. However, individual cell boundaries in the proximal tubules are not seen because of the complex interdigitations of the lateral cell walls. Also visible in the apical cytoplasm are numerous dense-staining **lysosomes (4, 8)**, which will break down the substances that are brought into the cytoplasm by the pinocytotic vesicles (2, 7). The apical cytoplasm also exhibits numerous **mitochondria (5)** and a section of the **nucleus (9)**.

1 Microvilli

2 Vesicles

3 Junctional complex

4 Lysosomes

5 Mitochondria

6 Microvilli

7 Vesicles

8 Lysosomes

9 Nucleus

FIGURE 18.6 ■ Ultrastructure of apical cell surface in the proximal convoluted tubule of the kidney. Courtesy of Dr. Rex A. Hess, Professor Emeritus, Comparative Biosciences, College of Veterinary Medicine, University of Illinois, Urbana, Illinois. ×8,000.

FIGURE 18.7 | Kidney: Scanning Electron Micrograph of Podocytes

This scanning electron micrograph illustrates the very unique and unusual appearance of the visceral epithelium of the glomerular capsule and the podocytes, which surround all the capillaries in the kidney glomeruli. The flattened **cell body** of the **podocyte (6)** extends thicker **primary processes (1, 3)** that surround the capillary walls. The primary processes (1, 3) give rise to the smaller **pedicles (2, 7)**, which interdigitate with similar pedicles from other podocytes around the capillaries. Between the pedicles (2, 6) are the tiny **filtration slits (5)**. Also visible are remnants of **proteinaceous debris (4)** that became lodged in the filtration slits (5) during blood filtration. Surrounding the podocytes in the renal corpuscle is the dark-appearing capsular space that would contain the glomerular filtrate in a functioning kidney.

FIGURE 18.8 | Kidney: Transmission Electron Micrograph of Podocyte and Glomerular Capillary

This transmission electron micrograph shows the association of a podocyte with glomerular capillaries in the renal corpuscle of kidney. The **nucleus (3)** and **cytoplasm** of the **podocyte (11)** are separated from the adjacent **basement membrane** of the **capillary (13)**. The larger **primary process** of the **podocyte (12)** extends from the podocyte cytoplasm (11) to surround the wall of the capillary. The smaller **pedicles (2, 5)** from the primary process of the podocyte (12) are attached to the basement membrane of the capillary (13). Between the individual pedicles (2, 5) are the **filtration slits (1)**. Separating the podocyte (3, 11) from the capillaries and adjacent podocytes is the clear **capsular space (4)**. In the **lumen of the capillary (6, 8)** are the **nucleus of an endothelial cell (10)** and sections of an **erythrocyte (7)** and a **leukocyte (9)**. In the lumen of the capillary (6, 8) are also visible tiny **fenestrations** in the endothelium (*arrowheads*).

1 Primary processes

2 Pedicles

3 Primary processes

4 Proteinaceous debris

5 Filtration slits

6 Cell body of podocyte

7 Pedicles

1.0 u

FIGURE 18.7 ■ Kidney: scanning electron micrograph of podocytes (visceral epithelium of glomerular [Bowman] capsule) surrounding the glomerular capillaries.

1 Filtration slits

2 Pedicles

3 Nucleus of podocyte

4. Capsular space

5 Pedicles

6 Lumen of capillary

7 Erythrocyte

8 Lumen of capillary

9 Leukocyte

10 Nucleus of endothelial cell

11 Cytoplasm of podocyte

12 Primary process of podocyte

13 Basement membrane of capillary

FIGURE 18.8 ■ Kidney: transmission electron micrograph of podocyte and adjacent capillaries in the renal corpuscle. ×6,500.

FIGURE 18.9 | Kidney Medulla: Papillary Region (Transverse Section)

The papilla in the kidney faces the minor calyx and contains the terminal portions of the collecting tubules, now called the **papillary ducts (3)**. The papillary ducts (3) exhibit large diameters and wide lumina and are lined with tall, pale-staining columnar cells. Also present in the papilla are the **straight (ascending) segments of the distal tubules (7, 10)** and the **straight (descending) segments of the proximal tubules (1, 6, 11)**. Note that these straight segments in the medulla are very similar to the corresponding convoluted tubules in the cortex. Interspersed among the ascending (7, 10) and descending straight tubules (1, 6, 11) are the transverse sections of the **thin segments of the loop of Henle (5, 8)** that resemble the **capillaries (4, 9)** or small **venules (2)**. The capillaries (4, 9) and the small venules (2) differ from the thin segments of the loop of Henle (5, 8) by thinner walls and by the presence of blood cells in their lumina.

The **connective tissue (12)** surrounding the tubules is more abundant in the papillary region of the kidney, and the papillary ducts (3) are spaced further apart.

FIGURE 18.10 | Kidney Medulla: Terminal End of Papilla (Longitudinal Section)

Several collecting ducts merge in the papilla of the kidney medulla to form large, straight tubules called the **papillary ducts (6)**, which are lined with a simple cuboidal or columnar epithelium. Openings of the numerous papillary ducts (6) at the tip of the papilla produce a sievelike appearance in the papilla that is called the area cribrosa. The contents from the papillary ducts (6) continue into the minor calyx that is adjacent to and surrounds the tip of each papilla.

In this illustration, the papilla is lined with a stratified **covering epithelium (7)**. At the area cribrosa, the covering epithelium (7) is usually a tall simple columnar type that is continuous with the papillary ducts (6).

Thin segments of the loops of Henle (3, 5) descend deep into the papilla and are identifiable as thin ducts with empty lumina. **Venules (1)** and the **capillaries (4)** of the vasa recta are usually identified by the presence of blood cells in their lumina. Surrounding the blood vessels (1, 4) and the papillary ducts (6) is the **renal interstitium (connective tissue) (2)**.

FUNCTIONAL CORRELATIONS 18.3	Collecting Tubules, Collecting Ducts, and Antidiuretic Hormone

Glomerular filtrate flows from the distal convoluted tubules to the **collecting tubules** and **collecting ducts**. Under normal conditions, these tubules are not permeable to water, and the urine remains dilute or hypotonic. However, during excessive water loss from the body or dehydration, **antidiuretic hormone (ADH)** is released from the posterior lobe (neurohypophysis) of the **pituitary gland** in response to increased blood osmolarity (decreased water). The released ADH causes the epithelium of collecting tubules and collecting ducts to become highly permeable to water. As a result, water leaves the collecting ducts and enters the hypertonic interstitium that was established by the thin loops of Henle and the surrounding capillary network, the vesa recta. Water in the interstitium is then collected or absorbed and returned to the general circulation via the peritubular capillaries and vasa recta, and the glomerular filtrate in the collecting ducts becomes hypertonic (highly concentrated) urine.

In the absence of ADH, the cells of the collecting tubules and ducts remain impermeable to water. Consequently, increased amount of water remains in the glomerular filtrate of the collecting ducts, resulting in dilute urine.

1 Straight (descending) segment of proximal tubule

2 Venules

3 Papillary ducts

4 Capillaries

5 Thin segments of the loop of Henle

6 Straight (descending) segment of proximal tubule

7 Straight (ascending) segment of distal tubule

8 Thin segments of the loop of Henle

9 Capillaries

10 Straight (ascending) segment of distal tubule

11 Straight (descending) segment of proximal tubule

12 Connective tissue

FIGURE 18.9 ■ Kidney medulla: papillary region (transverse section). Stain: hematoxylin and eosin. Medium magnification.

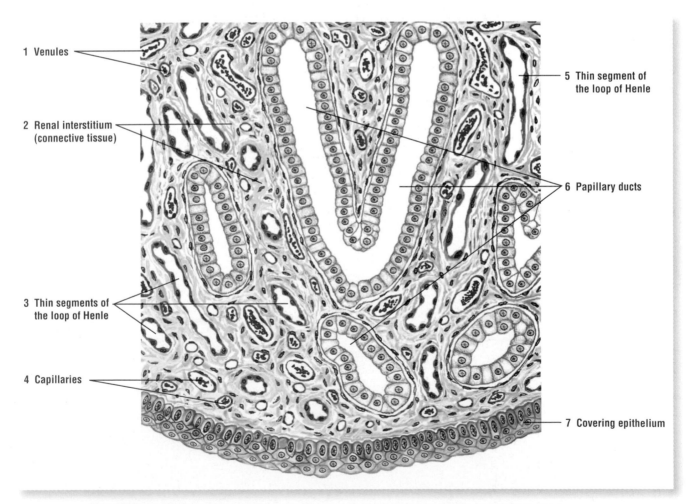

1 Venules

2 Renal interstitium (connective tissue)

3 Thin segments of the loop of Henle

4 Capillaries

5 Thin segment of the loop of Henle

6 Papillary ducts

7 Covering epithelium

FIGURE 18.10 ■ Kidney medulla: terminal end of papilla (longitudinal section). Stain: hematoxylin and eosin. Medium magnification.

FIGURE 18.11 | Kidney: Ducts of Medullary Region (Longitudinal Section)

The medullary region of the kidney consists primarily of various sized tubules, larger ducts, and blood vessels of the vasa recta. In this photomicrograph, different kidney tubules and blood vessels have been sectioned in a longitudinal plane. The tubules with large, light-staining cuboidal cells are the **collecting tubules (1)**. Adjacent to the collecting tubules (1) are tubules with darker-staining cuboidal cells. These are the **thick segments of the loop of Henle (2)**. Between the tubules are blood vessels of the **vasa recta (4)** and the **thin segments of the loop of Henle (3)**. Blood vessels of the vasa recta (4) can be distinguished from the thin segments of the loop of Henle (3) by the presence of blood cells in their lumina.

FIGURE 18.12 | Urinary System: Ureter (Transverse Section)

An undistended **lumen of the ureter (4)** exhibits numerous longitudinal mucosal folds formed by the muscular contractions. The wall of the ureter consists of mucosa, muscularis, and adventitia.

The ureter mucosa consists of **transitional epithelium (7)** and a wide **lamina propria (5)**. The transitional epithelium has several cell layers; the outermost layer is characterized by large cuboidal cells. The intermediate cells are polyhedral in shape, whereas the basal cells are low columnar, or cuboidal.

The lamina propria (5) contains fibroelastic connective tissue, which is denser with more fibroblasts under the epithelium and looser near the muscularis. Diffuse lymphatic tissue and occasional small lymphatic nodules may be observed in the lamina propria.

In the upper ureter, the muscularis consists of two muscle layers: an inner **longitudinal smooth muscle layer (3)** and a middle **circular smooth muscle layer (2)**; these layers are not always distinct. An additional third outer longitudinal layer of smooth muscle is found in the lower third of the ureter near the bladder.

The **adventitia (9)** blends with the surrounding fibroelastic connective tissue and **adipose tissue (1, 10)**, which contain numerous **arterioles (6), venules (8),** and small nerves.

1 Collecting tubules

2 Thick segments of the loop of Henle

3 Thin segment of the loop of Henle

4 Vasa recta

FIGURE 18.11 ■ Kidney: ducts of medullary region (longitudinal section). Stain: hematoxylin and eosin. ×130.

1 Adipose tissue

2 Circular smooth muscle layer

3 Longitudinal smooth muscle layer

4 Lumen of ureter

5 Lamina propria

6 Arteriole

7 Transitional epithelium

8 Venule

9 Adventitia

10 Adipose tissue

FIGURE 18.12 ■ Urinary system: ureter (transverse section). Stain: hematoxylin and eosin. Low magnification.

FIGURE 18.13 | Section of a Ureter Wall (Transverse Section)

This illustration shows a higher magnification of a ureter wall. The **transitional epithelium (7)** in an undistended ureter shows **mucosal folds (6)** and numerous layers with round cells. The superficial cells of the transitional epithelium (7) have a special **surface membrane (5)** that serves as an osmotic barrier between the urine and the underlying tissue. A thin basement membrane separates the epithelium from the loose **lamina propria (9)**.

The **muscularis (2, 8)** often appears as loosely arranged smooth muscle bundles surrounded by abundant connective tissue. The upper ureter has an inner **longitudinal smooth muscle layer (8)** and a middle **circular smooth muscle layer (2)**. A third longitudinal smooth muscle layer is found in the lower third of the ureter.

The **adventitia (4)** with **adipose cells (3)** merges with the connective tissue of the posterior abdominal wall to which the ureter is attached.

FIGURE 18.14 | Ureter (Transverse Section)

The ureter is a muscular tube that conveys urine from the kidneys to the bladder by the contractions of the thick, smooth muscle layers found in its wall. This low-magnification photomicrograph shows a ureter in transverse section. The mucosa of the ureter is highly folded and lined with a thick **transitional epithelium (1)**. Below the transitional epithelium (1) is the connective tissue **lamina propria (2)**. The muscularis of the ureter contains two smooth muscle layers: an **inner longitudinal layer (3)** and a **middle circular muscle layer (4)**. A third outer longitudinal layer (not shown) is added to the wall in the lower third of the ureter, near the bladder. A connective tissue **adventitia (6)**, with **blood vessels (5)** and **adipose tissue (7)**, surrounds the ureter.

1 Arteriole and venule

2 Circular smooth muscle layer

3 Adipose cells

4 Adventitia

5 Surface membrane

6 Mucosal fold

7 Transitional epithelium

8 Longitudinal smooth muscle layer

9 Lamina propria

FIGURE 18.13 ■ Section of a ureter wall (transverse section). Stain: hematoxylin and eosin. Medium magnification.

1 Transitional epithelium

2 Lamina propria

3 Inner longitudinal muscle layer

4 Middle circular muscle layer

5 Blood vessels

6 Adventitia

7 Adipose tissue

FIGURE 18.14 ■ Ureter (transverse section). Stain: iron hematoxylin and Alcian blue (IHAB). ×10.

FIGURE 18.15 | Urinary Bladder: Wall (Transverse Section)

The bladder has a thick muscular wall. The wall is similar to that of the lower third of the ureter, except for its thickness. In the wall are found three loosely arranged layers of smooth muscle, the inner longitudinal, middle circular, and the outer longitudinal layers. However, similar to the ureter, the distinct muscle layers are difficult to distinguish. The three layers are arranged in anastomosing **smooth muscle bundles (1)** between which is found the **interstitial connective tissue (2)**. In this illustration, the muscle bundles are sectioned in various planes (1), and the three distinct muscle layers are not distinguishable. The interstitial connective tissue (2) merges with the connective tissue of the **serosa (3)**. **Mesothelium (3b)** covers the **connective tissue of the serosa (3a)** and is the outermost layer. Serosa (3) lines the superior surface of the bladder, whereas its inferior surface is covered by the connective tissue adventitia, which merges with the connective tissue of adjacent structures.

The mucosa of an empty bladder exhibits numerous **mucosal folds (5)** that disappear during bladder distension. The **transitional epithelium (6)** is thicker than in the ureter and consists of about six layers of cells. The **lamina propria (7)**, inferior to the epithelium, is wider than in the ureters. The loose connective tissue in the deeper zone contains more elastic fibers. Numerous **blood vessels (4, 8)** of various sizes are found in the serosa (3), between the smooth muscle bundles (1), and in the lamina propria (8).

FIGURE 18.16 | Urinary Bladder: Contracted Mucosa (Transverse Section)

The mucosa from an empty and contracted urinary bladder wall is illustrated at a higher magnification. Here, the superficial cells of the **transitional epithelium (4)** are low cuboidal, or columnar, and appear dome shaped. Also, some superficial cells may be **binucleate (6)** (contain two nuclei). The outer **plasma membrane (5)** of the superficial cells in the epithelium is prominent. The deeper cells in the epithelium are round (4) and the basal cells more columnar (see also Fig. 4.7).

The subepithelial **lamina propria (3)** contains fine connective tissue fibers; numerous fibroblasts; and the blood vessels, a **venule and arteriole (2)**. The muscularis consists of three indistinct muscle layers that are visible as **smooth muscle bundles (1)** sectioned in longitudinal and transverse planes.

1 Smooth muscle bundles

2 Interstitial connective tissue

3 Serosa
  a. Connective tissue
  b. Mesothelium

4 Blood vessels

5 Mucosal folds

6 Transitional epithelium

7 Lamina propria

8 Blood vessels in lamina propria

FIGURE 18.15 ■ Urinary bladder: wall (transverse section). Stain: hematoxylin and eosin. Low magnification.

1 Smooth muscle bundles

2 Venule and arteriole

3 Lamina propria

4 Transitional epithelium

5 Outer plasma membrane

6 Binucleate cell

FIGURE 18.16 ■ Urinary bladder: contracted mucosa (transverse section). Stain: hematoxylin and eosin. Medium magnification.

FIGURE 18.17 | Urinary Bladder: Stretched Mucosa (Transverse Section)

When fluid fills the bladder, the **transitional epithelium (1)** changes its shape. Increased volume in the bladder appears to reduce the number of cell layers, the **surface cells (5)** appear squamous, and the thickness of the transitional epithelium (1) is reduced to about three layers. This is because the surface cells (5) flatten to accommodate the increasing surface area. In the stretched condition, the transitional epithelium (1) may resemble stratified squamous epithelium found in other regions of the body. Note also that the folds in the bladder wall disappear, and the **basement membrane (2)** is not folded. As in an empty bladder (Fig. 18.16) the underlying **connective tissue (6)** contains **venules (3)** and **arterioles (7)**. Below the connective tissue (6) are **smooth muscle fibers (4, 8)**, sectioned in cross (4) and longitudinal (8) planes.

FUNCTIONAL CORRELATIONS 18.4 | Urinary Bladder

The **urinary bladder** is a hollow organ with a thick muscular wall. Its main function is to store urine. Because the lumen of the bladder is lined with a **transitional epithelium**, the wall of the organ can stretch or enlarge (change shape) as the bladder fills with urine. When the bladder is empty, the thick transitional epithelium may exhibit five or six layers of cells. The superficial cells in the epithelium are cuboidal, large, dome shaped, and bulge into the lumen. When the bladder fills with urine, however, the transitional epithelium is stretched, and the cells in the epithelium appear thinner and squamous to accommodate the increased volume of urine.

The changes in the appearance and cell shapes in the transitional epithelium are due to the unique thickened regions in the plasma membrane of superficial cells called **plaques**. The plaques are connected to thinner, shorter, and more flexible **interplaque regions**. These structures act like "hinges," and, in an empty bladder, the interplaque regions allow the cell membrane to fold. When the bladder is filled with urine, these folds disappear, and the interplaque regions allow the cells to expand during full stretch. The plaques unfold and become part of the surface during stretching and flattening of the cells.

The exposed cell membrane of superficial cells in the transitional epithelium is also thicker. In addition, **desmosomes** and **occluding junctions** attach the lateral borders of the cells to each other. The plaques are impermeable to water, salts, and urine even when the epithelium is fully stretched. These unique properties of transitional epithelium in the urinary passages provide for an effective **osmotic barrier** between concentrated urine and the underlying connective tissue.

1 Transitional epithelium

2 Basement membrane

3 Venules

4 Smooth muscle (cross section)

5 Surface cells

6 Connective tissue

7 Arterioles

8 Smooth muscle (longitudinal section)

FIGURE 18.17 ■ Urinary bladder: stretched mucosa (transverse section). Stain: hematoxylin and eosin. Medium magnification.

Urinary System

The Kidney

- System consists of two kidneys, two ureters, a bladder, and a urethra
- Hilum contains renal artery, renal vein, and renal pelvis surrounded by renal sinus
- Darker outer region of kidney is cortex; lighter inner region is medulla
- Medulla contains numerous pyramids, which face the cortex at corticomedullary junction
- Round apex of each pyramid extends toward renal pelvis as renal papilla
- Cortex that extends on each side of renal pyramid constitutes the renal columns
- Each papilla is surrounded by a minor calyx that joins to form a major calyx
- Major calyces join to form funnel-shaped renal pelvis that narrows into muscular ureter
- Urine is formed as a result of blood filtration and absorption from and excretion into the filtrate
- Almost all filtrate is reabsorbed into the systemic circulation and about 1% is voided as urine
- Produces renin that regulates filtration pressure and erythropoietin for erythrocyte production

Uriniferous Tubules and Nephrons

- Functional unit of kidney is uriniferous tubule
- Consist of nephron and collecting duct

Nephrons of the Kidney

- Two types of nephrons: cortical nephrons in cortex and juxtamedullary nephrons in medulla
- Nephron is subdivided into renal corpuscle and renal tubules

Renal Corpuscle

- Blood is filtered in the glomerular capillaries of the corpuscle to form ultrafiltrate
- Consists of capillaries called glomerulus and double-layered glomerular (Bowman) capsule
- Visceral layer of capsule contains podocytes that invest fenestrated glomerular capillaries
- Podocytes exhibit primary processes from which arise smaller pedicles
- Pedicles form filtration slits around capillaries that are spanned by filtration slit diaphragm
- Parietal layer is lined with simple squamous epithelium of the glomerular capsule

- Between parietal and visceral layers is the capsular (urinary) space for glomerular filtrate
- At vascular pole, afferent and efferent arterioles enter and exit the renal corpuscle
- At opposite urinary pole, ultrafiltrate enters the proximal convoluted tubule

Blood Filtration

- In renal corpuscle, it is through glomerular capillaries
- Consists of capillary endothelium, basement membrane, and podocytes/pedicles
- Glomerular filtrate enters capsular space between parietal and visceral layers

Filtration Barrier in Glomerulus

- Glomerular endothelium is fenestrated and permeable except for blood cells and large proteins
- Basement membrane restricts molecules the size of albumin
- Slit diaphragms between pedicles contain the transmembrane protein nephrin
- Filtration slits responsible for glomerular permeability due to size-selective molecular filters

Renal Tubules

- From capsular space, glomerular filtrate enters renal tubules that extend to collecting ducts
- Initial tubule is the proximal convoluted tubule that starts at the urinary pole of renal corpuscle
- Loop of Henle consists of thick descending tubules, a thin loop, and thick ascending tubules
- Distal convoluted tubule ascends into kidney cortex and joins the collecting tubule
- Juxtamedullary nephrons have very long loops of Henle
- Collecting tubules are not part of nephron, but join larger collecting ducts to form papillary ducts
- Deep in medulla, papillary ducts are lined with columnar epithelium and exit in area cribrosa
- Medullary rays in cortex are collecting ducts, blood vessels, and straight portions of nephrons

Renal Blood Supply

- Renal artery divides in the hilus into segmental arteries that become interlobar arteries
- At corticomedullary junction, interlobar arteries branch into arcuate arteries

- Arcuate arteries form interlobular arteries from which arise afferent glomerular arterioles
- Glomerular arterioles form capillaries of glomeruli that exit renal corpuscles as efferent arterioles
- Efferent arterioles form peritubular capillaries and vasa recta in the medulla around kidney tubules

Kidney Cells and Kidney Tubules

Mesangial Cells

- Attached to capillaries in the renal corpuscle and serve important functions
- Produce extracellular matrix and provide structural support for glomerular capillaries
- Serve as phagocytes in glomerulus and phagocytose antigen–antibody complexes
- Function as macrophages and regulate blood pressure as a result of vasoactive receptors and contractility
- Extraglomerular cells form part of the juxtaglomerular apparatus

Kidney Cells

- Responsible for homeostasis of the body
- Involved in forming urine through filtration, absorption, and excretion
- Produce enzyme renin to maintain proper filtration pressure in glomeruli
- Synthesize erythropoietin to stimulate erythrocyte production in red bone marrow

Kidney Tubules

Proximal Convoluted Tubules

- Proximal convoluted tubules lined with brush border and absorb most of filtrate
- Basal infoldings of cell membrane contain numerous mitochondria and sodium pumps
- Mitochondria supply energy for ionic transport across cell membrane into the interstitium
- Absorb all glucose, proteins, and amino acids, almost all carbohydrates, and 75% to 85% of water
- Secrete metabolic waste, hydrogen, ammonia, dyes, and drugs into the filtrate for voiding
- Longer than distal convoluted tubules and more frequently seen in cortex near renal corpuscles

Loop of Henle

- In juxtamedullary nephrons, it produces hypertonic urine owing to the countercurrent multiplier system
- High interstitial osmolarity draws water from the filtrate as it flows through the loop

- Vasa recta capillaries take up water from interstitium and return it to systemic circulation

Distal Convoluted Tubules

- Shorter than proximal convoluted tubules, less frequent in cortex, and lack brush border
- Basolateral membrane shows infoldings and contains numerous mitochondria
- Under the influence of aldosterone, sodium ions actively absorbed from the filtrate
- Peritubular capillaries return ions to systemic circulation to maintain vital acid–base balance

Juxtaglomerular Apparatus

- Located adjacent to renal corpuscle and distal convoluted tubule
- Consists of juxtaglomerular cells, macula densa, and extraglomerular mesangial cells
- Juxtaglomerular cells are modified smooth muscle cells in afferent arteriole before entering glomerular capsule
- Main function is to maintain proper blood pressure for blood filtration in renal corpuscles
- Juxtaglomerular cells respond to stretching in the wall of afferent arterioles, as baroreceptors
- Macula densa is a group of modified distal convoluted tubule cells
- Macula densa responds to changes in sodium chloride concentration in glomerular filtrate
- Decreased blood pressure and ionic content causes release of enzyme renin by juxtaglomerular cells
- Renin release eventually causes plasma proteins to convert to angiotensin II, a powerful vasoconstrictor
- Angiotensin II stimulates release of aldosterone, which acts on the distal convoluted tubules
- Distal convoluted tubules absorb NaCl with water, increasing blood volume and pressure
- Distal convoluted tubule also eliminates hydrogen and potassium to maintain acid–base balance

Collecting Tubules, Collecting Ducts, and Antidiuretic Hormone

- Glomerular filtrate flows from distal convoluted tubules to collecting tubules and ducts
- During excessive water loss or dehydration, ADH is released from the pituitary gland
- ADH causes epithelium of collecting duct to become highly permeable to water
- Water that is retained in interstitium is collected by peritubular capillaries and vasa recta
- In the absence of ADH, increased water is retained in collecting ducts and urine is dilute

Ureter

- Lined with transitional epithelium and consists of mucosa, muscularis, and adventitia
- Upper part lined with inner longitudinal and middle circular smooth muscle layers
- Third longitudinal smooth muscle layer added in the lower third of the ureter
- Connective tissue adventitia surrounds the ureter

Bladder

- Thick muscular wall with three indistinct layers of smooth muscle
- Serosa lines superior surface and adventitia covers the inferior surface
- Transitional epithelium in empty bladder exhibits about six layers of cells
- When stretched, transitional epithelium appears stratified squamous
- Changes in epithelium caused by thicker plasma membrane of superficial cells and plaques
- Plaques act like hinges and allow cells to expand during stretching; cells become squamous
- Thicker plasma membrane and transitional epithelium provide osmotic barrier to urine

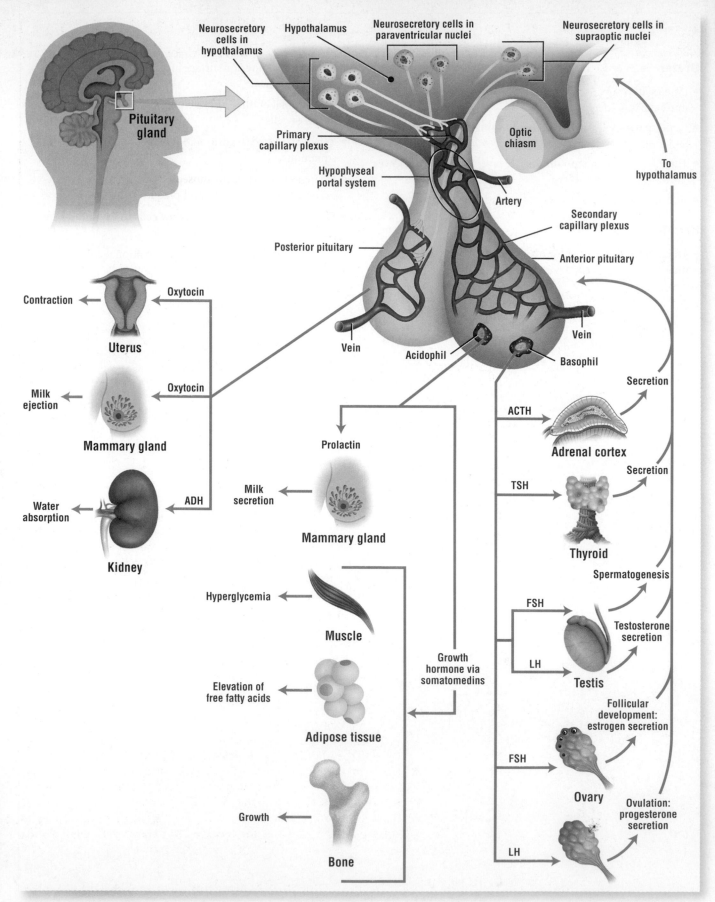

OVERVIEW FIGURE 19.1 ■ Hypothalamus and hypophysis (pituitary gland). A section of hypothalamus and hypophysis illustrates the neuronal, axonal, and vascular connections between the hypothalamus and the hypophysis. Also illustrated are the major target cells, tissues, and organs of the hormones that are produced by both the anterior (adenohypophysis) and posterior (neurohypophysis) pituitary gland. ACTH, adrenocorticotropic hormone; TSH, thyroid-stimulating hormone; FSH, follicle-stimulating hormone; LH, luteinizing hormone.

Endocrine System ▪

SECTION 1 Hormones and Pituitary Gland

The endocrine system consists of cells, tissues, and organs that synthesize and secrete products called **hormones**. The hormones are then released into the interstitial connective tissue from which the hormones pass directly into blood or lymph circulation. As a result, endocrine cells, tissues, glands, and organs are called **ductless** because they do not have excretory ducts for the release of their hormones. Furthermore, the cells in most endocrine tissues and organs are arranged into **cords** and **clumps** and are surrounded by an extensive **capillary network** that allows for more efficient transport of hormones.

Hormones produced by endocrine cells include polypeptides, proteins, steroids, amino acid derivatives, and catecholamines. Because hormones act at a distance from the site of their release, they enter the circulatory system to be transported to the **target organs**. Here, they influence the structure and the programmed function of the target organ cells in the organs by binding to and interacting with specific hormone receptors.

Hormone receptors can be located either on the cell membrane, in the cytoplasm, or in the nucleus of target cells. Nonsteroid receptors for protein and peptide hormones are usually located on cell surfaces because the hormones do not penetrate the cell membrane. Their interaction and activation by the hormone results in the production of intracellular molecules called **second messengers**, which is **cyclic adenosine monophosphate (cAMP)** for numerous hormones. cAMP then activates a specific sequence of enzymes and various cellular events of the cytoplasm and/or nucleus in specific response to the particular hormone.

Other receptors are **intracellular** and are usually localized in the **nucleus**. These receptors are activated by hormones that diffuse through cellular and nuclear membranes. Steroid hormones and thyroid hormones are soluble in lipids and can easily cross these membranes. Once inside the target cells, these steroid hormones combine with specific protein receptors. The resulting hormone–receptor complex binds in the nucleus to a particular DNA sequence that either activates or inhibits specific genes. The activated genes initiate the synthesis of messenger RNA, which enters the cytoplasm to initiate the production of new hormone-specific proteins. The new proteins induce cellular changes that are specifically associated with the influence of the particular hormone. The hormones that combine with the intracellular receptors do not use the second messenger. Instead, they directly influence **gene expression** of the affected cell.

Numerous organs in the body contain individual endocrine cells or endocrine tissues mixed with other tissues. Such mixed (endocrine-exocrine) organs are the pancreas, kidneys, reproductive organs of both sexes, placenta, and gastrointestinal tract. Endocrine cells and endocrine tissues are discussed with the specific exocrine organs in their respective chapters.

There are also complete endocrine organs or glands (Overview Fig. 19.1). These include the **hypophysis, or pituitary gland** (described below), **thyroid gland, adrenal (suprarenal) glands**, and **parathyroid glands** (described in Section 2).

Embryologic Development of Hypophysis (Pituitary Gland)

The pituitary gland, or hypophysis, is often called the master endocrine organ because it secretes many hormones that can influence the action of numerous peripheral tissues or organs in the body. However, the pituitary gland itself is controlled by the **hypothalamus** of the brain from which regulatory hormones are transported to the pituitary. To understand this functional relationship, it is important to understand the embryologic development of the pituitary gland.

The structure and function of the hypophysis reflect its dual embryologic origin. During embryonic development, the epithelium of the **pharyngeal roof** (oral cavity) forms an outpocketing called the **hypophyseal (Rathke) pouch**. As development proceeds, the hypophyseal pouch detaches from the oral cavity to become the cellular or glandular portion of the hypophysis, now called the **adenohypophysis (anterior pituitary)**. At the same time, the downgrowth from the developing brain (diencephalon) forms the neural portion of the hypophysis, called the **neurohypophysis (posterior pituitary)**. The two separately developed structures then unite to form a single pituitary gland, the hypophysis. The hypophysis remains attached to a ventral extension of the brain called the **hypothalamus**. A short neural stalk, called the **infundibulum**, is a neural pathway that attaches and connects the hypophysis to the hypothalamus. The neurons that are located in the hypothalamus control the release of hormones from the adenohypophysis as well as secrete hormones that are then transported to and stored in the neurohypophysis until needed.

After development, the hypophysis rests in a bony depression of the sphenoid bone of the skull called the **sella turcica** that is located inferior to the hypothalamus at the base of the brain.

Subdivisions of the Hypophysis

The epithelial-derived adenohypophysis has three subdivisions: pars distalis, pars tuberalis, and pars intermedia. The **pars distalis** is the largest part of the hypophysis. The **pars tuberalis** surrounds the neural stalk, or infundibulum. The **pars intermedia** is a thin cell layer between the pars distalis and the neurohypophysis. It represents the remnant of the hypophyseal (Rathke) pouch that becomes rudimentary in humans but prominent in other mammals.

The neurohypophysis, situated posterior to the adenohypophysis, also consists of three parts: median eminence, infundibulum, and pars nervosa. The **median eminence** is located at the base of the hypothalamus of the brain from which extends the pituitary stalk, or **infundibulum**. In the infundibulum is found a multitude of unmyelinated axons that extend from the neurons in the hypothalamus. The large portion of the neurohypophysis is the **pars nervosa**. This region contains the terminal ends of unmyelinated axons for the storage of hormones that have been secreted by the neurons in the hypothalamus. Surrounding the axons are the nonsecretory **pituicytes** that support and nourish the axons.

Vascular and Neural Connections of Hypophysis

Adenohypophysis

Because the adenohypophysis does not develop from the neural tissue, its connection to the **hypothalamus** of the brain is via a rich vascular network. **Superior hypophyseal arteries** from the internal carotid artery supply the pars tuberalis, median eminence, and infundibulum. These arteries form a **primary capillary plexus** in the median eminence at the base of the hypothalamus. Secretory neurons that are located in the hypothalamus synthesize hormones that have a direct influence on cell functions in the adenohypophysis. The axons from these neurons terminate on the fenestrated capillaries of the primary capillary plexus into which they release their hormones.

Small **hypophyseal portal venules** then drain the primary capillary plexus and deliver the blood with the hormones to a **secondary capillary plexus** that surrounds the cells in the pars distalis of the adenohypophysis. The venules that connect the primary capillary plexus of the hypothalamus with the secondary capillary plexus in the adenohypophysis form the **hypophyseal portal system**. To ensure efficient transport of hormones from the blood to the cells, the capillaries in the primary and secondary capillary plexuses are **fenestrated** (contain small pores).

Cells of the Adenohypophysis

The cells of the adenohypophysis were initially classified as **chromophobes** and **chromophils** based on the affinity of their cytoplasmic granules for specific stains. The pale-staining chromophobes are believed to be either degranulated chromophils with few granules or undifferentiated stem cells. The chromophils were further subdivided into **acidophils** and **basophils** because of their staining properties. Immunocytochemical techniques now identify these cells on the basis of their specific hormones. The adenohypophysis includes two types of acidophils, the **somatotrophs** and **mammotrophs**, as well as three types of basophils: **gonadotrophs**, **thyrotrophs**, and **corticotrophs**.

The hormones released from these cells are carried in the bloodstream to the target organs, where they bind to specific receptors that influence the structure and function of the target cells. Once the target cells are activated and release their secretory products, a **feedback mechanism** (positive or negative) controls the synthesis and release of these hormones by directly acting on cells in the adenohypophysis or neurons in the hypothalamus that have initially produced these hormones.

Neurohypophysis

In contrast to the adenohypophysis, the neurohypophysis has a direct neural connection with the brain. As a result, there are no neurons or hormone-producing cells in the neurohypophysis, and it remains connected to the brain by a multitude of unmyelinated axons and supportive cells, the pituicytes. The **neurons** (cell bodies) of these axons are located in the **supraoptic** and **paraventricular nuclei** (a collection of neurons) in the hypothalamus. The unmyelinated axons that extend from the hypothalamus into the neurohypophysis form the **hypothalamohypophyseal tract** and the bulk of the neurohypophysis. These axons also terminate near the fenestrated capillaries in the pars nervosa.

Neurons in the hypothalamus first synthesize the hormones that are released from the neurohypophysis. These hormones bind to the carrier glycoprotein **neurophysin** and are then transported from the hypothalamus down the axons by **axonal transport** to the neurohypophysis. Here, the hormones accumulate and are stored in the distended terminal ends of unmyelinated axons as **Herring bodies**. When needed, hormones from the neurohypophysis are directly released into the fenestrated capillaries of the pars nervosa by nerve impulses from the hypothalamus.

Supplemental micrographic images are available at **www.thePoint.com/Eroschenko12e** under Endocrine System.

FIGURE 19.1 | Hypophysis (Panoramic View, Sagittal Section)

The hypophysis (pituitary gland) consists of two major subdivisions: the adenohypophysis and neurohypophysis. The adenohypophysis is further subdivided into the **pars distalis (anterior lobe) (5)**, **pars tuberalis (7)**, and **pars intermedia (9)**. The neurohypophysis is divided into the **pars nervosa (11)**, **infundibulum (6)**, and the median eminence (not illustrated). The pars tuberalis (7) surrounds the infundibulum (6) and is visible above and below the infundibulum (6) in a sagittal section. The infundibulum (6) connects the hypophysis with the hypothalamus at the base of the brain.

The pars distalis (5) contains two main cell types: chromophobe cells and chromophil cells. The chromophils are subdivided into **acidophils (alpha cells) (4)** and **basophils (beta cells) (2)**, illustrated at a higher magnification in Figure 19.2.

The pars intermedia (9) and pars nervosa (11) form the posterior lobe of the hypophysis. The pars nervosa (11) consists primarily of unmyelinated axons and supporting pituicytes. A **connective tissue capsule (1, 10)** surrounds the pars distalis (5) and pars nervosa (11) portions of the gland.

The pars intermedia (9) is situated between the pars distalis (5) and the pars nervosa (11) and represents the residual lumen of the Rathke pouch. The pars intermedia (9) normally contains **colloid-filled vesicles (9a)** that are surrounded by the cells of the pars intermedia (9).

Both the pars distalis (5) and pars nervosa (11) are supplied by numerous **blood vessels (8)** and **capillaries (3)** of different sizes.

FIGURE 19.2 | Hypophysis: Sections of Pars Distalis, Pars Intermedia, and Pars Nervosa

At a higher magnification, numerous **sinusoidal capillaries (1)** and different cell types are visible in the **pars distalis**. **Chromophobe cells (2)** have a light-staining, homogeneous cytoplasm and are normally smaller than the chromophils. The cytoplasm of chromophils stains reddish in the **acidophils (3)** and bluish in the **basophils (4)**.

The **pars intermedia** contains **follicles (6)** and colloid-filled **cystic follicles (7)**. Follicles lined with basophils (8) are often present in the pars intermedia.

The **pars nervosa** is characterized by unmyelinated axons and the supportive **pituicytes (5)** with oval nuclei.

FUNCTIONAL CORRELATIONS 19.1 | Hormones of the Hypophysis

Hormones produced by neurons in the **hypothalamus** directly influence and control the synthesis and release of six specific hormones from the adenohypophysis. Most of the hormones are **releasing hormones** produced by neurons in the hypothalamus for each hormone that is released from the adenohypophysis. For two hormones, growth hormone (GH) and prolactin, **inhibitory hormones** are also produced. These releasing hormones are thyrotropin-releasing hormone, gonadotropin-releasing hormone, corticotropin-releasing hormone, and growth hormone–releasing hormone. The inhibitory hormones are **somatostatin**, which inhibits the release of GH, and **dopamine** (prolactin-inhibiting hormone), which inhibits the secretion of prolactin.

The releasing and inhibitory hormones secreted from the hypothalamic neurons are carried from the primary capillary plexus of the median eminence of the hypothalamus to the second capillary plexus in the adenohypophysis via the **hypophyseal portal system**. On reaching the adenohypophysis, the hormones bind to specific receptors on cells and either stimulate the cells to secrete and release a specific hormone into the circulation or inhibit this function.

In contrast, the neurohypophysis does not secrete hormones. Instead, the neurohypophysis stores and releases only two hormones when needed, **oxytocin** and **vasopressin** (antidiuretic hormone), that were synthesized in the hypothalamus by the neurons in the **paraventricular nuclei** and **supraoptic nuclei**. These hormones are then transported along unmyelinated axons and stored as tiny dilations in the axon terminals of the neurohypophysis as **Herring bodies** from which they are released into the capillaries of the par nervosa as needed. Herring bodies are visible with a light microscope.

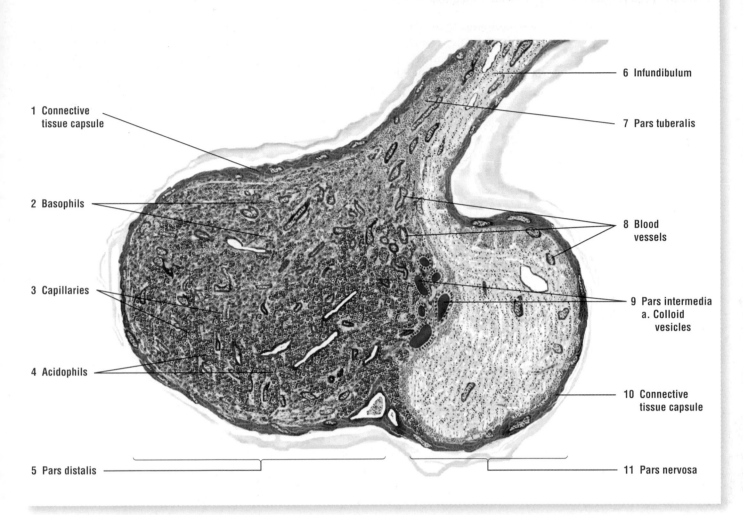

1 Connective tissue capsule

2 Basophils

3 Capillaries

4 Acidophils

5 Pars distalis

6 Infundibulum

7 Pars tuberalis

8 Blood vessels

9 Pars intermedia
   a. Colloid vesicles

10 Connective tissue capsule

11 Pars nervosa

FIGURE 19.1 ■ Hypophysis (panoramic view, sagittal section). Stain: hematoxylin and eosin. Low magnification.

Pars distalis   Pars intermedia   Pars nervosa

1 Sinusoidal capillaries

2 Chromophobe cells

3 Acidophils (alpha cells)

4 Basophils (beta cells)

5 Nuclei of pituicytes

6 Follicles (pars intermedia)

7 Cystic follicles (pars intermedia)

FIGURE 19.2 ■ Hypophysis: sections of pars distalis, pars intermedia, and pars nervosa. Stain: hematoxylin and eosin. Medium magnification.

FIGURE 19.3 | Hypophysis: Pars Distalis (Sectional View)

This illustration shows the two main populations of cells in the pars distalis of the adenohypophysis. The cells here are arranged in clumps. Between the clumps are seen the numerous **capillaries (5)**, **blood vessels (3)**, and thin **connective tissue fibers (6)** that separate the clumps. Cell types in the pars distalis can be identified with special fixation and the staining affinity of the cytoplasmic granules.

The **chromophobes (4)** usually exhibit pale nuclei and pale cytoplasm with poorly defined cell outlines. The aggregation of chromophobes in groups or clumps is seen in this illustration.

The **acidophils (2)** are more numerous and can be distinguished by their red-staining granules in the cytoplasm and blue nuclei.

The **basophils (1)** are less numerous and appear as cells that contain blue-staining granules in their cytoplasm. The degree of granularity and the stain density vary in different cells.

FIGURE 19.4 | Cell Types in the Hypophysis

Groups of different cell types of the hypophysis are illustrated at a higher magnification after modified Azan staining. The nuclei of all cells are stained orange-red.

The **chromophobes (a)** exhibit a clear and very light orange cytoplasm. The appearance of clear cytoplasm indicates that the cells do not have granules, and as a result, their cell boundaries are indistinct.

The cytoplasmic granules of **acidophils (b)** stain intensely red, and the cell outlines are distinct. A sinusoid capillary surrounds the acidophils.

The **basophils (c)** exhibit variable cell shapes and granules that vary in size.

The **pituicytes (d)** of the pars nervosa have variable cell shape and cell size. The small, orange-stained cytoplasm is diffuse and barely visible.

1 Basophils

2 Acidophils

3 Blood vessels

4 Chromophobes

5 Capillaries

6 Connective tissue fibers

FIGURE 19.3 ■ Hypophysis: pars distalis (sectional view). Stain: Azan. High magnification.

a. Chromophobes

b. Acidophils (alpha cells)

c. Basophils (beta cells)

d. Pituicytes

FIGURE 19.4 ■ Cell types in the hypophysis. Stain: modified Azan. Oil immersion.

FIGURE 19.5 | Hypophysis: Pars Distalis, Pars Intermedia, and Pars Nervosa

This higher-power photomicrograph illustrates the cellular pars distalis and pars intermedia of the adenohypophysis and the light-staining pars nervosa of the neurohypophysis. With this stain, different cell types can be identified in the pars distalis. The red-staining, or eosinophilic, cells are the **acidophils (5)**. The cells with bluish cytoplasm are the **basophils (4)**. The light, unstained cells scattered among the acidophils (5) and basophils (4) are the **chromophobes (7)**. The pars intermedia exhibits small cysts, or **vesicles (6),** filled with colloid.

The pars nervosa is filled with the unmyelinated, light-staining axons of secretory cells, whose cell bodies are located in the hypothalamus. Most of the red-staining nuclei in the pars nervosa are the supportive cell **pituicytes (2)**. Accumulations of the neurosecretory material at the end of the axon terminals in the pars nervosa are the irregular-shaped, red-staining structures called the **Herring bodies (3)**. Herring bodies (3) are closely associated with capillaries and **blood vessels (1)**. Surrounding the secretory cells and axon terminals in the neurohypophysis are blood vessels (1) and fenestrated capillaries.

FUNCTIONAL CORRELATIONS 19.2 | Cells and Hormones of the Adenohypophysis

ACIDOPHILS

Somatotrophs secrete **somatotropin**, also called growth hormone, or GH. This hormone targets the whole body and its general growth. It stimulates cellular metabolism, uptake of amino acids, and protein synthesis. Somatotropin also stimulates the liver to produce **somatomedins**, also called insulin-like growth factor 1 (IGF-1). These hormones increase proliferation of cartilage cells (chondrocytes) in the **epiphyseal plates** of developing or growing long bones to increase the bone length. There is also an increase in the growth of the skeletal muscle and increased release of fatty acids from the adipose cells for energy production by body cells. GH-inhibiting hormone, also called **somatostatin**, has an inhibitory effect on the release of GH from somatotrophs in the pituitary gland.

Mammotrophs produce the lactogenic hormone **prolactin** that stimulates the development of mammary glands during pregnancy. After parturition (birth), prolactin maintains milk production in the developed mammary glands during lactation. The release of prolactin from mammotrophs is inhibited by a prolactin release inhibitory hormone, also called **dopamine**.

BASOPHILS

Thyrotrophs secrete **thyroid-stimulating hormone (thyrotropin** or **TSH)**. TSH stimulates follicular cells in the thyroid gland to synthesize and secrete thyroglobulin and the hormones **thyroxin** and **triiodothyronine** from the thyroid gland.

Gonadotrophs secrete **follicle-stimulating hormone (FSH)** and **luteinizing hormone (LH)**. In females, FSH promotes growth and maturation of ovarian follicles and the subsequent **estrogen** secretion by developing follicles. In males, FSH promotes **spermatogenesis** in the testes and secretion of **androgen-binding protein** into seminiferous tubules by **Sertoli cells**. The androgen-binding protein maintains the needed concentration of testosterone in the seminiferous tubules to ensure proper spermatogenesis.

In females, LH in association with FSH induces **ovulation**, promotes the final maturation of ovarian follicles, and stimulates the formation of the **corpus luteum** after ovulation. LH also promotes the secretion of estrogen and progesterone from the corpus luteum. In males, LH maintains and stimulates the **interstitial cells** (of Leydig) in the testes to produce the hormone **testosterone**. As a result, LH is sometimes called interstitial cell–stimulating hormone.

Corticotrophs secrete **adrenocorticotropic hormone (ACTH)**. ACTH influences the function of the cells in **adrenal cortex**. ACTH also stimulates the synthesis and release of glucocorticoids from the zona fasciculata and zona reticularis of adrenal cortex.

PARS INTERMEDIA

In lower vertebrates (amphibians and fishes), the pars intermedia is well developed and produces **melanocyte-stimulating hormone (MSH)**. MSH increases skin pigmentation by causing the dispersion of melanin granules. In humans and most mammals, the pars intermedia is rudimentary.

1 Blood vessels

2 Pituicytes

3 Herring bodies

4 Basophils (beta cells)

5 Acidophils (alpha cells)

6 Vesicles

7 Chromophobes

FIGURE 19.5 ■ Hypophysis: pars distalis, pars intermedia, and pars nervosa. Stain: Mallory-Azan and orange G. ×80.

FUNCTIONAL CORRELATIONS 19.3	Cells and Hormones of the Neurohypophysis

OXYTOCIN

The two hormones, oxytocin and antidiuretic hormone (ADH), that are released from the neurohypophysis are synthesized in the supraoptic and paraventricular nuclei of the hypothalamus. The release of oxytocin is stimulated by vaginal and cervical distension before birth and nursing of the infant after birth. The main targets of **oxytocin** are the smooth muscles of the pregnant uterus. During labor, oxytocin is released to induce strong contractions of smooth muscles in the uterus, resulting in childbirth (parturition). After parturition, the suckling action of the infant on the nipple stimulates and activates the **milk-ejection reflex** in the lactating mammary glands. Afferent impulses from the nipple stimulate neurons in the hypothalamus, causing oxytocin release. Oxytocin then stimulates the contraction of **myoepithelial cells** around the alveoli and ducts in the lactating mammary glands, ejecting milk into the excretory ducts and the nipple.

ANTIDIURETIC HORMONE (VASOPRESSIN)

The main action of ADH is to increase **water permeability** in the **distal convoluted tubules** and **collecting ducts** of the kidney. As a result, more water is reabsorbed from the filtrate into the interstitium and retained in the body, creating more concentrated urine. A sudden decrease of blood pressure is also a stimulus for the release of ADH. It is believed that in large doses, ADH may cause smooth muscle contraction in arteries and arterioles. However, physiologic doses of ADH appear to have minimal effects on blood pressure.

CHAPTER 19 SUMMARY

SECTION 1 • Hormones and Pituitary Gland

- Consists of cells, tissues, and organs that produce blood-borne chemicals
- Consists of ductless glands, arranged in cords and clumps, and surrounded by capillaries
- Hormones enter connective tissue and then blood or lymphatic circulation
- Hormones interact with target organs that have specific receptors
- Hormone receptors located on cell membrane, in cytoplasm, or in nucleus
- Nonsteroid hormone receptors located on cell surface
- Proteins and polypeptide hormones use second messenger (cAMP) to activate responses
- Steroid and thyroid hormones that enter cells and influence gene expression in nucleus
- There are complete endocrine organs and mixed organs with endocrine cells and tissues

Embryologic Development of Hypophysis (Pituitary Gland)

- Has dual embryologic origin, epithelial and neural
- Epithelial portion develops from pharyngeal roof and Rathke pouch
- Pouch detaches and becomes the cellular portion, adenohypophysis (anterior pituitary)
- Downgrowth of brain forms the neural portion, neurohypophysis (posterior pituitary)
- Neurohypophysis remains attached to hypothalamus by a neural stalk, infundibulum
- Neurons in hypothalamus control release of hormones from adenohypophysis

Subdivisions of Hypophysis

- Adenohypophysis (anterior pituitary) has three subdivisions
- Pars distalis is the largest part
- Pars intermedia is remnant of the pouch and rudimentary in humans
- Pars tuberalis surrounds the neural stalk
- Neurohypophysis (posterior pituitary) consists of three parts
- Median eminence is located at the base of hypothalamus
- Infundibulum is the neural stalk that connects neurohypophysis to hypothalamus
- Pars nervosa is the largest portion that consists of unmyelinated axons and pituicytes

Vascular and Neural Connections of Hypophysis

Adenohypophysis

- Connection between hypothalamus of brain and adenohypophysis is vascular
- Superior hypophyseal arteries form fenestrated primary capillary plexus in median eminence
- Secretory neurons in hypothalamus terminate on capillary plexus and release hormones
- Hypophyseal venules connect to secondary capillary plexus in adenohypophysis, forming a hypophyseal portal system
- Hypothalamus produces releasing hormones and inhibitory hormones for cells in adenohypophysis
- Releasing or inhibitory hormones are carried via the portal system to cells in pars distalis
- Releasing hormones bind to specific receptors in cells of pars distalis

Cells and Hormones of Adenohypophysis

- Based on stains, there are three cell types: acidophils, basophils, and chromophobes
- Acidophils are subdivided into somatotrophs and mammotrophs
- Basophils are subdivided into thyrotrophs, gonadotrophs, and corticotrophs

Somatotrophs

- Secrete somatotropin or growth hormone for cell metabolism and general body growth
- Somatotropin also stimulates liver to produce somatomedins
- Somatomedins influence cartilage cells in epiphyseal plates to increase growth in length
- Somatostatin inhibits release of growth hormone from somatotrophs

Mammotrophs

- Produce prolactin that stimulates mammary gland development during pregnancy
- Prolactin maintains milk production after parturition
- Release of prolactin inhibited by inhibitory hormone called dopamine

Thyrotrophs

- Release thyroid-stimulating hormone that stimulates thyroid gland hormones
- Thyroid cells produce thyroglobulin, thyroxin, and triiodothyronine

Gonadotrophs

- Secrete both follicle-stimulating hormone and leuteinizing hormone
- In females, follicle-stimulating hormone stimulates follicular development, maturation, and estrogen production
- In males, follicle-stimulating hormone promotes spermatogenesis and androgen-binding protein secretion by Sertoli cells
- In females, luteinizing hormone induces follicular maturation, ovulation, and corpus luteum formation
- Corpus luteum secretes estrogen and progesterone
- In males, luteinizing hormone stimulates interstitial cells in testes to produce testosterone (androgens)

Corticotrophs

- Secrete adrenocorticotropic hormone to regulate adrenal cortex functions
- Feedback mechanism controls further synthesis and release of specific hormones
- Pars intermedia in humans is rudimentary; in lower vertebrates produces melanocyte-stimulating hormone

Neurohypophysis

- Does not have any secretory cells; secretory neurons are located in hypothalamus of brain
- Has a direct neural connection to hypothalamus via multitude of unmyelinated axons
- Contains axonal hypothalamohypophyseal tract and supportive cells pituicytes
- Neurons of axons located in supraoptic and paraventricular nuclei of hypothalamus
- Neurons synthesize hormones that are transported in and stored at axon terminals as Herring bodies
- Carrier glycoprotein neurophysin binds to hormones for transport to axon terminals
- Releases two hormones from axon terminals, oxytocin and antidiuretic hormone (vasopressin)

Oxytocin

- Release stimulated by vaginal and cervical distension during labor, and nursing infant
- Stimulates contraction of smooth uterine muscles during childbirth
- Activates milk ejection in lactating glands by stimulating contraction of myoepithelial cells

Antidiuretic Hormone

- Increases permeability to water in distal convoluted tubules and collecting ducts of kidney
- Creates more concentrated urine after water is reabsorbed from glomerular filtrate
- Is also released during decreased blood pressure and, in large doses, contracts arterial walls

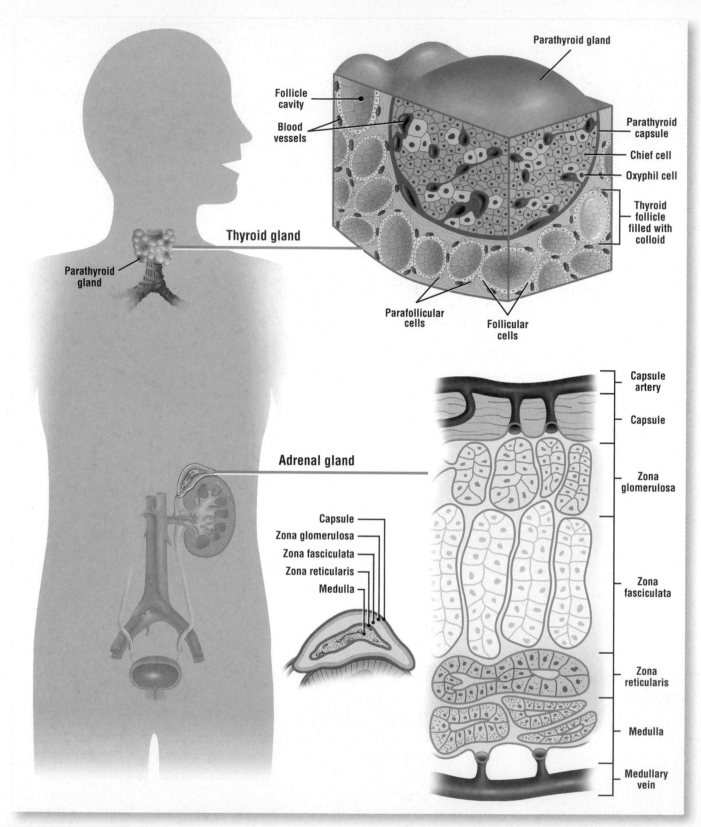

OVERVIEW FIGURE 19.2 ■ Thyroid gland, parathyroid gland, and adrenal gland. The microscopic organization and general location in the body of the thyroid, parathyroid, and adrenal glands are illustrated.

SECTION 2 Thyroid Gland, Parathyroid Glands, and Adrenal Gland

The location in the body and histologic appearance of the thyroid gland, parathyroid glands, and adrenal glands are illustrated in Overview Figure 19.2.

Thyroid Gland

The **thyroid gland** is located in the anterior neck inferior to the larynx. It is a single gland that consists of large right and left lobes, connected in the middle by an isthmus. Most endocrine cells, tissues, or organs are arranged in cords or clumps and store their secretory products within their cytoplasm. The thyroid gland is a unique endocrine organ in that its cells are arranged into spherical structures, called **follicles**, where the hormones are stored. Each follicle is lined with a single layer of follicular cells and surrounded by reticular fibers. The adjacent vascular network of capillaries surrounds the follicles for the easy entrance of thyroid hormones from the follicles into the bloodstream. The follicular epithelium can be simple squamous, cuboidal, or low columnar, depending on the state of activity of the thyroid gland.

Follicles are the structural and functional units of the thyroid gland. The cells that surround the follicles, the **follicular cells**, also called principal cells, synthesize, release, and store their product outside their cytoplasm, or extracellularly, in the lumen of the follicles as a gelatinous substance called **colloid**. Colloid is composed of **thyroglobulin**, an iodinated glycoprotein that is the inactive storage form of the thyroid hormones.

In addition to follicular cells, the thyroid gland also contains larger, pale-staining **parafollicular** cells. These cells are found either peripherally in the follicular epithelium or within the follicle. When parafollicular cells are located in the confines of a follicle, they are always separated from the follicular lumen by neighboring follicular cells.

Parathyroid Glands

Mammals generally have four **parathyroid glands**. These small oval glands are embedded on the posterior surface of the thyroid gland but are separated from the thyroid gland by a thin connective tissue **capsule**. Normally, one parathyroid gland is located on the superior pole and one on the inferior pole of each lobe of the thyroid gland. In contrast to the thyroid gland, the cells of the parathyroid glands are arranged into cords or clumps, surrounded by a rich network of capillaries, and normally they do not exhibit follicles that are seen in the adjacent thyroid gland.

There are two types of cells in the parathyroid glands: functional **principal**, or **chief, cells** and **oxyphil cells**. Oxyphil cells are larger, are found singly or in small groups, and are less numerous than the principal (chief cells). In routine histologic sections, these cells stain deeply acidophilic. On rare occasions, small colloid-filled follicles may be seen in the parathyroid glands.

Adrenal (Suprarenal) Glands

The **adrenal glands** are endocrine organs situated near the superior pole of each kidney. Each adrenal gland is surrounded by a dense irregular connective tissue capsule and embedded in the adipose tissue around the kidneys. The secretory portion of each adrenal gland consists of an outer **cortex** and an inner **medulla**. Although these two regions of the adrenal gland are located in one organ and are linked by a common blood supply, they have separate and distinct embryologic origins, structures, and functions.

Cortex

The adrenal cortex exhibits three concentric zones: the zona glomerulosa, zona fasciculata, and zona reticularis.

The **zona glomerulosa** is a thin zone inferior to the adrenal gland capsule. It consists of cells arranged in small clumps.

The **zona fasciculata** is intermediate and the thickest zone of the adrenal cortex. This zone exhibits vertical columns of one-cell thickness adjacent to straight capillaries. This layer is characterized by pale-staining cells owing to the increased presence of numerous lipid droplets.

The **zona reticularis** is the innermost zone that is adjacent to the adrenal medulla. The cells in this zone are arranged in cords or clumps.

In all three zones, the secretory cells are adjacent to fenestrated capillaries. The cells of these zones in the adrenal cortex produce three classes of steroid hormones: **mineralocorticoids, glucocorticoids**, and **sex hormones**.

Medulla

The medulla lies in the center of the adrenal gland. The cells of the adrenal medulla, also arranged in small cords, are modified postganglionic sympathetic neurons that have lost their axons and dendrites during development. Instead, they have become secretory cells that synthesize and secrete **catecholamines** (primarily epinephrine and norepinephrine). Preganglionic axons of the sympathetic neurons innervate the adrenal medulla cells, which are surrounded by an extensive capillary network. As result, the release of epinephrine and norepinephrine from the adrenal medulla is very efficient and under the direct control of the sympathetic division of the **autonomic nervous system**. Ganglion cells are also present in the adrenal medulla.

 Supplemental micrographic images are available at **www.thePoint.com/Eroschenko12e** under Endocrine System.

FIGURE 19.6 | Thyroid Gland: Canine (General View)

The thyroid gland is characterized by numerous and variable-sized **follicles (1, 10)** that are filled with an acidophilic secretory product called **colloid (1, 10)**. The follicles are usually lined with a simple cuboidal epithelium consisting of **follicular** (principal) **cells (5, 6)**. The **follicles (6, 9)** that are sectioned peripherally or tangentially do not exhibit follicular content and appear as separate cell clumps (6, 9). The follicular cells (5, 6) synthesize and secrete the colloid and the thyroid hormones. In routine histologic preparations, colloid often retracts from the follicular wall of the follicle (10).

Within the thyroid gland are also found another cell type called **parafollicular cells (11)**. These cells occur as single cells or in clumps on the periphery of the follicles. The parafollicular cells (11) stain somewhat lighter than the follicular cells (5) and are readily visible in the canine thyroid. Parafollicular cells (11) synthesize and secrete the hormone calcitonin.

Connective tissue **septa (8)** from the thyroid gland capsule extend into the gland's interior and divide the gland into lobules. Numerous blood vessels—**arterioles (3)**, **venules (4)**, and **capillaries (2)**—are seen in the connective tissue septa (8) and around individual follicles (2). A small amount of **interfollicular connective tissue (7)** is found between individual follicles.

FIGURE 19.7 | Thyroid Gland Follicles: Canine (Sectional View)

This higher magnification of a section of the thyroid gland shows greater detail of individual **thyroid follicles (7)** with secretory colloid material. The height of the **follicular cells (2, 6, 10)** depends on the function of the individual follicles. In highly active follicles, the epithelium is cuboidal (2, 10). In less active follicles, the epithelial cells appear flattened. All thyroid follicles (7) are filled with the secretory material, **colloid (7)**, some of which show **retraction (1)** from the follicular wall or **distortion (1)** as a result of chemicals used in slide preparation.

At a higher magnification, the location of **parafollicular cells (3, 11)** is seen to be adjacent to the follicular cells (2, 10) or in small clumps (3) adjacent to the thyroid follicles (7). The parafollicular cells (3, 11) are larger than the follicular cells (2, 10) and oval in shape with cytoplasm staining lighter than the cytoplasm of the follicular cells (2, 10). Although the parafollicular cells (3, 11) appear to be directly located on the follicular lumen, they are, instead, separated from the lumen by the processes of neighboring follicular cells (2, 10).

Surrounding the thyroid follicles (7), the follicular cells (2, 10), and the parafollicular cells (3, 11) is a thin **interfollicular connective tissue (9)** with numerous **blood vessels (5)** and **capillaries (4, 8)** that are very close to the individual follicles.

1 Follicles with colloid

2 Capillaries

3 Arteriole

4 Venule

5 Follicular cells

6 Follicular cells (tangential section)

7 Interfollicular connective tissue

8 Connective tissue septa

9 Follicle (tangential section)

10 Follicle with retracted colloid

11 Parafollicular cells

FIGURE 19.6 ■ Thyroid gland: canine (general view). Stain: hematoxylin and eosin. Low magnification.

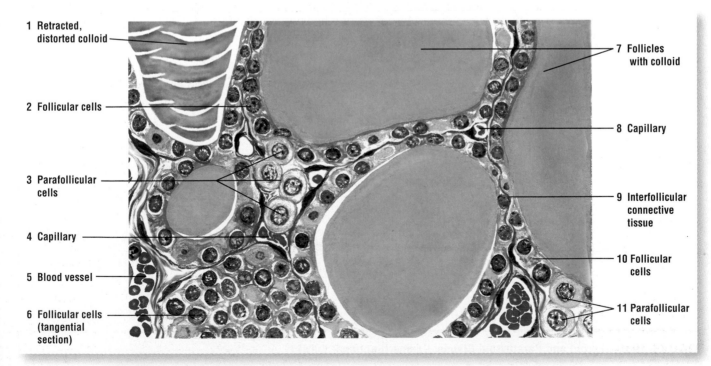

1 Retracted, distorted colloid

2 Follicular cells

3 Parafollicular cells

4 Capillary

5 Blood vessel

6 Follicular cells (tangential section)

7 Follicles with colloid

8 Capillary

9 Interfollicular connective tissue

10 Follicular cells

11 Parafollicular cells

FIGURE 19.7 ■ Thyroid gland follicles: canine (sectional view). Stain: hematoxylin and eosin. High magnification.

FUNCTIONAL CORRELATIONS 19.4 | Thyroid Gland

FORMATION OF THYROID HORMONES

The secretory functions of **follicular cells**, which are responsible for the production of thyroid hormones in the thyroid gland, are controlled by **thyroid-stimulating hormone (TSH)** released from the adenohypophysis. **Iodide** is an essential element for the production of the active thyroid hormones **triiodothyronine (T_3)** and **tetraiodothyronine, or thyroxine (T_4)**, that are released into the bloodstream by the thyroid gland.

Low levels of thyroid hormones in the blood stimulate the release of TSH from the adenohypophysis. In response to TSH stimulus, the follicular cells in the thyroid gland take up **iodide** into their cytoplasm from the circulation via the iodide pump located in the follicular basal cell membrane. Iodide is then oxidized to iodine in the follicular cells and transported into the follicular lumen that contains colloid material. In the follicular lumen, iodine combines with amino acid tyrosine groups to form **iodinated thyroglobulin**, of which the hormones (T_3 and T_4) are the principal products. T_3 and T_4 remain bound to the iodinated thyroglobulin in thyroid follicles in an inactive form until needed. TSH released from the adenohypophysis also stimulates the thyroid gland cells to release the thyroid hormones into the bloodstream.

RELEASE OF THYROID HORMONES

The release of thyroid hormones involves endocytosis (uptake) of thyroglobulin by follicular cells, hydrolysis of the iodinated thyroglobulin by lysosomal proteases, and release of the principal **thyroid hormones (T_3 and T_4)** at the base of follicular cells into the surrounding capillaries. Most of the released thyroid hormones are tightly bound to specific thyroxin-binding protein. The thyroid secretes greater quantities of T_4 than T_3 into the circulation; however, T_3 is physiologically much more potent than T_4. The presence of thyroid hormones in the general circulation accelerates the metabolic rate of the body and increases cell metabolism, growth, differentiation, and development throughout the body. In addition, thyroid hormones increase the rate of protein, carbohydrate, and fat metabolism.

PARAFOLLICULAR CELLS

The thyroid gland also contains **parafollicular cells**. These cells appear on the periphery of the follicular epithelium as single cells or as cell clusters between the follicles. Parafollicular cells are not part of thyroid follicles and are not in contact with colloid in the follicular lumen.

The parafollicular cells synthesize and secrete the hormone **calcitonin (thyrocalcitonin)** into capillaries, which regulates calcium metabolism in the body. The main function of calcitonin is to lower blood calcium levels in the body. This is primarily accomplished by inhibiting the resorptive action of **osteoclasts**, reducing calcium release, and increasing calcium deposition in bones. Calcitonin also promotes increased excretion of calcium and phosphate ions from the kidneys into the urine. The production and release of calcitonin by the parafollicular cells depends on increased blood calcium levels and is completely **independent** of the pituitary gland hormones. Thus, the secretion and release of calcitonin into the bloodstream is regulated by calcium levels through a simple **feedback** mechanism.

FIGURE 19.8 | Thyroid and Parathyroid Glands: Canine (Sectional View)

The **follicles (1)** filled with the secretory material colloid of the **thyroid gland (7)** are closely associated with the different cell types of the **parathyroid gland (9)**. Thin **connective tissue (3, 8)** septa from the surrounding glandular capsule extend into the thyroid gland to separate the parathyroid gland (9) cells from the thyroid gland (7) follicles. In the connective tissue (3, 8) are found larger blood vessels that eventually branch into numerous **capillaries (5)** to surround the parathyroid cells (9) as well as the follicles (1) in the thyroid gland (7).

The parathyroid gland (9) cells are arranged into anastomosing cords and clumps, instead of the follicles (1) filled with the secretory material colloid surrounded by **follicular cells (2)** of the thyroid gland (7). However, occasionally, an isolated small follicle with colloid material may be observed in the parathyroid gland. The parathyroid gland (9) contains two cell types: the **chief (principal) cells (4)** and the **oxyphil cells (6)**. The chief cells (4) of the parathyroid gland are the most numerous cells. They are round and have a pale, slightly acidophilic cytoplasm. In contrast, the oxyphil cells (6) are larger and less numerous than the chief cells (4) and exhibit an acidophilic cytoplasm with dark nuclei (6). The oxyphil cells (6) are found as single cells or in small clumps throughout the parathyroid gland (9); these cells increase in number with increasing age of the individual.

FIGURE 19.8 ■ Thyroid and parathyroid glands: canine (sectional view). Stain: hematoxylin and eosin. Low magnification.

FIGURE 19.9 | Thyroid Gland and Parathyroid Gland

This photomicrograph shows a section of parathyroid gland adjacent to the thyroid gland. A thin **connective tissue septum (3)** separates the two glands. Different size **follicles with colloid (1)** and lined with **follicular cells (2)** characterize the thyroid gland.

Instead of follicles, the parathyroid gland contains two cell types: **Chief cells (4)** are smaller and more numerous, whereas the **oxyphil cells (5)** are larger and less numerous and exhibit a highly eosinophilic cytoplasm. Numerous **blood vessels (6)** surround the secretory cells in both organs.

FUNCTIONAL CORRELATIONS 19.5 | Parathyroid Glands

The **chief cells** of the parathyroid glands produce **parathyroid hormone (parathormone)**. The main function of this hormone is to maintain proper calcium and phosphate levels in the extracellular body fluids by elevating calcium levels in the blood. This action is opposite, or antagonistic, to that of calcitonin, which is produced by parafollicular cells in the thyroid glands.

The release of parathyroid hormone indirectly stimulates differentiation and increases the activity of the **osteoclasts** in bones. However, because parathyroid hormone receptors are found on osteoprogenitor cells and osteoblasts, and not on osteoclasts, the osteoclasts are indirectly activated by the signaling mechanism from the osteoblasts. Parathyroid hormone initially targets **osteoblasts** that produce **receptor activator of nuclear factor κ B ligand (RANKL)**. Also, osteoclast precursors express receptor molecules called **receptor activator of nuclear factor κ B (RANK)**. The RANKL of osteoblasts directly interacts and controls osteoclast differentiation by activating the RANK on osteoclast precursors. Thus, the activation of the osteoclast–osteoblast/RANK–RANKL pathway becomes essential for the differentiation, proliferation, and activity of osteoclasts. This action leads to increased bone resorption and release of calcium and phosphates into the bloodstream, thereby raising and maintaining proper calcium levels. As the calcium concentration in the bloodstream increases, further production of parathyroid hormone is suppressed.

Parathyroid hormone also targets the kidneys and intestines. The distal convoluted tubules in the kidneys increase reabsorption of calcium from the glomerular filtrate and increase elimination of more phosphate, sodium, and potassium ions into urine. Parathyroid hormone also influences the kidneys to produce the hormone **calcitriol**, the active form of vitamin D, which results in increased calcium absorption from the gastrointestinal tract into the bloodstream.

The secretion and release of parathyroid hormone depends primarily on the concentration of calcium levels in the blood and not on any pituitary hormones. Thus, the secretion of parathyroid hormone is regulated by calcium levels through a simple **feedback** mechanism. Because parathyroid hormone maintains optimal levels of calcium in the blood, parathyroid glands are essential to life because calcium is utilized by different organs for many vital functions of the body.

The function of **oxyphil cells** in the parathyroid glands is presently not known, but they may represent old chief cells that are no longer secreting the parathyroid hormone.

1 Follicles with
  colloid

2 Follicular cells

3 Connective
  tissue septum

4 Chief cells

5 Oxyphil cells

6 Blood vessels

FIGURE 19.9 ■ Thyroid gland and parathyroid gland. Stain: hematoxylin and eosin. ×80.

FIGURE 19.10 | Adrenal (Suprarenal) Gland

The adrenal (suprarenal) gland consists of an outer **cortex (1)** and an inner **medulla (5)**, surrounded by a thick connective tissue **capsule (6)** that contains branches of adrenal blood vessels, veins, nerves (largely unmyelinated), and lymphatics. A **connective tissue septum** with a **blood vessel (2)** passes from the capsule (6) into the cortex. Other connective tissue septa carry the blood vessels to the medulla (5). Fenestrated sinusoidal **capillaries (8, 10)** and large **blood vessels (14)** are found throughout the cortex (1) and medulla (5).

The adrenal cortex (1) is subdivided into three concentric zones. Directly under the connective tissue capsule (6) is the outer **zona glomerulosa (7)**. The **cells (7)** in the zona glomerulosa (7) are arranged into ovoid groups or clumps and surrounded by numerous sinusoidal capillaries (8). The cytoplasm of these cells (7) stains pink and contains few lipid droplets.

The middle and the widest cell layer is the **zona fasciculata (3, 9)**. The **cells of the zona fasciculata (9)** are arranged in vertical columns, or radial plates. Because of the increased amount of lipid droplets in their cytoplasm, the cells of the zona fasciculata (9) appear light or vacuolated after a normal slide preparation. Sinusoidal capillaries (10) between the cell columns follow a similar vertical or radial course.

The third and the innermost cell layer is the **zona reticularis (4, 11)**. This cell layer borders on the adrenal medulla (5). The **cells (11)** of the zona reticularis (4) form anastomosing cords surrounded by sinusoidal capillaries.

The medulla (5) is not sharply demarcated from the cortex. The cytoplasm of the **secretory cells of the medulla (13)** appears clear. After tissue fixation in potassium bichromate, called the chromaffin reaction, fine brown granules become visible in the cells of the medulla. These granules indicate the presence of the catecholamines epinephrine and norepinephrine in the cytoplasm.

The medulla also contains **sympathetic neurons (12)** that are seen singly or in small groups. The neurons (12) exhibit a vesicular nucleus, prominent nucleolus, and a small amount of peripheral chromatin.

Sinusoidal capillaries drain the contents of the medulla (5) into the prominent medullary blood vessels (14).

FIGURE 19.10 ■ Adrenal (suprarenal) gland. Stain: hematoxylin and eosin. Low magnification.

FIGURE 19.11 | Adrenal (Suprarenal) Gland: Cortex and Medulla

This lower-magnification photomicrograph illustrates a section of the adrenal gland. The cortex is surrounded by a dense connective tissue **capsule (1)**. Beneath the capsule (1) is the **zona glomerulosa (2)**, containing irregular ovoid clumps of cells. The intermediate and widest zone is the **zona fasciculata (3)**. Here, the cells are arranged into light-staining, narrow cords, between which are found capillaries and fine connective tissue fibers. The innermost zone of the adrenal cortex is the **zona reticularis (4)**, in which the cells are arranged into groups of branching cords and clumps.

The adrenal **medulla (5)** is located adjacent to the zona reticularis (4). In the medulla (5), the cells are larger and also arranged into clumps. Large **blood vessels (6)** (veins) drain the medulla (5).

FUNCTIONAL CORRELATIONS 19.6 | Adrenal Gland Cortex and Medulla

ADRENAL GLAND CORTEX

The adrenal gland cortex is under the influence of the anterior pituitary gland hormone adrenocorticotropic hormone (ACTH). Cells of the adrenal gland cortex synthesize and release three types of steroids: mineralocorticoids, glucocorticoids, and androgens.

The cells of the **zona glomerulosa** in the adrenal cortex produce **mineralocorticoid hormones**, primarily **aldosterone** that is released into the fenestrated capillaries. Aldosterone release is initiated via the kidney **renin–angiotensin** pathway in response to decreased arterial filtration blood pressure and low levels of sodium in the glomerular filtrate. These changes are detected by the **juxtaglomerular apparatus** (juxtaglomerular cells in the afferent arteriole and macula densa in the distal convoluted tubule) located in the kidney cortex near the renal corpuscles.

Aldosterone has a major influence on fluid and electrolyte balance in the body, with the main target being the distal convoluted tubules in the kidneys. The primary function of aldosterone is to increase **sodium reabsorption** from the glomerular filtrate by cells in the distal convoluted tubules of the kidney and increase potassium excretion into urine. As water follows sodium, there is an increase in fluid volume in the circulation. As the blood pressure, blood volume, and electrolyte balance are restored to normal physiologic levels in response to aldosterone effects, the release of renin from the juxtaglomerular apparatus is decreased or stopped.

The cells of the zona fasciculata—and probably those of the zona reticularis—secrete **glucocorticoids**, of which **cortisol** and **cortisone** are the most important. Glucocorticoids are released into the circulation in response to stress. These steroids stimulate protein, fat, and carbohydrate metabolism, especially by increasing circulating blood **glucose** levels. Glucocorticoids also suppress immune and inflammatory responses by reducing the number of circulating lymphocytes from lymphoid tissues and decreasing their production of antibodies. In addition, cortisol suppresses the tissue response to injury by decreasing cellular and humoral immunity.

Although the cells of the zona reticularis are believed to produce sex steroids, they are mainly weak androgens and have little physiologic significance. Glucocorticoid secretions and the secretory functions of zona fasciculata and zona reticularis are regulated by feedback control from the pituitary gland and ACTH.

FUNCTIONAL CORRELATIONS 19.6 | Adrenal Gland Cortex and Medulla *(Continued)*

ADRENAL GLAND MEDULLA

The functions of the adrenal medulla are controlled by the hypothalamus through the sympathetic division of the autonomic nervous system. Cells in the adrenal medulla are called the **chromaffin cells** because they stain with chromium salts. These cells arise from neural crest, just like the postganglionic neurons of sympathetic and parasympathetic ganglia, and can, therefore, be considered as ganglion cells that lack dendrites and axons. They are activated by sympathetic axons in response to fear or acute emotional stress, causing them to release the catecholamines **epinephrine** and **norepinephrine**. The release of these chemicals prepares the individual for a "fight" or "flight" response, resulting in increased heart rate, increased cardiac output and blood flow, and a surge of glucose into the bloodstream from the liver for added energy. Catecholamines produce the maximal use of energy and physical effort to overcome the stress.

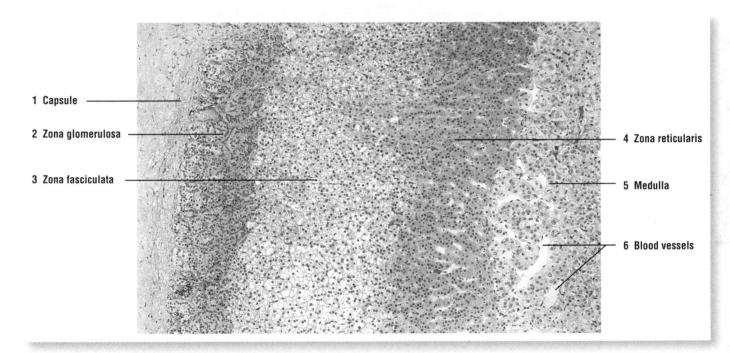

1 Capsule

2 Zona glomerulosa

3 Zona fasciculata

4 Zona reticularis

5 Medulla

6 Blood vessels

FIGURE 19.11 ■ Adrenal (suprarenal) gland: cortex and medulla. Stain: hematoxylin and eosin. ×25.

SECTION 2 • Thyroid Gland, Parathyroid Glands, and Adrenal Gland

Thyroid Gland

- Located in anterior neck region and consists of two large, connected lobes
- Consists of follicles surrounded by follicular cells that fill the lumen with colloid
- Colloid contains thyroglobulin, an iodinated inactive storage form of thyroid hormones
- Follicular cells controlled by thyroid-stimulating hormone
- Iodide is an essential element in the production of thyroid hormones
- Low levels of thyroid hormones stimulate the release of thyroid-stimulating hormone from adenohypophysis
- Iodide is taken up from blood, oxidized to iodine, and transported into follicular lumen
- Iodine combines with tyrosine groups to form iodinated thyroglobulin
- Triiodothyronine and tetraiodothyronine are main thyroid gland hormones
- Release of thyroid hormones involves endocytosis of thyroglobulin and hydrolysis of thyroglobulin
- Thyroid hormones bound to thyroxin-binding protein
- More tetraiodothyronine (T_4) is produced, but triiodothyronine is physiologically more potent than T_4
- Thyroid hormones increase metabolic rate, growth, differentiation, and body development
- Parafollicular cells are located in follicular peripheries of thyroid gland
- Parafollicular cells secrete calcitonin to lower blood calcium by inhibiting osteoclasts
- Parafollicular cells act independent of pituitary gland hormones, but depend on calcium levels

Parathyroid Glands

- Mammals have four glands situated on the posterior surface of thyroid
- Instead of follicles, cells arranged in cords or clumps surrounded by capillary clumps
- Two cell types: principal or chief cells and oxyphil cells
- Chief cells produce parathyroid hormone (parathormone) to maintain proper calcium
- Parathyroid hormone counterbalances calcitonin action
- Parathyroid hormone stimulates osteoclasts activity to release more calcium into blood
- Parathyroid hormone induces kidney and intestines to absorb and retain more calcium
- Release of hormone depends on calcium levels and not pituitary hormones
- Are essential to life owing to maintenance of proper calcium levels

- Function of oxyphil cells not presently known but may represent old chief cells

Adrenal Glands

- Located near superior pole of each kidney
- Have separate and distinct embryologic origin, structure, and function
- Covered with a connective tissue capsule and consist of outer cortex and inner medulla
- Fenestrated capillaries and large vessels throughout both regions
- Cortex shows three zones: zona glomerulosa, zona fasciculata, and zona reticularis

Cortex

- Under direct influence of adrenocorticotropic hormone from anterior pituitary gland
- Releases three steroid hormones: mineralocorticoids, glucocorticoids, and androgens
- Cells in zona glomerulosa secrete mineralocorticoids, primarily aldosterone
- Aldosterone release is caused by decreased arterial blood pressure and low sodium levels
- Juxtaglomerular apparatus in kidney initiates the renin–angiotensin pathway to increase blood pressure
- Aldosterone increases sodium reabsorption and increased water retention by distal convoluted tubules
- Increased fluid volume increases blood pressure and inhibits further release of aldosterone
- Cells of zona fasciculata secrete glucocorticoids, of which cortisol and cortisone are important
- Glucocorticoids are released in response to stress, increase metabolism and glucose levels, and suppress inflammatory responses
- Cells of zona reticularis produce weak androgens

Medulla

- Cells are modified postganglionic sympathetic neurons that became secretory
- Stain with chromium salts and are called chromaffin cells
- Medulla cells can be considered as ganglion cells without dendrites and axons
- Action controlled by sympathetic division of autonomic nervous system, not pituitary gland
- Cells contain catecholamines (epinephrine and norepinephrine) and respond to stress
- Prepares the individual for flight or fight response
- Cells activate maximal use of energy and physical effort

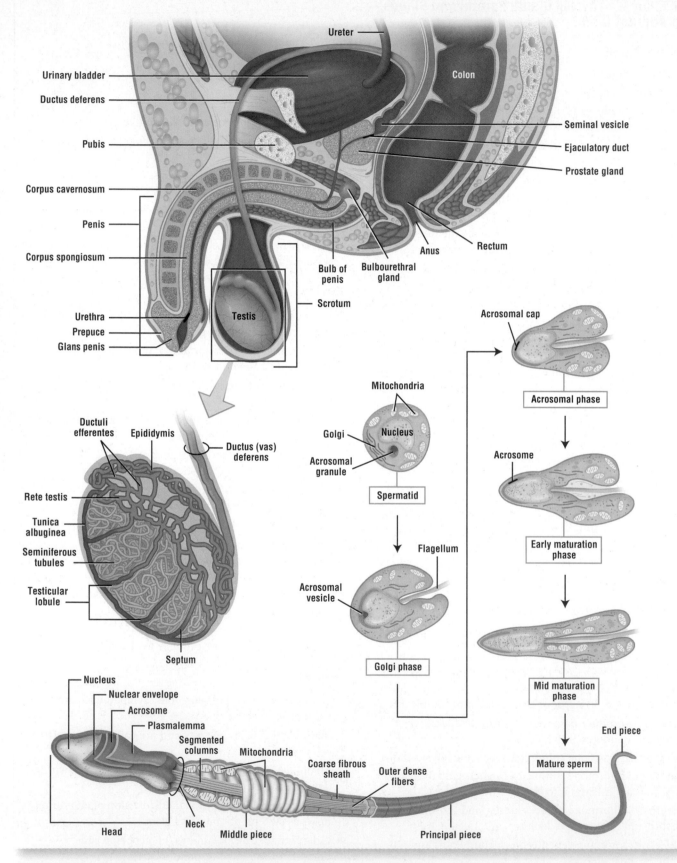

OVERVIEW FIGURE 20.1 ■ Location of the testes and the accessory male reproductive organs, with emphasis on the internal organization of the testis, the different phases of spermiogenesis, and the structure of a mature sperm.

CHAPTER 20

Male Reproductive System

SECTION 1 Testis

The male reproductive system consists of a pair of testes, numerous excurrent ducts, and different accessory glands that produce a variety of secretions that are added to sperm to form semen. The **testis** (plural, testes) contains spermatogenic **stem cells** that continuously divide to produce new generations of cells that are eventually transformed into **spermatozoa**, or **sperm**. From the testes, the sperm move through excurrent ducts to the **epididymis** for storage and maturation. During sexual excitation and ejaculation, sperm leave the epididymis via the **ductus (vas) deferens** and exit the reproductive system through the penile **urethra**.

The **accessory glands**—prostate gland, seminal vesicles, and bulbourethral glands—of the male reproductive system are discussed and illustrated in detail in Section 2.

Scrotum

The paired testes are located outside the body cavity in the **scrotum**. Here, the temperature of the testes is about 2°C to 3°C lower than normal body temperature. This lower temperature is vital for the normal functioning of the testes and **spermatogenesis**, or sperm production. In addition to the external location of the testes, perspiration and evaporation of sweat from the scrotal surface maintains the testes in a cooler environment. However, this lower temperature is not essential for hormone production by the testes.

Equally important in maintaining lower testicular temperature is the special arrangement of blood vessels that supply the testes. Testicular arteries that descend into the scrotum are surrounded by a complex plexus of veins that ascend from the testes and form the **pampiniform plexus**. Blood returning from the testes in the pampiniform plexus is cooler than the blood flowing in the testicular arteries toward the testes. By a **countercurrent heat-exchange mechanism**, arterial blood is cooled by venous blood before it enters the testes, helping to maintain a lower temperature in the testes.

Testes

A thick connective tissue capsule, the **tunica albuginea**, surrounds each testis. Posteriorly, the tunica albuginea thickens and extends inward into each testis to form the **mediastinum testis**. A thin connective tissue **septum** extends from the mediastinum testis and subdivides each testis into about 250 incomplete compartments or **testicular lobules**, each containing one to four highly coiled **seminiferous tubules**. Each seminiferous tubule is lined with a stratified **germinal epithelium**, containing proliferating **spermatogenic (germ) cells** and nonproliferating **supporting (sustentacular)**, or **Sertoli**, **cells**. In the seminiferous tubules, spermatogenic cells divide, mature, and are transformed into sperm (Overview Fig. 20.1).

Surrounding each seminiferous tubule are fibroblasts, muscle-like cells, nerves, blood vessels, and lymphatic vessels. In addition, between the seminiferous tubules are clusters of epithelioid cells, the **interstitial cells (of Leydig)**. These cells are steroid-secreting cells that produce the male sex hormone **testosterone**.

Formation of Sperm: Spermatogenesis

The process of sperm formation is called **spermatogenesis**. Included in this process are the mitotic divisions of spermatogenic cells that are located at the base of the seminiferous tubules. Spermatogenic cells are subdivided into type A spermatogonia and type B spermatogonia. Dark type A spermatogonia are stem cells that continue to divide and give rise to other dark and pale type A spermatogonia. Pale type A spermatogonia replicate themselves and give rise to type B cells. Type B cells proliferate by mitosis and give rise to **primary spermatocytes**, which undergo the **first meiotic division** to produce **secondary spermatocytes**. The secondary spermatocytes complete the **second meiotic division** and produce round **spermatids**. During these meiotic divisions, there is a reduction in the number of chromosomes and the amount of DNA in each cell. After the completion of the second meiotic division, the spermatids now contain 23 single chromosomes (22 + X or 22 + Y). Spermatids do not undergo any further divisions, but instead undergo extensive morphologic transformation of a conventional-appearing round cell into an elongated structure with a nucleus and a tail called the sperm, by a process called **spermiogenesis**. Upon fertilization of the egg by the sperm, the total normal number of chromosomes is restored to 46.

Once the spermatogenic cells in the germinal epithelium differentiate and begin to mature, they are held together by **intercellular bridges** during further development and differentiation. The intercellular bridges are only broken when the developed spermatids are released (spermiation) into the fluid-filled seminiferous tubules as fully formed sperm from the superficial tips of the supportive Sertoli cells.

Transformation of Spermatids: Spermiogenesis

Spermiogenesis is a complex morphologic process by which the spherical spermatids are transformed into elongated sperm cells. During spermiogenesis, the size and shape of the spermatids are altered, and the nuclear chromatin condenses. In the initial **Golgi phase**, small granules accumulate in the Golgi apparatus of the spermatid and form an **acrosomal granule** within a membrane-bound **acrosomal vesicle** adjacent to the nuclear envelope. The location of the acrosomal vesicle indicates the anterior region of the developing sperm. During the **acrosomal phase**, both the acrosomal vesicle and the acrosomal granule spread over the condensing spermatid nucleus at the anterior end of the spermatid as an **acrosome cap**. Also during this phase, centrioles migrate to the opposite or posterior pole of the spermatid and assemble the microtubules to form the sperm tail, or flagellum. The fully formed acrosome functions as a specialized type of **lysosome** and contains several hydrolytic enzymes, such as hyaluronidase and protease with trypsinlike activity, that assist the sperm in penetrating the cells (corona radiata) and the membrane (zona pellucida) that surround the ovulated oocyte at the time of fertilization. During the **maturation phases**, the spermatid head is embedded in the supportive Sertoli cell nucleus. Also, the plasma membrane moves posterior from the nucleus to cover the developing **flagellum** (sperm tail), which now extends into the lumen of the seminiferous tubule. The mitochondria at this time migrate to and form a tight sheath around the middle piece of the developed flagellum. The final maturation phase is characterized by the shedding of the excess, or **residual cytoplasm** of the spermatid and release of the sperm into the lumen of the seminiferous tubule. The supportive Sertoli cells then phagocytose the residual cytoplasm.

The mature sperm cell is composed of a **head** and an acrosome that surrounds the anterior portion of the nucleus, a **neck**, a **middle piece** characterized by the presence of a compact mitochondrial sheath, and a main or **principal piece** (see Overview Fig. 20.1).

Excurrent Ducts

Newly released sperm are not motile and pass from the seminiferous tubules into the fluid-filled intertesticular excurrent ducts that connect each testis with the overlying epididymis. These excurrent ducts consist of the **straight tubules** (tubuli recti) and the **rete testis**, the epithelial-lined spaces in the mediastinum testis. From the rete testis, the sperm enter approximately 12 short tubules, the **ductuli efferentes** (efferent ducts), which conduct sperm from the rete testis to the initial segment or the head of the **epididymis**.

SPERMATOGONIA

The two primary functions of the testes are the production of **sperm** (spermatogenesis) and the synthesis of the male sex hormone **testosterone**. Testosterone is an essential hormone for the development and maintenance of male sexual characteristics and normal functioning of the accessory reproductive glands.

The spermatogenic cells in the seminiferous tubules divide, differentiate, and produce sperm by a process called **spermatogenesis**. This process involves the following:

- Mitotic divisions of spermatogonia to form stem cells
- Formation of **primary** and **secondary spermatocytes** from spermatogenic cells
- **Meiotic divisions** of both primary and secondary spermatocytes to reduce the somatic chromosome numbers by one half and formation of **spermatids**, which are germ cells with only 23 single chromosomes (22 + X or 22 + Y)
- Morphologic transformation of round spermatids into mature, elongated sperm by a process called **spermiogenesis**

SUPPORTIVE SERTOLI CELLS

Sertoli cells are the supportive cells of the testes that are located among the spermatogenic cells in the seminiferous tubules. They perform numerous important functions in the testes, among which are the following:

- Physical support, protection, and nutrition of the developing spermatids
- Phagocytosis of excess cytoplasm (residual bodies) from the developing spermatids as well as degenerating germ cells
- Release of mature sperm, called **spermiation**, into the lumen of seminiferous tubules containing fluid produced by Sertoli cells
- Secretion of fructose-rich testicular fluid for the nourishment and transport of sperm to the excurrent ducts
- Production and release of androgen-binding protein (ABP) that binds to testosterone and increases the concentration of testosterone in the lumen of the seminiferous tubules that is necessary for spermatogenesis; ABP secretion is under the control of follicle-stimulating hormone (FSH) from the pituitary gland
- Secretion of the hormone inhibin, which suppresses the release of FSH from the pituitary gland
- Production and release of the anti-Müllerian hormone, also called Müllerian-inhibiting hormone, that suppresses the development of Müllerian ducts in the male and inhibits the development of female reproductive organs

BLOOD–TESTIS BARRIER

The adjacent cytoplasm of Sertoli cells are joined by occluding **tight junctions**, producing a **blood–testis barrier** that subdivides each seminiferous tubule into a **basal compartment** and an **adluminal compartment**. This important barrier segregates the spermatogonia from all successive stages of spermatogenesis in the adluminal compartment and excludes plasma proteins and bloodborne antibodies from the lumen of seminiferous tubules. The more advanced spermatogenic cells can be recognized by the body as foreign and cause an immune response. The blood–testis barrier protects developing cells from the immune system by restricting the passage of membrane **antigens** from developing sperm into the bloodstream. Thus, the blood–testis barrier prevents an autoimmune response to the individual's own sperm, antibody formation, and eventual destruction of spermatogenesis and induction of sterility. The blood–testis barrier also keeps harmful substances in the blood from entering the developing germinal epithelium.

The extratesticular duct that conducts the sperm to the penile urethra is the **ductus epididymis**, which is continuous with the **ductus (vas) deferens** and **ejaculatory ducts** in the prostate gland. During sexual excitation and ejaculation, strong contractions of the **smooth muscle** that surrounds the **ductus epididymis** expel the sperm (see Overview Fig. 20.1).

 Supplemental micrographic images are available at **www.thePoint.com/Eroschenko12e** under Male Reproductive System.

FIGURE 20.1 | Peripheral Section of Testis (Sectional View)

Each testis is enclosed in a thick, connective tissue capsule called the **tunica albuginea (1)**, internal to which is a vascular layer of loose connective tissue called the **tunica vasculosa (2, 8)**. The connective tissue extends inward from the tunica vasculosa (2, 8) into the testis to form the **interstitial connective tissue (3, 12)**. The interstitial connective tissue (3, 12) surrounds, binds, and supports the **seminiferous tubules (4, 6, 9)**. Extending from the mediastinum testis (see Fig. 20.7) toward the tunica albuginea (1) are thin fibrous **septa (7, 10)** (singular, septum) that divide the testis into compartments called lobules. Within each lobule are found one to four seminiferous tubules (4, 6, 9). The septa (7, 10) are not solid, and there is intercommunication between lobules.

Located in the interstitial connective tissue (3, 12) around the seminiferous tubules (4, 6, 9) are **blood vessels (13)**, loose connective tissue cells, and clusters of epithelial **interstitial cells (of Leydig) (5, 11)**. The interstitial cells (5, 11) are the endocrine cells of the testis and secrete the male sex hormone testosterone into the bloodstream.

The seminiferous tubules (4, 6, 9) are long, convoluted tubules in the testis that are normally observed cut in transverse (4), longitudinal (6), or tangential (9) planes of section. The seminiferous tubules (4, 6, 9) are lined with a stratified epithelium called the **germinal epithelium (14)**. The germinal epithelium (14) contains two cell types: the spermatogenic cells that produce sperm and the supportive Sertoli cells that nourish the developing sperm. The germinal epithelium (14) rests on the basement membrane of the seminiferous tubules (4, 6, 9) and its cells are illustrated in greater detail in Figures 20.2 through 20.5.

FIGURE 20.2 | Testis: Seminiferous Tubules (Transverse Section)

This photomicrograph illustrates a **seminiferous tubule (5)** and parts of adjacent seminiferous tubules. A thick germinal epithelium lines each seminiferous tubule (5).

The **dark type A (1a)** and the **pale type B (1b) spermatogonia (1)** are located in the base of the tubule. The **primary spermatocytes (2)** and **spermatids (7)** in different stages of maturation are embedded in the germinal epithelium closer to the lumen. The tails of the spermatids (7) protrude into the lumen of the seminiferous tubules (5). The supportive **Sertoli cells (6)** are located throughout the germinal epithelium.

Each seminiferous tubule (5) is surrounded by a fibromuscular interstitial **connective tissue (3)**. Here are found the testosterone-secreting **interstitial cells (4)**.

1 Tunica albuginea
2 Tunica vasculosa
3 Interstitial connective tissue
4 Seminiferous tubules
5 Interstitial cells (of Leydig)
6 Seminiferous tubule
7 Septum

8 Tunica vasculosa
9 Seminiferous tubule
10 Septum
11 Interstitial cells (of Leydig)
12 Interstitial connective tissue
13 Blood vessels
14 Germinal epithelium

FIGURE 20.1 ■ Peripheral section of testis (sectional view). Stain: hematoxylin and eosin. Low magnification.

1 Spermatogonia:
  a Dark type A
  b Pale type B

2 Primary spermatocytes

3 Connective tissue

4 Interstitial cells
5 Seminiferous tubule
6 Sertoli cells
7 Spermatids

FIGURE 20.2 ■ Testis: seminiferous tubules (transverse section). Stain: hematoxylin and eosin (plastic section). ×80.

FIGURE 20.3 | Testis: Spermatogenesis in Seminiferous Tubules (Transverse Section)

In examining a higher magnification of a **seminiferous tubule (8)** from a testis, different cell types and stages of spermatogenesis can be recognized. Each seminiferous tubule (8) is surrounded by an outer layer of connective tissue with **fibrocytes (11)** and an inner **basement membrane (3)**. Between each seminiferous tubule (8) are found the interstitial connective tissue with fibrocytes (11), numerous **blood vessels (5)**, nerves, lymphatic vessels, and the testosterone-producing **interstitial cells** (of Leydig) **(1, 12)**.

The stratified germinal epithelium of the seminiferous tubule (8) consists of supporting, or **Sertoli cells (6, 10)** and different **spermatogenic cells (7)**. Sertoli cells (6, 10) are slender, elongated cells with irregular outlines that extend from the basement membrane (3) to the lumen of the seminiferous tubule (8). The nuclei of Sertoli cells (6, 10) are ovoid, or elongated, and contain fine, sparse chromatin. A distinct and dense-staining nucleolus distinguishes Sertoli cells (6, 10) from the adjacent spermatogenic cells (7).

The immature spermatogenic cells, called the **spermatogonia (7)**, are adjacent to the basement membrane (3) of the seminiferous tubules (8). The spermatogonia (7) divide mitotically to produce several generations of cells. This illustration shows two types of spermatogonia: The **pale type A spermatogonia (7b)** have a light-staining cytoplasm and a round or ovoid nucleus with pale, finely granular chromatin; and the **dark type A spermatogonia (7a)** appear similar but with darker chromatin.

Type A spermatogonia (7a) serve as stem cells for the germinal epithelium and give rise to other type A and type B spermatogonia. The final mitotic division of type B spermatogonia produces **primary spermatocytes (2, 9)**.

The primary spermatocytes (2, 9) are the largest germ cells in the seminiferous tubules (8) and occupy the middle region of the germinal epithelium. Their cytoplasm contains large nuclei with coarse clumps or thin threads of chromatin. The first meiotic division of the primary spermatocytes (Fig. 20.5, I, 5) produces smaller secondary spermatocytes with less-dense nuclear chromatin (Fig. 20.5, I, 3). Because the secondary spermatocytes undergo a second meiotic division shortly after their formation, they are infrequently seen in the seminiferous tubules (8).

The second meiotic division produces **spermatids (4)** that are smaller cells than the primary or secondary spermatocytes (Fig. 20.5, I, 2, 3, 5). The spermatids (4) are grouped in the adluminal compartment of the seminiferous tubule (8) and are closely associated with supportive Sertoli cells (6, 10). In this illustration, the earlier and later stages of **developing spermatids (4)** are seen. The more mature spermatids (4, *upper leader*) are located in the periphery of the germinal epithelium with their tails extending into the lumen of the seminiferous tubule (8). The early spermatids (4, *lower leader*) are round with dense-staining round nuclei and are located deeper in the germinal epithelium. All developing spermatids (4) are embedded in the Sertoli cell (6, 10) cytoplasm and are grouped in the adluminal compartment of the seminiferous tubule (8). Here, the spermatids (4) eventually differentiate into sperm by a process called spermiogenesis and are released into seminiferous tubules (8) as sperm.

FIGURE 20.4 | Cross Section of Seminiferous Tubules Showing Supportive Sertoli Cells, Spermatogonia, and Spermatids in Different Stages of Development

This higher-magnification photomicrograph of testis tubules shows in greater detail the different cells in and around the seminiferous tubules. In the central tubule, the germinal epithelium contains the very prominent and largest cells, the **primary spermatocytes (3)**. In the right tubule are seen the developing round **early spermatids (10)** with dense, round nuclei. The central tubule contains the elongated and dense-staining nuclei of **late spermatids (6)** with their tails extending into the **lumen of the seminiferous tubule (5)**. At the base of the germinal epithelium are visible the **dark type A (4)** and **pale type A spermatogonia (7)**. Also visible in the seminiferous tubules are the very distinct **Sertoli cells (9, 12)** with oval nucleus and a characteristic dense-staining nucleolus. Sertoli cell cytoplasm extends from the base of the germinal epithelium to the lumen of the seminiferous tubule (5). Embedded within the Sertoli cell (9, 12) cytoplasm are the developing spermatocytes (3) and spermatids (6, 10). Surrounding the seminiferous tubules is a **basement membrane (11)** and the flattened connective tissue **fibrocytes (8)**. Located also between the seminiferous tubules are the testosterone-secreting **interstitial cells (of Leydig) (1, 13)**, some of which are located adjacent to a **capillary (2)**.

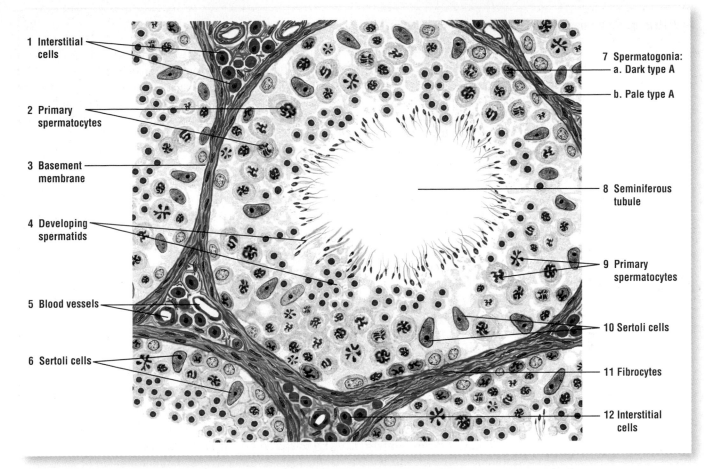

1 Interstitial cells
2 Primary spermatocytes
3 Basement membrane
4 Developing spermatids
5 Blood vessels
6 Sertoli cells

7 Spermatogonia:
a. Dark type A
b. Pale type A
8 Seminiferous tubule
9 Primary spermatocytes
10 Sertoli cells
11 Fibrocytes
12 Interstitial cells

FIGURE 20.3 ■ Testis: spermatogenesis in seminiferous tubules (transverse section). Stain: hematoxylin and eosin. Medium magnification.

1 Interstitial cell (of Leydig)
2 Capillary
3 Primary spermatocytes
4 Spermatogonium (dark type A)
5 Lumen of seminiferous tubule
6 Late spermatids
7 Spermatogonium (pale type A)

8 Fibrocytes
9 Sertoli cell
10 Early spermatids
11 Basement membrane
12 Sertoli cell
13 Interstitial cells (of Leydig)

FIGURE 20.4 ■ Cross section of seminiferous tubules showing supportive Sertoli cells, spermatogonia, and spermatids in different stages of development. Stain: hematoxylin and eosin. Plastic section. ×125.

FIGURE 20.5 | Primate Testis: Different Stages of Spermatogenesis

Three stages of spermatogenesis are illustrated from a section of the seminiferous tubule. In the left illustration (I), the large and distinct **primary spermatocytes (5)** divide to form smaller **secondary spermatocytes (3)**, which undergo rapid meiotic division to produce the **spermatids (1, 2)**. Both the early spermatids (2) and the more mature spermatids (1) become embedded deep in the supporting **Sertoli cell (4)** cytoplasm. Located at the base of the seminiferous tubule are the dark and **pale type A spermatogonia (6)**.

In the middle illustration (II), the **spermatids (7)** are near the lumen of the seminiferous tubule just before their release into the lumen. Also visible are the early, round **spermatids (8)** and the large **primary spermatocytes (9)** closely associated with the **Sertoli cells (10)**. Near the base of the seminiferous tubule are the **spermatogonia (11)**.

In the right illustration (III), the mature spermatids have been released as sperm (spermiation) into the seminiferous tubule, and the germinal epithelium contains only early **spermatids (8)**, **primary spermatocytes (9)**, **spermatogonia (11)**, and the supporting **Sertoli cells (10)**.

FIGURE 20.6 | Ultrastructure of a Sertoli Cell and Surrounding Cells

This ultrastructure image shows the base of the germinal epithelium in a seminiferous tubule. In the center are the **Sertoli cell cytoplasm (1)**, the distinctive **Sertoli cell nucleus (2)**, and the characteristic dense **Sertoli cell nucleolus (9)**. A section of an **early spermatid (7)** with the **Golgi complex (8)** is seen on the right of the Sertoli cell. A very distinct **junctional complex (3, 10)** between adjacent Sertoli cells forms the blood–testis barrier that separates the germinal epithelium into basal and adluminal compartments. Located below the Sertoli cell (1, 2, 9) is a thin **basal lamina (4)** adjacent to the thicker **basement membrane (11)**. On the other side of the basement membrane (11) is the **interstitial cell of Leydig (5)** completely filled with **smooth endoplasmic reticulum** and **mitochondria (12)** with round cristae. At the bottom left-hand corner is seen a section of cytoplasm and nucleus of what appears to be a **spermatogonium (6)** of an adjacent seminiferous tubule.

FIGURE 20.5 ■ Primate testis: different stages of spermatogenesis. Stain: hematoxylin and eosin. High magnification.

FIGURE 20.6 ■ Ultrastructure of a Sertoli cell and surrounding cells. Courtesy of Dr. Rex A. Hess, Professor Emeritus, Comparative Biosciences, College of Veterinary Medicine, University of Illinois, Urbana, Illinois. ×8,100.

FIGURE 20.7 | Seminiferous Tubules, Straight Tubules, Rete Testis, and Ductuli Efferentes (Efferent Ductules)

In the posterior region of the testis, the tunica albuginea extends into the testis interior as the **mediastinum testis (10, 16)**. In this illustration, the plane of section passes through the **seminiferous tubules (3, 5)**; the connective tissue and blood vessels of the mediastinum testis **(10, 16)**; and the excretory ducts, the **ductuli efferentes (efferent ductules) (9, 13)**.

A few seminiferous tubules **(3, 5)** are visible on the left side. The tubules **(3, 5)** are lined with spermatogenic epithelium and sustentacular Sertoli cells. The **interstitial connective tissue (4)** is continuous with the mediastinum testis **(10, 16)** and contains the steroid (testosterone)-producing **interstitial cells (of Leydig) (1)**. In the mediastinum testis **(10, 16)**, the seminiferous tubules **(3, 5)** terminate in the **straight tubules (2, 6)**. The straight tubules **(2, 6)** are short, narrow ducts lined with a cuboidal, or low columnar, epithelium that are devoid of spermatogenic cells.

The straight tubules **(2, 6)** continue into the **rete testis (7, 8, 12)** of the mediastinum testis **(10, 16)**. The rete testis **(7, 8, 12)** is an irregular, anastomosing network of tubules with wide lumina lined with a simple squamous to low cuboidal or low columnar epithelium. The rete testis **(7, 8, 12)** becomes wider near the ductuli efferentes (efferent ductules) **(9, 13)** into which the rete testis empties. The ductuli efferentes **(9, 13)** are straight but become highly convoluted in the head of the ductus epididymis. The ductuli efferentes **(9, 13)** connect the rete testis **(7, 8, 12)** with the epididymis (see Fig. 20.8). Some tubules in the rete testis **(12)** and ductuli efferentes **(9, 13)** contain accumulations of **sperm (11, 14)**.

The epithelium of the ductuli efferentes **(9, 13)** consists of groups of tall columnar cells that alternate with groups of shorter cuboidal cells. Because of the alternating cell heights, the lumina of the ductuli efferentes are uneven. The tall cells in the ductuli efferentes **(9, 13)** exhibit **cilia (15)**, and the cuboidal cells exhibit microvilli.

FUNCTIONAL CORRELATIONS 20.2 | Hormones of Male Reproductive Organs

Normal maintenance of spermatogenesis in adult testes depends on the stimulation of the testes by two hormones: **follicle-stimulating hormone (FSH)** and **luteinizing hormone (LH)**. The neurons in the hypothalamus of the brain secrete **gonadotropin-releasing hormone** that stimulates the **gonadotrophs** in the pituitary gland to synthesize and release LH. Normal spermatogenesis is dependent on the action of LH, which binds to LH receptors on **interstitial cells (of Leydig)** and stimulates them to synthesize the male hormone **testosterone**. FSH is also produced by gonadotrophs in the pituitary gland. FSH stimulates **Sertoli cells** to synthesize and release **androgen-binding protein (ABP)** into the seminiferous tubules. ABP combines with testosterone and increases its concentration in the seminiferous tubules, which then stimulates spermatogenesis. An increased concentration of testosterone in the seminiferous tubules is essential for proper spermatogenesis. In addition, the structure and function of the accessory reproductive glands, as well as the development and maintenance of male secondary sexual characteristics, are dependent on proper testosterone levels.

An excessive level of testosterone produces a negative feedback on the hypothalamic neurons by the hormone **inhibin** that is also secreted by the Sertoli cells. Inhibin produces inhibitory effects on the pituitary gland and suppresses or inhibits additional production of FSH.

FIGURE 20.8 | Ductuli Efferentes and Tubules of Ductus Epididymis

The **ductuli efferentes (1),** or efferent ductules, emerge from the mediastinum on the posterosuperior surface of the testis and connect the rete testis with the ductus epididymis. The ductuli efferentes are located in the **connective tissue (2, 12)** and form a portion of the head of the epididymis.

The lumen of the ductuli efferentes (1) exhibits an irregular contour because the lining epithelium consists of simple alternating groups of tall **ciliated** and shorter **nonciliated cells**. The basal surface of the tubules has a smooth contour. Located under the basement membrane is a thin layer of connective tissue (2) containing a thin **smooth muscle layer (5, 11)**. As the ductuli efferentes (1) terminate in the ductus epididymis, the lumina are lined with the **pseudostratified columnar epithelium (6, 8)** of the ductus epididymis (7).

The **ductus epididymis (3, 4)** is a long, convoluted tubule surrounded by connective tissue (2) and a thin smooth muscle layer (5, 11). A section through the ductus epididymis shows both **cross sections (3)** and **longitudinal sections (4)**. Some parts of the ductus contain mature **sperm (7)**.

The pseudostratified columnar epithelium (6, 8) consists of tall columnar **principal cells (9)** with long, nonmotile **stereocilia (8)** and small **basal cells (10)**.

1 Interstitial cells (of Leydig)
2 Straight tubules
3 Seminiferous tubules
4 Interstitial connective tissue
5 Seminiferous tubule
6 Straight tubule
7 Rete testis

8 Rete testis
9 Ductuli efferentes
10 Mediastinum testis
11 Sperm
12 Rete testis (with sperm)
13 Ductuli efferentes
14 Sperm
15 Cilia
16 Mediastinum testis

FIGURE 20.7 ■ Seminiferous tubules, straight tubules, rete testis, and efferent ductules (ductuli efferentes). Stain: hematoxylin and eosin. Low magnification (inset: high magnification).

1 Ductuli efferentes
2 Connective tissue
3 Cross sections of ductus epididymis
4 Longitudinal sections of ductus epididymis
5 Smooth muscle layer
6 Epithelium

7 Sperm
8 Pseudostratified columnar epithelium with stereocilia
9 Principal cells
10 Basal cells
11 Smooth muscle layer
12 Connective tissue

FIGURE 20.8 ■ Ductuli efferentes and tubules of ductus epididymis. Stain: hematoxylin and eosin. Left side, low magnification; right side, high magnification.

FIGURE 20.9 | Tubules of Ductus Epididymis (Transverse Section)

This photomicrograph illustrates the tubules of the ductus epididymis, some of which are filled with **sperm (1)**. The tubules of the ductus are lined with a **pseudostratified epithelium (2)**. The **principal cells (2a)** are tall columnar epithelium and are lined with **stereocilia (5)**, the long, branching microvilli. The **basal cells (2b)** are small and spherical and situated near the base of the epithelium. A thin layer of **smooth muscle (3)** surrounds each tubule. Adjacent to the smooth muscle layer (3) are cells and fibers of the **connective tissue (4)**.

FIGURE 20.10 | Ductus (Vas) Deferens (Transverse Section)

The ductus (vas) deferens exhibits a narrow and irregular lumen with **longitudinal mucosal folds (6)**, a thin mucosa, a thick muscularis, and an adventitia.

The lumen of the ductus deferens is lined with a **pseudostratified columnar epithelium (8)** with stereocilia. The epithelium of the ductus deferens is somewhat lower than in the ductus epididymis. The underlying thin **lamina propria (7)** consists of compact collagen fibers and a fine network of elastic fibers.

The thick muscularis consists of three smooth muscle layers: a thinner **inner longitudinal layer (1)**, a thick **middle circular layer (2)**, and a thinner **outer longitudinal layer (3)**. The muscularis is surrounded by **adventitia (5)** in which are found abundant **blood vessels (venule and arteriole) (4)**, and nerves. The adventitia (5) of the ductus deferens merges with the connective tissue of the spermatic cord.

1 Sperm

2 Pseudostratified epithelium

a. Principal cells

b. Basal cells

3 Smooth muscle

4 Connective tissue

5 Stereocilia

FIGURE 20.9 ■ Tubules of ductus epididymis (transverse section). Stain: hematoxylin and eosin (plastic section). ×50.

1 Inner longitudinal muscle layer

2 Middle circular muscle layer

3 Outer longitudinal muscle layer

4 Blood vessels (venule and arteriole)

5 Adventitia

6 Longitudinal mucosal folds

7 Lamina propria

8 Pseudostratified columnar epithelium

FIGURE 20.10 ■ Ductus (vas) deferens (transverse section). Stain: hematoxylin and eosin. Low magnification.

FIGURE 20.11 | Ampulla of the Ductus (Vas) Deferens (Transverse Section)

The terminal portion of the ductus deferens enlarges into an ampulla. The ampulla mainly differs from the ductus deferens in the structure of its mucosa.

The **lumen (3)** of the ampulla is larger than that of the ductus deferens. The mucosa also exhibits numerous irregular, branching **mucosal folds (4)** and deep **glandular diverticula, or crypts (1)** located between the folds that extend to the surrounding muscle layer. The secretory epithelium that lines the lumen (3) and the glandular diverticula (1) is simple columnar, or cuboidal. Below the epithelium is the **lamina propria (6)**.

The smooth muscle layers in the muscularis are similar to those in the ductus deferens. These consist of a thin **inner longitudinal muscle layer (7)**, a thick **middle circular muscle layer (8)**, and a thin **outer longitudinal muscle layer (9)**. Surrounding the ampulla is the connective tissue **adventitia (5)**.

FUNCTIONAL CORRELATIONS 20.3 | Excurrent Ducts of the Testes

DUCTULI EFFERENTES (EFFERENT DUCTULES)

The sperm leave the straight tubules and enter the rete testis. The motility of cilia in the **ductuli efferentes** creates a current that assists in transporting the fluid and sperm from the seminiferous tubules in the testes to the **ductus epididymis**. In addition, the contractility of the smooth muscle fibers that surround the ductules efferentes provides additional assistance to move the sperm into the ductus epididymis. The nonciliated cuboidal cells that also line the ductuli efferentes absorb most of the testicular fluid that was produced in the seminiferous tubules by Sertoli cells.

DUCTUS EPIDIDYMIS

The highly coiled ductus epididymis is the site for **accumulation, storage**, and further **maturation** of sperm. When sperm enter the epididymis, they are nonmotile and incapable of fertilizing an oocyte. However, during their passage through the convoluted tubules of the ductus epididymis, the sperm acquire motility, membrane receptors for zona pellucida proteins, maturation of the acrosome, and the ability to fertilize an oocyte. As are other functions of the male reproductive system, the maturation process of the sperm is dependent on the proper levels of testosterone.

The **principal cells** in the ductus epididymis are lined with long branching microvilli, or **stereocilia**, that continue to absorb testicular fluid that was not absorbed in the ductuli efferentes during the passage of sperm from the testes. In addition, the principal cells phagocytose abnormal or degenerating sperm cells and the remaining residual bodies that were not removed by the Sertoli cells in the seminiferous tubules. The principal cells in the ductus epididymis also produce a glycoprotein that **inhibits capacitation**, or the fertilizing ability of the sperm, until the sperm are deposited into the female reproductive tract.

Following the maturation of the sperm in the epididymis, the sperm must be activated within the female reproductive tract. This process is called **capacitation**, a process that produces structural and functional changes in the sperm that increases their affinity for fertilizing an oocyte. Following capacitation, the sperm can bind to sperm receptors on the zona pellucida of the ovulated oocyte. This causes an **acrosomal reaction** that allows the acrosomal enzymes to disperse the cells of the corona radiata that surround the ovulated oocyte, to digest the zona pellucida around the oocyte, and to fertilize the egg.

1 Glandular diverticula, or crypts

2 Epithelium

3 Lumen

4 Mucosal folds

5 Adventitia

6 Lamina propria

7 Inner longitudinal muscle layer

8 Middle circular muscle layer

9 Outer longitudinal muscle layer

FIGURE 20.11 ■ Ampulla of the ductus (vas) deferens (transverse section). Stain: hematoxylin and eosin. Low magnification.

SECTION 1 • Testis

- Consists of two testes that contain spermatogenic cells, which produce sperm
- Numerous excurrent ducts move sperm for storage and maturation into ductus epididymis
- During ejaculation, sperm leave system via ductus (vas) deferens and penile urethra
- Accessory glands include prostate, seminal vesicles, and bulbourethral glands

Scrotum

- Testes located outside the body cavity in scrotum whose temperature is 2°C to 3°C lower than the body temperature
- Lower temperature in scrotum due to sweat evaporation and pampiniform plexus
- Countercurrent heat-exchange mechanism cools arterial blood as it enters the testes

Testes

- Thick connective tissue tunica albuginea surrounds testes and forms mediastinum testis
- Thin connective tissue septa from mediastinum testis separate testis into testicular lobules
- Testicular lobules contain coiled seminiferous tubules lined with germinal epithelium
- Germinal epithelium contains spermatogenic cells and Sertoli (supportive) cells
- Between seminiferous tubules are testosterone-secreting interstitial cells (of Leydig)

Formation of Sperm: Spermatogenesis

- Includes mitotic divisions of spermatogenic cells to form type A and type B stem cells
- Type B spermatogenic cells give rise to primary spermatocytes, the largest cells in tubules
- Primary spermatocytes give rise to smaller secondary spermatocytes
- Meiotic divisions of spermatocytes reduce number of chromosomes and amount of DNA
- Secondary spermatocytes divide to form spermatids
- Spermatids do not divide and contain 23 single chromosomes (22 + X or 22 + Y)
- Spermatids undergo a morphologic transformation called spermiogenesis
- Spermatids connected by intercellular bridges until released as mature sperm into the tubules

Transformation of Spermatids: Spermiogenesis

- Size and shape of round spermatids altered, with condensation of nuclear chromatin

- On one side, acrosome granules in vesicle spread over the condensing nucleus as acrosome
- Acrosome contains hydrolytic enzymes needed to penetrate cells that surround the oocyte
- On the opposite side of acrosome, flagellum (tail) forms with mitochondria aggregating at middle piece
- Residual cytoplasm shed from spermatids and phagocytosed by Sertoli cells
- Mature sperm consists of head, neck, middle piece, and principal piece

Excurrent Ducts

- Released nonmotile sperm enter straight tubules and rete testis to ductuli efferentes
- Ductuli efferentes in mediastinum conduct sperm to head of ductus epididymis
- Epithelium lining ductuli efferentes is ciliated and nonciliated
- Cilia in ductuli efferentes move sperm and fluid from seminiferous tubules to ductus epididymis
- Nonciliated cells absorb much of the testicular fluid as it passes to ductus epididymis
- Ductus epididymis is continuous with ductus (vas) deferens that conducts sperm to penile urethra
- Smooth muscles around ductuli efferentes, ductus epididymis, and vas deferens contract to move sperm
- Pseudostratified epithelium with principal and basal cells lines ductuli efferentes and epididymis
- Stereocilia line the surface of cells in ductus epididymis and vas deferens
- Stereocilia absorb testicular fluid, and the principal cells phagocytose residual cytoplasm
- Principal cells in ductus epididymis also produce glycoprotein that inhibits sperm capacitation

Sertoli Cells

- Physical support, protection, nutrition, and release of mature sperm into tubules
- Secretion of fluid for sperm nutrition and transport of sperm to excurrent ducts
- Phagocytosis of residual cytoplasm of spermatids
- Secretion of androgen-binding protein to concentrate testosterone in tubules and testicular fluid for sperm transport
- Secretion of hormones inhibin and anti-Müllerian hormone

Blood–Testis Barrier

- Formed by tight junctions of adjacent Sertoli cells
- Separates seminiferous tubules in basal and adluminal compartments

- Protects developing sperm from autoimmune response and harmful materials

Male Hormones

- Spermatogenesis dependent on luteinizing and follicle-stimulating hormones produced by the pituitary gland
- Luteinizing hormone binds to receptors on interstitial cells and stimulates testosterone secretion
- Follicle-stimulating hormone stimulates Sertoli cells to produce androgen-binding hormone into seminiferous tubules to bind testosterone
- Testosterone in seminiferous tubules is vital for spermatogenesis and accessory gland function
- Sertoli cells produce inhibin, which inhibits FSH production from pituitary gland via negative feedback

SECTION 2 Accessory Reproductive Sex Glands

Seminal Vesicles, Prostate Gland, Bulbourethral Glands, and Penis

The accessory glands of the male reproductive system consist of paired **seminal vesicles**, paired **bulbourethral glands**, and a single **prostate gland**. These structures are directly associated with the male reproductive tract and produce numerous secretory products that mix with sperm to produce a fluid called **semen**. The penis serves as the copulatory organ, and the penile urethra serves as a common passageway for urine or semen.

The seminal vesicles are located posterior to the bladder and superior to the prostate gland. The excretory duct of each seminal vesicle joins the dilated terminal part of each ductus (vas) deferens, the **ampulla**, to form the **ejaculatory ducts**. The ejaculatory ducts enter and continue through the prostate gland to open into the **prostatic urethra**.

The prostate gland is located inferior to the neck of the bladder. The **urethra** exits the bladder and passes through the prostate gland as the **prostatic urethra**. In addition to the ejaculatory ducts, numerous excretory ducts from prostatic glands open into the prostatic urethra.

The bulbourethral glands are small, pea-sized glands located at the root of the **penis** and embedded in the skeletal muscles of the urogenital diaphragm; their excretory ducts terminate in the proximal portion of the **penile urethra**.

The **penis** consists of **erectile tissues**, the paired dorsal **corpora cavernosa** and a single ventral **corpus spongiosum** that expands distally into the **glans penis**. Because the penile urethra extends through the entire length of the corpus spongiosum, this portion of the penis is also called the **corpus cavernosum urethrae**. Each erectile body in the penis is surrounded by the connective tissue layer **tunica albuginea**.

The erectile tissues in the penis consist of irregular vascular spaces lined with a vascular endothelium. The trabeculae between these spaces contain collagen and elastic fibers and smooth muscles. Blood enters the vascular spaces from the branches of the **dorsal artery** and **deep arteries of the penis** and is drained by peripheral veins.

 Supplemental micrographic images are available at **www.thePoint.com/Eroschenko12e** under Male Reproductive System.

FIGURE 20.12 | Prostate Gland and Prostatic Urethra

The prostate gland is an encapsulated organ situated inferior to the neck of the bladder. The urethra that leaves the bladder and passes through the prostate gland is called the **prostatic urethra (1)**. A **transitional epithelium (6)** lines the lumen of the crescent-shaped prostatic urethra (1). Most of the prostate gland consists of small, branched tubuloacinar **prostatic glands (5, 11)**. Some of the prostatic glands (5, 11) contain solid secretory aggregations called **prostatic concretions (11)** in their acini. The prostatic concretions (11) appear as small red dots in this illustration. A characteristic **fibromuscular stroma (10)** with **smooth muscle bundles (4)**, mixed with collagen and elastic fibers, surrounds the prostatic glands (5, 11) and the prostatic urethra (1).

A longitudinal urethral crest of dense fibromuscular stroma without glands widens in the prostatic urethra (1) to form a smooth domelike structure called the **colliculus seminalis (7)**. The colliculus seminalis (7) protrudes into and gives the prostatic urethra (1) a crescent shape. On each side of the colliculus seminalis (7) are the **prostatic sinuses (2)**. Most excretory **ducts of the prostatic glands (9)** open into the prostatic sinuses (2).

In the middle of the colliculus seminalis (7) is a cul-de-sac called the **utricle (8)**. The utricle (8) often shows dilation at its distal end before it opens into the prostatic urethra (1). The thin mucous membrane of the utricle (8) is typically folded, and the epithelium is usually simple secretory or pseudostratified columnar type. Also, two **ejaculatory ducts (3)** open at the colliculus, one on each side of the utricle (8).

1 Prostatic urethra
2 Prostatic sinuses
3 Ejaculatory ducts
4 Smooth muscle bundles
5 Prostatic glands
6 Transitional epithelium
7 Colliculus seminalis
8 Utricle
9 Ducts of prostatic glands
10 Fibromuscular stroma
11 Prostatic glands with concretions

FIGURE 20.12 ■ Prostate gland and prostatic urethra. Stain: hematoxylin and eosin. Low magnification.

FIGURE 20.13 | Prostate Gland: Glandular Acini and Prostatic Concretions

A small section of the prostate gland from Figure 20.12 is illustrated at a higher magnification.

The size of the **glandular acini (1)** in the prostate gland is highly variable. The lumina of the acini are normally wide and typically irregular because of the protrusion of the epithelium-covered **connective tissue folds (10)**. Some of the glandular acini (1) contain proteinaceous **prostatic secretions (9)**. Other glandular acini (1) contain spherical **prostatic concretions (4, 6, 8)** that are formed by concentric layers of condensed prostatic secretions. The prostatic concretions (4, 6, 8) are characteristic features of the prostate gland acini. The number of prostatic concretions (4, 6, 8) increases with the age of the individual, and they may become calcified.

Although the **glandular epithelium (5)** is usually simple columnar or pseudostratified and the cells are light staining, there is considerable variation. In some regions, the epithelium may be squamous or cuboidal.

The **excretory ducts of the prostatic glands (2)** may often resemble the glandular acini (1). In the terminal portions of the ducts (2), the epithelium is usually columnar and stains darker before entering the urethra.

The **fibromuscular stroma (7)** is another characteristic feature of the prostate gland. **Smooth muscle bundles (3)** and the connective tissue fibers blend together in the stroma (7) and are distributed throughout the gland.

FIGURE 20.14 | Prostate Gland: Prostatic Glands With Prostatic Concretions

The parenchyma of the prostate gland consists of individual **prostatic glands (3)** that vary in size and shape. The glandular epithelium also varies from simple cuboidal or **columnar (2)** to pseudostratified epithelium. In older individuals, the secretory material of the prostatic glands (3) precipitates to form the characteristic dense-staining **prostatic concretions (1, 5)**. The prostate gland is also characterized by the **fibromuscular stroma (4)**. In this photomicrograph, the **smooth muscle fibers (4a)** in the fibromuscular stroma (4) are stained red, and the **connective tissue fibers (4b)** are stained blue.

1 Glandular acini

2 Excretory ducts of prostatic glands

3 Smooth muscle bundles

4 Prostatic concretion

5 Glandular epithelium

6 Prostatic concretion

7 Fibromuscular stroma

8 Prostatic concretion

9 Prostatic secretion

10 Connective tissue folds

FIGURE 20.13 ■ Prostate gland: glandular acini and prostatic concretions. Stain: hematoxylin and eosin. Medium magnification.

1 Prostatic concretion

2 Columnar epithelium

3 Prostatic glands

4 Fibromuscular stroma:

   a. Smooth muscle fibers

   b. Connective tissue fibers

5 Prostatic concretion

FIGURE 20.14 ■ Prostate gland: prostatic glands with prostatic concretions. Stain: Masson trichrome. ×64.

FIGURE 20.15 | Seminal Vesicle

The paired seminal vesicles are elongated glands located on the posterior side of the bladder. The excretory duct from each seminal vesicle joins the ampulla of each ductus deferens to form the ejaculatory duct, which then runs through the prostate gland to open into the prostatic urethra.

The seminal vesicle exhibits highly convoluted and irregular lumina. A cross section through the gland illustrates the complexity of the **primary mucosal folds (1)**. These folds branch into numerous **secondary mucosal folds (2)**, which frequently anastomose and form irregular cavities, chambers, or **mucosal crypts (7)**. The **lamina propria (6)** projects into and forms the core of the larger primary folds (1) and the smaller secondary folds (2). The folds extend far into the lumen of the seminal vesicle.

The glandular **epithelium (5)** of the seminal vesicles varies in appearance but is usually low pseudostratified and low columnar, or cuboidal.

The muscularis consists of an **inner circular muscle layer (3)** and an **outer longitudinal muscle layer (4)**. This arrangement of the smooth muscles is often difficult to observe because of the complex folding of the mucosa. The **adventitia (8)** surrounds the muscularis and blends with the connective tissue.

FIGURE 20.16 | Bulbourethral Gland

The paired bulbourethral glands are compound tubuloacinar glands. The fibroelastic capsule that surrounds these glands contains **connective tissue (3)**, smooth muscle fibers, and **skeletal muscle fibers (2, 7)** in the interlobular **connective tissue septum (5)**. Because the bulbourethral glands are located in the urogenital diaphragm, the skeletal muscle fibers (2, 7) from the diaphragm are present in the glands. Connective tissue septa (5) from the capsule (3) divide the gland into several lobules.

The secretory units vary in structure and size and resemble mucous glands. The glands exhibit either **acinar secretory units (6)** or **tubular secretory units (1)**. The secretory cells are cuboidal, low columnar, or squamous and light staining. The height of the epithelial cells depends on the functional state of the gland. The secretory product of the bulbourethral glands is primarily mucus.

Smaller **excretory ducts (4)** from the secretory units may be lined with secretory cells, whereas the larger excretory ducts exhibit pseudostratified or stratified columnar epithelium.

FUNCTIONAL CORRELATIONS 20.4 | Accessory Male Reproductive Glands

The secretory products from the seminal vesicles, prostate gland, and bulbourethral glands mix with sperm and form composite fluid **semen**. Semen provides the sperm with a liquid transport medium and nutrients. Semen also neutralizes the acidity of the male urethra and vaginal canal and activates the sperm after ejaculation.

The **seminal vesicles** produce a yellowish, viscous fluid that contains a high concentration of sperm-activating chemicals, such as **fructose**, the main carbohydrate component of semen. Fructose is metabolized by sperm and serves as the main **energy** source for sperm motility. Seminal vesicles produce most of the fluid found in semen.

The **prostate gland** produces a thin, watery, slightly acidic fluid, rich in citric acid, prostatic acid phosphatase, amylase, and prostate-specific antigen (PSA). The enzyme fibrinolysin in the fluid liquefies the congealed semen after ejaculation. PSA is very useful for the diagnosis of prostatic cancer because its concentration often increases in the blood during malignancy.

The **bulbourethral glands** produce a clear, viscid, mucuslike secretion that, during erotic stimulation, is released and serves as a lubricant for the penile urethra. During ejaculation, secretions from the bulbourethral glands precede other components of the semen.

1 Primary mucosal folds

2 Secondary mucosal folds

3 Inner circular muscle layer

4 Outer longitudinal muscle layer

5 Epithelium

6 Lamina propria

7 Mucosal crypts

8 Adventitia

FIGURE 20.15 ■ Seminal vesicle. Stain: hematoxylin and eosin. Low magnification.

1 Tubular secretory units

2 Skeletal muscle fibers (longitudinal section)

3 Connective tissue capsule

4 Excretory duct

5 Connective tissue septum

6 Acinar secretory units

7 Skeletal muscle fibers (transverse section)

FIGURE 20.16 ■ Bulbourethral gland. Stain: hematoxylin and eosin. High magnification.

FIGURE 29.17 | Human Penis (Transverse Section)

A cross section of the human penis illustrates the two dorsal **corpora cavernosa (15)** (singular, corpus cavernosum) and a single ventral **corpus spongiosum (21)** that form the body of the organ. The **urethra (9)** passes through the entire length of the penis in the corpus spongiosum (21). A thick connective tissue capsule called the **tunica albuginea (4)** surrounds the corpora cavernosa (15) and forms a **median septum (17)** between the two bodies. A thinner **tunica albuginea (8)** with smooth muscle fibers and elastic fibers surrounds the corpus spongiosum (21).

All three cavernous bodies (15, 21) are surrounded by loose connective tissue called the **deep penile** (Buck) **fascia (5, 16)**, which, in turn, is surrounded by the connective tissue of the **dermis (10)** located below the stratified squamous keratinized epithelium of the **epidermis (11)**. Strands of smooth muscle of the **dartos tunic (7), nerves (2), sebaceous glands (20)**, and peripheral blood vessels are located in the dermis (10).

Trabeculae (19) with collagenous, elastic, nerve, and smooth muscle fibers surround and form the core of the **cavernous sinuses** (veins) **(18, 22)** in the corpora cavernosa (15) and corpus spongiosum (21). The cavernous sinuses (18) of the corpora cavernosa (15) are lined with endothelium and receive blood from the **dorsal arteries (1, 14)** and **deep arteries (3)** of the penis. The deep arteries (3) branch in the corpora cavernosa (15) and form the **helicine arteries (6)**, which empty directly into the cavernous sinuses (18). The cavernous sinuses (22) in the corpus spongiosum (21) receive blood from the bulbourethral artery, a branch of the internal pudendal artery. Blood leaving the cavernous sinuses (18, 22) exits mainly through the **superficial vein (12)** and the **deep dorsal vein (13)**.

As the urethra (9) passes the base of the penis, it is lined with a pseudostratified or stratified columnar epithelium. As the urethra exits the penis, the epithelium changes to stratified squamous. The urethra (9) also shows invaginations called urethral lacunae (of Morgagni) with mucous cells. Branched tubular urethral glands (of Littre) located below the epithelium open into these recesses. These glands are shown at a higher magnification in Figure 20.18.

FIGURE 20.18 | Penile Urethra (Transverse Section)

The penile urethra extends the entire length of the penis and is surrounded by the **corpus spongiosum (9)**. This illustration shows a transverse section through the **lumen of the penile urethra (3)** and the surrounding corpus spongiosum (9). The lining of this portion of the urethra is a pseudostratified or stratified **columnar epithelium (2)**. A thin underlying **lamina propria (5)** merges with the surrounding connective tissue of the corpus spongiosum (9).

Numerous irregular outpockets or **urethral lacunae (4)** with mucous cells are found in the lumen of the penile urethra (3). The urethral lacunae (4) are connected with the branched mucous **urethral glands (of Littre) (6, 7)** located in the surrounding connective tissue of the corpus spongiosum (9) and found throughout the length of the penile urethra. The ducts from the urethral glands (6) open into the lumen of the penile urethra (3).

The corpus spongiosum (9) consists of **cavernous sinuses (1, 10)** lined with endothelial cells and separated by connective tissue **trabeculae (8)** that contain smooth muscle fibers and collagen fibers. Numerous **blood vessels (arteriole and venule) (11)**, supply the corpus spongiosum. The internal structure of the corpus spongiosum (9) is similar to that of the corpora cavernosa described in Figure 20.17.

1 Dorsal artery
2 Nerves
3 Deep arteries
4 Tunica albuginea
5 Deep penile fascia
6 Helicine arteries
7 Dartos tunic
8 Tunica albuginea
9 Urethra
10 Dermis
11 Epidermis

12 Superficial dorsal vein
13 Deep dorsal vein
14 Dorsal artery
15 Corpora cavernosa
16 Deep penile fascia
17 Median septum
18 Cavernous sinuses
19 Trabeculae
20 Sebaceous glands
21 Corpus spongiosum
22 Cavernous sinuses

FIGURE 20.17 ■ Human penis (transverse section). Stain: hematoxylin and eosin. Low magnification.

1 Cavernous sinuses
2 Columnar epithelium
3 Lumen of penile urethra
4 Urethral lacunae
5 Lamina propria
6 Urethral glands (of Littre) and duct

7 Urethral gland (of Littre)
8 Trabeculae
9 Corpus spongiosum
10 Cavernous sinuses
11 Blood vessels (arteriole and venule)

FIGURE 20.18 ■ Penile urethra (transverse section). Stain: hematoxylin and eosin. Low magnification.

SECTION 2 • Accessory Reproductive Glands

Seminal Vesicles

- Located posterior to the bladder and superior to prostate gland
- Excretory ducts join with the ampulla of vas deferens to form ejaculatory ducts
- Ejaculatory ducts continue through prostate gland to open into prostatic urethra
- Produce fluid with sperm-activating fructose, the main energy source for sperm motility
- Produce most of the fluid found in semen

Prostate Gland

- Located inferior to the neck of the bladder
- Urethra exits bladder and passes through prostate as prostatic urethra
- Excretory ducts from the prostatic glands enter the prostatic urethra
- Transitional epithelium lines the prostatic urethra
- Characterized by fibromuscular stroma and prostatic concretions in the glands

- Produces watery secretions with numerous chemicals, including prostate-specific antigen

Bulbourethral Glands

- Small glands located at the root of penis and in the skeletal muscle of urogenital diaphragm
- Excretory ducts enter the proximal part of penile urethra
- Produce mucuslike secretion that serves as a lubricant for penile urethra

Penis

- Consists of erectile tissue or vascular spaces lined with endothelium
- Erectile corpora cavernosa is located on dorsal side and corpus spongiosum on ventral side
- Tunica albuginea surrounds the erectile bodies
- Dorsal artery and deep artery supply erectile bodies with blood

OVERVIEW FIGURE 21.1 ■ The anatomy of the female reproductive organs is presented in detail, with emphasis on the ovary and the sequence of changes during follicular development, culminating in ovulation and corpus luteum formation. In addition, the changes in the uterine wall during the menstrual cycle are correlated with pituitary hormones and ovarian functions. GnRH, gonadotropin-releasing hormone; FSH, follicle-stimulating hormone; LH, luteinizing hormone.

CHAPTER 21

Female Reproductive System

SECTION 1   Ovary and Uterus—An Overview

The human female reproductive system consists of paired internal **ovaries**, paired **uterine (fallopian) tubes**, and a single **uterus**. Inferior to the uterus and separated by the **cervix** is the **vagina**. Because **mammary glands** are associated with the female reproductive system, their histologic structure and function are illustrated and discussed in this chapter.

During reproductive life, the human female internal reproductive organs exhibit cyclic monthly changes in both structure and function. These changes constitute the **menstrual cycle**. The appearance of the initial menstrual cycle in a sexually maturing individual is called **menarche**. When the menstrual cycles become irregular and eventually cease, this phase of female reproduction is **menopause**.

The menstrual cycle is primarily controlled by two hormones secreted by the adenohypophysis of the anterior pituitary gland, **follicle-stimulating hormone (FSH)** and **luteinizing hormone (LH)**, and by two ovarian steroid hormones, **estrogen** and **progesterone**, respectively. The release of FSH and LH from the pituitary gland is controlled by the **gonadotropin-releasing hormone (GnRH)** secreted by neurons in the hypothalamus (Overview Fig. 21.1).

The individual organs of the female reproductive system perform numerous important functions. These include the secretion of female sex hormones (estrogen and progesterone) for the development of female sexual characteristics, production of oocytes, providing suitable environment for the fertilization of the oocytes in the uterine (fallopian) tube, transportation of the embryo to the uterus and its implantation, nutrition and development of the fetus during pregnancy, and nutrition of the newborn.

In humans, a mature ovarian follicle ovulates and releases an immature egg called the **oocyte** into the uterine tube approximately every 28 days. The oocyte remains viable in the female reproductive tract for about 24 hours, after which the oocyte degenerates if it is not fertilized. The transformation or maturation of the immature oocyte into a mature egg or ovum occurs at the time of **fertilization**, when the sperm, with the release of the hydrolytic enzymes from the acrosome during acrosomal reaction, dissolves the surrounding cell layers and penetrates the zona pellucida of the oocyte.

Ovaries and Development of Follicles

Each ovary is a flattened, ovoid structure located deep in the pelvic cavity. One section of the ovary is attached to the **broad ligament** by a peritoneal fold called the **mesovarium** and another section to the uterine wall by an **ovarian ligament**. The ovarian surface is covered by a single layer of cells called the **germinal epithelium** that overlies the dense, irregular connective tissue **tunica albuginea**. Located below the tunica albuginea is the **cortex** of the ovary. The ovarian follicles are located in the connective tissue of the cortex. Deep to the cortex is the highly vascularized, connective tissue core of the ovary, the **medulla**. There is no distinct boundary line between the cortex and medulla, and these two regions blend together.

During embryonic development, **primordial germ cells** migrate from the yolk sac and colonize the embryonic gonadal ridges. Here, the germ cells differentiate into **oogonia** through the process of mitosis and then enter the first phase of **meiotic** division without completing it. The germ cells become arrested in this state of development and are now called **primary oocytes.**

Primordial follicles are also formed during fetal life and consist of a primary oocyte surrounded by a single layer of squamous follicular cells. Beginning at puberty and under the influence of pituitary hormones, some selected primordial follicles grow and enlarge to become **primary, secondary**, and large **mature follicles**, which can span the cortex and extend deep into the medulla of the ovary.

The cortex of a mature ovary is normally filled with numerous ovarian follicles in various stages of development. In addition, the ovary may contain a large **corpus luteum** of a previously ovulated follicle and a **corpus albicans** of a degenerated corpus luteum. Also, most ovarian follicles in various stages of development (primordial, primary, secondary, and maturation) may undergo a process of degeneration called **atresia**, which are then phagocytosed by macrophages. Follicular atresia is common in an ovary. It occurs before birth and continues throughout the reproductive period of the individual.

Uterine (Fallopian) Tubes

Each uterine tube is about 12 cm long and extends from the ovaries to the uterus. One end of the uterine tube penetrates and opens into the uterus; the other end opens into the peritoneal cavity near the ovary. The uterine tubes are normally divided into four continuous regions. The region closest to the ovary is the funnel-shaped **infundibulum**. Extending from the infundibulum are slender, fingerlike processes called **fimbriae** (singular, fimbria) located close to the ovary. Continuous with the infundibulum is the second region, the **ampulla**, the widest and longest portion. The **isthmus** is short and narrow and joins each uterine tube to the uterus. The last portion of the uterine tube is the **interstitial (intramural) region**. It passes through the thick uterine wall to open into the uterine cavity.

Uterus

The human uterus is a pear-shaped organ with a thick muscular wall. The **body** or **corpus** forms the major portion of the uterus. The rounded upper portion of the uterus located above the entrance of the uterine tubes is called the **fundus**. The lower, narrower, and terminal portion of the uterus located below the body or corpus is the **cervix**. The cervix protrudes and opens into the vaginal canal.

The wall of the uterus is composed of three layers: an outer **perimetrium** lined with serosa or adventitia, a thick smooth muscle layer called the **myometrium,** and an inner **endometrium**. The endometrium is lined with a simple epithelium that descends into a lamina propria to form numerous **uterine glands**.

The endometrium is normally subdivided into two functional layers, the luminal **stratum functionalis** and the basal **stratum basalis**. In a nonpregnant female, the superficial functionalis layer with the uterine glands and blood vessels is sloughed off, or shed, during **menstruation**, leaving the intact deeper basalis layer with the basal remnants of the uterine glands—the source of cells for the regeneration of a new functionalis layer. The arterial supply to the endometrium plays an important role during the menstrual phase of the menstrual cycle.

Uterine arteries in the broad ligament give rise to the **arcuate arteries** that penetrate and assume a circumferential course in the myometrium of the uterus. Arcuate vessels give rise to **straight** and **spiral arteries** that supply the endometrium of the uterus. The straight arteries are short and supply the basalis layer of the endometrium, whereas the spiral arteries are long and coiled and supply the surface or functionalis layer of the endometrium. In contrast to the straight arteries, spiral arteries are highly sensitive to hormonal changes in the blood during menstrual cycles. Decreased blood levels of the ovarian hormones estrogen and progesterone during the menstrual cycle results in the degeneration and then shedding of the stratum functionalis, resulting in menstruation.

Supplemental micrographic images are available at **www.thePoint.com/Eroschenko12e** under Female Reproductive System.

FUNCTIONAL CORRELATIONS 21.1 | Ovaries, Follicles, and Their Development

Beginning at puberty and during the reproductive years of the individual, the ovaries exhibit structural and functional changes during each menstrual cycle, which lasts an average of 28 days. These changes involve numerous phases in ovarian function. Different follicles exhibit growth, and some mature. In other follicles, the developing oocyte completes the first meiotic division and is ovulated as a secondary oocyte from a mature dominant follicle. Following ovulation, a corpus luteum is formed, and, without fertilization and implantation of a developing embryo, the corpus luteum degenerates and forms a connective tissue corpus albicans. The initiation and activation of the developmental phase of primordial follicular growth in the ovaries is believed to be **independent** of gonadotropin stimulation but, instead, is dependent on local growth factors. However, the pituitary hormones follicle-stimulating hormone (FSH) and luteinizing hormone (LH) are responsible for the later stages of follicular development, maturation, ovulation of oocytes, and production of the hormones estrogen and progesterone. In healthy follicles that are not undergoing atresia, further development and maturation depends on FSH and LH stimulation.

The first half of the menstrual cycle lasts about 14 days and involves the growth of a small number of primordial ovarian follicles. At this time, FSH is the principal circulating gonadotrophic hormone, and, at this stage, the growing follicles express receptors for FSH, which are located on the surrounding granulosa cells. FSH controls the growth and maturation of ovarian follicles and initially stimulates the development of **theca interna cells** around the follicular peripheries. Later in development, LH stimulates the theca interna cells to produce **androgenic steroid precursors**. The androgenic precursors diffuse into the follicles, where the **granulosa cells** of the follicles, in response to FSH, convert them into **estrogen** with the **aromatase** enzyme. Estrogen then stimulates the granulosa cells to proliferate and increase the follicular size. As the follicles develop and mature, the circulating levels of estrogen in the blood rise. Under normal conditions, only one developing follicle becomes dominant and will reach maturity to ovulate an oocyte, whereas all the others will degenerate or become **atretic**. The dominant follicle also becomes less dependent on FSH, and it produces a hormone called **inhibin**, which, along with estrogen, inhibits the release of FSH from the pituitary gland. Increased levels of estrogen inhibit the release of gonadotropin-releasing hormone from the hypothalamus and decrease the release of FSH from the pituitary gland. This decreased level of FSH induces atresia in other follicles that started to develop.

At midcycle, or shortly before ovulation, estrogen levels reach a peak and produce a positive feedback on the pituitary gland. This peak causes a sharp surge of LH hormone from the adenohypophysis of the pituitary gland, with a concomitant smaller release of FSH hormone. Increased blood levels of both LH and FSH cause the following changes in the ovary:

- Completion of the **first meiotic division** of the oocyte just before ovulation with the liberation of a **secondary oocyte** into the uterine tube
- Final **maturation** of the mature ovarian follicle and **ovulation** (rupture) of a secondary oocyte at about the 14th day of the cycle
- Collapse of the ovulated mature follicle and the luteinization or modification of the granulosa lutein cells and theca lutein cells that surrounded the oocyte
- Transformation of the postovulatory mature follicle into the corpus luteum, a temporary functioning endocrine organ
- Vascularization of the corpus luteum and, in response to LH, production of increased amounts of progesterone and estrogen by the luteal cells

Final maturation, or the second meiotic division of the secondary oocyte, occurs only when it is fertilized by sperm. The liberated secondary oocyte remains viable in the female reproductive tract for about 24 hours before it begins to degenerate without completing the second meiotic division.

FIGURE 21.1 | Ovary: Different Stages of Follicular Development (Panoramic View)

This low-magnification image illustrates a sagittal section of an ovary and all the various forms of follicular development that would normally be seen in different functional periods of the ovary.

The ovary is covered by a single layer of low cuboidal or squamous cells called the **germinal epithelium (11)**, which is continuous with the **mesothelium (13)** of the visceral peritoneum. Beneath the germinal epithelium (11) is a dense, connective tissue layer called the **tunica albuginea (15)**.

The ovary has a peripheral **cortex (10)** and a central **medulla (8)**, in which are found numerous blood vessels, nerves, and lymphatics. In addition to the follicles, the cortex (10) contains fibrocytes with collagen and reticular fibers. The medulla (8) is a typical dense irregular connective tissue that is continuous with the **mesovarium (23)** ligament that suspends the ovary. Larger **blood vessels in the medulla (8)** distribute smaller vessels to all parts of the ovarian cortex. The mesovarium (23) is covered by the germinal epithelium (11) and peritoneal mesothelium (13).

Numerous ovarian follicles, especially the smaller types, are seen in various stages of development in the stroma (connective tissue) of the cortex (10). The most numerous follicles are the **primordial follicles (19)**, which are located in the periphery of the cortex (10) and inferior to the tunica albuginea (15). The primordial follicles (19) are the smallest and simplest in structure. They are surrounded by a single layer of squamous follicular cells. The primordial follicles (19) contain the immature, small primary oocyte, which gradually increases in size as the follicles develop into primary, secondary, and mature follicles. Before the ovulation of the mature follicle, all developing follicles contain a **primary oocyte (2, 12, 21)**.

Smaller follicles with cuboidal, columnar, or stratified cuboidal cells that surround the primary oocytes (12) are called **primary follicles (12)**. As the follicles increase in size, a fluid, called liquor folliculi (follicular liquid), begins to accumulate between the follicular cells, now called the **granulosa cells (5)**. The fluid areas eventually coalesce to form a fluid-filled cavity, called the **antrum (4, 20)**. Follicles with antral cavities are called **secondary (antral) follicles (21)**. These follicles (21) are larger and are situated deeper in the cortex (10). All larger follicles, including primary follicles (12), secondary follicles (21), and **mature follicles** exhibit a granulosa cell layer (5), a **theca interna (6)**, and an outer connective tissue layer, the **theca externa (7)**.

The largest ovarian follicle is the **mature follicle**. It exhibits the following structures: a large antrum (4) filled with liquor folliculi (follicular fluid); **a cumulus oophorus (1)**, the mound on which the primary oocyte (2) is situated; a **corona radiata (3)**, the cell layer that is attached directly to the primary oocyte (2); **granulosa cells (5)** that surround the antrum (4); the inner layer theca interna (6); and the outer theca externa (7).

After ovulation, the large follicle collapses and transforms into a temporary endocrine organ, the **corpus luteum (16)**. The granulosa cells (5) of the follicle are transformed into light-staining **granulosa lutein cells (17)**, and the theca interna (6) cells become the darker-staining **theca lutein cells (18)** of the functioning corpus luteum (16). If fertilization and implantation do not occur, the corpus luteum (16) regresses, degenerates, and ultimately turns into a connective tissue scar called the **corpus albicans (9, 14)**. This illustration shows a recent larger corpus albicans (9) and an older smaller corpus albicans (14).

Most ovarian follicles do not attain maturity. Instead, they undergo degeneration (atresia) at all stages of follicular growth and become **atretic follicles (22)**, which eventually are replaced by the connective tissue.

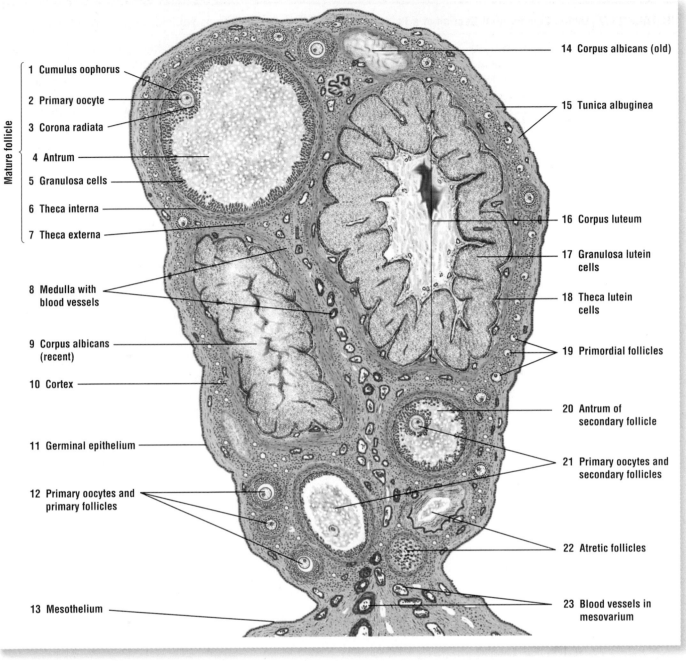

Mature follicle

1 Cumulus oophorus

2 Primary oocyte

3 Corona radiata

4 Antrum

5 Granulosa cells

6 Theca interna

7 Theca externa

8 Medulla with blood vessels

9 Corpus albicans (recent)

10 Cortex

11 Germinal epithelium

12 Primary oocytes and primary follicles

13 Mesothelium

14 Corpus albicans (old)

15 Tunica albuginea

16 Corpus luteum

17 Granulosa lutein cells

18 Theca lutein cells

19 Primordial follicles

20 Antrum of secondary follicle

21 Primary oocytes and secondary follicles

22 Atretic follicles

23 Blood vessels in mesovarium

FIGURE 21.1 ■ Ovary: different stages of follicular development (panoramic view). Stain: hematoxylin and eosin. Low magnification.

FIGURE 21.2 | Ovary: Longitudinal Section of a Feline (Cat) Ovary Showing Numerous Follicles and Corpora Lutea

This low-magnification photomicrograph shows a section of a feline (cat) ovary. The surface of the ovary is covered with a low cuboidal, or squamous **germinal epithelium (1),** that continues with the **mesothelium (6)** of the visceral peritoneum. The mesothelium (6) covers the dense connective tissue of the suspensory ligament of the ovary, the **mesovarium (8).** Numerous blood vessels, lymphatic vessels, and nerves enter and supply the ovarian **medulla (7)** through the mesovarium (8). Located directly under the germinal epithelium is the dense connective tissue **tunica albuginea (2)** that encloses the entire ovary. Below the tunica albuginea (2) is the cortex of the ovary. Here are seen numerous, light-staining, small **primordial follicles (4).** Deeper in the cortex are visible developing **primary follicles (5)** and numerous larger **antral follicles (9)** that are filled with liquor folliculi (follicular fluid). The large mature follicles that ovulated have been transformed into temporary **corpora lutea (3)** in which the follicular wall of the mature follicles collapsed on the former antral cavity. The granulosa cells that surrounded the antral cavity are transformed into the granulosa lutein cells of the corpora lutea (3).

FIGURE 21.3 | Ovary: A Section of an Ovary Showing the Ovarian Cortex with Developing Follicles

This higher-magnification photomicrograph shows a section of an ovarian cortex and its contents. Covering the surface of the ovary is a thin layer of cuboidal cells of the **germinal epithelium (1).** Beneath the layer of germinal epithelium (1) is the thicker layer of dense connective tissue **tunica albuginea (5).** Just under the tunica albuginea (5) is the connective tissue of the **ovarian cortex (8)** in which are found numerous **primordial follicles (2)** that are surrounded by flat follicular cells. A larger **primary follicle (4)** with a **primary oocyte (3)** is surrounded by stratified cuboidal granulosa cells. Also visible are other **primary follicles (6)** with cuboidal follicular cells. On the right side of the image is a larger follicle with what appears to be disorganized granulosa cells in the antrum and some denser-staining cell with pycnotic nuclei. This appears to be an **atretic follicle (7).**

1 Germinal epithelium
2 Tunica albuginea
3 Corpora lutea
4 Primordial follicles
5 Primary follicles
6 Mesothelium
7 Medulla
8 Mesovarium
9 Antral follicles

FIGURE 21.2 ■ Ovary: longitudinal section of a feline (cat) ovary showing numerous follicles and corpora lutea. Stain: Mallory-Azan. ×6.5.

1 Germinal epithelium
2 Primordial follicles
3 Primary oocyte
4 Primary follicle
5 Tunica albuginea
6 Primary follicles
7 Atretic follicle
8 Cortex

FIGURE 21.3 ■ Ovary: a section of ovarian cortex and developing follicles. Stain: hematoxylin and eosin. ×64.

FIGURE 21.4 | Ovary: Ovarian Cortex and Primary and Primordial Follicles

The ovarian surface is covered by a cuboidal **germinal epithelium (10)**. Located directly beneath the germinal epithelium (10) is a layer of dense connective tissue called the **tunica albuginea (16)**. Numerous **primordial follicles (14, 17)** are located in the cortex below the tunica albuginea (16). Each primordial follicle (14, 17) is surrounded by a single layer of squamous **follicular cells (17)**. As the follicles grow larger, the follicular cells (17) of the primordial follicles (14, 17) change to cuboidal, or low columnar, and the follicles are now called **primary follicles (4, 11)**. The developing oocytes (4, 13) also have a large eccentric **nucleus (7, 13)** with a conspicuous nucleolus.

In primary (growing) follicles (4, 11), the follicular cells proliferate by **mitosis (3)** and form layers of cuboidal cells called the **granulosa cells (8, 12)** that surround the primary oocytes (4, 13). A single layer of the granulosa cells that surround the oocyte forms the **corona radiata (5)**.

Between the corona radiata (5) and the oocyte appears the noncellular glycoprotein layer called the **zona pellucida (6)**. The stromal cells that surround the follicular cells now differentiate into the **theca interna (9)** layer that is located adjacent to the granulosa cells (8, 12). A thin basement membrane (not shown) separates the granulosa cells (8, 12) from the theca interna (9) cells.

Many primordial, developing, or mature follicles exhibit degeneration, die, and are lost through a process called atresia. A degenerating **atretic follicle (1)** is illustrated in the upper left corner of the illustration. Numerous blood vessels, such as a **capillary (2)**, surround the developing follicles and are found in the **connective tissue of the cortex (15)**.

FIGURE 21.5 | Ovary: Primordial and Primary Follicles

This photomicrograph shows different types of follicles in the cortex of an ovary. The immature **primordial follicles (2)** consist of a primary **oocyte (3)** surrounded by a layer of simple squamous **follicular cells (1, 7)**. As the primordial follicles (2) grow to become **primary follicles (4)**, the layer of simple squamous follicular cells around the oocyte changes to a cuboidal layer. In a larger **primary follicle (8)**, the follicular cells have proliferated into a stratified layer around the oocyte called **granulosa cells (11)**. A prominent layer of glycoprotein, the **zona pellucida (10)**, develops between the granulosa cells (11) and the immature **oocyte (9)**.

The cells around the developing follicles also organize into two distinct cell layers: the inner hormone-secreting **theca interna (12)** and the outer connective tissue layer **theca externa (13)**. The theca interna (12) and theca externa (13) are separated from the granulosa cells (11) by a thin **basement membrane (6)**. Surrounding the follicles in the cortex are the cells and fibers of the **connective tissue (5)**.

1 Atretic follicle
2 Capillary
3 Mitosis of follicular cells
4 Primary follicle with a primary oocyte
5 Corona radiata
6 Zona pellucida
7 Nucleus of a primary oocyte
8 Granulosa cells
9 Theca interna

10 Germinal epithelium
11 Primary follicle
12 Granulosa cells
13 Nucleus of a primary oocyte
14 Primordial follicles
15 Connective tissue of the cortex
16 Tunica albuginea
17 Follicular cells of primordial follicles

FIGURE 21.4 ■ Ovary: ovarian cortex and primordial and primary follicles. Stain: hematoxylin and eosin. Low magnification.

1 Follicular cells
2 Primordial follicles
3 Oocyte
4 Primary follicles
5 Connective tissue
6 Basement membrane

7 Follicular cells
8 Primary follicle
9 Oocyte
10 Zona pellucida
11 Granulosa cells
12 Theca interna
13 Theca externa

FIGURE 21.5 ■ Ovary: primordial and primary follicles. Stain: hematoxylin and eosin. ×64.

FIGURE 21.6 | Ovary: Maturing Ovarian Follicle in Feline (Cat) Ovary

This medium-magnification micrograph shows a maturing ovarian follicle in a feline ovary. A large area that has been filled with liquor folliculi is the **antrum (3)**, displacing the **primary oocyte (10)** on one side of the follicle. Surrounding the oocyte is a faint glycoprotein layer, the **zona pellucida (9)**. The primary oocyte (10) rests on the **cumulus oophorus (11)**, a mound of cells that also exhibits separation due to accumulation of **intercellular follicular fluid (12)**. The cells that surround the oocyte form the **corona radiata (5),** although, in this image, the separation between the oocyte and the corona radiata is abnormally enlarged due to the chemical fixation process. The cells that surround the antrum (3) are the **granulosa cells (4)**. They are separated by a thin **basement membrane (6)** from the surrounding connective tissue cells that have been altered to form the inner and more secretory epithelioid type of cells, the **theca interna (2)** layer and the outer connective tissue layer, the **theca externa (8)**. On the right side of the maturing follicle are the light-staining **interstitial cells (7)**, which represent the remnants of the theca interna cells (2) that persist as individual cells or as a group of cells in the ovarian cortex following follicular atresia. Also visible near the follicle is the dense **connective tissue (1)** of the ovarian cortex.

FIGURE 21.7 | Ovary: Primary Oocyte and Wall of a Mature Follicle

This more detailed illustration of a mature follicle shows the primary oocyte, the surrounding cells, and the mound on which it is located. During the growth of the follicles, fluid begins to accumulate between the granulosa cells that surround the oocyte, forming a fluid-filled cavity, the antrum. The follicle is called a secondary follicle when the antrum is present.

This figure illustrates the **cytoplasm** and **nucleus** of a **primary oocyte (3)** and the wall of a fluid-filled mature follicle. A local thickening of the **granulosa cells (5)** on one side of the follicle surrounds the primary oocyte (3) and projects into the **antrum (4, 7)** of the follicle. Here, the granulosa cells form a hillock (mound) called the **cumulus oophorus (8)**. The single layer of granulosa cells (5) that are located immediately adjacent to the primary oocyte (3) forms the **corona radiata (1)**. Between the corona radiata (1) and the cytoplasm of the primary oocyte (3) is a prominent, acidophilic-staining glycoprotein, the **zona pellucida (2)**.

The granulosa cells (5) surround the antrum (4, 7) and secrete follicular fluid that fills the antrum cavity. Smaller isolated accumulations of the fluid also occur among the granulosa cells (5) as **intercellular follicular fluid (6, 9)**.

The basal row of granulosa cells (5) rests on a thin **basement membrane (10)** that separates the granulosa cells (5) from the cells of the **theca interna (11)**, an inner layer of vascularized, secretory cells of the follicle. Surrounding the cells of the theca interna (11) is the **theca externa (12)** layer that blends with the **connective tissue (13)** of the ovarian cortex.

1 Connective tissue
2 Theca interna
3 Antrum
4 Granulosa cells
5 Corona radiata
6 Basement membrane
7 Interstitial cells
8 Theca externa
9 Zona pellucida
10 Primary oocyte
11 Cumulus oophrus
12 Intercellular follicular fluid

FIGURE 21.6 ■ Ovary: maturing ovarian follicle in feline (cat) ovary. Stain: Mallory-Azan. ×45.

1 Corona radiata
2 Zona pellucida
3 Cytoplasm and nucleus of a primary oocyte
4 Antrum
5 Granulosa cells
6 Intercellular follicular fluid
7 Antrum
8 Cumulus oophorus
9 Intercellular follicular fluid
10 Basement membrane
11 Theca interna
12 Theca externa
13 Connective tissue

FIGURE 21.7 ■ Ovary: primary oocyte and wall of a mature follicle. Stain: hematoxylin and eosin. High magnification.

FIGURE 21.8 | Corpus Luteum (Panoramic View)

At a higher magnification, the corpus luteum is a collapsed and folded mass of glandular epithe-lium, primarily consisting of **theca lutein cells (5)** and **granulosa lutein cells (6)**. Theca lutein cells (5) extend along the **connective tissue septa (3)** into the folds of the corpus luteum.

The **theca externa (2)** cells form a poorly defined capsule around the corpus luteum that also extends inward with the connective tissue septa (3) into folds.

The center of the corpus luteum or the **former follicular cavity (9)** contains remnants of follicular fluid, serum, blood cells, and loose **connective tissue with blood vessels (7)** from the theca externa that has proliferated and extended into the layers of the glandular epithelium. The connective tissue (7) also covers the inner surface of the granulosa lutein cells (6) and then spreads throughout the core of the corpus luteum. Some corpora lutea may contain a postovula-tory **blood clot (8)** in the former follicular cavity (9).

The **connective tissue of the cortex (1)** that surrounds the corpus luteum contains numer-ous **blood vessels (4)**.

FIGURE 21.9 | Corpus Luteum: Theca Lutein Cells and Granulosa Lutein Cells

The granulosa **lutein cells (6)** represent the hypertrophied former granulosa cells of the mature follicle and constitute the highly folded mass of the corpus luteum. The granulosa lutein cells (6) are large, have large vesicular nuclei, and stain lightly owing to lipid inclusions. The **theca lutein cells (1, 7)** (the former theca interna cells) are located external to the granulosa lutein cells (6) on the periphery of the glandular epithelium. The theca lutein cells (1, 7) are smaller than the granulosa lutein cells (6), and their cytoplasm stains darker. Also, the nuclei of theca lutein cells (1, 7) are smaller and darker.

The **theca externa (2)** with numerous blood vessels, **venule and arteriole (4)** and **capillaries (5)**, invades the granulosa lutein cells (6) and theca lutein cells (1, 7). A fine **connective tissue septum with fibrocytes (3)** penetrates the theca lutein cells (1, 7). The fibrocytes (3) in the septum between the theca lutein cells (1, 7) can be identified by their elongated and flattened appearance.

1 Connective tissue of the cortex

2 Theca externa

3 Connective tissue septa

4 Blood vessels in the connective tissue

5 Theca lutein cells

6 Granulosa lutein cells

7 Connective tissue with blood vessels

8 Blood clot

9 Former folicular cavity

FIGURE 21.8 ■ Corpus luteum (panoramic view). Stain: hematoxylin and eosin. Low magnification.

1 Theca lutein cells

2 Theca externa

3 Connective tissue septum with fibrocytes

4 Venule and arteriole in theca externa

5 Capillaries

6 Granulosa lutein cells

7 Theca lutein cells

FIGURE 21.9 ■ Corpus luteum: theca lutein cells and granulosa lutein cells. Stain: hematoxylin and eosin.

FIGURE 21.10 | Human Ovary: A Section of Corpus Luteum and Corpus Albicans

This low-magnification micrograph shows a section of a human ovary. On the left side is a section of the highly folded wall of the corpus luteum that consists of the hypertrophied and lighter-staining **granulosa lutein cells (3, 5)** and the surrounding darker-staining **theca lutein cells (1, 4)** that are located peripherally and between the folds of the granulosa lutein cells (3, 5) of the corpus luteum. Surrounding the corpus luteum is the dark-staining and dense connective tissue layer of the **theca externa (2)**. On the right side of the figure is the blue-staining connective tissue scar of the corpus luteum, the **corpus albicans (7)**. Above the corpus albicans (7) is the light-staining and **degenerating corpus luteum (6)**. Between the corpus luteum and the corpus albicans (7) is the highly vascular dense **connective tissue (9)** with different sizes of **blood vessels (8)**.

FUNCTIONAL CORRELATIONS 21.2 | Corpus Luteum

After the ovulation of a mature follicle and the liberation of a secondary oocyte into the infundibulum of the uterine tube, the wall of the ruptured follicle collapses and becomes highly folded. At this time, the ovary enters the **luteal phase**. During this phase, luteinizing hormone (LH) secretion induces hypertrophy and transformation of the granulosa cells and theca interna cells of the ovulated follicle into **granulosa lutein cells** and **theca lutein cells**, respectively. These changes transform the ovulated follicle into a temporary endocrine tissue, the corpus luteum. LH continues to stimulate and regulate the cells of the corpus lutein to secrete **estrogen** and large amounts of **progesterone**. High levels of estrogen and progesterone further stimulate the development of the **uterus** and mammary glands in anticipation of the implantation of a fertilized egg and pregnancy.

Rising levels of estrogen and progesterone produced by the corpus luteum exert an inhibitory effect on the further release of follicle-stimulating hormone (FSH) and LH, influencing both the neurons in the hypothalamus and gonadotrophs in the adenohypophysis. This effect prevents further ovulation.

If the ovulated secondary oocyte is not fertilized, the corpus luteum continues to secrete its hormones for about another 12 days and then begins to regress. After its regression, it is called the **corpus luteum of menstruation**, which eventually becomes a nonfunctional structure that becomes a connective tissue scar called the **corpus albicans**. With the decreased functions of the corpus luteum, estrogen and progesterone levels decline, affecting the blood vessels in the endometrium of the uterus and resulting in the shedding of the stratum functionalis of the endometrium in the menstrual flow.

As the corpus luteum ceases function, the inhibitory effects of estrogen, progesterone, and inhibin on the hypothalamus and pituitary gland cells are removed. As a result, FSH is again released from the adenohypophysis, initiating a new ovarian cycle of follicular development and maturation.

CORPUS LUTEUM AND PREGNANCY

If fertilization of the oocyte and implantation of the embryo occurs, the corpus luteum increases in size and becomes the **corpus luteum of pregnancy**. The hormone **human chorionic gonadotropin (hCG)**, secreted by the trophoblast cells of the

FUNCTIONAL CORRELATIONS 21.2 | Corpus Luteum *(Continued)*

developing placenta in the implanting embryo, continues to stimulate luteal functions of the corpus luteum and prevents its regression. The influence of hCG is similar to that produced by LH from the pituitary gland and extends its function of progesterone secretion. As a result, the corpus luteum of pregnancy persists for several months. As the pregnancy progresses, however, the function of the corpus luteum gradually diminishes and is taken over by the **placenta**. The placenta functions as a temporary endocrine organ and assumes the dominant role of secreting sufficient amounts of estrogen and progesterone to maintain the pregnancy until parturition.

1 Theca lutein cells
2 Theca externa
3 Granulosa lutein cells
4 Theca lutein cells
5 Granulosa lutein cells
6 Degenerating corpus luteum
7 Corpus albicans
8 Blood vessels
9 Connective tissue

FIGURE 21.10 ■ Human ovary: a section of corpus luteum and corpus albicans. Stain: Mallory-Azan. ×10.5.

FIGURE 21.11 | Uterine Tube: Ampulla with Mesosalpinx Ligament (Panoramic View, Transverse Section)

The paired, muscular uterine (fallopian) tubes extend from the proximity of the ovaries to the uterus. On one end, the infundibulum opens into the peritoneal cavity adjacent to the ovary. The other end penetrates the uterine wall to open into the interior of the uterus. The uterine tubes conduct the ovulated oocyte toward the uterus.

The ampulla is the longest part of the tube and is normally the site of fertilization. The mucosa of the ampulla exhibits the most extensive **mucosal folds (8)**. These folds (8) form an irregular **lumen** in the **uterine tube (7)** that produces deep grooves between the folds (8). These folds become smaller as the uterine tube nears the uterus.

The mucosa of the uterine tube consists of simple columnar ciliated and nonciliated **epithelium (6)** that overlies the loose connective tissue **lamina propria (9)**. The muscularis consists of two smooth muscle layers, an **inner circular layer (5)** and an **outer longitudinal layer (4)**. The **interstitial connective tissue (10)** is abundant between the muscle layers, and as a result, the smooth muscle layers (4, 5)—especially the outer layer (4)—are not distinct. Numerous **venules (3)** and **arterioles (2)** are visible in the interstitial connective tissue (10). The **serosa (11)** of the visceral peritoneum forms the outermost layer on the uterine tube, which is connected to the **mesosalpinx ligament (1)** of the superior margin of the broad ligament.

FIGURE 21.12 | Uterine Tube: Mucosal Folds

A higher magnification of the mucosal folds of the uterine tube shows that the lining epithelium consists of **ciliated cells (3)** and nonciliated **peg (secretory) cells (1)**. The ciliated cells (3) are most numerous in the infundibulum and ampulla of the uterine tube. The beat of the cilia is directed toward the uterus. Under the epithelium is seen a prominent **basement membrane (2)** and the **lamina propria (4)** with numerous **blood vessels (5)**. The lamina propria (4) is a cellular, loose connective tissue with fine collagen and reticular fibers.

During the early proliferative phase of the menstrual cycle and under the influence of estrogen, the ciliated cells (3) undergo hypertrophy, exhibit cilia growth, and become predominant. In addition, there is an increase in the secretory activity of the nonciliated peg cells (1). The epithelium of the uterine tube shows cyclic changes, and the proportion of ciliated and nonciliated cells varies with the stages of the menstrual cycle.

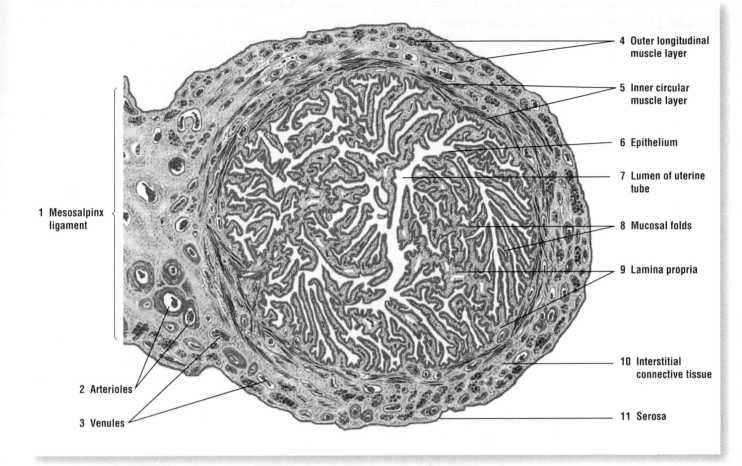

1 Mesosalpinx ligament

2 Arterioles

3 Venules

4 Outer longitudinal muscle layer

5 Inner circular muscle layer

6 Epithelium

7 Lumen of uterine tube

8 Mucosal folds

9 Lamina propria

10 Interstitial connective tissue

11 Serosa

FIGURE 21.11 ■ Uterine tube: ampulla with mesosalpinx ligament (panoramic view, transverse section). Stain: hematoxylin and eosin. Low magnification.

1 Peg (secretory) cells

2 Basement membrane

3 Ciliated cells

4 Lamina propria

5 Blood vessels

FIGURE 21.12 ■ Uterine tube: mucosal folds. Stain: hematoxylin and eosin. High magnification.

FIGURE 21.13 | Uterine Tube: Lining Epithelium

This high-magnification photomicrograph illustrates a section of the uterine tube wall with complex mucosal folds that are lined with a **simple columnar epithelium (2)**.

The luminal epithelium consists of two cell types, the **ciliated cells (5)** and the nonciliated **peg cells (6)** with apical bulges that extend above the cilia. A thin **basement membrane (1)** separates the luminal epithelium (2) from the underlying vascularized **connective tissue (4)** that forms the core of the mucosal folds. A portion of the **inner circular smooth muscle (3)** layer that surrounds the uterine tube is visible in the periphery on the left side of the illustration.

FUNCTIONAL CORRELATIONS 21.3 | Uterine Tubes

The uterine tubes perform several important reproductive functions. Just before ovulation and rupture of the mature follicle, the fingerlike **fimbriae** of the infundibulum that are very close to the ovary begin to sweep its surface to capture the released oocyte. This function is accomplished by gentle **peristaltic contractions** of smooth muscles in the uterine tube wall and fimbriae. In addition, the heavily ciliated cells on the fimbriae surfaces create a current toward the uterus that guides the released oocyte into the infundibulum of the uterine tube. The cilia action and the muscular contractions in the wall of the uterine tube transport the captured oocyte, or fertilized egg, through the remaining regions of the uterine tube toward the uterus.

The uterine tubes also serve as the site of oocyte **fertilization**, which normally occurs in the upper region of the **ampulla**. The nonciliated (peg) cells in the uterine tube are secretory and contribute important nutritive material for the oocyte, the initial development of the fertilized ovum, and the embryo. The uterine secretions also maintain the viability of sperm in the uterine tubes and allow them to undergo **capacitation**, a complex biochemical and structural process that activates the sperm and enables them to fertilize the released oocyte. The fertilization triggers the ovulated secondary oocyte to undergo the **second meiotic division** to produce an ovum that can now be fertilized by the sperm.

When the sperm reaches the secondary oocyte, it is surrounded by cells that form a protective layer around it called the **corona radiata**, which the sperm must first penetrate. In order to fertilize the oocyte, the sperm must also penetrate the surrounding **zona pellucida** and bind to zona pellucida receptors to complete capacitation. This binding triggers the **acrosome reaction**, which releases the hydrolytic enzymes from the acrosome on the sperm nucleus into the zona pellucida to allow for the passage of sperm into the oocyte. As the sperm penetrates the oocyte, a **cortical reaction** is produced that blocks **polyspermy**, a barrier around the zona pellucida that allows the penetration of only one sperm to fertilize the egg.

The epithelium in the uterine tubes exhibits changes that are associated with the ovarian cycle. The height of the uterine tube epithelium is at its maximum during the follicular phase, at which time the ovarian follicles are maturing and circulating levels of estrogen are high.

1 Basement
  membrane

4 Connective
  tissue

5 Ciliated cells

6 Peg cells

2 Simple columnar
  epithelium

3 Inner circular
  smooth muscle

FIGURE 21.13 ■ Uterine tube: lining epithelium. Stain: hematoxylin and eosin (plastic section). ×130.

FIGURE 21.14 | Uterus: Proliferative (Follicular) Phase

The surface of the **endometrium** is lined with a simple columnar **epithelium (1)** overlaying the thick **lamina propria (2)**. The lining epithelium (1) extends down into the connective tissue of the lamina propria (2) and forms long, tubular **uterine glands (4)**. In the proliferative phase, the uterine glands (4) are usually straight in the superficial portion of the endometrium but may exhibit branching in the deeper regions near the myometrium. As a result, numerous uterine glands (4) are seen in cross section.

The wall of the uterus consists of three layers: the inner endometrium (1 to 4), a middle layer of smooth muscle **myometrium (5, 6),** and the outer serous membrane perimetrium (not illustrated). The endometrium is further subdivided into two zones or layers: a narrow, deep **basalis layer (8)** adjacent to the myometrium (5) and the **functionalis layer (7)**, a wider, superficial layer above the basalis layer (8) that extends to the lumen of the uterus.

During the menstrual cycle, the endometrium exhibits morphologic changes that are directly correlated with ovarian function. The cyclic changes in a nonpregnant uterus are divided into three distinct phases: the proliferative (follicular) phase, the secretory (luteal) phase, and the menstrual phase.

In the proliferative phase of the cycle and under the influence of ovarian estrogen, the stratum functionalis (7) increases in thickness, and the uterine glands (4) elongate and follow a straight course to the surface. Also, the **coiled (spiral) arteries (3)** (in cross section) are primarily seen in the deeper regions of the endometrium. The lamina propria (2) in the upper regions of the endometrium is cellular and resembles mesenchymal tissue. The connective tissue in the **basalis layer (8)** is more compact and appears darker in this illustration. The endometrium continues to develop during the proliferative phase as a result of the increasing levels of estrogen secreted by the developing ovarian follicles.

The endometrium is situated above the myometrium (5, 6), which consists of compact bundles of **smooth muscle (5, 6)** separated by thin strands of **interstitial connective tissue (9)** with numerous **blood vessels (10)**. As a result, the muscle bundles are seen in cross, oblique, and longitudinal sections.

1 Lining epithelium

2 Lamina propria

3 Coiled arteries

4 Uterine glands

5 Smooth muscle (longitudinal)

6 Smooth muscle (cross section)

7 Functionalis layer

8 Basalis layer

9 Interstitial connective tissue

10 Blood vessels

Endometrium

Myometrium

FIGURE 21.14 ■ Uterus: proliferative (follicular) phase. Stain: hematoxylin and eosin. Low magnification.

FIGURE 21.15 | Uterus: Secretory (Luteal) Phase

The secretory (luteal) phase of the menstrual cycle is initiated after the ovulation of the mature follicle. The additional changes in the endometrium are caused by the influence of both estrogen and progesterone that is secreted by the functioning corpus luteum. As a result, the **functionalis layer (1)** and **basalis layer (2)** of the endometrium become thicker owing to increased **glandular secretion (5)** and edema in the **lamina propria (6)**.

The epithelium of the **uterine glands (5, 8)** undergoes hypertrophy (enlarges) as a result of increased accumulation of the secretory product (5, 8). The uterine glands (5, 8) also become highly coiled (tortuous), and their lumina become dilated with nutritive **secretory material (5)** rich in carbohydrates. The **coiled arteries (7)** continue to extend into the upper portion of the endometrium (functionalis layer) (1) and become prominent because of their thicker walls.

The alterations in the surface **columnar epithelium (4)**, uterine glands (5), and lamina propria (6) characterize the functionalis layer (1) of the endometrium during the secretory or luteal phase of the menstrual cycle. The basalis layer (2) exhibits minimal changes. Below the basalis layer is the **myometrium (3)** with **smooth muscle bundles (10)**, sectioned in both longitudinal and transverse planes, and **blood vessels (9)**.

1 Functionalis layer

2 Basalis layer

3 Myometrium

4 Columnar epithelium

5 Uterine glands (with secretion)

6 Lamina propria (with edema)

7 Coiled arteries

8 Uterine glands (hypertrophied and tortuous)

9 Blood vessel

10 Smooth muscle bundles

FIGURE 21.15 ■ Uterus: secretory (luteal) phase. Stain: hematoxylin and eosin. Low magnification.

FIGURE 21.16 | Uterine Wall (Endometrium): Secretory (Luteal) Phase

This low-magnification photomicrograph illustrates a section of the endometrium during the secretory (luteal) phase of the menstrual cycle. The thick and lighter area of the endometrium is the **stratum functionalis (1)**. The darker and deeper endometrium is the **stratum basalis (2)**. The **uterine glands (3)** during the secretory phase are coiled (tortuous) and secrete glycogen-rich nutrients into their lumina.

Surrounding the uterine glands (3) is the highly cellular **connective tissue (4)**. The light, empty spaces in the connective tissue (4) layer are caused by increased edema in the endometrium. Below the stratum basalis (2) is the smooth muscle layer **myometrium (5)** of the uterine wall.

1 Stratum
  functionalis

2 Stratum basalis

3 Uterine glands

4 Connective tissue

5 Myometrium

FIGURE 21.16 ■ Uterine wall (endometrium): secretory (luteal) phase. Stain: hematoxylin and eosin. ×10.

FIGURE 21.17 | Uterus: Menstrual Phase

If fertilization of the ovum and implantation of the embryo do not occur, the uterus enters the menstrual phase, and much of the preparatory changes made for implantation in the endometrium are lost. During the menstrual phase, the **endometrium** in the **functionalis layer (1)** degenerates and is sloughed off. The shed endometrium contains fragments of disintegrated stroma, **blood clots (7)**, and uterine glands. Some of the intact **uterine glands (2)** are filled with **blood (6)**. In the deeper layers of the endometrium, the **basalis layer (4)**, the **bases of the uterine glands (9)** remain intact during the shedding of the functionalis layer and the menstrual flow.

The endometrial stroma of most of the functionalis layer contains aggregations of erythrocytes (7) that have been extruded from the torn and disintegrating blood vessels. In addition, the endometrial stroma exhibits the infiltration of lymphocytes and neutrophils.

The basalis layer (4) of the endometrium remains unaffected during this phase. The distal (superficial) portions of the **coiled arteries (3, 8)** become necrotic, whereas the deeper parts of these vessels remain intact.

FUNCTIONAL CORRELATIONS 21.4 | Uterus

The endometrium exhibits cyclic changes in its structure and function in response to the ovarian hormones **estrogen** and **progesterone**. The uterine changes are associated with impending implantation and nourishment of the developing embryo. Secretion of progesterone by the functioning corpus luteum prepares the uterus for **implantation** of the embryo, formation of the placenta, and creation of a suitable environment for the development and maturation of the offspring. However, if fertilization of the oocyte and implantation of the embryo do not occur, blood vessels in the endometrium deteriorate and rupture, and the **functionalis layer** of endometrium is **shed** as part of the menstrual flow or discharge. With each menstrual cycle during the reproductive period of the individual, the endometrium passes through three successive phases, the proliferative, secretory, and menstrual phase, with each phase gradually passing into the next.

The **proliferative (preovulatory, follicular) phase** is characterized by rapid growth and development of the endometrium. The resurfacing and growth of the endometrium during the proliferative phase closely coincides with the rapid growth of **ovarian follicles** and their increased production of **estrogen**. This phase starts at the end of the menstrual phase, or about day 5, and continues to about day 14 of the cycle. Increased mitotic activity of the connective tissue in the **lamina propria** and in basal remnants of the **uterine glands** in the **basalis layer** of the endometrium produces new cells and ground substance that begin to cover the raw surface of the uterine mucosa that was denuded or shed during menstruation. The resurfacing of the mucosa produces a new functionalis layer of the endometrium. As the functionalis layer thickens, the uterine glands proliferate, lengthen, and become closely packed. The **spiral arteries** begin to grow toward the endometrial surface and begin to show light coiling.

The **secretory (postovulatory, luteal) phase** begins shortly after ovulation on about day 15 and continues to about day 28 of the cycle. This phase is dependent on the functional corpus luteum that was formed after ovulation and the secretion of **progesterone** and **estrogen** by the lutein cells (granulosa lutein and theca lutein cells). During the postovulatory secretory phase, the endometrium thickens and accumulates fluid, becoming **edematous** (increased fluid retention). In addition, the uterine glands

1 Disintegrating stratum
   functionalis

2 Uterine glands

3 Coiled arteries

4 Lamina propria
   of stratum basalis

5 Myometrium

6 Blood in disintegrating
   uterine glands

7 Blood clots in lamina
   propria

8 Coiled arteries

9 Intact uterine glands
   of stratum basalis

FIGURE 21.17 ■ Uterine wall: menstrual phase. Stain: hematoxylin and eosin. Low
magnification.

FUNCTIONAL CORRELATIONS 21.4 | Uterus *(Continued)*

undergo hypertrophy and become tortuous, and their lumina become filled with secretions rich in **nutrients**, especially **glycoproteins** and **glycogen**. The spiral arteries in the endometrium also lengthen, become more coiled, and extend almost to the surface of the endometrium. The changes seen in this phase are due primarily to hypertrophy of the glandular epithelium, increased vascularity, and edema in the endometrium.

The **menstrual (menses) phase** of the cycle begins when the ovulated oocyte is not fertilized, and no implantation occurs in the uterus. Reduced levels of circulating progesterone (and estrogen), as a result of the regressing corpus luteum, initiate this phase. Decreased levels of these hormones induce intermittent constrictions of the walls of the spiral arteries and interruption of blood flow to the functionalis layer of the endometrium, whereas the blood flow to the basalis layer remains uninterrupted. These constrictions deprive the functionalis layer of oxygenated blood and produce transitory **ischemia**, causing necrosis (degeneration) of cells in the walls of blood vessels and degeneration of the functionalis layer in the endometrium. After extended periods of vascular constriction, the spiral arteries dilate, resulting in the rupture of their necrotic walls and hemorrhage (bleeding) into the stroma. The necrotic functionalis layer then detaches from the rest of the endometrium. Blood, uterine fluid, stromal cells, secretory material, and epithelial cells from the functionalis layer mix to form the **menstrual flow**, which lasts about 5 days.

The shedding of the functionalis layer of the endometrium continues until only the raw surface of the basalis layer is left. At the end of the menstrual cycle, the stratum basalis portion of the endometrium consists of a thin layer of connective tissue and the basal parts of the uterine glands. The remnants of uterine glands in this stratum basalis layer serve as the source of new cells for regenerating the next functionalis layer. Rapid proliferation of cells in the glands of the basalis layer, under the influence of rising estrogen levels during the proliferative phase, resurface and restore the lost stratum functionalis layer of the endometrium and prepare the uterus for the next phase of the menstrual cycle.

SECTION 1 • Ovary and Uterus

The Female Reproductive System—Overview

- Consists of paired ovaries, uterine tubes, and a single uterus
- Uterus separated from vagina by cervix
- Organs exhibit cyclic monthly changes in the form of a menstrual cycle
- Start of first cycle is the menarche and ending of cycles is the menopause
- Cycles controlled by follicle-stimulating hormone and luteinizing hormone and ovarian estrogen and progesterone
- Follicle-stimulating hormone and luteinizing hormone release controlled by gonadotropin-releasing hormone
- Immature oocyte released about every 28 days into uterine tube

Ovaries and Development of Follicles

- Germinal epithelium overlies connective tissue tunica albuginea
- Consist of an outer cortex and inner medulla, without distinct boundaries
- During embryonic development, oogonia divide by mitosis in gonadal ridges
- Oogonia enter first meiotic division and remain as primary oocytes in primordial follicles
- At puberty, primordial follicles can grow to become primary, secondary, and mature follicles
- Ovarian follicles can undergo degeneration or atresia at any stage of development
- Primordial follicles with primary oocyte are surrounded by squamous follicular cells
- Primordial follicles: initiation of development and activation is independent of gonadotropin stimulation
- Primary follicles exhibit simple cuboidal or stratified granulosa cell layers
- Secondary follicles exhibit liquid accumulations between granulosa cells or antrum
- Largest follicles are mature, span the cortex, and extend into medulla
- In maturing follicles, oocytes are located on the mound cumulus oophorus
- Theca interna and theca externa are visible in larger, developing follicles
- Primary oocytes are surrounded by zona pellucida and corona radiata cells in follicles

- Follicle-stimulating hormone and luteinizing hormone are responsible for later development, maturation, and ovulation of follicles
- During first half of the menstrual cycle and during follicular growth, follicle-stimulating hormone is the principal hormone
- Follicle-stimulating hormone controls later growth of follicles and stimulates estrogen production from follicles
- Luteinizing hormone stimulates theca interna cells to produce androgenic steroid precursors
- Androgenic steroid precursors converted to estrogen by aromatase in granulosa cells
- One follicle becomes dominant, less dependent on follicle-stimulating hormone (FSH) and inhibits further FSH release
- Decreased follicle-stimulating hormone levels induce atresia in other developing follicles
- At midcycle, estrogen levels peak, induce a positive feedback, and cause the surge of luteinizing hormone
- Follicle-stimulating hormone and luteinizing hormone release cause final maturation and ovulation of the dominant, mature follicle
- At ovulation, first meiotic division is completed, and a secondary oocyte is released
- Ovulation site on mature follicle is the thinned cell area called stigma
- Ovulated follicle collapses, is vascularized, and becomes temporary corpus luteum
- Completion of second meiotic division occurs only when oocyte is fertilized by sperm
- Oocyte is viable for about 24 hours before it degenerates if not fertilized
- Interstitial cells in ovary are remnants of theca interna cells after follicular atresia

Corpus Luteum

- Forms after ovulation and liberation of secondary oocyte
- Luteinizing hormone induces hypertrophy and luteinization of granulosa cells and theca interna cells
- Luteinizing hormone causes liberation of estrogen and increased amounts of progesterone
- Without fertilization, it is active for about 12 days before regression
- Regression eventually leads to connective scar tissue corpus albicans

- After regression, inhibitory effects of estrogen and progesterone are removed
- Follicle-stimulating hormone and luteinizing hormone are again released to start a new cycle of ovarian follicular development
- If fertilization occurs, corpus luteum becomes corpus luteum of pregnancy
- Human chorionic gonadotropin produced by trophoblasts stimulates corpus luteum
- Persists during pregnancy until the placenta produces estrogen and progesterone
- The placenta takes over corpus luteum functions and becomes temporary endocrine organ

Uterine Tubes

- Extend from ovaries into the uterus and exhibit four continuous regions
- Infundibulum with fimbriae of the uterine tube located adjacent to the ovary
- Mucosa consists of extensive folds and forms irregular lumen
- Epithelium is simple columnar with ciliated and nonciliated secretory (peg) cells
- Ciliated cells create a current toward uterus and become predominant in proliferative phase
- Secretory cells provide nutrition for oocyte, fertilized ovum, and developing embryo
- Uterine tube secretions maintain sperm and enhance capacitation of sperm
- Smooth muscles provide peristaltic contractions to help capture ovulated oocyte
- Epithelium exhibits changes associated with ovarian cycle
- Sperm binds to zona pellucida, completes capacitation, and triggers acrosome reaction

- Acrosome reaction releases hydrolytic enzymes, and cortical reaction blocks polyspermy

Uterus

- Consists of body, fundus, and cervix
- Wall consists of outer perimetrium, middle myometrium, and inner endometrium
- Endometrium is divided into stratum functionalis and stratum basalis
- During monthly menstrual cycles, stratum functionalis is shed with menstrual flow
- Endometrium morphology responds to estrogen and progesterone and ovarian functions
- Proliferative phase starts at the end of menstrual phase after estrogen release
- Ovarian estrogen induces endometrial growth and formation of a new stratum functionalis
- Secretory phase starts after ovulation and corpus luteum formation
- Estrogen and increased progesterone levels induce uterine gland secretion of nutrients
- Spiral arteries extend and reach the surface of endometrium
- Menstrual phase starts when the ovulated oocyte is not fertilized and no implantation occurs
- Spiral arteries are highly sensitive to declining hormone levels and constrict intermittently
- Ischemia destroys the walls of blood vessels and the stratum functionalis
- Dilation of spiral arteries ruptures walls, detaches functionalis, and causes menstruation
- Stratum basalis remains intact and is not shed during menstruation; blood flow is not interrupted
- Stratum basalis serves as the source of cells for regenerating a new stratum functionalis

SECTION 2 Cervix, Vagina, Placenta, and Mammary Glands

Cervix and Vagina

The cervix is located in the lower part of the uterus that projects into the vaginal canal as the **portio vaginalis**. A narrow **cervical canal** passes through the cervix. The opening of the cervical canal that directly communicates with the uterus is the **internal os** and, with the vagina, the **external os**. Unlike the functionalis layer of the uterine endometrium, the cervical mucosa undergoes only minimal changes during the menstrual cycle and is not shed during menstruation. The cervix contains numerous branched **cervical glands** that exhibit altered secretory activities during the different phases of the menstrual cycle. The amount and type of mucus secreted by the cervical glands change during the menstrual cycle as a result of different levels of ovarian hormones.

The **vagina** is a fibromuscular structure that extends from the cervix to the vestibule of the external genitalia. Its wall has numerous folds and consists of an inner **mucosa**, a middle **muscular layer**, and an outer connective tissue **adventitia**. The vagina does not have any glands in its wall, and its lumen is lined with a **nonkeratinized stratified squamous epithelium**. Mucus produced by cells in the **cervical glands** lubricates the vaginal lumen. Loose fibroelastic connective tissue and a rich vasculature constitute the lamina propria that overlies the smooth muscle layers of the organ. Like the cervical epithelium, the vaginal lining is not shed during the menstrual flow.

Placenta

The **placenta** is a temporary organ that is formed when the developing embryo, now called a **blastocyst**, attaches to and implants in the endometrium of the uterus. The placenta consists of a **fetal portion**, formed by the **chorionic plate** and its **branching chorionic villi**, and a **maternal portion**, formed by the **decidua basalis** of the endometrium. Fetal and maternal blood comes into close proximity in the villi of the placenta. Exchange of nutrients, electrolytes, hormones, antibodies, gaseous products, and waste metabolites takes place as the blood passes over the villi. Fetal blood enters the placenta through a pair of **umbilical arteries**, passes into the villi, and returns through a single **umbilical vein**.

Mammary Glands

The adult mammary gland is a compound **tubuloalveolar gland** that consists of about 20 lobes. All lobes are connected to **lactiferous ducts** that open at the **nipple**. The lobes are separated by connective tissue partitions and adipose tissue.

The resting or inactive mammary glands are small, consist primarily of **ducts**, and do not exhibit any developed or secretory alveoli. Inactive mammary glands also exhibit slight cyclic alterations during the course of the menstrual cycle. Under estrogenic stimulation, the secretory cells increase in height, lumina appear in the ducts, and a small amount of secretory material is accumulated.

 Supplemental micrographic images are available at **www.thePoint.com/Eroschenko12e** under Female Reproductive System.

FIGURE 21.18 | Cervix, Cervical Canal, and Vaginal Fornix (Longitudinal Section)

The cervix is the lower part of the uterus. This figure illustrates a longitudinal section through the cervix, the endocervix or **cervical canal (5)**, a portion of the **vaginal fornix (8)**, and the **vaginal wall (10)**.

The cervical canal (5) is lined with a tall, mucus-secreting columnar **epithelium (2)** that is different from the uterine epithelium, with which it is continuous. The cervical epithelium also lines the highly branched and tubular **cervical glands (3)** that extend at an oblique angle to the cervical canal (5) into the **lamina propria (12)**. Some of the cervical glands may become occluded and develop into small **glandular cysts (4)**. The connective tissue in the lamina propria (12) of the cervix is more fibrous than in the uterus. Blood vessels, nerves, and occasional **lymphatic nodules (11)** may be seen.

The lower end of the cervix, the **os cervix (6)**, bulges into the lumen of the **vaginal canal (13)**. The columnar epithelium (2) of the cervical canal (5) abruptly changes to nonkeratinized stratified squamous **epithelium** to line the vaginal portion of the cervix called the **portio vaginalis (7)** and the external surface of the vaginal fornix (8). At the base of the fornix, the epithelium (7) of the vaginal cervix turns back to become the **vaginal epithelium (9)** of the vaginal wall (10).

The smooth muscles of the **muscularis (1)** extend into the cervix but are not as compact as the muscles in the body of the uterus.

| FUNCTIONAL CORRELATIONS 21.5 | Cervix |

The cervical mucosa does not undergo extensive changes during the menstrual cycle. However, the cervical glands exhibit functional changes during the menstrual cycle that influence sperm passage through the cervical canal. During the **proliferative phase** of the menstrual cycle, the secretion from the cervical glands is thin and watery. This type of secretion in the cervical canal allows for easier passage of sperm from the vagina through the cervix into the uterus. However, during the **secretory (luteal) phase** of the menstrual cycle and increased progesterone secretions, as well as during pregnancy, the cervical gland secretions change and become highly viscous, forming a **mucus plug** in the cervical canal. The mucus plug serves as an important protective measure that hinders the further passage of sperm and microorganisms from the vagina into the body of the uterus. Thus, the cervical glands in the cervical canal perform an important protective function initially in assisting the passage of sperm to fertilize the oocyte and later in protecting the developing embryo in the uterus.

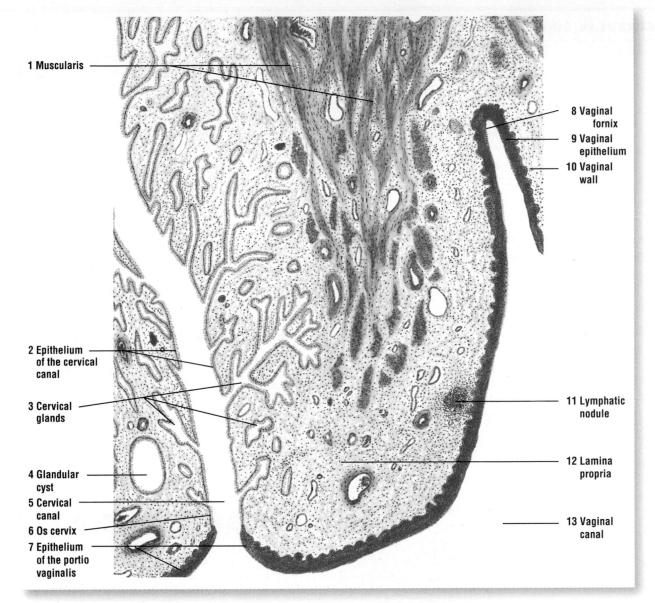

1 Muscularis

8 Vaginal fornix

9 Vaginal epithelium

10 Vaginal wall

2 Epithelium of the cervical canal

3 Cervical glands

4 Glandular cyst

5 Cervical canal

6 Os cervix

7 Epithelium of the portio vaginalis

11 Lymphatic nodule

12 Lamina propria

13 Vaginal canal

FIGURE 21.18 ■ Cervix, cervical canal, and vaginal fornix (longitudinal section). Stain: hematoxylin and eosin. Low magnification.

FIGURE 21.19 | Vagina (Longitudinal Section)

The vaginal mucosa is irregular and shows **mucosal folds (1)**. The surface epithelium of the vaginal canal is noncornified **stratified squamous (2)**. The underlying connective tissue **papillae (3)** are prominent and indent the epithelium.

The **lamina propria (7)** contains dense, irregular connective tissue with elastic fibers that extend into the muscularis layer as **interstitial fibers (10)**. Diffuse **lymphatic tissue (8)**, **lymphatic nodules (4)**, and small **blood vessels (9)** are in the lamina propria (7).

The muscularis of the vaginal wall consists predominantly of **longitudinal bundles (5a)** and oblique bundles of **smooth muscle (5)**. The **transverse bundles (5b)** of the smooth muscle are less numerous but more frequently found in the inner layers. The interstitial connective tissue (10) is rich in elastic fibers. **Blood vessels (11)** and nerve bundles are abundant in the **adventitia (6, 12)**.

FIGURE 21.20 | Glycogen in Human Vaginal Epithelium

Glycogen is a prominent component of the vaginal epithelium, except in the deepest layers, where it is minimal or absent. During the follicular phase of the menstrual cycle, glycogen accumulates in the vaginal epithelium, reaching its maximum level before ovulation. Glycogen can be demonstrated by iodine vapor or iodine solution in mineral oil (Mancini method); glycogen stains a reddish purple.

The vaginal specimens in illustrations (a) and (b) were fixed in absolute alcohol and formaldehyde. The amount of glycogen in the vaginal epithelium is illustrated during the **interfollicular phase (a)**. During the **follicular phase (b)**, glycogen content increases in the intermediate and superficial cell layers.

The tissue sample in illustration (c) is from the same specimen as in (b) but was fixed by the Altmann-Gersh method (freezing and drying in a vacuum). This method produces less tissue shrinkage and illustrates more glycogen and its diffuse distribution in the vaginal epithelium during the **follicular phase (c)**.

FUNCTIONAL CORRELATIONS 21.6 | Vagina

The wall of the vagina consists of the mucosa, a smooth muscle layer, and an adventitia. There are no glands in the vaginal mucosa. The surface of the vaginal canal is kept moist and lubricated by secretions produced by the **cervical glands**.

The vaginal epithelium exhibits minimal changes during each menstrual cycle. During the proliferative (follicular) phase of the menstrual cycle and owing to increased estrogen stimulation, the vaginal epithelium increases in thickness. In addition, estrogen stimulates the vaginal cells to synthesize and accumulate increased amounts of **glycogen** as these cells migrate toward the vaginal lumen, into which they are shed, or desquamated. Bacterial flora in the vagina metabolizes glycogen into **lactic acid**, which increases acidity in the vaginal canal to protect the organ against microorganisms or pathogenic invasion.

Microscopic examination of cells collected (scraped) from the vaginal and cervical mucosae, called a **Pap smear**, provides highly valuable diagnostic information of clinical importance. Cervicovaginal Pap smears are routinely examined for early detection of pathologic changes in the epithelium of these organs that may lead to cervical cancer.

1 Mucosal folds

2 Stratified squamous epithelium

3 Connective tissue papillae

4 Lymphatic nodule

5 Smooth muscles:
   a. Longitudinal bundles

   b. Transverse bundles

6 Adventitia

7 Lamina propria

8 Lymphatic tissue

9 Blood vessels

10 Interstitial connective tissue

11 Blood vessels

12 Adventitia

FIGURE 21.19 ■ Vagina (longitudinal section). Stain: hematoxylin and eosin. Low magnification.

a. Interfollicular phase   b. Follicular phase   c. Follicular phase

FIGURE 21.20 ■ Glycogen in human vaginal epithelium. Stain: Mancini iodine technique. Medium magnification.

FIGURE 21.21 | Vaginal Exfoliate Cytology (Vaginal Smear) During Different Reproductive Phases

Vaginal exfoliate cytology (vaginal smear) is closely correlated with the ovarian cycle. The presence of certain cell types in the smear permits the recognition of the follicular activity during normal menstrual phases or after hormonal therapy. Also, exfoliate cytology together with cells from the endocervix provides a very important source of information for the early detection of cervical or vaginal cancers.

This figure illustrates cells in vaginal smears obtained during different menstrual cycles, early pregnancy, and menopause. A combination of hematoxylin, orange G, and eosin azure facilitates the recognition of different cell types. In most phases, the surface squamous cells show small, dark-staining pyknotic nuclei and an increased amount of cytoplasm.

Figure (**a**) illustrates vaginal cells collected during the **postmenstrual phase** (fifth day of the menstrual cycle). The **intermediate cells (1)** from the intermediate cell layers (precornified superficial vaginal cells) predominate. In addition, a few **superficial acidophilic (2)** cells and leukocytes are present.

Figure (**b**) represents a vaginal smear collected during the **ovulatory phase** (14th day) of the menstrual cycle. There is a scarcity of **intermediate cells (8)** and an absence of leukocytes. The large **superficial acidophilic cells (9)** characterize this phase. This smear characterizes the results of the high estrogenic stimulation normally observed before ovulation. The superficial acidophilic cells (8) mature with increased estrogen levels and become acidophilic. A similar type of smear is seen when a menopausal woman is treated with high doses of estrogen.

Figure (**c**) represents a vaginal smear collected during the **luteal (secretory) phase** and represents the effects of increased levels of progesterone. The large **intermediate cells (3)** with folded borders aggregate into clumps and characterize the smear. **Superficial acidophilic cells (4)** and leukocytes are scarce.

Figure (**d**) represents a vaginal smear taken during the **premenstrual phase**. This stage is characterized by a predominance of grouped **intermediate cells (10)** with folded borders, an increase in the number of the **neutrophils (11)**, a scarcity of the **superficial acidophilic cells (12)**, and an abundance of mucus.

Figure (**e**) illustrates a vaginal smear taken during **early pregnancy**. The cells exhibit dense groups or **conglomerations (5)** of predominantly **intermediate cells (6)** with folded borders. **Superficial acidophilic cells (7)** and neutrophils are scarce.

The vaginal smear collected during menopause in Figure (**f**) is different from all other phases. The **intermediate cells (13)** are scarce, whereas the predominant cells are the oval **basal cells (14)**. Also, **neutrophils (15)** are in abundance. Menopausal smears are variable and depend on the stage of the menopause and the estrogen levels.

FUNCTIONAL CORRELATIONS 21.7	Cellular Characteristics of Vaginal Cytology (Smear)

The superficial **acidophilic cells** of the vaginal epithelium appear flat and irregular in outline, measuring about 35 to 65 μm in diameter; exhibit small pyknotic nuclei; and contain cytoplasm that is stained light red (acidophilic) or orange.

The **intermediate cells** are flat like the superficial cell but are somewhat smaller, measuring 20 to 40 μm in diameter, and show a basophilic blue-green cytoplasm. The nuclei are somewhat larger than those of the superficial cells and are often vesicular. The intermediate cells are also elongated with folded borders and elongated, eccentric nuclei.

The larger **basal cells** are from the basal layers of the vaginal epithelium. All basal cells are oval, measure from 12 to 15 μm in diameter, and exhibit large nuclei with prominent chromatin. Most of these cells exhibit basophilic staining.

1 Intermediate cells

2 Superficial acidophilic cells

a. Postmenstrual phase

8 Intermediate cells

9 Superficial acidophilic cells

b. Ovulatory phase

3 Intermediate cells

4 Superficial acidophilic cells

c. Luteal (secretory) phase

10 Intermediate cells

11 Neutrophils

12 Superficial cell

d. Premenstrual phase

5 Conglomeration

6 Intermediate cells

7 Superficial acidophilic cell

e. Early pregnancy

13 Intermediate cell

14 Basal cells

15 Neutrophils

f. Menopause

FIGURE 21.21 ■ Vaginal exfoliate cytology (vaginal smear) during different reproductive phases. Stain: hematoxylin, orange G, and eosin azure. Medium magnification.

FIGURE 21.22 | Vagina: Surface Epithelium

This higher-magnification photomicrograph illustrates the vaginal epithelium and the underlying connective tissue. The surface epithelium is **stratified squamous nonkeratinized (1)**. Most of the superficial cells in vaginal epithelium appear empty owing to increased accumulation of glycogen in their cytoplasm. During histologic preparation of the organ, the glycogen was extracted by chemicals.

The **lamina propria (2)** contains dense, irregular connective tissue. The lamina propria lacks glands but contains numerous **blood vessels (4)** and **lymphocytes (3)**.

1 Stratified squamous nonkeratinized epithelium

2 Lamina propria

3 Lymphocytes

4 Blood vessels

FIGURE 21.22 ■ Vagina: surface epithelium. Stain: hematoxylin and eosin. ×50.

FIGURE 21.23 | Human Placenta (Panoramic View)

The upper region of the figure illustrates the fetal portion of the placenta, which includes the **chorionic plate (1)** and the **chorionic villi (2, 10, 12, 14)**. The maternal part of the placenta is the **decidua basalis (15)** of the endometrium that lies directly beneath the fetal placenta. The **amniotic surface (8)** is lined with a **simple squamous epithelium (8)**, below which is the **connective tissue (1)** of the chorion (1). Inferior to the connective tissue layer (1) are the **trophoblast cells (9)** of the chorion (1). The trophoblasts (9) and the underlying connective tissue (1) form the chorionic plate (1).

The **anchoring chorionic villi (2, 14)** arise from the chorionic plate (1), extend to the uterine wall, and attach to the **decidua basalis (15)**. Numerous **floating villi (chorion frondo-sum) (3, 10, 12)**, sectioned in various planes, extend in all directions from the anchoring villi (2). These villi "float" in the **intervillous space (11)**, which is bathed in **maternal blood (11)**.

The maternal portion of the placenta, the decidua basalis (15), contains anchoring villi (14), large **decidual cells (5)**, and a typical connective tissue stroma. The decidua basalis (15) also contains the basal portions of the **uterine glands (6)**. The **maternal blood vessels (13)** in the decidua basalis (15) are recognized by their size or by the presence of blood cells in their lumina. A **maternal blood vessel (4)** can be seen opening directly into the intervillous space (11).

A portion of the smooth muscle **myometrium (7)** of the uterine wall is visible in the left corner of the illustration.

1 Chorionic plate with connective tissue

2 Anchoring chorionic villi

3 Chorionic frondosum

4 Maternal blood vessel opening into intervillous space

5 Decidual cells

6 Basal uterine glands

7 Myometrium

8 Epithelium of amniotic surface

9 Trophoblasts

10 Floating chorionic villi

11 Intervillous space with maternal blood

12 Floating chorionic villi

13 Maternal blood vessels

14 Anchoring villi

15 Decidua basalis

FIGURE 21.23 ■ Human placenta (panoramic view). Stain: hematoxylin and eosin. Low magnification.

FIGURE 21.24 | Chorionic Villi: Placenta During Early Pregnancy

The **chorionic villi (6)** from a placenta during early pregnancy are illustrated at a higher magnification. The trophoblast cells of the embryo give rise to the embryonic portion of the placenta. The chorionic villi (6) arise from the chorionic plate and become surrounded by the trophoblast epithelium that consists of an outer layer of the darker-staining **syncytiotrophoblasts (1, 10)** and an inner layer of lighter-staining **cytotrophoblasts (2, 9)**.

The core of each chorionic villus (6) contains mesenchyme, or embryonic connective tissue, and contains two cell types, the fusiform **mesenchyme cells (8)** and the darker-staining **macrophage (Hofbauer cell) (4)**. The **fetal blood vessels (3, 7)**, branches of the umbilical arteries and veins, are located in the core of the chorionic villi (6) and contain fetal nucleated erythroblasts, although nonnucleated cells can also be seen. The **intervillous space (11)** is bathed by **maternal blood cells (5)** and nonnucleated erythrocytes.

FIGURE 21.25 | Chorionic Villi: Placenta at Term

The chorionic villi are illustrated from a placenta at term. In contrast to the chorionic villi in the placenta during pregnancy, the chorionic epithelium in the placenta at term is reduced to only a thin layer of **syncytiotrophoblasts (1)**. The connective tissue in the villi is differentiated with more fibers and **fibroblasts (4)** and contains large, round **macrophages (Hofbauer cells) (5)**. The villi also contain mature blood cells in the **fetal blood vessels (2)** that have increased in complexity during pregnancy. The **intervillous space (6)** is surrounded by **maternal blood cells (3)**.

FUNCTIONAL CORRELATIONS 21.8 | Placenta

The placenta is an organ that performs an important function in regulating the **exchange** of different substances between the maternal and fetal circulation during pregnancy. One side of the placenta is attached to the uterine wall, and on the other side, it is attached to the fetus via the umbilical cord. Maternal blood enters the placenta through blood vessels located in the endometrium and is directed to the **intervillous spaces**, where it continually bathes the surface of the **chorionic villi**, which contain vessels through which flows the fetal blood. Chorionic villi are separated from the intervillous space by double layers of trophoblast cells (syncytiotrophoblasts and cytotrophoblasts) that surround the chorionic villi. These structures form the **placental barrier**. In the intervillous space, metabolic waste products, carbon dioxide, hormones, and water are passed from the fetal circulation to the maternal circulation. Oxygen, nutrients, vitamins, electrolytes, hormones, immunoglobulins (antibodies), metabolites, and other substances pass in the opposite direction. Maternal blood leaves the intervillous spaces through the endometrial veins. The maternal and fetal blood does not mix, and the placental barrier ensures this separation.

The placenta also serves as a temporary—yet major—**endocrine organ** that produces numerous essential hormones for the maintenance of pregnancy. **Placental cells (syncytial trophoblasts)** secrete the hormone **human chorionic gonadotropin (HCG)** shortly after the implantation of the fertilized ovum. In humans, HCG appears in urine within 10 days of pregnancy, and its presence can be used to determine **pregnancy** with commercial kits. HCG is similar to luteinizing hormone in structure and function, and it maintains the **corpus luteum** in the maternal ovary during the early stages of pregnancy. HCG also stimulates the corpus luteum to continue to produce estrogen and progesterone, the two hormones that are essential for maintaining pregnancy. The placenta also secretes **chorionic somatomammotropin**, a glycoprotein hormone that exhibits both **lactogenic** (mammary gland stimulation) and general **growth-promoting** functions.

As pregnancy proceeds, the placenta gradually takes over the production of estrogen and progesterone from the corpus luteum and produces sufficient amounts of progesterone to maintain the pregnancy until birth. The placenta also produces

FUNCTIONAL CORRELATIONS 21.8 | Placenta *(Continued)*

relaxin, a hormone that softens the cervix and the fibrocartilage in the pubic symphysis to widen the pelvic canal for impending birth. In some mammals, the placenta also secretes **placental lactogen**, a hormone that promotes growth and development of the maternal mammary glands.

1 Syncytiotrophoblasts
2 Cytotrophoblasts
3 Fetal blood vessels
4 Macrophage (Hofbauer cell)
5 Maternal blood cells
6 Chorionic villi
7 Fetal blood vessel
8 Mesenchymal cells
9 Cytotrophoblasts
10 Syncytiotrophoblasts
11 Intervillous space

FIGURE 21.24 ■ Chorionic villi: placenta during early pregnancy. Stain: hematoxylin and eosin. High magnification.

1 Syncytiotrophoblasts
2 Fetal blood vessels
3 Maternal blood cells
4 Fibroblasts
5 Macrophages (Hofbauer cells)
6 Intevillous space

FIGURE 21.25 ■ Chorionic villi: placenta at term. Stain: hematoxylin and eosin. High magnification.

FIGURE 21.26 | Inactive Mammary Gland

The inactive mammary gland is characterized by an abundance of connective tissue and by a scarcity of the glandular elements. Some cyclic changes in the mammary gland may be seen during the menstrual cycles.

A glandular **lobule (1)** consists of small tubules or **intralobular ducts (4, 7)** lined with a cuboidal or a low columnar epithelium. At the base of the epithelium are the contractile **myoepithelial cells (6)**. The larger **interlobular ducts (5)** surround the lobules (1) and the intralobular ducts (4, 7).

The intralobular ducts (4, 7) are surrounded by loose **intralobular connective tissue (3, 8)** that contains fibroblasts, lymphocytes, plasma cells, and eosinophils. Surrounding the lobules (1) is a dense **interlobular connective tissue (2, 10)** containing blood vessels, a **venule and arteriole (9)**.

The mammary gland consists of 15 to 25 lobes, each of which is an individual compound tubuloalveolar type of gland. Each lobe is separated by dense interlobar connective tissue. A lactiferous duct independently emerges from each lobe at the surface of the nipple.

FIGURE 21.27 | Mammary Gland: Micrograph of Inactive Mammary Gland

An inactive, or immature, mammary gland consists primarily of undeveloped glandular ducts and dense irregular connective tissue. The **interlobular connective tissue (4)** is located between the glandular **lobules (3)** and the **intralobular connective tissue (7)** between the **intralobular ducts (1)**. A larger **interlobular duct (6)** is located outside the lobules (3). Surrounding the intralobular (1) and interlobular (6) ducts are the contractile **myoepithelial cells (2, 5)**.

1 Lobule

2 Interlobular
connective tissue

3 Intralobular
connective tissue

4 Intralobular ducts

5 Interlobular ducts

6 Myoepithelial cells

7 Intralobular ducts

8 Intralobular
connective tissue

9 Venule and arteriole

10 Interlobular
connective tissue

FIGURE 21.26 ■ Inactive mammary gland. Stain: hematoxylin and eosin. Left side, medium magnification; right side, high magnification.

1 Intralobular ducts

2 Myoepithelial cell

3 Lobule

4 Interlobular
connective tissue

5 Myoepithelial cell

6 Interlobular duct

7 Intralobular
connective tissue

FIGURE 21.27 ■ Mammary gland: micrograph of inactive mammary gland. Stain: hematoxylin and eosin. ×102.

FIGURE 21.28 | Mammary Gland During Proliferation and Early Pregnancy

In preparation for milk secretion (lactation), the mammary gland undergoes extensive structural changes. During the first half of the pregnancy, the intralobular ducts undergo rapid proliferation and form terminal buds that differentiate into **alveoli (2, 7)**. At this stage, most of the alveoli are empty, and it is difficult to distinguish between the small **intralobular excretory ducts (10)** and the alveoli (2, 7). The intralobular excretory ducts (10) appear more regular with a more distinct epithelial lining. The intralobular excretory ducts (10) and the alveoli (2, 7) are lined with two layers of cells, the luminal epithelium and a basal layer of flattened **myoepithelial cells (8)**.

A loose **intralobular connective tissue (1, 9)** surrounds the alveoli (2, 7) and the ducts (10); a denser connective tissue with **adipose cells (6)** surrounds the individual lobules and forms **interlobular connective tissue septa (3)**. The **interlobular excretory ducts (4, 11)**, lined with taller columnar cells, course in the interlobular connective tissue septa (3) to join the larger **lactiferous duct (5)** that is usually lined with a low pseudostratified columnar epithelium. Each lactiferous duct (5) collects the secretory product from the lobe and transports it to the nipple.

FIGURE 21.29 | Mammary Gland During Activation and Early Development

The activated mammary gland exhibits well-developed secretory **alveoli (3)** and branching **intralobular ducts (6)**. Both the alveoli (3) and the intralobular ducts (6) are lined with a simple cuboidal epithelium and contain secretory products. Surrounding both the alveoli (3) and the intralobular ducts (6) are **myoepithelial cells (7)**. Located between the alveoli (3) and the intralobular ducts (6) are small **blood vessels (5)**. Individual glandular lobules are separated by narrow and dense **connective tissue septa (4)**, whereas the **interlobular connective tissue (1)** and the **intralobular connective tissue (2)** are thinner and less dense.

1 Intralobular connective tissue

2 Alveoli

3 Interlobular connective tissue septa

4 Interlobular excretory ducts

5 Lactiferous duct

6 Adipose cells

7 Alveoli

8 Myoepithelial cells

9 Intralobular connective tissue

10 Intralobular excretory ducts

11 Interlobular excretory duct

FIGURE 21.28 ■ Mammary gland during proliferation and early pregnancy. Stain: hematoxylin and eosin. Left side, medium magnification; right side, high magnification.

1 Interlobular connective tissue

2 Intralobular connective tissue

3 Alveoli

4 Connective tissue septa

5 Blood vessels

6 Intralobular excretory duct

7 Myoepithelial cells

FIGURE 21.29 ■ Mammary gland during activation and early development. Stain: hematoxylin and eosin. ×85.

FIGURE 21.30 | Mammary Gland During Late Pregnancy

A small section of a mammary gland with lobules, connective tissue, and excretory ducts is illustrated at lower *(left)* and higher *(right)* magnification. During pregnancy, the glandular epithelium is prepared for lactation. The alveolar cells become secretory, and the **alveoli (2, 8)** and the **ducts (1, 7, 13)** enlarge. Some of the alveoli (2) contain a secretory product (2, upper leader). However, the secretion of milk by the mammary gland does not begin until after parturition (birth). Because the **intralobular excretory ducts** (1) of the mammary gland also contain secretory material, the distinction between alveoli and ducts is difficult.

As pregnancy progresses, the amount of **intralobular connective tissue (4, 11)** decreases, while the amount of **interlobular connective tissue (3, 9)** increases because of the enlargement of the glandular tissue. Surrounding the alveoli are flattened **myoepithelial cells (10, 12)**, which are more visible in the higher magnification on the right. Located in the interlobular connective tissue (3, 9) are the **interlobular excretory ducts (7, 13), lactiferous ducts (14)** with secretory product in their lumina, various types of **blood vessels (5)**, and **adipose cells (6)**.

FIGURE 21.31 | Mammary Gland During Lactation

This illustration of a mammary gland shows in greater detail the structure of individual alveoli during lactation at both lower *(left)* and higher *(right)* magnification.

A lactating mammary gland exhibits a large number of distended **alveoli** filled with **secretions** and **vacuoles (1, 5, 9)**. Some of the alveoli (1) show irregular **branching (1)**. Because of the increased size of the glandular epithelium (alveoli) and increased presence of **adipose cells (10)**, the **interlobular connective tissue (3, 7)** is reduced when compared to the morphology of the inactive gland (Figs. 21.26 and 21.27)

During lactation, the histology of individual alveoli varies. Not all of the alveoli exhibit secretory activity. The active alveoli (1, 5, 9) are lined with a low epithelium and filled with milk that appears as eosinophilic (pink) material with large vacuoles of dissolved fat droplets (1, 5, 9). Some alveoli accumulate secretory product in their cytoplasm, and their apices appear vacuolated, or light staining, because of the removal of fat during tissue preparation. Other alveoli in the lactating mammary gland can appear **inactive (4)** with empty lumina lined with a taller epithelium.

Surrounding the alveoli in the mammary gland are the **myoepithelial cells (8)** that are present between the alveolar cells and the basal lamina. When the plane of section passes at just the right level, the myoepithelial cells (8, upper leader) can be seen surrounding the secretory alveoli in a basketlike fashion. When the myoepithelial cells contract around the alveoli, the milk is expelled into the **interlobular excretory ducts (2, 6)** that are embedded in the connective tissue septa that also contain numerous adipose cells (10).

1 Intralobular duct
2 Alveoli
3 Interlobular connective tissue
4 Intralobular connective tissue
5 Blood vessels
6 Adipose cells

7 Interlobular excretory duct
8 Alveolus
9 Interlobular connective tissue
10 Myoepithelial cell
11 Intralobular connective tissue
12 Myoepithelial cell
13 Interlobular excretory ducts
14 Lactiferous duct

FIGURE 21.30 ■ Mammary gland during late pregnancy Stain: hematoxylin and eosin. Left side, medium magnification; right side, high magnification.

1 Branching alveoli
2 Interlobular excretory duct
3 Interlobular connective tissue
4 Inactive alveoli
5 Active alveoli with secretions

6 Interlobuar excretory duct
7 Interlobular connective tissue
8 Myoepithelial cells
9 Active alveoli
10 Adipose cells

FIGURE 21.31 ■ Mammary gland during lactation. Stain: hematoxylin and eosin. Left side, medium magnification; right side, high magnification.

FIGURE 21.32 | Lactating Mammary Gland

This photomicrograph illustrates a lobule of a lactating mammary gland that is separated from the adjacent lactating lobule by a thin layer of **connective tissue (5)**. The lactating mammary gland contains **alveoli (2, 3)** with the **secretory product (6)** (milk) and separated by thin connective tissue septa (5). Some of the alveoli (3) are single, whereas others are branching alveoli (2). All the alveoli eventually drain into larger excretory ducts that deliver the milk to the lactiferous ducts in the nipple. The mammary glands contain large amounts of **adipose tissue (1, 4)** during lactation.

FUNCTIONAL CORRELATIONS 21.9 | Mammary Glands

Before puberty, the mammary glands are undeveloped and consist primarily of branched **interlobular ducts** that open at the nipple. In males, the mammary glands remain undeveloped. In females, mammary glands enlarge during puberty because of stimulation by estrogen and progesterone during menstrual cycles. As a result, adipose tissue and connective tissue accumulate and grow. Also, branching of the ducts in the mammary glands increases, and numerous secretory alveoli are formed.

The mammary glands remain inactive until pregnancy. During pregnancy, the mammary glands undergo increased growth owing to the continuous and prolonged stimulatory actions of estrogen and progesterone. As a result, the mammary glands become structurally and functionally mature. Estrogen and progesterone hormones are initially produced by the corpus luteum of the ovary and later by cells in the placenta. In addition, further growth of the mammary glands depends on the pituitary hormone **prolactin, placental lactogen**, and **adrenal corticoids**. These hormones stimulate the intralobular ducts of the mammary glands to rapidly proliferate, branch, and form numerous **alveoli**. The alveoli then undergo hypertrophy and become active sites of **milk production** during the lactation period. All alveoli become surrounded by contractile **myoepithelial cells**.

When the individual is born (parturition) and pregnancy ends, the mammary gland alveoli initially produce a fluid called **colostrum** that is rich in proteins, vitamins, minerals, and antibodies (IgA), which provide the newborn with some immunity. Unlike milk, however, colostrum contains little lipid. Milk is not produced until a few days after parturition. The hormones estrogen and progesterone from the corpus luteum and placenta suppress milk production by mammary alveoli until their levels decrease.

After parturition and elimination of the placenta, the hormones that inhibited milk secretion (estrogen and progesterone) are eliminated, and the mammary glands begin active secretion of milk. As the pituitary hormone **prolactin** activates milk secretion, the production of colostrum ceases. During nursing of the newborn, tactile stimulation of the nipple by the suckling infant promotes further release of prolactin and prolonged milk production.

In addition, tactile stimulation of the nipple by the infant initiates the **milk ejection reflex** that causes the release of the hormone **oxytocin** from the neurohypophysis of the pituitary gland. Oxytocin causes the contraction of myoepithelial cells around the secretory alveoli and excretory ducts in the mammary glands, resulting in milk ejection from the mammary glands toward the nipple.

Decreased nursing and suckling by the infant soon results in the cessation of milk production and eventual regression of the mammary glands to an inactive state.

1 Adipose tissue

2 Branching alveoli

3 Secretory alveoli

4 Adipose tissue

5 Connective tissue

6 Secretory product

FIGURE 21.32 ■ Lactating mammary gland. Stain: hematoxylin and eosin. ×75.

SECTION 2 • Cervix, Vagina, Placenta, and Mammary Glands

Cervix

- Located between uterus and vagina, with cervical canal passing into uterus
- Undergoes minimal change during menstrual cycle
- Cervical glands exhibit altered secretory activities, depending on menstrual cycle
- During proliferative phase, secretion is watery to allow sperm passage into uterus
- During secretory phase, secretion is viscous, forms a plug, and protects uterus

Vagina

- Extends from cervix to external genitalia
- Does not have glands, is lined with stratified epithelium, and is lubricated by cervical glands
- Epithelium thickens after estrogenic stimulation but is not shed during menstrual cycles
- Glycogen accumulates during proliferative phase and, after metabolism, becomes acidic
- Vaginal exfoliate cytology (vaginal smear) is closely correlated with the ovarian cycle
- Follicular activity can be determined by predominant cell type in the smear
- Smears of surface epithelium are highly valuable for detecting cervical or vaginal cancers

Placenta

- The fetal portion includes the chorionic plate and its villi
- Maternal part includes the decidua basalis layer of endometrium
- Anchoring villi arise from chorionic plate and attach to decidua basalis
- Maternal blood enters intervillous space to bathe villi that contain fetal blood
- Regulates exchange of vital substances between maternal and fetal circulations
- Cells secrete the hormone human chorionic gonadotropin shortly after pregnancy
- Human chorionic gonadotropin appears in urine and is used for pregnancy tests
- Human chorionic gonadotropin stimulates corpus luteum to secrete estrogen and progesterone and other substances
- Takes over function of corpus luteum until birth

Mammary Glands

- Before puberty, they consist primarily of lactiferous ducts that open at the nipple
- Inactive glands contain connective tissue and ducts, surrounded by myoepithelial cells
- Estrogen and progesterone induce growth in females, forming tubuloalveolar glands
- Development also depends on prolactin, placental lactogen, and adrenal corticoids
- During pregnancy, ducts branch, enlarge, and form terminal buds with alveoli
- Late in pregnancy, alveoli contain some secretory products, but not milk
- At the end of pregnancy, alveolar secretion is colostrum, rich in proteins and antibodies
- During lactation, some alveoli are distended with secretory material containing more fat
- After placenta eliminated, prolactin activates milk secretion
- Suckling of nipple releases oxytocin, causing myoepithelial contraction and milk release

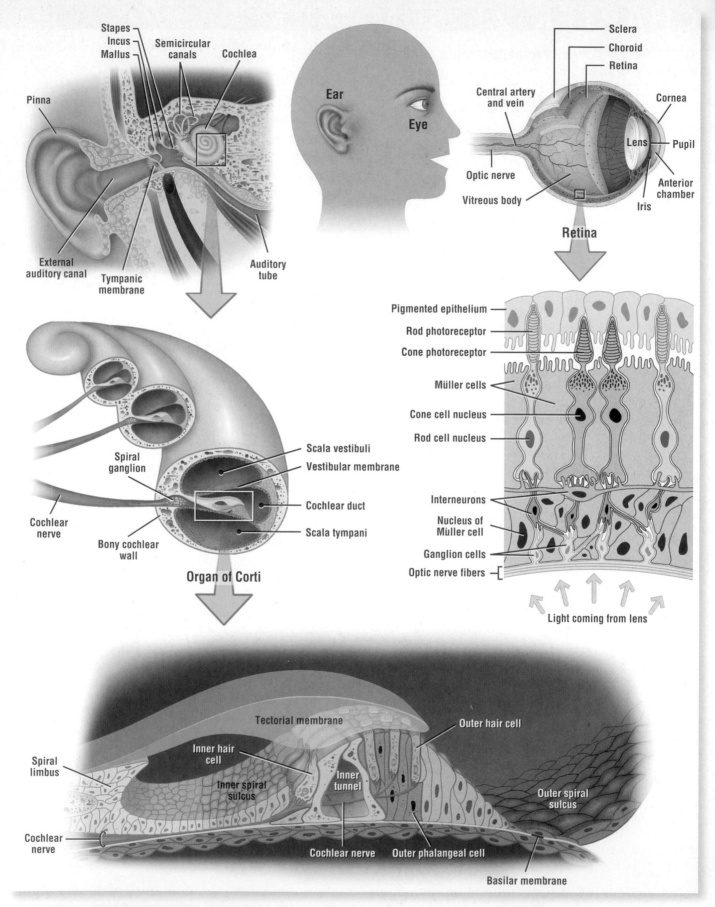

Ear

Eye

Stapes
Incus
Mallus
Semicircular canals
Cochlea
Pinna
External auditory canal
Tympanic membrane
Auditory tube

Sclera
Choroid
Retina
Central artery and vein
Cornea
Lens
Pupil
Optic nerve
Anterior chamber
Vitreous body
Iris

Retina

Spiral ganglion
Scala vestibuli
Vestibular membrane
Cochlear nerve
Cochlear duct
Bony cochlear wall
Scala tympani

Organ of Corti

Pigmented epithelium
Rod photoreceptor
Cone photoreceptor
Müller cells
Cone cell nucleus
Rod cell nucleus
Interneurons
Nucleus of Müller cell
Ganglion cells
Optic nerve fibers

Light coming from lens

Tectorial membrane
Outer hair cell
Spiral limbus
Inner hair cell
Inner spiral sulcus
Inner tunnel
Outer spiral sulcus
Cochlear nerve
Cochlear nerve
Outer phalangeal cell
Basilar membrane

OVERVIEW FIGURE 22.1 ■ The internal structures of the eye and the ear are illustrated, with emphasis on the cells that constitute the photosensitive retina and the hearing organ of Corti.

CHAPTER 22

Organs of Special Senses: Visual and Auditory Systems

SECTION 1 Visual System

In the visual system, the eye is a highly specialized organ for perception of form, light, and color. The eyes are located in protective cavities within the skull, called **orbits**. Each eye contains a protective cover to maintain its shape, a lens for focusing, photosensitive cells that respond to light stimuli, and numerous cells that process visual information. The visual impulses from the photosensitive cells are then conveyed to the brain via the axons that leave the eye in the **optic nerve**.

Layers in the Eye

Each eyeball is surrounded by three distinct layers. The outer fibrous layer consists of cornea and sclera, in the middle is the vascular layer, and the inner layer is the sensory retina.

Cornea and Sclera

On the anterior sixth of the eyeball, the fibrous **sclera** is modified into a transparent **cornea**, through which light rays enter the eye. The posterior five sixths of the sclera is an opaque outer layer of dense connective tissue that extends from the cornea to the optic nerve. The inner layer of the sclera is located adjacent to the **choroid**, which contains different types of connective tissue fibers and connective tissue cells, including macrophages and melanocytes.

Vascular Layer (Uvea)

Internal to the sclera is the middle or vascular layer (**uvea**). This layer consists of three parts: a densely pigmented layer called the **choroid**, a **ciliary body**, and an **iris**. Choroid is the highly pigmented dark brown layer with melanocytes that is located between the sclera and the light-sensitive retina. Located in the choroid are numerous blood vessels that nourish the photoreceptor cells in the retina and structures of the eyeball.

Retina

The innermost lining of the posterior chamber of the eye is the **retina** that is in contact with the highly vascular choroid. The posterior three quarters of the retina is a **photosensitive** region. It consists of **rods, cones**, and various **interneurons**—cells that are stimulated by and respond to light. The photosensitive part of the retina terminates in the anterior region of the eye, called the **ora serrata**. This **nonphotosensitive** part of the retina continues forward in the eye to line the inner part of the ciliary body and the posterior region of the iris.

Chambers in the Eye

The eye also contains three chambers.

- The **anterior chamber** is a space located between the cornea, iris, and lens.
- The **posterior chamber** is a small space situated between the iris, ciliary process, zonular fibers, and lens. The zonular fibers radiate from the ciliary process and insert into the lens capsule. This forms the suspensory ligaments of the lens that anchor it in the eyeball.
- The **vitreous chamber** is a larger, posterior space that is situated behind the lens and zonular fibers and is surrounded by the retina.

Chamber Contents: Aqueous Humor and Vitreous Body

The anterior and posterior chambers of the eye are filled with a clear, watery fluid called the **aqueous humor**. This fluid is continually produced by the epithelial cells of the **ciliary process** located behind the iris in the posterior chamber. Aqueous humor circulates from the posterior chamber to the anterior chamber, where it is drained by veins.

The large vitreous chamber is filled with a transparent gelatinous substance called the **vitreous body**. The contents of the vitreous body are primarily water with some soluble proteins. The fluid component of the vitreous body is called the **vitreous humor**.

Photosensitive Parts of the Eye

The photosensitive retina contains numerous cell types organized into numerous and distinct cell layers. The layer that is sensitive to light contains cells called **rods** and **cones**. These cells are stimulated by light rays that pass through the lens. Leaving the retina are **afferent** (sensory) **axons** (nerve fibers) that conduct light impulses from the retina via the **optic nerve** to the brain for visual interpretation.

The posterior region of the eye also contains a yellowish pigmented spot called the **macula lutea**. In the center of the macula lutea is a depression called the **fovea**. The fovea is devoid of photoreceptive rods and blood vessels. Instead, the fovea contains a dense concentration of photosensitive cones (Overview Fig. 22.1).

 Supplemental micrographic images are available at **www.thePoint.com/Eroschenko12e** under Organs of the Special Senses.

FIGURE 22.1 | Eyelid (Sagittal Section)

The exterior layer of the eyelid is composed of thin skin (left side). The **epidermis (4)** consists of stratified squamous epithelium with papillae. In the **dermis (6)** are **hair follicles (1, 3)** with associated **sebaceous glands (3)** and **sweat glands (5)**.

The interior layer of the eyelid is a mucous membrane called the **palpebral conjunctiva (15)**. It lies adjacent to the eyeball. The lining epithelium of the palpebral conjunctiva (15) is low stratified columnar with a few goblet cells. The stratified squamous epithelium (4) of the thin skin continues over the margin of the eyelid and then merges into the stratified columnar of the palpebral conjunctiva (15).

The thin lamina propria of the palpebral conjunctiva (15) contains both elastic and collagen fibers. Beneath the lamina propria is a plate of dense, collagenous connective tissue called the **tarsus (16)** in which are found large, specialized sebaceous glands called the **tarsal (meibomian) glands (17)**. The secretory acini of the tarsal glands (17) open into a **central duct (19)** that runs parallel to the palpebral conjunctiva (15) and opens at the margin of the eyelid.

The free end of the eyelid contains **eyelashes (10)** that arise from large, long **hair follicles (9)**. Associated with the eyelashes (10) are small **sebaceous glands (11)**. Between the hair follicles (9) of the eyelashes (10) are large **sweat glands (of Moll) (18)**.

The eyelid contains three sets of muscles: the palpebral portion of the skeletal muscle, called the **orbicularis oculi (8)**; the skeletal **ciliary muscle (of Riolan) (20)** in the region of the hair follicles (9), the eyelashes (10), and the tarsal glands (17); and smooth muscle called the **superior tarsal muscle (of Müller) (12)** in the upper eyelid.

The connective **tissue (7)** of the eyelid contains **adipose cells (2), blood vessels (14)**, and **lymphatic tissue (13)**.

1 Hair follicle

2 Adipose cells

3 Sebaceous gland
(of hair follicle)

4 Epidermis

5 Sweat glands

6 Dermis

7 Connective tissue

8 Orbicularis oculi

9 Hair follicle (of eyelash)

10 Eyelashes

11 Sebaceous gland (of eyelash)

12 Superior tarsal
muscle (of Müller)

13 Lymphatic tissue

14 Blood vessels

15 Palpebral conjunctiva

16 Tarsus

17 Tarsal (meibomian) glands

18 Sweat glands (of Moll)

19 Central duct (of tarsal glands)

20 Ciliary muscle (of Riolan)

FIGURE 22.1 ■ Eyelid (sagittal section). Stain: hematoxylin and eosin. Low magnification.

FIGURE 22.2 | Lacrimal Gland

The lacrimal gland consists of several lobes that are separated into discrete lobules by the **connective tissue (2)** septa that contain **nerves (4), adipose cells (6),** and **blood vessels (9).** The lacrimal gland is a serous compound gland that resembles the salivary glands in lobular structure and **tubuloalveolar acini (8)** that vary in size and shape. The well-developed **myoepithelial cells (1, 5)** surround the individual secretory acini (8) of the gland.

A small **intralobular excretory duct (7),** lined with a simple cuboidal or columnar epithelium, is located between the tubuloalveolar acini (8). The larger **interlobular excretory duct (3)** is lined with two layers of low columnar cells, or pseudostratified epithelium.

FIGURE 22.3 | Cornea (Transverse Section)

The cornea is a thick, transparent, nonvascular structure of the eye. The anterior surface of the cornea is covered with a **stratified squamous corneal epithelium (1)** that is nonkeratinized and consists of five or more cell layers. The basal cell layer is columnar and rests on a thin basement membrane that is supported by a thick, homogeneous **anterior limiting (Bowman) membrane (4).** The underlying **corneal stroma (substantia propria) (2)** forms the body of the cornea. It consists of parallel bundles of **collagen fibers (5)** and layers of flat **fibroblasts (6).**

The **posterior limiting (Descemet) membrane (7)** is a thick basement membrane that is located at the posterior portion of the corneal stroma (2). The posterior surface of the cornea that faces the anterior chamber of the eye is covered with a simple squamous epithelium called the **posterior epithelium (3),** which is also the corneal endothelium.

1 Myoepithelial cells

2 Connective tissue septa

3 Interlobular excretory duct

4 Nerve

5 Myoepithelial cells

6 Adipose cells

7 Intralobular excretory duct

8 Tubuloalveolar acini

9 Blood vessels

FIGURE 22.2 ■ Lacrimal gland. Stain: hematoxylin and eosin. Medium magnification.

1 Stratified squamous corneal epithelium

2 Corneal stroma (substantia propria)

3 Posterior epithelium

4 Anterior limiting (Bowman) membrane

5 Collagen fibers

6 Fibroblasts

7 Posterior limiting (Descemet) membrane

FIGURE 22.3 ■ Cornea (transverse section). Stain: hematoxylin and eosin. Medium magnification.

FIGURE 22.4 | Whole Eye (Sagittal Section)

The eyeball is surrounded by three major concentric layers: an outer, tough fibrous connective tissue layer composed of the **sclera (18)** and **cornea (1)**; a middle layer or uvea composed of the highly vascular, pigmented **choroid (7)**, the **ciliary body (consisting of ciliary processes and ciliary muscle) (4, 14, 15)**, and the **iris (13)**; and the innermost layer composed of the photosensitive **retina (8)**.

The sclera (18) is a white, opaque, tough connective tissue layer composed of densely woven collagen fibers. The sclera (18) maintains the rigidity of the eyeball and appears as the "white" of the eye. The junction between the cornea and sclera occurs at the transition area called the **limbus (12)**, located in the anterior region of the eye. In the posterior region of the eye, where the **optic nerve (10)** emerges from the ocular capsule, is the transition site between the sclera (18) of the eyeball and the connective tissue **dura mater (23)** of the central nervous system.

The choroid (7) and the ciliary body (4, 14, 15) are adjacent to the sclera (18). In a sagittal section of the eyeball, the ciliary body (4, 14, 15) appears triangular in shape and is composed of the smooth **ciliary muscle (14)** and the **ciliary processes (4, 15)**. The fibers in the ciliary muscle (14) exhibit longitudinal, circular, and radial arrangements. The folded and highly vascular extensions of the ciliary body constitute the ciliary processes (4, 15) that attach to the equator of the **lens (16)** by the suspensory ligament or **zonular fibers (5)** of the lens. Contraction of the ciliary muscle (14) reduces the tension on the zonular fibers (5) and allows the lens (16) to assume a convex shape.

The **iris (13)** partially covers the lens and is the colored portion of the eye. The circular and radial smooth muscle fibers form an opening in the iris called the **pupil (11)**.

The interior portion of the eye in front of the lens is subdivided into two compartments: the **anterior chamber (2)** located between the iris (13) and the cornea (1) and the **posterior chamber (3)** located between the iris (13) and the lens (16). Both the anterior (2) and posterior (3) chambers are filled with a watery fluid called the aqueous humor. The large posterior compartment in the eyeball located behind the lens is the **vitreous body (19)**. It is filled with a gelatinous material, the transparent vitreous humor.

Behind the ciliary body (4, 14, 15) is the **ora serrata (6, 17)**, the sharp, anteriormost boundary of the photosensitive portion of the retina (8). The retina (8) consists of numerous cell layers, one of which contains the light-sensitive cells—the rods and cones. Anterior to the ora serrata (6, 17) lies the nonphotosensitive portion of the retina that continues forward in the eyeball to form the inner lining of the ciliary body (4, 14, 15) and posterior part of the iris (13). The histology of the retina is presented in greater detail in Figures 22.6 and 22.7.

In the posterior wall of the eye is the **macula lutea (20)** and the **optic papilla (9)** or the optic disk. The macula lutea (20) is a small, yellow-pigmented spot, as seen through an ophthalmoscope, with a shallow central depression called the **fovea (20)**. The fovea (20) is the area of greatest visual acuity in the eye. The center of the fovea (20) is devoid of rod cells and blood vessels. Instead, the fovea contains a high concentration of cone cells.

The optic papilla (9) is the region where the **optic nerve (10)** leaves the eyeball. The optic papilla (9) lacks the light-sensitive rods and the cones and constitutes the "blind spot" of the eye.

The outer sclera (18) is adjacent to the orbital tissue and contains loose connective tissue, **adipose cells (21)** of the orbital fatty tissue, nerve fibers, **blood vessels (22)**, lymphatics, and glands.

FIGURE 22.5 | Posterior Eyeball: Sclera, Choroid, Optic Papilla, Optic Nerve, Retina, and Fovea (Panoramic View)

This higher-magnification illustration shows a section of the retina in the posterior region of the eyeball. Visible here are the pigmented **choroid (7)** with its numerous blood vessels and the connective tissue layer **sclera (8)**. A distinct shallow depression in the retina represents the **fovea (5)**, which primarily consists of the light-sensitive **cones (6)**. In the rest of the retina are visible the **rods** and **cones (3)**, the different cell and fiber layers of the retina, and **fibers** of the **optic nerve (1)**. The optic nerve fibers (1) converge in the posterior region of the eyeball to form the **optic papilla (2)** and the **optic nerve (4)**, which exits the eyeball.

The specific cell and fiber layers that constitute the rest of the photosensitive retina are illustrated and described at a higher magnification in Figures 22.6 and 22.7.

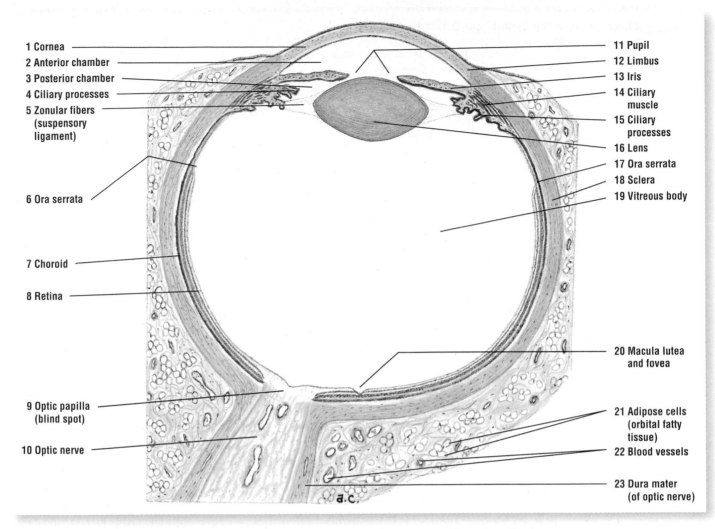

1 Cornea
2 Anterior chamber
3 Posterior chamber
4 Ciliary processes
5 Zonular fibers (suspensory ligament)
6 Ora serrata
7 Choroid
8 Retina
9 Optic papilla (blind spot)
10 Optic nerve

11 Pupil
12 Limbus
13 Iris
14 Ciliary muscle
15 Ciliary processes
16 Lens
17 Ora serrata
18 Sclera
19 Vitreous body
20 Macula lutea and fovea
21 Adipose cells (orbital fatty tissue)
22 Blood vessels
23 Dura mater (of optic nerve)

FIGURE 22.4 ■ Whole eye (sagittal section). Stain: hematoxylin and eosin. Low magnification.

1 Fibers of the optic nerve
2 Optic papilla
3 Rods and cones
4 Optic nerve

5 Fovea
6 Cones
7 Choriod
8 Sclera

FIGURE 22.5 ■ Posterior eyeball: sclera, choroid, optic papilla, optic nerve, retina, and fovea (panoramic view). Stain: hematoxylin and eosin. Medium magnification.

FIGURE 22.6 | Layers of the Choroid and Retina (Detail)

The inner layer of the connective tissue **sclera (10)** is located adjacent to the choroid. The choroid is subdivided into several layers: the **suprachoroid lamina with melanocytes (11)**, the **vascular layer (1)**, the **choriocapillaris layer (12)**, and the transparent limiting membrane or glassy (Bruch) membrane.

The suprachoroid lamina (11) consists of fine collagen fibers, a network of elastic fibers, fibroblasts, and numerous melanocytes. The vascular layer (1) of the choroid contains medium-sized and large **blood vessels (1)**. In the loose connective tissue between the blood vessels (1) are large, flat **melanocytes (2)** that impart a dark color to this layer. The choriocapillaris layer (11) contains a network of capillaries with large lumina. The innermost layer of the choroid, the glassy (Bruch) membrane, lies adjacent to the **pigment epithelium cells (3)** of the retina and separates the choroid and retina (see Fig. 22.7).

The outermost layer of the retina contains the pigment epithelium cells (3). The basement membrane of the pigment epithelium cells (3) forms the innermost layer of the glassy (Bruch) membrane of the choroid. The cuboidal pigment epithelium cells (3) contain melanin (pigment) granules in their cytoplasm.

Adjacent to the pigment epithelium cells (3) is a photosensitive layer of slender **rods (4)** and thicker **cones (5)**. These cells are situated next to the **outer limiting membrane (6)** that is formed by the processes of supportive neuroglial cells called Müller cells.

The outer **nuclear layer (13)** contains the **nuclei of rods (4, 7)** and **cones (5, 7)** and the outer processes of Müller cells. In the **outer plexiform layer (14)** are found the axons of rods and cones (4, 5) that synapse with the dendrites of bipolar cells and horizontal cells that connect the rods (4) and cones (5) to the **ganglion cell layer (8)**. The **inner nuclear layer (15)** contains the nuclei of bipolar, horizontal, amacrine, and neuroglial Müller cells. The horizontal and amacrine cells are association cells. In the **inner plexiform layer (16)**, the axons of bipolar cells synapse with the dendrites of the ganglion (8) and amacrine cells.

The ganglion cell layer (8) contains the cell bodies of ganglion cells and neuroglial cells. The dendrites from the ganglion cells synapse in the inner plexiform layer (16).

The optic **nerve fiber layer (17)** contains the axons of the ganglion cells (8) and the inner fibers of Müller cells. Axons of ganglion cells (8) converge toward the optic disk and form the optic nerve fiber layer (17). The terminations of the inner fibers of Müller cells expand to form the **inner limiting membrane (9)** of the retina.

Blood vessels of the retina course in the optic nerve fiber layer (17) and penetrate as far as the inner nuclear layer (15). Numerous blood vessels in various planes of section can be seen in this layer (unlabeled).

FIGURE 22.7 | Eye: Layers of Retina and Choroid (Detail)

This high-magnifications photomicrograph illustrates the layers of the photosensitive retina. The **choroid (1)** is a vascular outer layer with loose connective tissue and pigmented melanocytes. The choroid (1) layer is situated adjacent to the outermost retinal layer—the single-cell, **pigment epithelium (2)** layer. The light-sensitive **rods and cones (3)** form the next layer, which is separated from the dense **outer nuclear layer (4)** by a thin **outer limiting membrane (5)**. Deep to the outer nuclear layer (4) is a clear area of synaptic connections. This is the **outer plexiform layer (6)**.

The dense layer of cell bodies of the integrating neurons forms the **inner nuclear layer (7)**, which is adjacent to the clear **inner plexiform layer (8)**. In the inner plexiform layer (8), the axons of the integrating neurons form synaptic connections with axons of the neurons that form the optic tract. The cell bodies of the optic tract neurons form the **ganglion cell layer (9)**, and their afferent axons form the light-staining **optic nerve fiber layer (10)**. The innermost layer of the retina is the inner **limiting membrane (11)**, which separates the retina from the vitreous body of the eyeball.

1 Blood vessels in choroid
2 Melanocytes
3 Pigment cells of retina
4 Rods
5 Cones
6 Outer limiting membrane
7 Nuclei of rods and cones
8 Ganglion cell layer
9 Inner limiting membrane

10 Sclera
11 Suprachoroidal layer with melanocytes
12 Choriocapillary layer
13 Outer nuclear layer
14 Outer plexiform layer
15 Inner nuclear layer
16 Inner plexiform layer
17 Optic nerve fiber layer

FIGURE 22.6 ■ Layers of choroid and retina (detail). Stain: hematoxylin and eosin. High magnification.

1 Choroid
2 Pigment epithelium
3 Rods and cones
4 Outer nuclear layer

5 Outer limiting membrane
6 Outer plexiform layer
7 Inner nuclear layer
8 Inner plexiform layer
9 Ganglion cell layer
10 Optic nerve fiber layer
11 Inner limiting membrane

FIGURE 22.7 ■ Eye: layers of retina and choroid. Stain: Masson trichrome. ×100.

FIGURE 22.8 | Section of Posterior Eyeball Showing Retina with Fovea Depression

At the posterior region of the eyeball, the retina exhibits a shallow depression, or an indentation. This region is called the **fovea**. Here, the retina does not exhibit any blood vessels, most of the retinal layers are reduced, and almost all photoreceptor cells in the depression are cones. On each side of the depression are visible the more expanded retinal layers. The dense-staining layers of **ganglion cells (1)**, the **inner nuclear layer (2)**, the **outer nuclear layer (3)**, and the **pigment epithelium (8)** adjacent to the dense-staining **choroid (4)** layer are readily visible. Similarly, the light-staining **inner plexiform layer (5), outer plexiform layer (6)**, and the layer of photoreceptors **rods and cones (7)** adjacent to the pigment epithelium (8) are also clearly visible. Surrounding the periphery of the eyeball is the dense connective tissue of the **sclera (9)**.

FIGURE 22.9 | Optic Papilla (Optic Disk), Optic Nerve, and the Section of Retina in the Posterior Region of the Eyeball

Located in the posterior region of the eyeball is the site where **retinal axons (5)** from the ganglion cells of the retina converge to form a solid **optic nerve**. Here, the optic nerve penetrates the connective tissue **sclera (3)** and leaves the eyeball. Where the optic nerve leaves the eyeball is the **optic disk (optic papilla)**. This area of the optic disk is completely insensitive to light because it lacks the photoreceptor cells and is, therefore, considered a blind spot in the eye. The axons in the optic nerve convey the stimulatory signals from the eyes to the brain for the interpretation of light sensations. After leaving the eyeball, the optic nerve in the orbit of the skull is surrounded by the meninges of the brain, which include the **pia mater (7)**, a **subarachnoid space (6)**, and a thick connective tissue **dura mater (8)**. This low-magnification micrograph also shows different dark-staining cellular and light-staining layers of the **retina (1)** and the adjacent, dense-staining **choroid (2).** Surrounding the exterior of the eyeball are the clear-staining cells of the **adipose tissue (4)**.

FIGURE 22.8 ■ Section of posterior eyeball showing retina with depression fovea. Stain: hematoxylin and eosin. ×17.

FIGURE 22.9 ■ Optic papilla (optic disk), optic nerve, and the section of retina in the posterior region of the eyeball. Stain: hematoxylin and eosin. ×10.5.

FIGURE 22.10 | Section of Posterior Retina with the Yellow Pigment of Macula Lutea

With special stains, it is possible to see the yellowish area of the macula lutea in the posterior region of the retina. The macula lutea is a small yellow area that immediately surrounds the retinal depression (fovea) and is also closely located to the optic disk in the posterior region of the eyeball. This micrograph image shows the yellow color of the macula lutea that is due to the accumulated **yellow pigment (xanthophyll) (7)** in the ganglion cells from the fovea. The **ganglion cell layer (2)** and the **retinal axons (1)** that pass in the area of the macula lutea are displaced laterally off the fovea so that the light can pass unimpeded directly to the very sensitive cone cells in the center of the fovea. With this stain are also visible the different layers of the retina, such as the ganglion cell layer (2), the **inner plexiform layer (8)**, the **inner nuclear layer (3)**, the **outer plexiform layer (9)**, the **outer nuclear layer (4)**, and the very distinct layer of the photoreceptors cells—the **rods and cones (10)**. Barely visible is the **pigment epithelium (5)** layer that is adjacent to the dense-staining **choroid (6)**. Surrounding the retina is the connective tissue **sclera (11)**.

FUNCTIONAL CORRELATIONS 22.1 | Eye

SECRETIONS (TEARS)

Each eyeball is covered on its anterior surface with thin **eyelids** and fine hairs, **eyelashes**, located on the margins of the eyelids. Eyelids and eyelashes protect the eyes from foreign objects and excessive light. Situated above each eye is a secretory **lacrimal gland** that continually produces **lacrimal secretions**, or **tears**. Blinking spreads the lacrimal secretion across the outer surface of the eyeball and the inner surface of the eyelid. The lacrimal secretion contains numerous proteins, mucus, salts, and the antibacterial enzyme **lysozyme**. Lacrimal secretions clean, protect, moisten, and lubricate the surface of the eye (conjunctiva and cornea).

The **tarsal glands** produce a secretion that forms an oily layer on the surface of the tear film. This functions in preventing the evaporation of the normal tear layer. The **sweat glands (of Moll)** produce and empty their secretions into the follicles of the eyelashes.

AQUEOUS HUMOR

Aqueous humor is the product of the ciliary epithelium of the **ciliary process** in the eye. This watery fluid flows into the anterior and posterior chambers of the eye between the cornea and lens. Aqueous humor bathes the nonvascular **cornea** and **lens** and also supplies them with nutrients and oxygen.

VITREOUS BODY

The vitreous chamber of the eye is located behind the lens and contains a gelatinous substance called the **vitreous body**, a transparent colorless gel that consists mainly of water. In addition, the vitreous body contains small amounts of hyaluronic acid, very thin collagen fibers, glycosaminoglycans, and some proteins. The vitreous body transmits incoming light, is nonrefractive with respect to the lens, contributes to the intraocular pressure and shape of the eyeball, and holds the retina in place against the pigmented layer of the eyeball.

RETINA

The photosensitive retina contains three types of neurons, distributed in different layers: photoreceptive **rods** and **cones, bipolar cells**, and **ganglion cells**. The rods and cones are receptor neurons essential for vision. They synapse with the bipolar cells, which then connect the receptor neurons with the ganglion cells. The afferent axons that leave the ganglion cells converge posteriorly in the eye at the **optic papilla** (optic disk) and leave the eye as the **optic nerve**. The optic papilla is also called the **blind spot** of the eye because this area lacks photoreceptor cells and only contains axons.

FUNCTIONAL CORRELATIONS 22.1 | Eye *(Continued)*

Because the rods and cones are situated adjacent to the **choroid layer** of the retina, light rays must first pass through the ganglion and bipolar cell layers to reach and activate the photosensitive rods and cones. The **retinal pigmented layer** of the choroid next to the retina absorbs light rays and prevents them from reflecting back through the retina and producing glare. In addition, these cells phagocytose worn-out outer components of both rods and cones, which are continually shed in renewal processes. The retinal pigment layer also stores vitamin A, a rhodopsin precursor that initiates visual stimulation. Retinal pigmented epithelial cells utilize vitamin A to form visual pigment molecules for both rods and cones.

RODS AND CONES

The rods are highly sensitive to light and function best in dim or **low light**, such as at dusk or at night. In the dark, a visual pigment called **rhodopsin** is synthesized and accumulates in the rod cells, which initiates the visual stimulus when it interacts with light. In contrast, the cones are less sensitive to low light, but respond best to **bright light**. Cones are also essential for high visual acuity and **color vision.** The cones contain the visual pigment **iodopsin** that responds maximally to the colors red, green, or blue of the color spectrums that trigger a visual response. Absorption and interaction of light rays with these pigments cause transformations in the pigment molecules. This action excites the rods and/or cones and produces a nerve impulse for vision.

At the posterior region of the eye is a shallow depression in the retina where the blood vessels do not pass over the photosensitive cells. This thin region is called the **fovea**, and its center contains only the **cone cells**. The visual axis of the eye directly passes through the fovea. As a result, light rays fall directly on and stimulate the tightly packed cones in the center of fovea. For this reason, the fovea in the eye produces the greatest **visual acuity** and the sharpest **color discrimination**. Immediately adjacent to and surrounding the depression fovea is the **macula lutea**, a small area that appears yellow in the retina. The yellow color of the surrounding macula is due to the presence and accumulation of the yellow pigment **xanthophyll** in the laterally located ganglion cells of the fovea.

1 Retinal axons
2 Ganglion cell layer
3 Inner nuclear layer
4 Outer nuclear layer
5 Pigment epithelium
6 Choroid
7 Yellow pigment (xanthophyll)
8 Inner plexiform layer
9 Outer plexiform layer
10 Rods and cones
11 Sclera

FIGURE 22.10 ■ Section of posterior retina with the yellow pigment of macula lutea. Stain: gold and yellow. ×100.

SECTION 1 • Visual System

- Eyes are located in protective orbits in the skull
- Visual images are conveyed from eye to brain via optic nerves

Layers in the Eye

- Sclera is the outer layer of eye and is composed of dense connective tissue
- Internal to sclera is the middle or vascular layer uvea that nourishes the retina and the eyeball
- Uvea consists of pigmented choroid, ciliary body, and iris
- Retina is the innermost lining of eye; posterior three quarters of retina is photosensitive
- Retina terminates anteriorly at ora serrata, which is a non-photosensitive part of retina

The Whole Eye

- Sclera maintains the rigidity of the eyeball and is the white of the eye
- Anteriorly, sclera is modified into transparent cornea through which light enters eye
- Choroid and ciliary body are adjacent to sclera
- Ciliary processes from ciliary body attach lens by suspensory ligament or zonular fibers
- Iris partially covers the lens and is the colored part of the eye
- Radial smooth muscle forms an opening in the iris, called the pupil

Chambers of the Eye

- Anterior chamber located between cornea, iris, and lens
- Posterior chamber is a small space between iris, ciliary process, zonular fibers, and lens
- Vitreous chamber is a large posterior space behind lens and zonular fibers, surrounded by retina

Photosensitive Parts of the Eye

- Rods and cones in the retina are sensitive to light
- Afferent axons leave retina and conduct impulses from eye to brain for interpretation

Secretions (Tears)

- Each eyeball is covered with an eyelid, which contains sebaceous glands and sweat glands (of Moll)
- Above each eyeball is the lacrimal gland, which produces lacrimal secretions or tears
- Myoepithelial cells surround secretory acini in lacrimal gland

- Tears contain mucus, salts, and antibacterial enzyme lysozyme
- Sebaceous (tarsal) gland secretions form an oily layer on the surface of tear film

Chamber Contents—Aqueous Humor and Vitreous Body

- Produced by ciliary epithelium of the eye and fills both the anterior and posterior chambers
- Bathes nonvascular cornea and lens; supplies them with nutrients and oxygen

Vitreous Body

- Vitreous chamber located behind lens and contains transparent gelatinous substance called vitreous body
- Consists mainly of water and water-soluble proteins
- Transmits incoming light, is nonrefractive, and contributes to intraocular pressure of eyeball
- Holds retina in place against pigmented layer of the eyeball

Retina

- Contains three types of neurons distributed in different layers
- Rods and cones are receptor neurons essential for vision that synapse with bipolar cells
- Bipolar cells connect to ganglion cells, from which axons converge posteriorly at optic papilla
- Area of optic papilla contains only axons of optic nerve and is the blind spot
- Light rays pass through all cell layers to activate rods and cones
- Pigmented layer of choroid next to retina absorbs light and prevents reflection

Choroid

- Divided into suprachoroid lamina, vascular layer, and choriocapillaris layer
- Suprachoroid layer contains connective tissue fibers and numerous melanocytes
- Vascular layer contains numerous blood vessels and melanocytes
- Choriocapillaris layer contains capillaries with large lumina
- Innermost layer of choroid is glassy membrane and lies adjacent to pigment cells
- Pigment cells separate choroid from retina and perform important functions

- Pigment cells are phagocytic, store vitamin A, and form visual pigments for rods and cones

Rods and Cones

- Rods are highly sensitive to light, function in low light, and synthesize visual pigment rhodopsin

- Cones are sensitive to bright light, essential for visual acuity and color vision

- Cones are most sensitive to red, green, or blue color spectrums and contain visual pigment iodopsin

- Interaction of light with visual pigments transforms their molecules and excites rods and cones

- Pigment xanthophyll accumulates in ganglion cells of macula lutea

- Fovea is in the center of macula lutea and devoid of rods and blood vessels

- Fovea contains a high concentration of the photosensitive cones

- Fovea produces greatest visual acuity and sharpest color discrimination

SECTION 2 Auditory System

The **auditory system** consists of three major parts: the external ear, the middle ear, and the inner ear. The ear is a specialized organ that contains structures responsible for hearing, balance, and maintenance of equilibrium.

External Ear

The auricle, or **pinna**, of the **external ear** gathers sound waves from the external environment and directs them through the **external auditory canal** interiorly to the eardrum or **tympanic membrane,** from which the sound is directed to the middle ear.

Middle Ear

The **middle ear** is a small, air-filled cavity called the **tympanic cavity**. It is located in and protected by the temporal bone of the skull. The **tympanic membrane** separates the external auditory canal from the middle ear. Located in the middle ear are three very small bones: the **auditory ossicles** consisting of the **stapes, incus**, and **malleus.** These bones are attached to the tympanic membrane and to the cochlea of the inner ear; also in the middle ear is the **auditory (eustachian) tube**. The sound waves vibrate the tympanic membrane and are then transmitted through the auditory ossicle bones to the inner ear. The cavity of the middle ear also communicates with the nasopharynx region of the head via the auditory tube. The presence of the auditory tube allows for the equalization of air pressure on both sides of the tympanic membrane during swallowing or blowing the nose.

Inner Ear

The inner ear lies deep in the temporal bone of the skull. It consists of small, communicating cavities and canals of different shapes. These cavities, the **semicircular canals, vestibule**, and **cochlea**, are collectively called the **osseous**, or bony, **labyrinth**. All sections of the bony labyrinth are filled with **perilymph**, a fluid that is rich in sodium and similar in composition to the cerebrospinal fluid of the central nervous system. Located within the bony labyrinth is the **membranous labyrinth** that consists of a series of interconnected, thin-walled compartments filled with fluid called **endolymph**.

Cochlea

The organ specialized for receiving and transmitting sound (hearing) is found in the inner ear in the structure called the cochlea. It is a spiral bony canal that resembles a snail's shell. The cochlea makes three turns on itself around a central bony pillar called the **modiolus**.

Interiorly, the cochlea is partitioned into three channels: **vestibular duct (scala vestibuli), tympanic duct (scala tympani)**, and **cochlear duct (scala media)**. Located within the cochlear duct on the **basilar membrane** are specialized receptor cells that detect sound; this is the hearing **organ of Corti**. This organ consists of numerous auditory receptor cells, or **hair cells**, and several supporting cells that respond to different sound frequencies. The hair cells contain long, stiff **stereocilia** and project into the fluid-filled cochlear duct. The auditory stimuli (sounds) are carried away from the receptor hair cells via afferent axons of the **cochlear nerve** to the brain for interpretation. A **tectorial membrane** overlies the organ of Corti.

Vestibular Functions

The organ of vestibular functions is responsible for **balance** and **equilibrium.** It is found in the **utricle, saccule**, and three **semicircular canals**.

 Supplemental micrographic images are available at **www.thePoint.com/Eroschenko12e** under Organs of the Special Senses.

FIGURE 22.11 | Inner Ear: Cochlea (Vertical Section)

This low-magnification image illustrates the labyrinthine characteristics of the inner ear. The **osseous**, or **bony**, **labyrinth** of the **cochlea (14, 16)** spirals around a central axis of a spongy bone called the **modiolus (15)**. Located within the modiolus (15) are the **spiral ganglia (7)**, which are composed of numerous bipolar afferent (sensory) neurons. The dendrites from these **bipolar neurons (7)** extend to and innervate the hair cells that are located in the hearing apparatus called the **organ of Corti (12)**. The axons from these afferent neurons join and form the **cochlear nerve (13)**, which is located in the modiolus (15).

The osseous labyrinth (14, 16) of the inner ear is divided into two major cavities by the **osseous (bony) spiral lamina (6)** and the **basilar membrane (9)**. The osseous spiral lamina (6) projects from the modiolus (15) about halfway into the lumen of the cochlear canal. The basilar membrane (9) continues from the osseous spiral lamina (6) to the **spiral ligament (11)**, which is a thickening of the connective tissue of the periosteum on the **outer bony wall** of the **cochlear canal (8)**.

The cochlear canal (8) is subdivided into two large compartments: the lower **tympanic duct (scala tympani) (4)** and the upper **vestibular duct (scala vestibuli) (2)**. The separate tympanic duct (4) and vestibular duct (2) continue in a spiral course to the apex of the cochlea, where they communicate through a small opening called the **helicotrema (1)**.

The **vestibular** (Reissner) **membrane (5)** separates the vestibular duct (2) from the **cochlear duct (scala media) (3)** and forms the roof of the cochlear duct (3). The vestibular membrane (5) attaches to the spiral ligament (11) in the outer bony wall of the cochlear canal (8). The sensory cells for sound detection are located in the organ of Corti (12), which rests on the basilar membrane (9) of the cochlear duct (3). A **tectorial membrane (10)** overlies the cells in the organ of Corti (12) (see also Figs. 22.12 through 22.14).

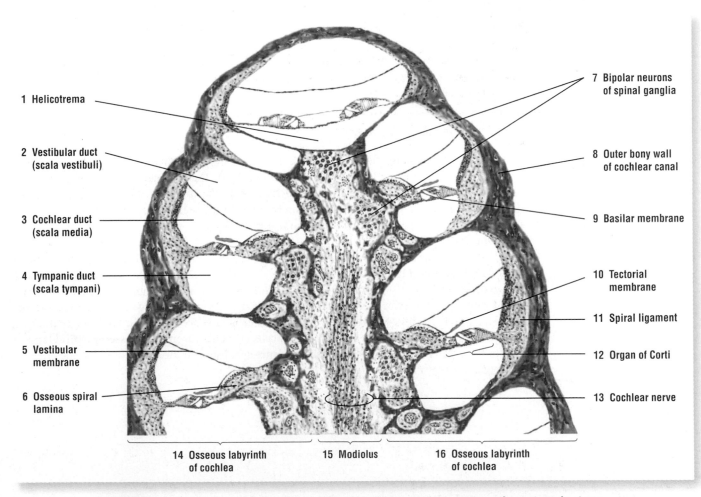

1 Helicotrema

2 Vestibular duct (scala vestibuli)

3 Cochlear duct (scala media)

4 Tympanic duct (scala tympani)

5 Vestibular membrane

6 Osseous spiral lamina

7 Bipolar neurons of spinal ganglia

8 Outer bony wall of cochlear canal

9 Basilar membrane

10 Tectorial membrane

11 Spiral ligament

12 Organ of Corti

13 Cochlear nerve

14 Osseous labyrinth of cochlea

15 Modiolus

16 Osseous labyrinth of cochlea

FIGURE 22.11 ■ Inner ear: cochlea (vertical section). Stain: hematoxylin and eosin. Low magnification.

FIGURE 22.12 | Inner Ear: Cochlear Duct (Scala Media) and the Hearing Organ of Corti

This illustration shows in more detail the **cochlear duct (scala media) (9)** and the hearing **organ of Corti (13)** and its associated cells at a higher magnification.

The outer wall of the cochlear duct (9) is formed by a vascular area called the **stria vascularis (15)**. The stratified epithelium covering the stria vascularis (15) contains an intraepithelial capillary network that was formed from the blood vessels that supply the connective tissue in the **spiral ligament (17)**. The spiral ligament (17) contains collagen fibers, pigmented fibroblasts, and numerous blood vessels.

The roof of the cochlear duct (9) is formed by a thin **vestibular (Reissner) membrane (6)**, which separates the cochlear duct (9) from the **vestibular duct (scala vestibuli) (7)**. The vestibular membrane (6) extends from the spiral ligament (17) in the outer wall of the cochlear duct (9) that is located at the upper extent of the stria vascularis (15) to the thickened periosteum of the **osseous spiral lamina (2)** near the **spiral limbus (1)**.

The spiral limbus (1) is a thickened mass of periosteal connective tissue of the osseous spiral lamina (2) that extends into and forms the floor of the cochlear duct (9). The spiral limbus (1) is covered by an **epithelium (5)** that appears columnar and is supported by a lateral extension of the osseous spiral lamina (2). The lateral extracellular extension of the spiral limbus epithelium (5) beyond the spiral limbus (1) forms the **tectorial membrane (10)**, which overlies the **inner spiral tunnel (8)** and a portion of the organ of Corti (13).

The **basilar membrane (16)** is a vascularized connective tissue that forms the lower wall of the cochlear duct (9). The organ of Corti (13) rests on the fibers of the basilar membrane (16) and consists of the sensory **outer hair cells (11)**, supporting cells, associated inner spiral tunnel (8), and an **inner tunnel (12)**.

The afferent fibers of **the cochlear nerve (4)** from the bipolar cells located in the **spiral ganglion (3)** course through the osseous spiral lamina (2) and synapse with outer hair cells (11) in the organ of Corti (13).

FIGURE 22.13 | Inner Ear: Cochlear Duct and the Organ of Corti

This higher-magnification photomicrograph illustrates the inner ear with the cochlear canal and the hearing **organ of Corti (8)** in the **bony cochlea (1, 9)**. The cochlear canal is subdivided into the **vestibular duct** (scala vestibuli) **(10), cochlear duct** (scala media) **(3)**, and **tympanic duct** (scala tympani) **(14)**. A thin, **vestibular membrane (2)** separates the cochlear duct (3) from the scala vestibuli (10). A thicker **basilar membrane (7)** separates the cochlear duct (3) from the tympanic duct (scala tympani) (14).

The basilar membrane (7) extends from the connective tissue **spiral ligament (6)** to a thickened **spiral limbus (11)**. The basilar membrane (7) supports the organ of Corti (8) with its sensory **hair cells (5)** and supportive cells. Extending from the spiral limbus (11) is the **tectorial membrane (4)**. The tectorial membrane (4) covers a portion of the organ of Corti (8) and the hair cells (5). The sensory bipolar **spiral ganglion cells (13)** are located in the bony cochlea (1, 9). The afferent axons from the spiral ganglion cells (13) pass through the **osseous spiral lamina (12)** to the organ of Corti (8) where their dendrites synapse with the hair cells (5) in the organ of Corti (8).

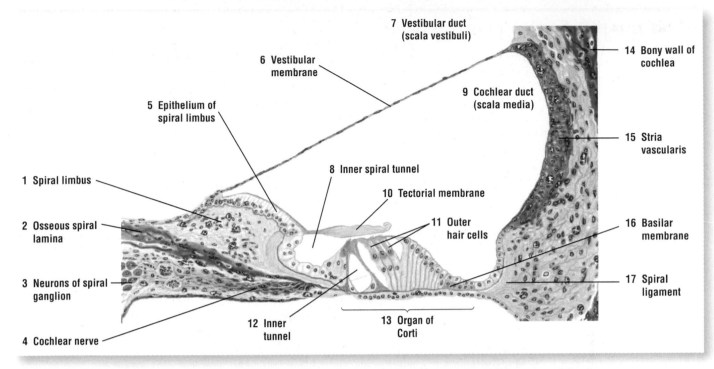

7 Vestibular duct
(scala vestibuli)

6 Vestibular
membrane

5 Epithelium of
spiral limbus

9 Cochlear duct
(scala media)

14 Bony wall of
cochlea

15 Stria
vascularis

8 Inner spiral tunnel

10 Tectorial membrane

1 Spiral limbus

11 Outer
hair cells

2 Osseous spiral
lamina

16 Basilar
membrane

3 Neurons of spiral
ganglion

17 Spiral
ligament

4 Cochlear nerve

12 Inner
tunnel

13 Organ of
Corti

FIGURE 22.12 ■ Inner ear: cochlear duct (scala media) and the hearing organ of Corti. Stain: hematoxylin and eosin. Medium magnification.

1 Bony cochlea

2 Vestibular
membrane

3 Cochlear duct

4 Tectorial
membrane

5 Hair cells

6 Spiral ligament

7 Basilar membrane

8 Organ of Corti

9 Bony cochlea

10 Vestibular duct
(scala vestibuli)

11 Spiral limbus

12 Osseous spiral
lamina

13 Spiral ganglion
cells

14 Tympanic duct
(scala tympani)

FIGURE 22.13 ■ Inner ear: cochlear duct and the organ of Corti. Stain: hematoxylin and eosin. ×30.

FIGURE 22.14 | Inner Ear: Organ of Corti in the Cochlear Duct

This micrograph enlarges the image in Figure 22.13 and shows greater detail of the cochlea and the surrounding cells in the inner ear. The micrograph focuses primarily on the **cochlear duct (2)** and the cells and structures in the **organ of Corti (14)** that is situated on the **basilar membrane (6)**. Visible in the organ of Corti (14) are the **outer hair cells (12)**, the **inner tunnel (13)**, and the **outer tunnel (5)** that separates the cells in the hearing organ. Superior to the outer hair cells (12) is the **tectorial membrane (4)**, with the **inner spiral tunnel (11)** located inferior to the tectorial membrane (4). The thin **vestibular membrane (8)** separates the **vestibular duct** (scala vestibuli) **(1)** from the cochlear duct (2). Facing the cochlear duct (2) is the vascularized **stria vascularis (3)** that overlies the connective tissue **spiral ligament (7)**. The vestibular membrane (8) attaches to the **spiral limbus (9)** under which are found the axons of the **cochlear nerve (10)**.

FUNCTIONAL CORRELATIONS 22.2 | Inner Ear

COCHLEA

The cochlea of the inner ear contains the auditory **organ of Corti**. Sound waves that enter the ear and pass through the **external auditory canal** vibrate the **tympanic membrane**. These vibrations activate the three bony **ossicles** (stapes, incus, and malleus) in the middle ear, which then transmit these vibrations across the air-filled **middle ear**, or **tympanic cavity**, to the fluid-filled **inner ear**. The sounds vibrate the **basilar membrane** on which are located the sensitive receptor cells for hearing, the hair cells of the organ of Corti. The vibrations of the basilar membrane due to the sound and the shearing, or bending motion, between the hairs (stereocilia) in the hair cells and the overlying **tectorial membrane** activate neurotransmitters at the base of sensitive **hair cells** in the organ of Corti. The deflections of the stereocilia on the hair cells convert this mechanical displacement into **nerve impulses**.

Impulses for sound pass along the afferent axons of bipolar **ganglion cells** located in the **spiral ganglia** of the inner ear. The axons from the spiral ganglia join to form the **auditory (cochlear) nerve**, which carries the impulses from the sensitive cells in the organ of Corti to the brain for sound interpretation.

VESTIBULAR APPARATUS

The vestibular apparatus consists of the **utricle, saccule**, and **semicircular canals**. These sensitive organs respond to linear or angular accelerations or movements of the head. Sensory inputs from the vestibular apparatus initiate the very complex neural pathways that activate specific skeletal muscles that correct balance and equilibrium and restore the body to its normal position.

1 Vestibular duct

2 Cochlear duct

3 Stria vascularis

4 Tectorial membrane

5 Outer tunnel

6 Basilar membrane

7 Spiral ligament

8 Vestibular membrane

9 Spiral limbus

10 Cochlear nerve

11 Inner spiral tunnel

12 Outer hair cells

13 Inner tunnel

14 Organ of Corti

FIGURE 22.14 ■ Inner ear: organ of Corti in the cochlear duct. Stain: hematoxylin and eosin. ×50.

- Ear is specialized for hearing, balance, and maintenance of equilibrium

External Ear

- Auricle, or pinna, gathers sound waves and directs them through external auditory canal
- Sound waves reach eardrum or tympanic membrane

Middle Ear

- Contains a small, air-filled cavity called tympanic cavity in temporal bone of the skull
- Tympanic membrane separates external auditory canal from middle ear
- Contains three very small bones, the auditory ossicles: stapes, incus, and malleus
- Contains auditory (Eustachian) tube that communicates with nasopharynx
- Auditory tube equalizes air pressure on both sides of tympanic membrane

Inner Ear

- Lies deep in the temporal bone of the skull
- Consists of semicircular canals, vestibule, and cochlea, which is called bony labyrinth
- In bony labyrinth is the membranous labyrinth, a series of compartments filled with fluid

- All sections of bony labyrinth filled with fluid perilymph
- Membranous labyrinth filled with fluid endolymph

Cochlea

- Located in inner ear; receives and transmits sound
- Spiral canal that makes three turns around central bony pillar called modiolus
- Embedded in modiolus is the spiral ganglion composed of bipolar afferent neurons
- Interiorly partitioned into vestibular duct (scala vestibuli), tympanic duct (scala tympani), and cochlear duct (scala media)
- Cochlear duct contains receptor or hair cells in the hearing organ of Corti
- Sound waves vibrate tympanic membrane, which activates the bony ossicles in the middle ear
- Bony ossicles transmit vibrations to inner ear and vibrate basilar membrane
- Organ of Corti is located on basilar membrane; vibrations stimulate hair cells in the organ
- Hair cells (stereocilia displacement) in the organ of Corti convert mechanical vibrations into nerve impulses
- Impulses pass along afferent nerves in spiral ganglia of inner ear to cochlear nerve and brain

OSPE Questions

Brijesh Kumar*

For a student, the practical knowledge of histology can be tested by spot examination or objective structured practical examination (OSPE). Unlike in spot examination, where students are asked to identify the histological slide and write few points of identification, in OSPE, more detailed and specific histological, functional, and clinical knowledge is assessed. In a typical OSPE, there are several stations (like spot exam) and each station has a slide and its related questions. Students are expected to answer the question within a fixed time duration.

Listed below are few slides from the book given as OSPEs for the student to identify and answer the questions for each slide.

FIGURE A.1

Q1. Identify the type of epithelium in the above slide.

Q2. Identify the structure marked as 1.

Q3. Mention the main function of the structures marked as 2 and 3.

---

*Assistant Professor, Department of Anatomy, Oman Medical College, Oman.

Q1. Identify the slide.

Q2. Identify the structure marked as 1.

Q3. Mention the cell responsible for the synthesis of the structure marked as 1.

FIGURE A.2

Q1. Identify the structure marked as 1.

Q2. Identify the structure marked as 2 and mention its function.

Q3. Identify the structures marked as 3.

FIGURE A.3

Q1. Identify the slide.

Q2. Identify the structure marked as 1.

Q3. Identify the structures marked as 2 and mention the structure receding in it.

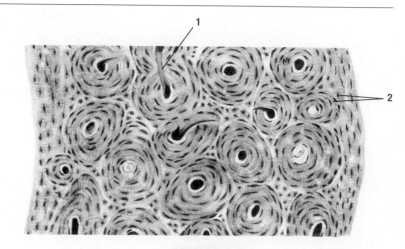

FIGURE A.4

Q1. Identify the slide.

Q2. Mention the function of the structures marked as 1.

Q3. Identify the structure marked as 2.

FIGURE A.5

Q1. Identify the slide.

Q2. Identify the structures marked as 1.

Q3. Mention the function of the structures marked as 2.

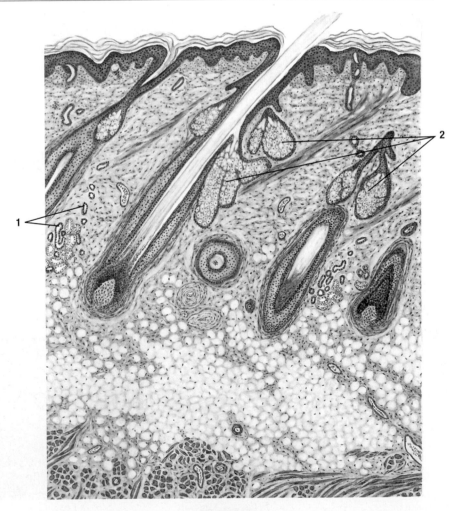

FIGURE A.6

Q1. Identify the slide.

Q2. Mention the type of epithelium marked as 1 and 2.

Q3. Identify the structures marked as 3.

FIGURE A.7

Q1. Identify the structures marked as 1 and 2.

Q2. Mention the different types of cells present in the structure marked as 3.

FIGURE A.8

Q1. Identify the slide.

Q2. Identify the structures marked as 1 and 2.

Q3. Mention the main function of the structures marked as 3.

FIGURE A.9

Q1. Identify the slide.

Q2. Identify the structures marked as 1 and 2.
Mention the functions of each.

FIGURE A.10

Q1. Identify the slide.

Q2. Identify the structure marked as 1.

Q3. Mention the different types of cells present
in the structure marked as 2.

FIGURE A.11

Q1. Identify the structure marked as 1. Mention the lining epithelium of it.

Q2. Mention the types of cells lining the structure marked as 2.

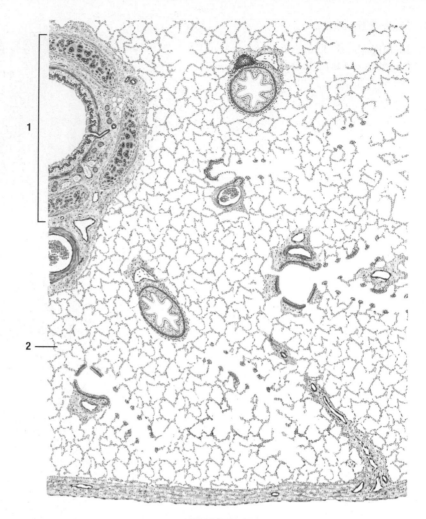

FIGURE A.12

Q1. Identify the slide.

Q2. Mention the function of the cells marked as 1.

Q3. Mention the function of the cells marked as 2.

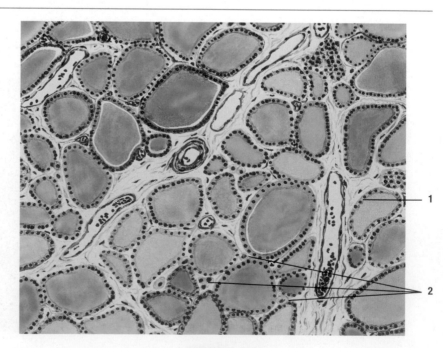

FIGURE A.13

Q1. Identify the structure marked as 1.

Q2. Identify the structures marked as 2.

Q3. Mention the function of the structure marked as 3.

FIGURE A.14

Q1. Identify the layer marked as 1.

Q2. Mention the types of cells in the layer marked as 2.

Q3. Mention the function of the layer marked as 3.

FIGURE A.15

Q1. Identify the slide.

Q2. Identify the structure marked as 1.

Q3. Mention the function of the cells marked as 2.

FIGURE A.16

Q1. Identify the slide.

Q2. Identify the structure marked as 1.

Q3. Identify the structure marked as 2.

FIGURE A.17

Q1. Identify the slide.

Q2. Mention the lining epithelium.

Q3. Identify the structure marked as 1.

FIGURE A.18

Q1. Mention the lining epithelium.

Q2. Identify the structure marked as 1.

Q3. Identify the structure marked as 2.

FIGURE A.19

Q1. Mention the main constituents of the structure marked as 1.

Q2. Mention the main constituents of the structure marked as 2.

FIGURE A.20

Note: Page numbers in *italics* indicate figure.